Greene and Mathieson's
The Voice and Its Disorders

6th Edition

LESLEY MATHIESON DipCST, FRCSLT

Visiting Lecturer in Voice Pathology, University of Reading

U.S. CONSULTANT: R.J. BAKEN PhD
The New York Eye & Ear Infirmary, New York

W

WHURR PUBLISHERS
LONDON AND PHILADELPHIA

Sixth edition © 2001 Whurr Publishers Ltd
Fifth edition published 1989 by
Whurr Publishers Ltd
19b Compton Terrace, London N1 2UN, England and
325 Chestnut Street, Philadelphia PA 19106, USA

British Library Cataloguing in Publication Data
A catalogue record for this book is available from the British
Library.

ISBN: 1 86156 196 2

Therapeutic procedures are constantly developing in the
field of voice pathology. Every effort has been made in this
book to describe voice therapy intervention strategies clearly,
to draw the reader's attention to some of the main
contraindications for their use and to highlight some of the
unsatisfactory methods of carrying out procedures. It is the
responsibility of those who carry out treatments for voice
disorders, however, to ensure that they are appropriately
qualified to carry out such treatment, that they are fully
aware of information which contraindicates certain types of
intervention in each case and that they make their own
assessment of the appropriateness of any intervention for a
particular patient.

Printed and bound in the UK by Athenaeum Press Ltd,
Gateshead, Tyne & Wear

Greene and Mathieson's
The Voice and Its Disorders

6th Edition

Contents

Preface to 6th edition

The first edition of *The Voice and Its Disorders* was published in 1957. There were very few books on this subject at that time and Margaret C.L. Greene OBE, FRCSLT made a major contribution to the literature by writing a book which encapsulated her knowledge and experience. It became a standard text on the subject and the success of the first edition led her to write three more editions, all well received. In the 1980s she invited me to be her co-author for the 5th edition, which was published twelve years ago. The 6th edition has been extensively re-written and my perspective, like Margaret Greene's, is that of a speech-language pathologist specialising in the treatment of individuals with voice disorders who also lectures to undergraduates, postgraduates and to my peers.

When the last edition was published, the use of sophisticated instrumentation for visualising the larynx was steadily becoming more widespread and was presaging a change in the clinical practice of many laryngologists and speech-language pathologists. Enlightened clinicians of both disciplines became aware of the importance of working together in order to determine causative factors and to decide upon the most suitable treatments. They realised that collaboration enabled more soundly based clinical decisions to be made and that by learning from each other their own skills developed. Throughout the 1990s, more readily available computer software for acoustic analysis contributed to objective voice measurement. Although limited equipment budgets may restrict the amount and type of instrumentation which can be purchased, the concept of working collaboratively is fundamental to good clinical practice in this area and it is regrettable that this is still not the case in some centres. During the last decade, the potential for definitive diagnoses and successful treatment of clinical voice disorders has increased considerably in many clinics throughout the world as a result of the developments in laryngoscopic examination and working practices. It is now incumbent upon those of us working in the field of clinical voice disorders, as in other specialities, to provide the evidence of the efficacy of our intervention.

Although these developments are welcome and to be encouraged, the development of a significant clinical tool – the voice pathologist's own vocal skills – has taken a retrograde step during the last decade. In the UK, most university courses have eliminated practical voice work for speech pathologists, although in other countries, such as Sweden, it is recognised as essential. The voice pathologist's vocal skills should provide a model for modifying vocal behaviour during treatment. It is also by experiencing an extensive range of vocal behaviours and how to adapt and control them, that the clinician gains insight into the processes through which he or she is trying to guide the patient. The acquisition of these vocal skills by the voice pathologist is beyond the remit of this book but is an essential foundation for successful voice therapy. How can we expect to elicit changes in vocal behaviour from others that we cannot produce ourselves? If such experiential learning needs to be made academically respectable, it can be closely linked to the study of vocal tract biomechanics and to acoustic and aerodynamic measurement.

I have received support, generosity and kindness from numerous sources while I have been writing this edition and I acknowledge the continued contribution of those who provided input to the 5th edition. Formal acknowledgments are made throughout the text but my personal thanks are due to many people. I am extremely grateful for the wisdom, guidance, sensitivity and humour of Dr Ron Baken who agreed to take on the task of U.S. Consultant to this edition. His meticulous review of the draft manuscript was invaluable and his encouraging e-mails helped me to persevere. I am also indebted to Mr Julian McGlashan for generously providing many of the laryngeal images and for inviting me to spend a day with him to dissect larynges. My thanks are also due to Professor Adrian Fourcin for his enthusiastic involvement in producing laryngograph images derived from his collaboration with Julian McGlashan.

I received prompt and unfailingly generous responses from Dr Charles N Ford and Dr Marc Bouchayer allowing me to reproduce their photographs of vocal fold sulci as well as from Dr Barbara Jacobson who kindly agreed to reproduction of the Voice Handicap Index, for which I am most grateful. I would also like to thank Professor Martin J Ball and Professor David M Howard for giving permission to reproduce their material.

My clinical experience has been developed immeasurably by working with Mr Ram Dhillon for many years and, more recently, with Mr John Rubin. I am grateful to them both for sharing their knowledge and insights so readily. My thanks are also due to Ram Dhillon for allowing me to reproduce figures from his book.

I have valued enormously the encouragement of my friends and colleagues Dr Eva Carlson and Christina Shewell, who have always been so positive about the work in hand, and Annette Fernholz and Claire Holmes for so willingly reviewing early drafts of the manuscript. I am greatly indebted to Marion Finney for her meticulous production of the many tables in the manuscript and for the maintenance of my sanity throughout the entire process.

Finally, my gratitude is due to my husband, Ian, for his support of a wife who has been welded to a computer late at night for so long, and to our sons, Mark and John, whose humour and encouragement have helped to keep the task in perspective.

Lesley Mathieson
Chalfont St Giles
Buckinghamshire
England
February 2001

Preface to 5th edition

After the publication of the fourth edition in 1980 the last thing that was envisaged was another edition of *The Voice and Its Disorders*. However, as a decade progressed, far from falling into oblivion, requests for the book increased. These requests came mainly from qualified speech therapists confronted with the problems of planning and executing treatment for dysphonia.

Undergraduate speech therapists are given theoretical understanding of voice production and voice pathology in addition to important clinical experience. This alone is not sufficient preparation for their therapeutic role. They have little practical instruction in the production of their own voices which is an essential requirement for real insight into the perception and clinical treatment of dysphonic patients. Whilst we have explored theories and the latest research and instruments which can be used in objective assessment, we have been at pains to emphasise the practical approach to the rehabilitation of the dysphonic patient. We have asked ourselves, 'What do we do with this patient?'. The answers can often be found in the case histories we have quoted which endeavour to explain the problem and the measures which helped.

In the first edition (1957) the preface began thus: 'The chief motive in writing this book was the desire to provide a guide to treatment of voice disorders, simple yet comprehensive enough to serve not only speech therapists but doctors and laryngologists, and, more especially, those in many countries of the world where speech therapy is unknown and unpractised.' We have included therefore some pathologies not encountered in the Western World but still endemic in the less developed countries where such conditions as diphtheria and syphilis of the larynx still occur.

At risk of being over-repetitive we would like to comment here on a point frequently made in the text. No machine can replace the expertise and empathy of the experienced speech therapist. Increasingly sophisticated instrumentation for the analysis of vocal function and for monitoring response to treatment gives us interesting new insights but it is only one aspect of intervention. Effective therapy is soundly based upon clinical experience and is comprised of an amalgam of watching and of listening to the voice and the complaints of the dysphonic patient. It is linked into a network of anatomical, physiological, neurological, cultural and pathological cues, and presents a holistic picture against which particular acoustic measurement falls into proper perspective. To speech therapists without the instrumentation we describe we wish to extend the consolation that we have also worked extensively in situations where it has been unavailable. This lack has not prevented us from providing successful voice therapy to a large number of patients.

We must acknowledge our appreciation of all those who have helped us over some of our worries with advice and discussion. Not least we must thank all those writers of excellent books and papers encapsulating their research and the wisdom of their experience which we acknowledge in our references throughout the text. Particular thanks must be made to Eva Carlson who has been most generous in providing laryngograph waveforms and analyses.

We are greatly indebted to Mr D. Garfield Davies, FRCS, Director of the Ferens Institute of Otolaryngology, The University College and Middlesex Hospital School of Medicine, London who provided many photographs and diagrams of the larynx to illustrate pathological conditions of the vocal folds. He helped in their selection and gave invaluable advice and encouragement.

We also wish to thank Dr Frances MacCurtain for giving permission to reproduce the xeroradiographs of our patients.

We are indebted to Brüel and Kjaer Ltd in Denmark and the UK and to Kay Elemetrics Corporation in the USA for providing an excellent selection of slides and photographs from which we were able to choose suitable illustrations.

Finally, we must thank Mark Mathieson who organised our disk filing system and wrote appropriate computer programs for producing flow charts, waveforms and index lists, while convincing us that sanity could prevail.

Margaret Greene, Wingrave
Lesley Mathieson, Chalfont St Giles
June 1989

Phonetic symbols used in the text

Vowels

/i/	as in <u>i</u>t
/i:/	as in <u>ea</u>t
/e/	as in b<u>e</u>d
/æ/	as in <u>a</u>t
/a:/	as in <u>ar</u>m
/ɜ:/	as in h<u>er</u>
/ə/	as in supp<u>er</u>
/ʌ/	as in c<u>u</u>t
/ɒ/	as in n<u>o</u>t
/u:/	as in p<u>oo</u>l

Consonants

/m/	as in <u>m</u>e
/n/	as in <u>n</u>o
/ŋ/	as in si<u>ng</u>
/p/	as in <u>p</u>ea
/b/	as in <u>b</u>at
/t/	as in <u>t</u>o
/d/	as in <u>d</u>ay
/k/	as in <u>c</u>at
/g/	as in <u>g</u>o
/f/	as in <u>f</u>it
/v/	as in <u>v</u>im
/θ/	as in <u>th</u>ink
/ð/	as in <u>th</u>at
/r/	as in <u>r</u>ed
/j/	as in <u>y</u>et
/s/	as in <u>s</u>o
/z/	as in <u>z</u>oo
/ʃ/	as in <u>sh</u>oe
/tʃ/	as in <u>ch</u>at
/dʒ/	as in <u>j</u>am
/ʒ/	as in lei<u>s</u>ure
/h/	as in <u>h</u>e

Diphthongs

/au/	as in h<u>ou</u>se
/ei/	as in d<u>ay</u>
/aɪ/	as in l<u>ie</u>

In memory of my parents
Marion and Jack Glass

'I thank you for your voices, thank you.
Your most sweet voices'

Coriolanus Act 2 III
Shakespeare

Introduction

This book is about the voice, voice disorders and their remediation. It is intended for those professionals who are involved in the treatment of abnormal voices and for students who are developing their skills in this area. It is primarily directed at speech-language pathologists, but will also be of interest to laryngologists who are keen to develop insight into the processes and methods of voice therapy that can be used both as a primary treatment route and as an essential adjunct to laryngeal surgery. All professionals involved with voice-disordered individuals in a medical setting should find relevant information in this book. Some chapters will be informative for voice professionals working in non-medical settings, e.g. voice and singing teachers, who would like to expand their understanding of the anatomy and physiology of normal voice as well as to develop awareness of vocal pathologies that merit referral for laryngeal examination.

The text is divided into three parts. The five chapters of the first section are concerned with normal voice. Chapter 1 provides an overview of the role of the voice in human communication. This sociopsychological perspective might be regarded by some readers as a slightly incongruous bedfellow for the chapters on the anatomy, physiology and acoustics of phonation that follow in the same section. It is included because the appreciation of the many aspects of the voice that contribute to oral communication should enable clinicians to develop some insight into what the voice-disordered patient has lost in losing normal vocal function. By understanding the functional and psychological roles of normal voice, it is to be hoped that clinicians working in this field are able to investigate and treat the patient's condition with sensitivity and full regard for the individual's difficulties and needs. The remaining chapters in the first section describe the vocal tract, the production of normal voice, and the ways in which both change throughout the individual's lifetime. This information about normal structure and function provides the foundation for Parts II and III, and the reader may find it helpful to return to these earlier chapters for reference when reading the later sections.

The second part of the book describes the various categories of voice disorders, each aetiological category in a separate chapter. Such clear divisions are rarely the reality in any discipline and the area of voice disorders is no exception. Voice disorders tend to overlap in the way in which they present and neatly separated chapters are used purely for organisational purposes. It has to be remembered that most individuals with a voice disorder attempt to compensate for the problem. As a result, there may be a hyperfunctional element of a voice disorder that results primarily from a structural abnormality of the vocal tract, for example. It is also important to bear in mind that having a voice disorder can be stressful and that this can affect its presentation, although the primary cause might not be psychological. This section aims to provide the reader not only with factual information about each condition, but also with some indication of the many strands of information that need to be explored in the assessment of each patient. It is a truism, but worth remembering, that voice clinicians do not deal purely with voice disorders but with people who have voice disorders.

The final part deals with the assessment and treatment options that may be employed in treating voice disorders. These chapters reflect two of the important developments over the last two decades. First, the technology that is now available for viewing the larynx and making acoustic measurements has transformed treatment by providing objective information that is fundamental to making decisions about methods of treatment and to providing feedback during treatment. It has also contributed to the fact that laryngologists, voice therapists, speech scientists and other voice professionals work together more closely now than ever before in many centres. In the best centres throughout the world, patients are assessed in multidisciplinary voice clinics. The specialist speech-language pathologist (or voice therapist) is an integral part of the medical team, working closely with the laryngologist, and is increasingly involved in the assessment, diagnostic and decision-making processes which are fundamental to planning treatment, whether medical, surgical, therapeutic or a combination of all three. A multidisciplinary approach helps to ensure that the complexities of any voice disorder are comprehensively evaluated. The different but combined perspectives of the contributing disciplines, particularly laryngology and speech-language pathology, are essential and complementary in providing good care for these patients. A coordinated team approach can help to avoid unnecessary surgery, for example, but will also indicate when surgery is essential. The concept of close coordination between members of the team involved in treating voice disorders is implicit in this book.

The second, more recent, development is the emphasis on evidence-based practice. Clinicians are increasingly expected to prove that their clinical intervention is effective and to base their treatment on proven techniques. As a result, day-to-day practice is more concerned with analysing the processes of intervention and measuring treatment outcomes than in the past. Consequently, clinicians have to consider which instrumental procedures and assessment protocols can provide the most useful baselines from which progress and outcomes can be measured. Studies of the effectiveness of voice therapy and the most useful techniques are accumulating but are frequently difficult to compare because timeframes of treatment are not described in detail. Many of the most frequently used treatment approaches are described in the final section of this book. The clinical experience of voice therapists and laryngologists is that these methods can be effective, but further studies are essential if this impression is to be convincingly substantiated.

Finally, there is the dilemma about the nomenclature of the clinician who carries out voice therapy. The speech-language pathologist (or therapist) who specialises in treating clinical voice disorders may be described as a 'voice pathologist' or 'voice therapist' in some centres. The term 'voice pathologist' probably incorporates most effectively all the elements of the role (including analysis and assessment), whereas 'therapist' implies treatment alone. This title recognises the speech-language pathologist's specialisation in voice disorders and is arguably more logical for patients with voice disorders who consider their speech and language to be normal. The use of various terms in this book reflects the global reality and attempts to avoid the tedium of constant repetition of one title.

Part I
Normal voice

1 CHAPTER

Communicative functions of the voice: an overview

The human voice fulfils a number of roles in the process of oral communication, as well as contributing to the way in which individuals relate to each other. It is essential for clinicians who treat patients with voice disorders to have some understanding of the range of the communicative functions of the voice in order to comprehend the effects of vocal impairment on the individual. The multiple roles of the voice described in this chapter demonstrate the importance of its subtle, as well as its more obvious, aspects. When any aspect of vocal function is impaired, the speaker's communicative effectiveness is reduced.

It is generally recognised that the human voice makes a major contribution to the audibility of verbal communication. Most people have lost their voices at some time and remember the difficulty of trying to make themselves heard, even in quiet settings. It is also generally accepted that voices tend to be identifiable as belonging to particular individuals and can be recognised, like faces, although this is not entirely true. The functions of the voice are much more extensive than this, however, and it is through the voice that considerable information about the speaker is conveyed to the listener. The speaker is frequently unaware that the voice is potentially so revealing and that what is heard and perceived also depends on the listener's experience and sensitivity. A speech-language pathologist or linguist, for example, will be aware of nuances that may evade the non-professional. Throughout life, emotions are reflected in the voice and aspects of the personality are revealed. Infant vocalisation progresses to babbling as a preliminary to speech, and the intonation patterns of the home language are absorbed and form musical patterns which gradually incorporate words and phrases. As the social and emotional boundaries of a child's life expand, the voice absorbs characteristics of the socioeconomic groups encountered, and the peculiarities of regional dialect and social class. In adulthood, the voice eventually provides an amalgam of personal information.

Inferences from vocal behaviour

Even when it might be regarded as neutral, a voice constantly transmits information about the speaker. Even more is revealed as it changes in different social contexts and reflects responses and attitudes to situations encountered. Vocal behaviour is one aspect of the total image – a composite of dress, grooming, posture, gesture and facial expression – presented by an individual. Individuals rarely think about how to use their voices, unless the situation particularly demands care, although they frequently consider what to say. Yet everything has to be said in a certain way, in a certain tone of voice, at a certain pitch and at a certain loudness (Tannen, 1995). It is perhaps surprising, therefore, that 'the voice' has not generally been considered an element of the individual that can be 'groomed' or manipulated for everyday communication. Articulation, language structure and content, accent and dialect are all the subjects of formal instruction, but development of vocal skills has largely remained the territory of voice and singing teachers who teach actors, singers and public speakers. Although this tuition addresses many aspects of vocal function, it is related to the speaker's or singer's ability to perform the adopted role effectively. It has been known for many years by sociolinguists, however, that listeners draw inferences from the voice regarding sex, age, intelligence, regional and socioeconomic origins, education and occupation (Ryan, Giles and Sebastian, 1982). Recently, politicians, businesses and others have become aware of the importance of the inferences that listeners draw from the various aspects of the speaker's voice and this is influencing training patterns for an increasing number of people. As yet, it is probably unusual for individuals to consider trying to alter their voices aesthetically for everyday life, in the way that they would go to a gym for a more beautiful body. Attempts to achieve a more desirable accent is routine in some cultures, but it is unusual for most people to attempt to make their communication skills more effective by changing subtle aspects of vocal behaviour.

A cross-disciplinary approach and the study of various attitudes in social settings is recognised as necessary in any comprehensive evaluation of communicative behaviour (Edwards, 1982). This is the core construct of sociolinguistics that provides an integrative approach to social psychology. The aspects of voice from which inferences are drawn are known as paralinguistic features; they run parallel to the linguistic message and are important for placing it in context. This introduction to vocal function will be directed broadly into these two areas – paralinguistic and linguistic – although in practice the two aspects are not always clearly defined, and they frequently overlap and fuse.

Voice permanence

The distinctive vocal characteristics by which each person is identifiable are dependent to some extent on anatomical features, but they are also determined by habitual settings of the vocal tract.

ANATOMICAL FEATURES

The configuration of the vocal tract of each individual is unique. It imparts the particular vocal quality that distinguishes one individual from another and that contributes to identification of the speaker. These anatomical features of the vocal tract result in the permanent voice quality over which there is little control and which cannot be completely suppressed or disguised.

VOCAL SETTINGS

Superimposed on the permanent anatomical voice features are many possible 'voice settings'. These are the muscular adjustments of the vocal tract, which are learned unconsciously in the family and, later on, in the school, social, professional or occupational group. They affect the timbre of the voice as well as determining the characteristic levels of volume and pitch. As they are habitual, there is no awareness of them in the majority of speakers, although they can be controlled by the individual. It is this aspect of the voice that impersonators manipulate when imitating the voice of a well-known personality. The settings can be assumed and imitated and are peculiar to different groups within regional and local populations. An interesting illustration of this is the evidence that suggests that many American males have learned to use a lower part of the pitch range than British males (Giles and Powesland, 1975) (see 'Contact ulcers', page 172).

The sociolinguistic implications of an individual's speech patterns are acknowledged in the literature, but these usually relate to articulatory patterns rather than to the voice itself. For example, the class-conscious British detect the background of a speaker very readily (Scherer and Giles, 1979). It is agreed that 'received pronunciation' (RP) is the most prestigious standard accent in Britain (Kramarac, 1982), with high status and competence connotations, placing speakers in a socially superior position to those with apparently less advantageous antecedents. Conversely, some speakers consciously reject RP because they do not want to be perceived as members of an élitist and privileged group. The English are reputed to be the most class-conscious race in Europe, whereas Americans acknowledge regional differences of accent but are less likely to perceive them as important markers of social class. In Italy, a Tuscan accent is quite different from that of the north or south. It is appreciated for its beauty but does not place these Italians on a higher social plane, although it has great cultural status.

Studies of the voice and social grouping are less common, however, and appear to be less frequently considered. A study in Edinburgh (Scherer and Giles, 1979) produced results showing a correlation between social status and voice settings. Higher social status was associated with more 'creaky' phonation, whereas lower social status revealed voices with more whispering and harshness. It is suggested by some writers that future academic success can be predicted by voice pitch and range. Scherer and Giles (1979) cite a study by Freuder, Brown and Lambert in which teachers evaluating young school children judged slow speech at a low pitch to be indicative of school failure. This study was confirmed by Edwards (1982). It was found that the academically successful pupils of low socioeconomic status did actually use higher pitch, less volume and more appropriate intonation than their unsuccessful peers. The judgement of an individual's abilities and intelligence from the voice is obviously highly dubious. Some teachers and many other members of society unconsciously hold stereotyped and often negative views of certain ethnic and social groups.

PARALINGUISTIC FEATURES

In contrast to the long-term nature of the anatomy and voice settings that combine to make voice permanence, there are paralinguistic features of the voice that change with emotion. These result from changes in tension in the vocal folds and the vocal tract which, in turn, affect vocal features. Shades of feeling are reflected in the voice and are inextricably linked with the verbal message and may override it. These features are recognised as timbre, tone of voice or vocal quality. Crystal (1980) refers to them as voice qualifiers. Such changing vocal settings are difficult to measure, but it is universally recognised that voices change 'colour' with changing emotion. This is reflected in the way a remark is delivered rather than how it is worded: *It wasn't what she said but the way that she said it that made me mad. I know perfectly well what he meant although he didn't say it in so many words.* An impartial judge may be totally bewildered by the feelings of bitterness and aggression that arise between the protagonists and by the way in which innocent words can be misinterpreted. Inevitably, changes in articulation are associated with vocal variation; increases in tension in the vocal tract, for example, may manifest themselves in the tongue and lips as well as in the muscles of the larynx.

In more subtle emotional contexts, feelings such as sadness, disappointment, happiness, love and joy are reflected in the voice. The sincerity and empathy of a speaker are conveyed to the listener, and words not sincerely felt may be recognised as false. The paralinguistic features of voice allow us to communicate feeling without being explicit when it would be difficult or socially inappropriate to make an overt statement. Siegman (1987) suggests that, in this way, we can express feelings without taking full responsibility for them. Although paralinguistic features usually emerge unconsciously, it is also possible for them to be consciously manipulated in order to make them appropriate to the situation or to influence the listener to the speaker's advantage.

Social group differences

Paralinguistic features of voice are not necessarily interpreted correctly between individuals of different ethnic groups. Scherer and Giles (1979) observed, for instance, that West Indians in normal calm conversation will suddenly alter pitch and increase loudness of the voice for emphasis. This may be interpreted as an angry outburst by those of other groups, and emphatic speech may be incorrectly regarded as angry or aggressive. The potential dangers to relationships between different ethnic and social groups are obvious.

Personality indicators

Inferences can be drawn from the voice about a speaker's personality, although the same inference is not necessarily made by each listener. For example, relatively high vocal pitch may indicate positive aspects of personality such as competence, dominance and assertiveness to one listener, but another may conclude that the speaker is nervous and deceitful (Street and Hopper, 1982). There seems to be a general assumption that a speaker is dynamic and extrovert if the pitch shows marked variability. A loud voice can also indicate extroversion but, if the voice is inappropriately loud, it may signal insensitivity to the situation and embarrass the listener (Street and Hopper, 1982). Addington (1968) says that nasality is strongly linked to negative attributes such as unattractiveness and neuroticism.

Psychiatrists recognise the voices of anxiety, depression and despair. Moses (1954) emphasised the vocal symptoms exhibited by distressed individuals. Ostwald (1963) noted the importance of listening to different vocal qualities such as a more 'hollow tone' and a flatter intonation than the 'robust' voice. There is evidence that it is the frequency range of a voice that has the most powerful effect on listener judgements of the speaker's emotional status (Scherer, 1995). A wide frequency range expresses high arousal, whether negative or positive, whereas a narrow frequency range is perceived as sadness or neutrality. Low vocal pitch in association with slow speech is recognised as indicating depression and breathy, irregular voice accompanying rapid speech may indicate anxiety (Gudykunst, 1986).

The voice, therefore, can indicate who we are and how we are feeling. It is one of the most informative clues about any individual. As a result, changes in the voice as a result of illness or injury make the speaker feel at a disadvantage, because it is realised intuitively that the voice might be conveying erroneous messages about important aspects of the personality. A 'beautiful' speaking voice, on the other hand, encourages positive responses from the listener and could be regarded as enhancing the perception of the speaker's personal attributes. What constitutes the 'beautiful' voice is debatable and probably varies from one culture to another.

Voice loudness

Loudness is a parameter of voice that varies from one individual to another and will vary at different times within the same individual, according to the emotional or linguistic content of the communication. There appear to be differences of voice volume between the sexes, with men generally talking more loudly, although women are more likely to compensate for external noise by increasing vocal intensity (Scherer and Giles, 1979). It is suggested that both sexes tend to talk more loudly to members of the opposite sex in general conversation, although the quiet voices of a close relationship maintain intimacy.

The ability to vary vocal volume allows the speaker considerable control over the behaviour of others. Increasing loudness is an effective way of establishing the speaker's turn in a conversation and will also deter the intervention of other speakers. Margaret Thatcher's dominant role in the House of Commons demonstrated this publicly, but increased vocal volume has a similar effect in other contexts. The loud voice used for commanding, calling, warning and attracting attention cannot be ignored by the listener very easily, whereas the whisper or very quiet voice signals the appropriate behaviour for the listener. In anger, the amplitude of the voice may be the dominant feature in communicating the heartfelt message.

Non-verbal communication

A description of paralinguistic aspects of voice is not complete without acknowledging the part played by non-verbal communication, or body language, which is also a significant paralinguistic feature. From the purely physiological perspective, some body postures modify the tensions and dimensions of the vocal tract and so affect the sound of the voice. The relatively immobile face of the depressed individual or one who is being inscrutable reduces the extent of mouth opening during speech. As a result, the sound of the voice is different from when the same individual is relaxed and outgoing. Similarly, the vocal note itself will be affected by the head posture of the pompous individual whose chin is depressed and retracted.

Vocal behaviour tends to be integrated with non-verbal communication and to vary in similar ways. Facial, hand and arm gestures, and body postures vary between individuals and between social and ethnic groups. There are also differences in each individual's vocal and non-verbal behaviour according to mood and the relative degree of formality of a situation. In general, both are less animated when an individual is depressed or very relaxed, or when the occasion is particularly formal. Even complete lack of both facial expression and active body gesture is an aspect of communication as is the monotonous voice. The posture of participants in a job interview, for instance, marks the dominant role of the employer and the submissive role of the applicant. The former may lean back in his chair and the latter sit stiffly erect or lean forward, ingratiatingly. The questions and answers, of course, guide the conversation (Cappella and Street, 1985) but allied to this are the vocal undertones. The quality of the voices vary according to levels of confidence and anxiety. The posture, eye contact or avoidance, head movement, shifting or fidgeting all play a part. However, during conversation some individuals model their own behaviour on that of the person to whom they are talking, particularly if they are in agreement. This behaviour was referred to by Argyle (1970) as 'response matching' and can also apply to vocal behaviour. The voice is inevitably affected by vocal tract gestures arising from some of the physical changes of non-verbal communication.

Set patterns of social conduct greatly influence communication and enable individuals to influence attitudes and change them radically. Kalin (1982) has reviewed the social significance of speech in medical, legal and social settings, and the 'set' registers that maintain dominant and subservient roles and that differ greatly in colloquial contexts. Manipulation of attitude can reassure and antagonise: empathy can be established or confidence and trust destroyed. This aspect of communication is of considerable importance for the clinician in establishing rapport with the patient. It is crucial to successful rehabilitation (Morris, 1985) and to the clinician's success in relating to colleagues.

Linguistic vocal features

SEGMENTAL PHONOLOGY

The voice is an integral part of individual phonemes and in this context is part of the structure of pronunciation, as opposed to the system of language (Abercrombie, 1967; Grunwell, 1982). It can be analysed and described in relation to each phonological segment. Coordination of phonation with articulation is essential; if phonemes that should be voiced are produced without voice, and vice versa, word meaning is changed. For instance, in the words 'fleece' and 'fleas' the positions of the articulators are identical; the only distinguishing factor is that the final phoneme is voiced in 'fleas' and voiceless in 'fleece'.

NON-SEGMENTAL PHONOLOGY (SUPRASEGMENTAL PHONOLOGY)

The voice plays a crucial role in the linguistic conveyance of meaning in non-segmental phonology. This can be considered separately from the para-linguistic aspects which convey the emotional context of the message previously described. In non-segmental phonology, voice contributes to 'linguistic contrastivity' (Crystal, 1981), which is based on the variables of pitch, stress, tempo, rhythm and pause, collectively known as prosody. Intelligible speech is dependent not only on the accuracy of articulation and on an audible voice, but also on phonation that can fulfil the requirements of normal prosody.

The prosodic system of language is learned very early and appears in the infant's vocalisations before the first words. The system is difficult, if not impossible, to acquire after childhood. It is deviant prosody that immediately identifies a foreigner to the native of the language, however perfect vocabulary, syntax and semantic proficiency may be. Incorrect stress and loss of natural rhythm can render speech almost incomprehensible. Crystal (1981, 1982) provides many examples of prosodic contrasts in conversational and colloquial speech, and has devised the Prosody Profile (PROP) for describing this aspect of linguistic disability.

The flexibility of the normal voice allows the pitch changes that constitute intonation patterns, an important aspect of suprasegmental phonology. The rises and falls of the vocal pitch clarify the language of the message and can even indicate what is to follow. Crystal (1981) has described five major functions of intonation:

1.   Intonation has a grammatical role. For example, it marks the end of sentences and clauses. In English, the end of a sentence that is a

statement is frequently indicated by a falling intonation pattern. The sentence 'We're going out' (⎯⎯⌍), in which a falling pattern is used, indicates what we are going to do. The same words and structure become a question, asking if we are going out, when rising intonation is used at the end of the sentence (We're going out? ⎯⎯⌃). During the past 10-15 years, there has been a growing trend in younger English speakers to use rising intonation at the end of a statement. The effect is confusing for listeners who are not used to this pattern. If the statement 'I went out last night' is said with a rising intonation and becomes 'I went out last night' (⎯⎯⌃), the listener might draw the conclusion that the speaker does not know whether or not he or she went out and is asking for confirmation. Sometimes this pattern is misinterpreted as reflecting general uncertainty. In reality, the speaker is signalling that an account of the event is about to follow and really means 'Did you know, or do you remember, that I went out last night?' as a precursor to recounting what happened. This change in intonation patterns is observed in the USA, Australia and Britain and is an interesting example of the constant development and modification of communicative behaviour, sometimes viewed by older people as an example of declining standards.

2. A further grammatical role of intonation is to make contrasts, such as those between past and present (e.g. 'I saw him **yesterday** not **today**') and between positive and negative (e.g. Is the answer **yes** or **no**?). The change in intonation for the key words will frequently be accompanied by a change in loudness so that together they stress the important words in the sentence.

3. The semantic role of intonation is probably most dramatically demonstrated in tonal languages, such as Chinese languages, in which the same word has different meanings according to the intonation pattern. In English, its semantic role occurs when it is used to draw attention to certain information, particularly if it is new. For example, the sentence 'Jim is in the car' (⎯⎯⌍) said with a falling intonation pattern is a relatively unambiguous statement of fact. On the other hand, '**Jim** is in the car' tells the listener that it is Jim rather than Tom or Bob who is in the car. The intonation on the key word 'Jim' might rise if there is an element of surprise, or fall if there is some disappointment that it is Jim rather than Tom or Bob. The intonation can also vary if the speaker wants to indicate that Jim has come by car rather than on foot: 'Jim is in the **car**'.

4. The social role is apparent in the way intonation is used to manipulate conversation. It is unconsciously recognised that certain patterns

encourage a response whereas others indicate that the speaker regards the interaction as finished. Rising or falling pitch can indicate that the speaker is ready for the listener to speak. Intonation will also frequently reveal the attitude of the speaker concerning the subject matter of the utterance, so that uncertainty or confidence is readily recognised.

5. The psychological function of intonation affects the performance of the listener. By varying its pattern and relevant aspects of prosody, the speaker can influence attitude, recall, comprehension and other parameters of communication in conversational contexts.

Summary

The functions of the voice can be classified into three categories (see Figure 1.1). The voice makes speech and language audible, it has a paralinguistic role and a linguistic role. It is more than a means of communicating verbal messages clearly, however, as Locke (1995) has pointed out. He comments that there are many social interactions where the linguistic content of what is said is relatively unimportant but in which speech becomes a series of vocal gestures by which we demonstrate our friendliness, sincerity and sense of humour. In many circumstances, we use the voice and speech to interact rather than to inform. The voice serves as a powerful conveyor of personal identity, emotional state, education and social status. It is because the voice fulfils so many functions that its impairment or loss can be so distressing. Voice is a fundamental element of verbal communication, suffusing all parameters of human speech and the unique self we present to the world.

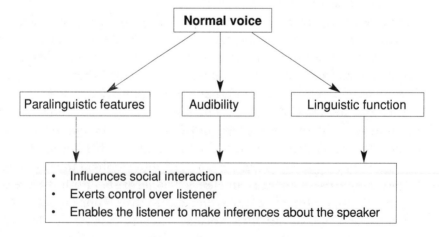

Figure 1.1 The role of normal voice in social interaction.

The larynx and upper respiratory tract

This chapter, together with Chapter 3, describes the anatomy and physiology of the vocal tract in which the vocal note is generated and subsequently modified to produce the sound heard by the listener. The parameters of the voice, and the way in which the vocal folds adapt to produce them, are discussed in Chapter 4.

The **respiratory system** consists of the **upper respiratory tract** and the **lower respiratory tract**. The upper respiratory tract includes the **larynx, oropharynx, oral cavity** and **nasal cavities**. The lower respiratory tract consists of the **trachea, bronchi** and **lungs**. Together, the upper and lower respiratory tracts comprise the **vocal tract** and are functionally interdependent. Modifications to one system will affect the function of the other immediately. The tract above the vocal folds is known as the **supraglottic tract** and, below the vocal folds, the **subglottic vocal tract** (Figure 2.1).

The larynx

The larynx is situated in the neck at the level of the third to sixth cervical vertebrae (C3–C6) and extends from the base of the tongue to the trachea. It lies anterior to the **oesophagus**, to which it is attached by the **cricopharyngeal sphincter muscle** at the level of the fifth vertebra (C5). The larynx is continuous with the **trachea** (windpipe) below and the **pharynx** above. It consists of a framework of cartilages bound together by ligaments, membranes and muscles. Housed within the laryngeal frame are the two **vocal folds**, which constitute the vibrator that generates the voice. The larynx is an **air passage**, a **sphincteric device** and an **organ of phonation** (Williams et al., 1995).

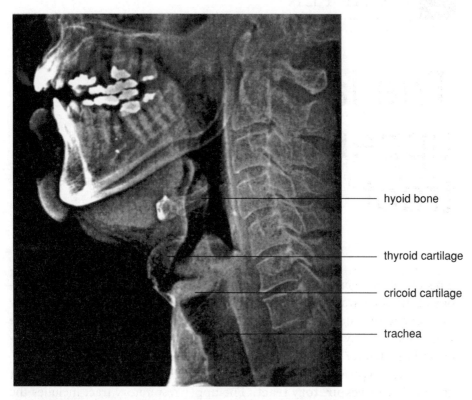

Figure 2.1 Normal vocal tract (phonating on /iː/) (Xeroradiograph reprinted by permission of the late Dr. Frances MacCurtain).

HYOID BONE

The hyoid is a U-shaped bone from which the larynx is suspended. It is generally considered to be part of the larynx because it is an important point of attachment for the larynx, which follows its vertical excursions in deglutition and phonation.

LARYNGEAL CARTILAGES (FIGURE 2.2)

There are nine laryngeal cartilages: three unpaired (**cricoid, thyroid, epiglottis**) and three paired (**arytenoids, corniculates, cuneiforms**).

Cricoid cartilage

The cricoid cartilage is the lowest laryngeal cartilage and forms an inflexible ring at the top of the trachea. It is shaped like a signet ring, narrow anteriorly and broad and flat posteriorly. It has articular facets on its lateral aspects for the inferior horns of the thyroid cartilage and, on its superior border, for the arytenoid cartilages.

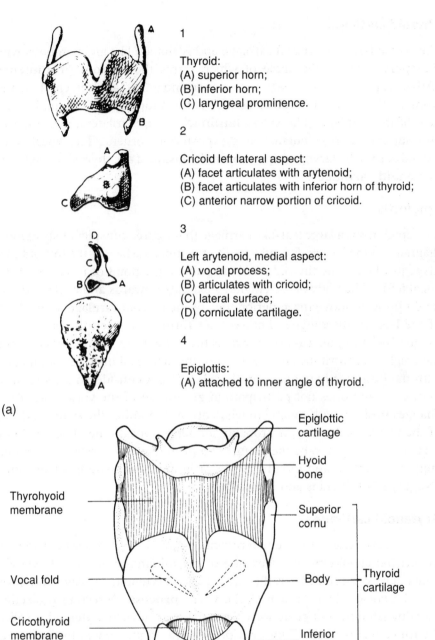

1

Thyroid:
(A) superior horn;
(B) inferior horn;
(C) laryngeal prominence.

2

Cricoid left lateral aspect:
(A) facet articulates with arytenoid;
(B) facet articulates with inferior horn of thyroid;
(C) anterior narrow portion of cricoid.

3

Left arytenoid, medial aspect:
(A) vocal process;
(B) articulates with cricoid;
(C) lateral surface;
(D) corniculate cartilage.

4

Epiglottis:
(A) attached to inner angle of thyroid.

(a)

Epiglottic cartilage

Hyoid bone

Thyrohyoid membrane

Superior cornu

Vocal fold

Body

Thyroid cartilage

Cricothyroid membrane

Inferior cornu

Cricoid cartilage

Tracheal rings

(b)

Figure 2.2 Laryngeal cartilages.

Reprinted from 'Ear, Nose and Throat' Dhillon R.S., East C.A., page 55, 1994, by permission of the publisher Churchill Livingstone

Thyroid cartilage

This is the largest laryngeal cartilage and is shaped like an open book with the spine in front, the angle of which forms the **thyroid prominence** (Adam's apple). This is a 90° angle in men and a 120° angle in children and women. The **thyroid notch** can be felt at the midpoint of the superior surface of the cartilage. The sides (**laminae**) are quadrilateral with inferior and superior horns (**cornu**) at the posterior corners. The vocal folds extend across the laryngeal space from the inside of the thyroid angle to the **arytenoid cartilages**.

Epiglottis

The epiglottis is a large leaf-like cartilage that figures conspicuously in most diagrams of the larynx. It is attached to the inner surface of the thyroid cartilage just below the thyroid notch and above the point of insertion of the vocal folds. The body of the epiglottis extends upwards and backwards, so that it projects above the superior edge of the thryoid cartilage, to the level of the base of the tongue. The recesses formed between the base of the tongue and the epiglottis are known as the **valleculae**. During swallowing, the epiglottis contributes to occlusion of the laryngeal inlet, in conjunction with the posterior hypopharyngeal wall. It is not considered important in phonation and does not participate in generation of the vocal note. As it changes position with tongue movements and modifies the shape and size of the pharyngeal cavity, it probably influences vocal tone. The epiglottic cartilage is thought to be the vestige of a primitive olfactory system associated with sniffing and monitoring scent in animals, possibly while eating (Negus, 1949; Perkins and Kent, 1986).

Arytenoid cartilages

The concave bases of these two pyramid-shaped cartilages articulate with the cricoid shoulders on either side of the midline by means of synovial joints. The projection from the base of each arytenoid cartilage anteriorly into the vocal fold is known as the **vocal process**. A second projection pointing laterally and posteriorly from the base of each arytenoid is called the **muscular process**. This provides a point of attachment for the lateral and posterior cricoarytenoid muscles (see Figure 2.7 on page 22). The posterior curved surface of the arytenoid cartilage receives the fibres of the transverse and oblique arytenoid muscles.

The movements of the arytenoid cartilages are complex and include sliding across the cricoid cartilage in addition to rotation (Von Leden and Moore, 1961; Citardi, Gracco and Sasaki, 1995). On **adduction** of the vocal processes the arytenoids move **medially, inferiorly** and **posteriorly**, whereas on **abduction** they move **laterally, superiorly** and **posteriorly** (Hirano et al., 1991). As Tucker (1993) points out, the movement of the arytenoids on the cricoarytenoid joints appears to produce a rotary action. In reality, a much more complex movement takes place because of the characteristics of the cricoarytenoid joint. The articular surfaces on the cricoid lamina are orientated in a slightly posterior direction and are biconcave when seen from above. The articular surfaces on the underside of the arytenoid cartilage are also biconcave. Consequently, the apparent rotation of the arytenoids is caused by the sliding effect both in an anteroposterior direction and in the lateromedial direction.

Corniculate and cuneiform cartilages

The corniculate cartilages are tiny, conical structures at the apex of each arytenoid cartilage. The small cuneiform cartilages support the edges of the aryepiglottic folds which run bilaterally from the arytenoid cartilages to the base of the epiglottis. There is considerable normal variation of these cartilages which are not necessarily present in all individuals. Normal people frequently deviate from the idealised illustrations of anatomy textbooks. In many instances these variations have no clinical significance.

LARYNGEAL MEMBRANES

Thyrohyoid membrane

This **external** laryngeal membrane arises from the superior border of the thyroid cartilage and is inserted into the superior edge of the hyoid bone.

Fibroelastic internal laryngeal membrane

Beneath the laryngeal mucosa lies the fibroelastic laryngeal membrane, which consists of upper and lower parts:

- The upper part is the **quadrangular membrane**, which is rather poorly defined. It extends between the arytenoid cartilages and the sides of the epiglottis.
- The lower part is the **cricothyroid ligament**, which is also known as the **cricovocal ligament** or **conus elasticus**. This membrane arises from the inner surface of the cricoid arch. It passes medially and superiorly to insert on the vocal ligaments, which form the free margin of the vocal folds.

LARYNGEAL MUSCLES

Laryngeal function is dependent on the **intrinsic laryngeal muscles,** which **move the laryngeal cartilages in relation to each other,** and the **extrinsic laryngeal muscles,** which **alter the position of the larynx in the neck** (Figures 2.3–2.8).

Intrinsic laryngeal muscles (Table 2.1 and Figure 2.7)

The intrinsic laryngeal muscles are named according to their attachment to the laryngeal cartilages. They do not affect the spatial relationship of the larynx to the rest of the neck, but rather adduct, abduct, lengthen, shorten and alter the tension of the vocal folds. The muscles are all paired except the transverse arytenoid muscle which is a single muscle.

Thyroarytenoid muscles

The thyroarytenoid muscles constitute the body of each vocal fold. They are of unique and complex structure, as has been shown by Hirano's investigations using high-speed photography and morphological dissection of

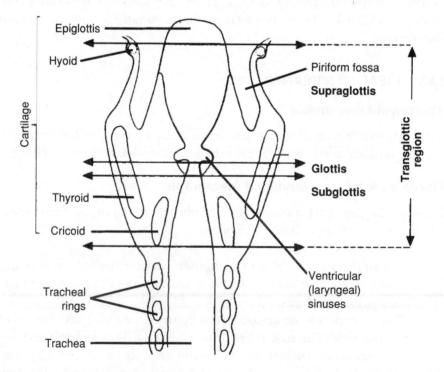

Figure 2.3 Coronal section of larynx: posterior view.
Reprinted from 'Ear, Nose and Throat' Dhillon R.S., East C.A., page 55, 1994, by permission of the publisher Churchill Livingstone

Table 2.1 Intrinsic laryngeal muscles

Coordinated function:
1 Adduct and abduct vocal folds
2 Determine vibratory characteristics
3 Determine cross-sectional contour of vocal folds

Muscle	Attachments	Function
Thyroarytenoid	Thyroid cartilage to arytenoid vocal processes	Adduct true vocal folds Shorten, tense, thicken true vocal folds Adduct false vocal folds
Posterior cricoarytenoid	Posterior part of cricoid cartilage to arytenoid muscular process	Abduct vocal folds
Lateral cricoarytenoid	Lateral edge of cricoid cartilage to arytenoid muscular process	Adduct vocal folds
Interarytenoid muscles:		
• Oblique arytenoids • Transverse arytenoid		Approximate arytenoid cartilages
• Aryepiglotticus	Connect arytenoid cartilages to epiglottis	Pulls epiglottis down over laryngeal orifice
Cricothyroid muscle	Cricoid cartilage to thyroid cartilage	Weak vocal fold adduction Thin, lengthen vocal folds Sharpen vocal fold free edges

the muscle (Hirano, 1974). The thyroarytenoid muscles are attached to the interior angle of the thyroid cartilage where they are fixed adjacent to each other. The point where they join anteriorly is called the **anterior commissure**. The thyroarytenoid muscles extend posteriorly to the anterior surfaces of the vocal processes of the arytenoid cartilages. The free margins of the vocal folds confront each other across a triangular space called the **glottis** (also known as the glottic aperture or rima glottidis). The parts of the vocal tract above and below the vocal folds are known, therefore, as the supra- and subglottic vocal tract, respectively. Each thyroarytenoid muscle has a superior, lateral portion and an inferior, medial portion.

False vocal folds

The superior portion of the thyroarytenoid muscle forms the **false vocal fold** (also known as the ventricular fold or vestibular fold). Normally, the false vocal folds are not directly involved in phonation, but approximate during swallowing to make a firm valve or seal. The area from the laryngeal inlet to the ventricular folds is called the **laryngeal vestibule**. There is a space

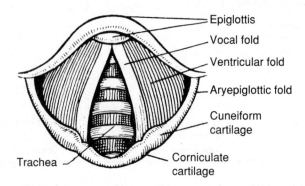

Epiglottis

Vocal fold

Ventricular fold

Aryepiglottic fold

Cuneiform
cartilage

Trachea

Corniculate
cartilage

Figure 2.4 Laryngoscopic view of a laryngeal interior.

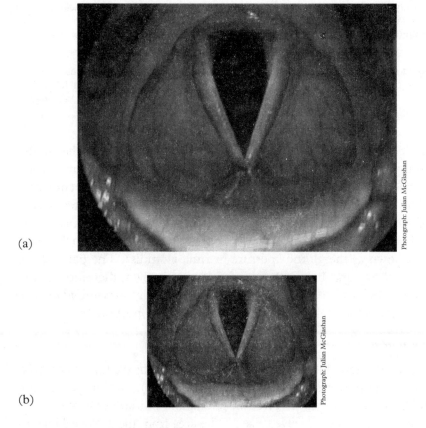

(a)

(b)

Figure 2.5 (a) Normal vocal folds at rest; (b) adult male vocal folds: actual size.

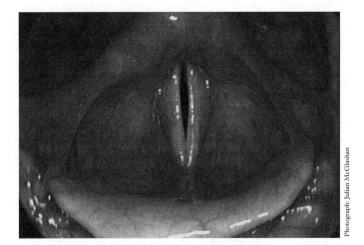

Photograph: Julian McGlashan

Figure 2.6 Normal vocal folds during phonation: modal voice.

between the false vocal fold and the true vocal fold called the **laryngeal ventricle** or **ventricle of Morgagni**. This ventricle extends upwards to form the **laryngeal saccule** in which 60–70 mucous glands are found in the submucosa (Williams et al., 1995). The saccule is separated from the internal surface of the thyroid cartilage by the thyroepiglottic muscle which, on contraction, compresses the saccule so that its secretions are expressed on to the vocal folds. This mucus protects the surface of the vocal folds from the effects of friction and drying, and so facilitates vibration of the vocal fold mucosa during phonation.

Vocal folds (Figures 2.3–2.6)

The lower portion of the thyroarytenoid muscle (the **vocalis muscle**) forms the muscular body of the true **vocal fold** (also known as the vocal cord). ('Vocal fold' is the preferred term because it describes the structure more accurately. The term 'vocal cords', however, is still used by many otorhinolaryngologists and others.) The free edges of the two folds are covered with a superficial membranous layer of squamous epithelium and interwoven in the layers below are elastic and collagenous fibres of the vocal ligaments. The folds are white in appearance and contrast with the red false folds when viewed from above. (A more detailed discussion of the mucous membrane covering the vocalis muscle appears on page 28.)

The function of the thyroarytenoid muscles is adduction of true and false vocal folds. The vocalis fibres shorten, tense and thicken the vocal folds and so alter their vibratory characteristics (Citardi, Gracco and Sasaki, 1995).

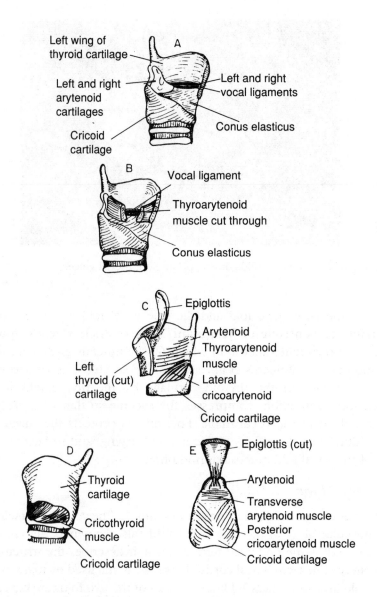

Figure 2.7 Intrinsic laryngeal muscles.

Posterior cricoarytenoid muscles

These muscles originate in the broad outer surface of the cricoid cartilage and are inserted into the muscular processes of the arytenoid cartilages. They abduct and pull upwards and backwards the vocal processes of the arytenoids, thus elongating the vocal folds. They are the major **abductors** of the vocal folds (Last, 1984).

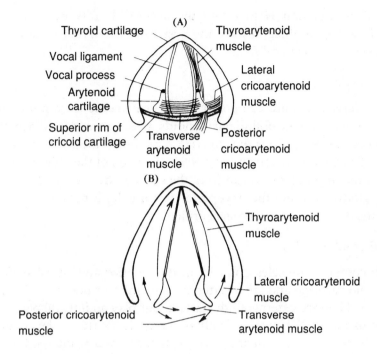

Figure 2.8 Transverse view of laryngeal muscles and actions.

Zemlin, Davis and Gaza (1984), in a study of the fine morphology of the posterior cricoarytenoids, resolved a long-standing disagreement of the exact function of the muscle and contradictions in the electromyographic results of many researchers. There are two separate bundles of muscle which have separate tendons. Therefore, there are two muscles, not one, forming each posterior cricoarytenoid muscle. One muscle has oblique fibres and the other is composed of vertical and lateral fibres. The horizontal fibres rotate the arytenoids on their axes and swing the vocal processes outwards. The vertical fibres draw the arytenoids away from each other by pulling down, laterally, on the sloping upper border of the cricoid lamina. The net result of the action of the whole muscle is rotation and separation of the arytenoids. The existence of a dual muscle action is of particular relevance in the variable positions assumed by the vocal folds in paralysis of the recurrent laryngeal nerve (see page 312).

Their function is vocal fold abduction and lengthening.

Lateral cricoarytenoid muscles

These muscles originate along the superior and lateral borders of the cricoid cartilage and pass back obliquely to the outside corner of the arytenoid cartilages.

Their function is to rotate the arytenoids forwards and slightly inwards, acting as antagonists to the posterior cricoarytenoid muscles and as adductors of the vocal folds.

Interarytenoid muscles

The interarytenoids are composed of the **transverse arytenoid muscle**, which is single, and the **oblique arytenoids**, which are a crossed pair of muscles (Tucker, 1987a). Their function is to approximate the arytenoid cartilages.

The **aryepiglotticus** muscle is an extension of the oblique arytenoid muscle, the fibres of which run from the apex of the arytenoid to attach to the epiglottis, forming the **aryepiglottic fold**. Its function is to pull the epiglottis down over the laryngeal orifice.

Cricothyroid muscles

The cricothyroid muscles originate in the anterior and lateral surfaces of the cricoid cartilage and are inserted into the inferior border of the thyroid cartilage. They are external to the larynx, but play an integral part in vocal fold adjustments. When the cricothyroid muscle contracts, the cricoid cartilage pivots, rising in front and lowering behind. As a result, the vocal folds are brought into a paramedian position and are stretched, lengthened and thinned. The free edges of the folds become sharp as their four layers are stiffened while, at the same time, the posterior cricoarytenoid muscles brace back the arytenoid cartilages. The cricothyroid muscles are the most important muscles for raising frequency and achieve this in conjunction with the lateral cricoarytenoids and the thyroarytenoids (Hirose and Sawashima, 1981; Hollien, 1983a, 1983b). Their functions are:

- to thin and lengthen vocal folds
- to sharpen free edges of the vocal folds
- as weak adductors of vocal folds.

A cautionary remark is appropriate here. Although each muscle performs a particular action, in reality the intrinsic laryngeal muscles participate together in a finely coordinated, harmonious and rhythmic mechanical system that controls muscle posture in relation to subglottic air pressure (Citardi, Gracco and Sasaki, 1995). There is evidence that vocal fold abduction during speech, for example, is the result of activation of the posterior cricoarytenoid in coordination with the suppression of interarytenoid activity (Lofqvist and Yoshioka, 1980), whereas vocal fold adduction requires simultaneous contraction of the interarytenoid, the lateral cricoarytenoid and the thyroarytenoid (Hirose, 1977). Similarly, a normal vocal fold can be increased 50% in length by the combined action of the cricothyroid and posterior cricoarytenoid muscles (Williams et al., 1995). Changes in upper airway pressure have been shown to affect laryngeal muscle activity, with the cricothyroid muscle showing marked response to such stimulation (Woodson et al., 1991).

Extrinsic laryngeal muscles (Table 2.2, Figures 2.9 and 2.10)

The extrinsic laryngeal muscles (excluding the sternothyroid muscle) alter the position of the larynx in the neck via their attachment to the hyoid bone from which the thyroid cartilage is suspended. (Changes of laryngeal position may cause changes within the larynx which modify vocal fold oscillation.) They can be classified according to both position and function. The **suprahyoid** muscles **elevate** the larynx and the **infrahyoid** muscles **depress** the larynx.

Table 2.2 Extrinsic laryngeal muscles

Muscle	Attachments	Function
Suprahyoid muscles (laryngeal elevators)		
Digastric	Mastoid process to chin	Depresses mandible Elevates hyoid bone
Stylohyoid	Styloid bone to hyoid bone	Elevates hyoid bone and draws it backwards
Mylohyoid	Mandible to hyoid bone	Elevates floor of mouth in first stage of deglutition Elevates hyoid bone Depresses mandible
Geniohyoid	Mandible to hyoid bone	Elevates hyoid bone and pulls it forward Depresses mandible
Infrahyoid muscles (laryngeal depressors)		
Sternohyoid	Sternum to hyoid bone	Depresses hyoid bone
Sternothyroid	Sternum to thyroid cartilage	Draws larynx down
Omohyoid	1 Superior portion: sternal tendon to hyoid bone 2 Inferior portion: scapula to sternal tendon	Depresses hyoid bone
Thyrohyoid	Thyroid cartilage to hyoid bone	Pulls hyoid bone and thyroid cartilages together

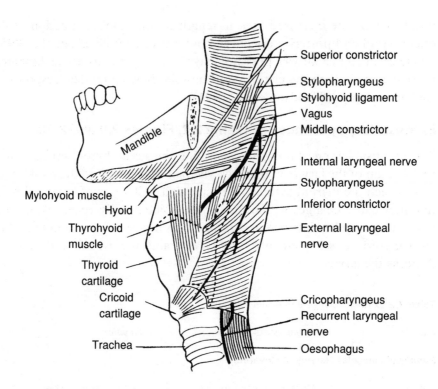

Mandible

Mylohyoid muscle
Hyoid
Thyrohyoid
muscle
Thyroid
cartilage
Cricoid
cartilage
Trachea

Superior constrictor
Stylopharyngeus
Stylohyoid ligament
Vagus
Middle constrictor

Internal laryngeal nerve
Stylopharyngeus
Inferior constrictor
External laryngeal
nerve

Cricopharyngeus
Recurrent laryngeal
nerve
Oesophagus

Figure 2.9 Extrinsic laryngeal muscles and nerve supply.

Suprahyoid muscles (laryngeal elevators) (Figure 2.10)

Digastric

The anterior and posterior bellies of each digastric muscle lie below the mandible and extend from the mastoid processes (behind the ears) to the chin.

Their function is to depress the mandible and elevate the hyoid bone; they also assist in supporting the floor of the mouth.

Stylohyoid

These muscles extend from the styloid process to the hyoid bone.

Their function is to elevate the hyoid bone and draw it backwards, resulting in elongation of the floor of the mouth.

Mylohyoid

These muscles form a flat, triangular sheet which is attached to the whole length of the mylohyoid line of the mandible. They extend from the mandible to the hyoid bone.

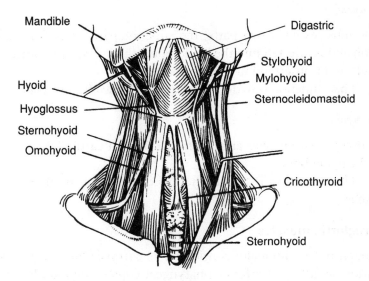

Figure 2.10 Suprahyoid and infrahyoid muscles.

Their function is to elevate the floor of the mouth in the first stage of deglutition. They might also elevate the hyoid bone and depress the mandible (Williams et al., 1995).

Geniohyoid

The geniohyoid muscles arise from the mandible and insert into the hyoid bone.

Their function is to elevate the hyoid bone and pull it forwards. They act partly as an antagonist to the stylohyoid. When the hyoid bone is fixed, the geniohyoid muscle depresses the mandible.

Infrahyoid muscles (laryngeal depressors)

Sternohyoid

The sternohyoid muscles arise from the sternum (breastbone) and are inserted into the hyoid bone.

Their function is to depress the hyoid bone after it has been elevated.

Sternothyroid

The sternothyroid muscles also arise from the sternum, but they are inserted into the thyroid cartilage.

Their function is to draw the larynx down after it has been elevated during swallowing or phonation. During production of low notes in singing, this downward traction is exerted against a relatively fixed hyoid bone (Williams et al., 1995).

Omohyoid

These muscles have two parts: the superior part arises from the sternal tendon and is inserted into the hyoid bone; the inferior part arises from the scapula and is inserted into the sternal tendon.

Their function is to depress the hyoid bone after it has been elevated.

Thyrohyoid

The thyrohyoid muscles arise from the thyroid cartilage and are inserted into the hyoid bone.

Their function is to pull the hyoid bone and the thyroid cartilages together.

Supraglottic muscles

Although not traditionally considered as extrinsic laryngeal muscles, the superior, middle and inferior pharyngeal constrictor muscles *(see below)* and the extrinsic tongue muscles (*styloglossus, genioglossus* and *hyoglossus*) also affect laryngeal position and spatial relations.

Superficial and lateral cervical muscles

Of the various superficial muscles in the neck, the most obvious are the **sternocleidomastoids** which descend obliquely across the side of the neck. They are particularly prominent when contracted in effortful phonation and can give rise to considerable discomfort in a hyperfunctional speaker. Inferiorly, each muscle has a clavicular and sternal attachment. Superiorly, each is attached to the lateral surface of the mastoid process by a strong tendon.

VOCAL FOLD HISTOLOGY

The true vocal folds are highly elastic and have a complex histological structure (Hirano and Sato, 1993) which contributes to the extraordinary versatility of the voice and its wide range of pitch, volume and quality. The vocal fold is composed of five layers (Figure 2.11):

1.   The integument (outer layer) of the vocal fold is mainly **ciliated columnar epithelium** but the medial edge, which is designed to withstand the impact stresses of phonation, is covered by **stratified squamous epithelium**. The shape of the vocal fold is maintained by the integument.
     Beneath this epithelial cover there are three layers of connective tissue which compose the **lamina propria**.

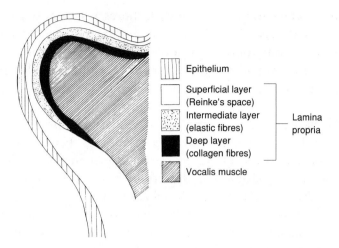

Figure 2.11 Histological structure of vocal folds.

2. The **superficial** or **top layer** of the lamina propria consists of a loose fibrous matrix which Hirano (1974, 1981) likens to gelatin. This is **Reinke's space**, which vibrates most markedly during phonation (Hirano and Kiminori, 1993). It can become oedematous in pathological conditions such as laryngitis or vocal abuse.

3. The second or **intermediate layer** of the lamina propria consists of elastic fibres which resemble soft rubber bands. The amount of elastin varies between men and women.

4. Finally, the third or **deep layer** consists of collagenous fibres, which Hirano and Kiminori (1993) compare with cotton threads.

The intermediate and deep layers are known as the **transition** (Kahane, 1986) and these layers form the vocal ligament. The boundary between the superficial and intermediate layers is well defined, but there is less clear definition between the intermediate and deep layers (Hirano and Bless, 1993). The layer structure varies in thickness throughout the vocal fold length and is constructed in a way that reduces any mechanical damage that might be caused by vibration at the ends of the folds. The lamina propria in men is usually thicker than that in women. It is possible that this results partly from a larger amount of the substance called hyaluronic acid in the vocal folds of men (Hammond et al., 1997) and might account for why women are more susceptible to conditions resulting from trauma to the vocal fold mucosa, such as vocal nodules. The fibres and small vessels in the lamina propria run parallel to the edge of the vocal fold.

5. **The vocalis muscle**: the muscle fibres run almost parallel to the vocal fold edge. The vocalis can shorten and thicken the fold and effect rounding of the lips of the glottis by contraction whereas the cover and lamina propria are slack. Contraction also stiffens the vocal folds in an action that is independent of the vocal fold length.

The various layers of the vocal fold are morphologically distinct (Hirano, 1981; Gray, Hirano and Sato, 1993) and therefore differ in their vibratory characteristics. The layers can be divided in terms of function into the **cover**, the **transition** and the **body**. Table 2.3 illustrates how this mechanical division relates to the histology of the vocal fold. The chief role of the vocalis muscle is to control the shape of the fold and to provide the appropriate degree of tonicity to allow normal vibration to take place (Hiroto, 1981; Perkins and Kent, 1986). The mucous membrane vibrates more than the vocalis muscle during phonation, moving in a wave from the inferior to the superior margins of the vocal fold (see page 70). The mechanical properties of the vocalis muscle are controlled actively by the muscle itself, as well as passively by the other laryngeal muscles, whereas those of the lamina propria are passively controlled by the laryngeal muscles.

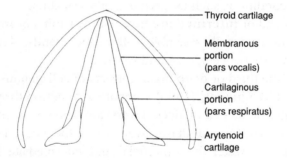

Thyroid cartilage

Membranous portion (pars vocalis)

Cartilaginous portion (pars respiratus)

Arytenoid cartilage

Figure 2.12 Vocal folds: membranous and cartilaginous portions.

Table 2.3 Vocal fold: body-cover

Functional layer	Histological layer
Cover	Epithelium Superficial layer of lamina propria
Transition	Intermediate and deep layers of lamina propria
Body	Vocalis muscle

The complexity of the simultaneous patterns of vibration during phonation, and their interrelationship, are the subject of extensive research (Bless and Abbs, 1983; Stevens and Hirano, 1981; Baer, Sasaki and Harris, 1991). The developing fields of computer modelling and high-speed photography are making significant contributions to the understanding of laryngeal biomechanics (Farley and Barlow, 1994; Titze, 1995; Schutte, Švec and Sram, 1998).

Hormonal target cells have been identified in the larynx. Ferguson, Hudson and McCarty (1987), and Narbaitz, Stumpf and Sar (1980) reported oestrogen and progesterone receptors in the vocalis muscle and a lower number in the lamina propria. None was found in the epithelium. The effects of hormones on the larynx and the voice are not fully understood but their action clearly causes significant changes (see Chapter 5).

Divisions of the vocal folds (Figure 2.12)

Traditionally, on being viewed from above, the vocal folds have been considered to be divided into thirds. The anterior two-thirds are known as the **membranous portion** (traditionally *pars vocalis*) and the posterior one-third as the **cartilaginous portion** (traditionally *pars respiratus*). Hirano (1991) points out that this ratio is really 3:2 not 2:1.

Membranous portion

The membranous portion of the vocal fold is highly elastic, mobile and active in phonation.

It is in the middle of this portion that the greatest excursions occur, because of position and structure.

Cartilaginous portion

The posterior third is that part into which the vocal process of the arytenoid cartilage penetrates. This cartilaginous part does not participate in phonatory vibration except in the deepest notes when the whole fold enacts a rolling motion.

Laryngeal spaces

The **laryngeal vestibule** and **ventricle** in the interior of the larynx have been described above. In addition to these spaces, there are two further lateral spaces known as the **pyriform sinuses** (or fossae) which lie between the interior surface of the thyroid cartilage laminae and the aryepiglottic folds. The mucous membrane lining the normal, healthy larynx and vocal tract is always moist. This lubrication is provided by the mucous glands in the ventricle and **laryngeal saccule** (see above). The dryness and irritation caused by infection, atmospheric changes and certain emotions are uncomfortable and have noticeable effects on the voice. In a dry atmosphere, the mucous membrane overlying the vocal folds becomes drier and its normal undulations are reduced (Hiroto, 1981).

LARYNGEAL INNERVATION

Phonation is dependent on the integrated functioning of many elements of the central and peripheral nervous systems (CNS and PNS). No part of the nervous system is self-contained or able to function independently of any other. Although the motor and sensory tracts serving the larynx (see below) are relatively well understood, the way in which phonation is initiated and controlled continues to be the subject of neurological research. In addition to the cortical loci associated with voluntary phonation, there is evidence of subcortical representation which is responsible for reflex laryngeal function and involuntary phonation (Aronson, 1990). Research has shown that a region of the midbrain, the periaqueductal grey matter (PAG), is a crucial site for mammalian voice production (Davis et al., 1996). It appears to have more than one important role in this process: not only is it involved in the production of emotional or involuntary sounds, it also appears to generate specific respiratory and laryngeal motor patterns fundamental to human speech and singing. Davis et al. conclude that the patterned muscle activity corresponding to the major categories of voiced and voiceless sound production are represented in the PAG. The role of the PAG might also include integration of cortical and subcortical aspects of language with basic respiratory and laryngeal motor patterns by which speech is produced (Larson, 1985; Davis, Zhang and Bandler, 1993; Zhang et al., 1994; Zhang, Bandler and Davis, 1995). The motor activity for vocalisation appears to be integrated through a projection from the PAG to a column of neurons known as the nucleus retroambigualis (NRA). The NRA appears to play a significant role in generating respiratory pressure and laryngeal adduction, which occurs in both vocalisation and vegetative manoeuvres, such as coughing.

Larson (1985) has suggested that the cortical mechanisms involved in vocalisation and speech may have a role in modulating the subcortical systems that are involved in involuntary, or vegetative, phonation such as crying. It is possible that these are the mechanisms for coordinating timing, pitch and intensity fluctuations with the segmental and suprasegmental aspects of speech and language. There is also evidence arising from clinical cases that the frontal lobes and other cerebral structures are important in the integrated neurological systems required for phonation (see Chapter 10). Coordinated, symmetrical, laryngeal function is essential for normal voice.

Upper motor and sensory neurons (Figures 2.13 and 2.14)

The neural pathways for voluntary vocalisation arise in the precentral gyrus of the motor cortex in both cerebral hemispheres, and fibres descend as part of the corticobulbar tract, which is part of the **pyramidal system** or 'direct activation' tract. On reaching the medulla, some fibres of the corticobulbar tracts take a direct pathway, remaining on the same side of the body throughout their route. These fibres synapse with the ipsilateral tenth cranial nerve (vagus) nucleus and subsequently with lower motor neurons without interruption. Other fibres decussate (cross-over) and change sides at the bulbar level to synapse with the contralateral vagal nucleus. The vagal nuclei, in the nucleus ambiguus within the reticular formation of the medulla, lie in a group of cells also containing the ninth and eleventh cranial nerve elements. They are influenced by both the pyramidal and extrapyramidal systems (see below). Motor and sensory tracts from both cerebral hemispheres, the basal ganglia and the cerebellum extending to the cranial nerve nuclei in the brain stem are known as **upper motor** and **sensory tracts**.

The indirect neurons of the pyramidal tract have multiple off-shoots and synapses with the basal ganglia and reticular formation in the brain stem. They appear to contribute to temporospatial orientation while the direct system is related to discrete movement. The upper motor neurons do not govern isolated muscles, but groups of muscles. The frontobulbar portions of the pyramidal tracts connect with cranial nerves IX–XII (as well as I–VIII), thus controlling articulation, phonation and respiration.

The **extrapyramidal system** refers to tracts other than the pyramidal tracts and includes the basal ganglia in the cerebral hemispheres, the substantia nigra and subthalamic nucleus in the upper brain stem, the cerebellum and the thalamus, among other structures. The basal ganglia consist of the corpus striatum and its associated nuclei, and the caudate and lenticular nuclei. The latter is divided into the putamen and the globus pallidus. The **cerebellum** has an integrating and controlling role over movements that arise in other parts of the motor system. It regulates the force, speed, range, timing and direction of movements throughout the body so that excesses are inhibited. The extrapyramidal system influences the pyramidal tract, the function of which is to regulate the muscle tone required for posture and for changing position. It is also involved in the automatic component of skilled voluntary movement. The specific function of each of these elements of the extrapyramidal system with respect to phonation is unknown, but phonation may be influenced adversely by neurological conditions involving these structures (see Chapter 10).

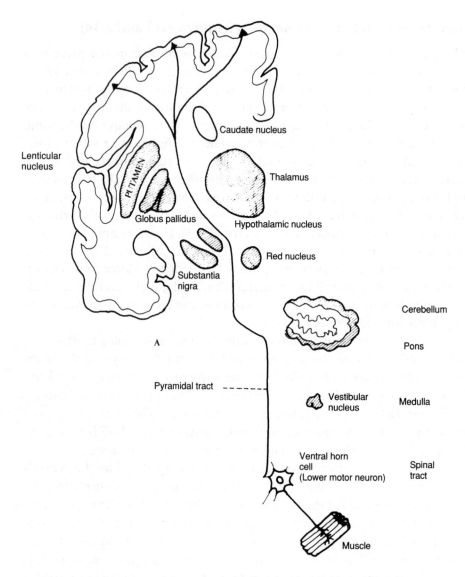

Figure 2.13 Upper motor neuron pathway (corticospinal tract).

Lower motor and sensory neurons

The nerve fibres originating in the cranial nerve nuclei form the lower motor neuron pathway. The right and left vagus nerves, which they form, provide ipsilateral innervation to the larynx. The neural 'commands' that travel down to the cranial nerve nuclei are largely responsible for what is ultimately transmitted to the laryngeal muscles via the lower motor neuron pathways. These 'commands' are fashioned by complex interaction of, and constant remodelling by, many cortical, basal ganglia and brain-stem influences.

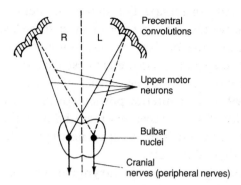

Figure 2.14 Connections from both hemispheres of upper motor neurons with bulbar nuclei.

The **vagus nerve** (cranial nerve X) provides all the **innervation** to the intrinsic laryngeal muscles and the **sensory** structures of the larynx. It also supplies the pharynx, palate, trachea, bronchi, lungs, heart, external ear and parts of the gastrointestinal tract. Some of the fibres of the vagus originate in the medulla in the nucleus ambiguus whereas others originate at a higher level. Fibres from the upper section of the nucleus ambiguus join the glossopharyngeal nerve (cranial nerve IX) and those from the inferior portion join the accessory nerve (cranial nerve XI) (Gray, 1949). Cranial nerves IX, X and XI are so intimately connected in the medulla that all the muscles supplied by them are frequently involved either equally or progressively in medullary lesions. For this reason, Walshe (1952) grouped them together in pathological conditions affecting the nucleus ambiguus in what he termed the 'glossopharyngeal–accessorius complex'. Nuclear lesions of the vagus may, therefore, be associated with paralysis of the palate, tongue and larynx.

The vagus forms a flat cord from its many united filaments and leaves the skull through the jugular foramen, passing vertically down the neck within the carotid sheath. It branches to form the **superior laryngeal nerve (SLN)**, the **recurrent laryngeal nerve (RLN)** and the **pharyngeal nerve**.

- The **superior laryngeal nerve** branches off from the vagus at the ganglion nodosum (inferior ganglion) below the level of the jugular foramen, and subdivides into the **internal** and **external superior laryngeal nerves**. The **internal branch** of the superior laryngeal nerve consists of both sensory and parasympathetic secretomotor fibres which supply glands within the tissue above the level of the vocal folds. This branch of the SLN, in turn, divides into three branches supplying the valleculae, the epiglottis and the pyriform sinus (or pyriform fossa). The density of nerve endings providing sensory innervation appears to be greatest at the laryngeal inlet as part of the protective mechanism for the respiratory system. The laryngeal surface of the epiglottis has the greatest sensory innervation whereas the vocal folds have a lower density of sensory fibres (Sasaki and Weaver, 1997). The anterior portions of the vocal folds also have a lower density of touch receptors than the posterior half. The **external branch** of the superior laryngeal nerve provides the motor supply to the cricothyroid muscle.

- The **left** and **right recurrent laryngeal nerves** provide the motor supply to all the intrinsic laryngeal muscles except the cricothyroid muscle, which is innervated by the external branch of the SLN. The recurrent laryngeal nerves contain both adductor and abductor fibres (Sasaki and Weaver, 1997). They differ significantly with regard to their origin and pathway. The right RLN arises from the main trunk of the vagus in front of the subclavian artery and the left RLN arises from the vagus at the arch of the aorta round which it winds before ascending to the larynx. On account of its extensive course, the left recurrent nerve is more liable to injury than the right, and is especially vulnerable to pressure from aortic aneurysm and intrathoracic masses. It is also easily injured during thyroidectomy and thoracic surgery. The left vocal fold is affected twice as frequently as the right by laryngeal paralysis. The recurrent laryngeal nerves on both sides ascend the groove between the trachea and oesophagus for a variable distance in different individuals. Then they divide into anterior and posterior branches before entering the larynx behind the cricothyroid articulation (Figure 2.15). The RLN provides the sensory supply to the glottis and subglottis (Figure 2.16).

- The **pharyngeal nerve** descends between the internal and external carotid arteries to supply the **middle pharyngeal constrictor muscle**. Its fibres subsequently join with the glossopharyngeal and external laryngeal nerves, together with branches from the sympathetic trunk, to form the **pharyngeal plexus**. The pharynx and all the muscles of the soft palate, except the tensor palati, are supplied by fibres from the pharyngeal plexus.

Cranial nerves V (trigeminal), VII (facial) and XII (hypoglossal), and cervical spinal nerves C1–C3 provide the motor supply for the extrinsic laryngeal muscles. Figure 2.17 gives a diagrammatic representation of the laryngeal nerve supply.

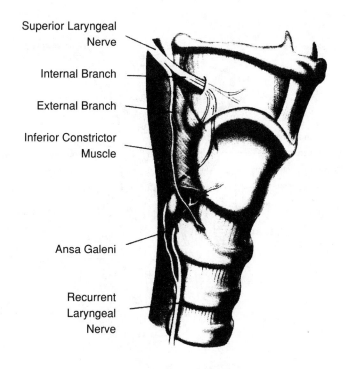

Superior Laryngeal
Nerve

Internal Branch

External Branch

Inferior Constrictor
Muscle

Ansa Galeni

Recurrent
Laryngeal
Nerve

Figure 2.15 Distribution of the vagus nerve to the larynx (lateral view).

Laryngeal mechanoreceptors

The extrinsic and intrinsic muscles of the larynx, as already described, are under voluntary cortical control. They are responsible for the pre-phonatory tuning that precedes phonation and is followed by the phasic, tonic and volitional contractions, and also by maintenance of length, tension, bulk and position of the vocal folds (Bowden, 1972). However, the phonatory modulations that take place in speech happen so rapidly that it seems that such fine tuning cannot be cortically regulated (Wyke, 1983). The linguistic demands of intonation, phonemic differentiations and emotional nuances in quality would appear to be regulated by an independent subcortical reflex neural system.

Free fibrils and terminal filaments enclosed in capsules constitute the receptor end-organs (the **mechanoreceptors**) embedded in the laryngeal tissues at sites sensitive to muscle stretch and airflow pressures. Some are involved in protecting the airway whereas others contribute to the control of phonation (Garrett and Larson, 1991). Wyke (1967, 1969, 1972) postulated that mechanoreceptors are found in three sites.

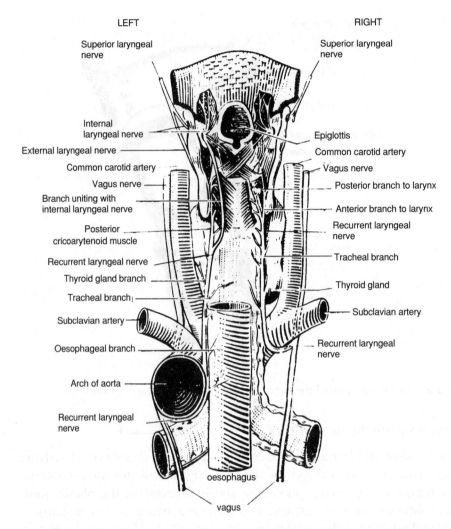

LEFT   RIGHT

Superior laryngeal   Superior laryngeal
nerve   nerve

Internal
laryngeal nerve   Epiglottis
External laryngeal nerve   Common carotid artery
Common carotid artery   Vagus nerve
Vagus nerve   Posterior branch to larynx
Branch uniting with   Anterior branch to larynx
internal laryngeal nerve
Posterior   Recurrent laryngeal
cricoarytenoid muscle   nerve
Recurrent laryngeal nerve   Tracheal branch
Thyroid gland branch
Tracheal branch   Thyroid gland
Subclavian artery   Subclavian artery
Oesophageal branch   Recurrent laryngeal
                                                 nerve
Arch of aorta

Recurrent laryngeal
nerve

oesophagus

vagus

Figure 2.16 Posterior view of the larynx showing the distribution of the left and right laryngeal nerves.

1. The mucosal lining of the larynx (**subglottic mucosal mechanoreceptors**): the corpuscular nerve endings in the subglottic mucous membrane covering the surface of the vocal folds are particularly numerous and sensitive to the stimuli of muscle stretch, air pressure level, liquid and touch (Garrett and Larson, 1991). They discharge impulses into the afferent fibres of the vagus.

2. The capsules of the articulatory joints (**articular mechanoreceptors**): the existence and function of this group remain controversial.

3. The extrinsic and laryngeal muscles (**myotatic mechanoreceptors**). The tone of the laryngeal muscles depends on the myotatic reflex,

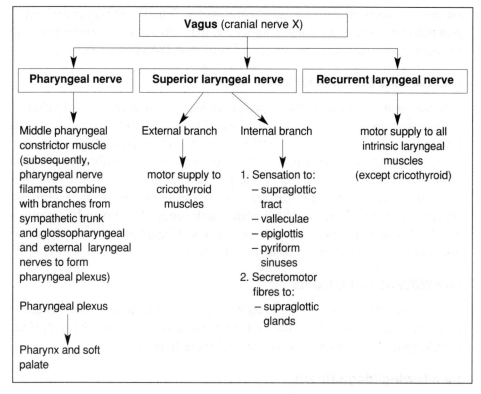

Note: Vagus supplies: Gastrointestinal tract, External ear, Heart, Lungs, Bronchi, Trachea, Pharynx, Palate, Larynx.

Figure 2.17 Diagrammatic representation of laryngeal nerve supply.

which is a function of the muscle spindles. The laryngeal muscles contain a large number of muscle spindles.

Stimulation of all categories of laryngeal mechanoreceptors initiates activity in the larynx, which presumably ensures that the vocal folds are stabilised and return to their pre-set pattern after displacement by the expiratory airstream. This process, by monitoring the tonicity and position of the vocal folds, enables necessary adjustments to be made instantaneously and accurately. Although it would seem inevitable that there must ultimately be integration of this servosystem with other control systems during phonation, Wyke stated that this process is independent of auditory feedback.

The hypothesis concerning the reflex mechanoreceptor system has been chiefly promoted by the research of Wyke who has applied the concept to voice pathology. However, although other researchers in the field affirm the histological proof regarding the presence of mechanoreceptors in the larynx, their precise function remains a matter of controversy. Whether stimuli in the laryngeal mucosa, muscles and joints can operate in isolation, and control aspects of laryngeal motor activity, remains open to question (Kirchner, 1983).

LARYNGEAL BLOOD SUPPLY

The larynx is supplied by the superior laryngeal, cricothyroid and inferior laryngeal arteries. The vascular network of the vocal folds is adapted for a vibrating structure; there is a marked decrease in volume of blood in the vocal fold while it is vibrating, so that circulation and metabolism are not disturbed (Mihashi et al., 1981). Very small blood vessels come into the vocal fold edge from either the anterior or posterior end of the membranous vocal fold and run roughly parallel to the edge (Hirano and Kiminori, 1993). There is no blood supply to the vocal ligaments, hence the pale appearance of normal vocal folds on laryngoscopy.

LARYNGEAL FUNCTIONS

The primary function of the larynx is to protect the airway. The intrinsic and extrinsic laryngeal muscles coordinate to effect efficient valving during **swallowing, breathing, phonation** and **weight-bearing**.

Swallowing (deglutition)

During swallowing, the primary function of the larynx is to prevent food and liquid entering the airway. This is achieved by means of the sphincteric action of the aryepiglottic folds and the true and false vocal folds, which occurs simultaneously with elevation of the larynx (Logemann, 1983a). Laryngeal elevation is important in controlling pressures and the function of the cricopharyngeal sphincter, in order that the bolus can pass into the oesophagus (Mendelsohn and McConnel, 1987). The process of swallowing can be divided into the **oral stage** and the **pharyngeal stage**. The oral stage is under voluntary control and consists of the **oral preparatory stage** and the **oral transport stage** (Perlman, 1994). The food bolus is manipulated by the tongue and broken down before being propelled towards the oropharynx. The pharyngeal stage of swallowing is a reflex activity which is initiated as the bolus reaches the back of the tongue. During this process, the glottis is closed by adduction of the arytenoids and contraction of the lateral cricoarytenoid muscles, false vocal folds and true vocal folds. Vocal fold adduction during swallowing is thought to average approximately 2.3 seconds (Perlman, 1994). The airway is also protected by the epiglottis, which covers the laryngeal entrance and directs the bolus in two parts into the valleculae and the pyriform sinuses. The two columns of the divided bolus meet at the upper border of the cricopharyngeus muscle which relaxes to allow the bolus to enter the oesophagus (Lund, 1990).

Coughing

Coughing is the process by which material is expelled from the airway. It is preceded by rapid inspiration, followed by forceful closure of both the vocal and vestibular folds. Air pressure is then built up below the adducted folds as the diaphragm ascends spasmodically, until the folds separate explosively and mucus or foreign material is expelled. Expiratory effort against a closed glottis such as this is known as the Valsalva manoeuvre (Slonim and Hamilton, 1976).

Effort closure

Laryngeal structure has evolved in order to contain intrathoracic pressure, so as to provide a stable fulcrum for the upper limbs. During any form of exertion involving use of the arms, the vocal folds are firmly adducted, preventing expulsion of air and collapse of the chest walls, thus providing a fixed origin for the arm and shoulder muscles. This fact is clinically important in that damage to the vocal fold mucosa can occur in individuals who work out with weights, and individuals who have undergone laryngectomy (see Chapter 17) may have difficulty with weight-bearing activities because of their inability to close the glottis.

   Effort closure of the larynx also occurs during childbirth and defaecation as the abdominal contents are compressed by the abdominal muscles in order to achieve expulsion.

Respiration

When the larynx is at rest and respiration quiet, the vocal folds abduct on inspiration and slightly adduct on expiration. They move up and down slightly in sympathy with the outflow and inflow of respiratory air, whereas the larynx descends on inspiration and ascends on expiration (Tucker, 1993). The folds are drawn wide apart to a position of full abduction in forceful inspiration (see also Chapter 3).

Phonation

The vocal note is generated by pulmonic air (air from the lungs) as it is exhaled between the adducted vocal folds. The vocal folds working together, therefore, constitute a vibrator that is activated by the excitor, the exhaled air. The production of the vocal note at this point is the result of the repeated vibratory movement of the vocal folds known as **vocal fold oscillation**. The mobility and deformability of the vocal fold determine the ease with which vocal fold vibration can be initiated (Titze, 1994b). The biomechanics of phonation are discussed in detail in Chapter 4.

Pharynx

The larynx is continuous above with the pharynx, which is a muscular tube extending from the cricoid cartilage below to the base of the skull above. It varies in length from person to person, but is generally estimated at between 13 cm and 14 cm long. Above, it is continuous with the nasal cavity and opens into the oral cavity anteriorly. Below, it leads into the laryngeal inlet anteriorly and the oesophagus posteriorly.

PHARYNGEAL CONSTRICTOR MUSCLES

The pharynx (Figure 2.18) is described in three parts – **nasopharynx**, **oropharynx** and **hypopharynx** – which are bounded by the superior, middle and inferior constrictor muscles respectively.

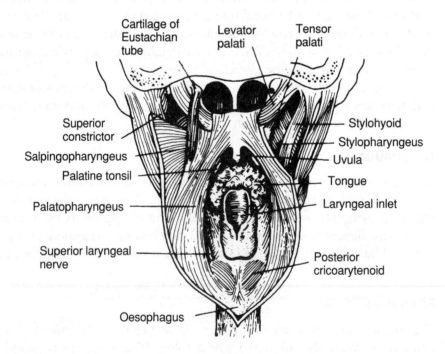

Figure 2.18 Dissection of pharynx, showing the muscles of the soft palate in relation to tongue and larynx.

- The **superior pharyngeal constrictor muscle** forms the uppermost section of the pharynx and on contraction assists, together with the levator palati, sphincteric closure of the nasopharyngeal port. Fritzell (1969) found both muscles to be consistently active in speech. The superior constrictor also assists movement of the pharyngeal walls medially.
- The **middle pharyngeal constrictor muscle**: The upper fibres of this muscle in the shape of a cone overlap the lower fibres of the superior constrictor muscle.
- The **inferior pharyngeal constrictor muscle** is composed of superior and inferior portions. The superior portion is the **thyropharyngeus muscle** which arises from the thyroid cartilage and which is inserted into the pharynx. The inferior portion forms the **cricopharyngeus muscle**. The cricopharyngeal fibres are in contraction at rest and thus ensure that air does not enter the oesophagus during respiration (Logemann, 1983a). It relaxes in order to allow the food bolus into the oesophagus.

The pharyngeal constrictor muscles decrease the circumference of the pharynx on contraction and assist in swallowing (see above). The dimensions of the pharynx also change according to the prevailing emotional state. The constrictor muscles may tighten sufficiently for the individual to be 'choked with emotion' or to feel a 'lump in the throat' when near to tears. These involuntary pharyngeal responses have a marked effect on voice quality. The importance of the pharynx to voice quality is acknowledged by singers who stress the importance of an 'open throat'. A short and capacious pharynx is possibly advantageous in singing (Van den Berg, 1962; Sundberg, 1974). Henderson (1954), in a description of the pharyngeal cavity of the English contralto Kathleen Ferrier, stated that it was so capacious that it could easily accommodate a moderately sized apple.

Oral cavity (Figure 2.19)

The oral cavity opens anteriorly from the oropharynx. The tongue, jaws (**maxilla** and **mandible**) and soft palate enclose the oral cavity. The lips form the inlet and the **faucial arches** form the outlet posterior to the oropharynx (Figure 2.20). Between the anterior and posterior faucial arches, the **tonsils** are housed in the tonsillar sinuses. The **adenoidal pad** is in the nasopharynx. The roof of the oral cavity is composed of the **hard** and **soft palates**. The enlargement of the oral cavity, which is so important to the quality of the fundamental vocal note, is achieved by the **temporomandibular joint** (TMJ) which enables the mandible to be lowered and

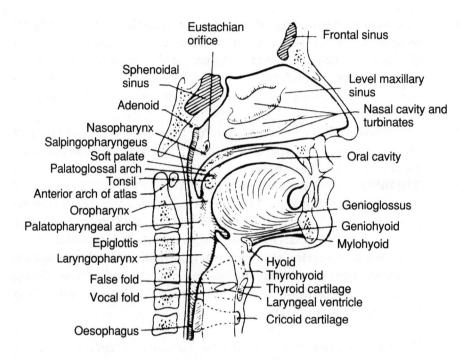

Figure 2.19 Sagittal section through nose, mouth, pharynx and larynx to show relative position of organs of articulation, resonance and phonation.

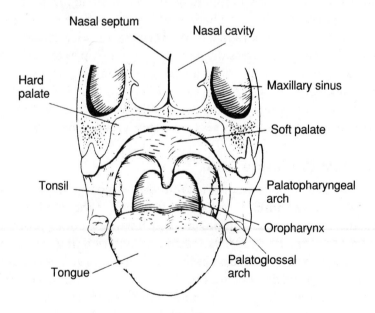

Figure 2.20 Oral view of palate and faucial arches.

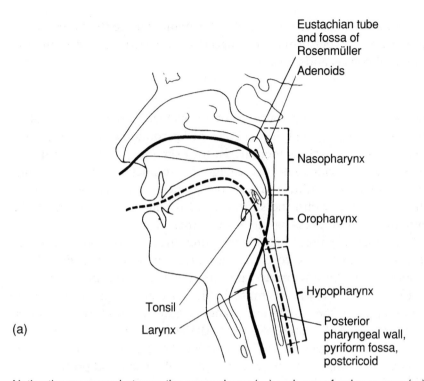

Notice the crossover between the upper airway (—) and upper food passages (---)

Reprinted from 'Ear, Nose and Throat' Dhillon R.S., East C.A., page 54, 1994, by permission of the publisher Churchill Livingstone

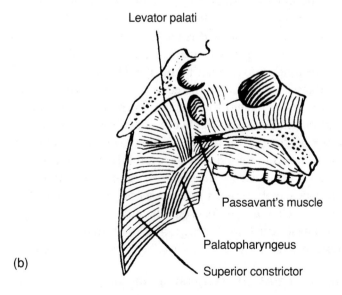

Figure 2.21 Muscles of the nasopharyngeal isthmus.

raised. The articulators are responsible for manipulating the bolus during deglutition and for performing the necessary phonetic gestures for pronunciation of vowels and consonants.

Lips

The lips are important in pronunciation of bilabial /p, b, m, w/ and labiodental /f, v/ phonemes. Varying degrees of lip-rounding, protruding and spreading achieve vowel distinctions as, for example: /u:, i:/. The muscles of the lips can be divided into two categories: sphincter muscles and dilator muscles. The **orbicularis oris** is the sphincteric muscle, which encircles the oral orifice within the substance of the lips. It is responsible for lip-rounding and compressing the lips together.

A number of paired muscles radiating out from the orbicularis oris muscle act as dilators and account for the extreme mobility of the lips (Table 2.4). Fibres from the **buccinator** muscle (*buccina* = trumpet) blend and form part of the orbicularis oris muscle. The buccinator muscle arises from the outer margins of the maxilla and mandible and its fibres form the muscle layer of the cheek. At the angle of the mouth the fibres decussate, those from below entering the upper lip and those from above entering the lower lip. The buccinator compresses the cheeks against the teeth and protrudes the lips. Table 2.4 summarises the lip muscles and their function.

Tongue

The tongue's primary function is for swallowing, but it is also the most important articulator of consonants and vowels. Its intrinsic muscles, including the **genioglossus, geniohyoid** and **mylohyoid muscles,** form an intricate network of superior and inferior, transverse, vertical and longitudinal fibres. These muscles anchor the tongue posteriorly to the hyoid bone and anteriorly to the mandible, but otherwise the tongue is free to move in the oral cavity. Tongue movements are closely related to vertical movements of the larynx because of their common attachment to the hyoid bone. The tongue is able to assume a vast number of shapes. It is divided down the centre by a fibrous septum (raphé) and is attached to the floor of the mouth by the **frenum.**

The movements of the back of the tongue change the shape and patency of the oropharynx which, besides being essential in the articulation of vowels and diphthongs, also affects the voice quality. A relaxed tongue opens up the oropharyngeal outlet and retraction of the tongue narrows it. Lowering the mandible and the tongue increases the size of the oral cavity.

Soft palate (velum) and palatopharyngeal sphincter

The soft palate is designed primarily to prevent regurgitation of food down the nose. In swallowing, it is elevated as the tongue passes the food bolus into the

Table 2.4 Function of the lip muscles

Sphincter muscle of the lips	Attachments	Function
Orbicularis oris	Fibres encircle oral orifice within the lips	Lip-rounding Compresses lips together
	Some fibres arise near the midline from the maxilla above and the mandible below	
	Other fibres arise from the deep surface of the skin and pass obliquely to the mucous membrane lining the inner surface of the lips	
	Many fibres derive from buccinator muscle	

Dilator muscles of the lips	Attachments	Function
	The dilator muscles radiate out from the lips	
	They arise from the bone and fascia around the oral aperture and converge to be inserted in the lips	
Levator labii superioris alaeque nasi		Raises and everts the upper lip
Levator labii superioris		Raises and everts the upper lip
Zygomaticus minor		Elevates lip, exposing maxillary teeth Curls upper lip in smiling
Zygomaticus major		Draws angle of mouth upwards and laterally (as in laughing)
Levator anguli oris		Raises angle of mouth
Risorius		Involved in many facial movements (not associated with laughter more than any other muscles)
Depressor anguli oris		Draws angle of mouth downwards and laterally
Depressor labii inferioris		Draws lower lip downwards and laterally
Mentalis		Raises lower lip

pharynx. When the mouth is shut, the palate is lowered and closes the oropharyngeal outlet, permitting nasal breathing at rest. It is an entirely muscular flap attached to the hard palate anteriorly and hanging free posteriorly, terminating in the uvula. In conjunction with the posterior and lateral walls of the pharynx, the elevated soft palate forms the **palatopharyngeal sphincter** which is also known as the **velopharyngeal sphincter**. Occasionally, the posterior nasopharyngeal wall can be seen to bulge forward at the point of closure with the soft palate, or just below. This bulge is called **Passavant's pad** and seems to arise from the circular fibres of the superior pharyngeal constrictor muscle, which originate in the velum and form a true sphincter on contraction (Bzoch, 1989). The purpose of Passavant's pad is controversial, however, as many observers report that it is too low to contribute to palatopharyngeal closure. It has been noted that Passavant's pad is frequently observed in individuals with cleft palate and it has been suggested that this is the result of increased activity in an attempt to close the palatopharyngeal port (Bzoch, 1989).

The palate is elevated in the articulation of vowels and consonants except in the case of nasal consonants /m, n, ŋ/. Calnan (1953) noted that throughout speech the velum is raised and ready to make pharyngeal contact. It 'kneels' against the posterior pharyngeal wall but often fails to make a complete seal even during normal speech, which shows no sign of hypernasality or nasal escape (see page 231). The rise and fall of the velum can be inspected as the vowel /a:/ is articulated. The extent of palatal elevation varies during speech and at times it may be above or below the level of the hard palate. McWilliams, Morris and Shelton (1984) undertook a comprehensive survey of research concerning the mechanism of the velopharyngeal sphincter. They pointed out that interest in the 1950s and 1960s focused on elevation of the palate but, subsequently, improved imaging techniques allowed researchers to investigate the role of the lateral pharyngeal walls (Pigott, 1977). Hirschberg (1986) has also reviewed velopharyngeal insufficiency.

The soft palate is composed of several paired muscles, some fibres of which are inserted in the tongue and others in the pharynx (Table 2.5).

The nose and paranasal sinuses

The nasal cavity is divided into two chambers by the central nasal septum and communicates with the nasopharynx posteriorly. The paranasal sinuses drain into the nasal chambers which are divided laterally by three turbinates or conchae. The nasal chambers are lined with ciliated mucous membrane for shunting mucus and also warming and filtering inspired air, a necessary form of air-conditioning, as Negus (1957a) described it. Specialised olfactory mucosa high in the nose is the basis of the sense of

Table 2.5 Muscles of the soft palate

Muscles	Attachments	Function
Tensor palati muscles	Arise in the anterior wall of the cartilaginous Eustachian tube to form the palatal aponeurosis to which the other palatal muscles are attached	Involved in opening the Eustachian tube in yawning and swallowing (McWilliams, Morris and Shelton, 1984 Maintain equalisation of air pressure within the eustachian tubes, with external air pressure
Uvula muscles	Fibres descend from the palatal aponeurosis and meet in the uvula	On contraction, the paired muscles raise a ridge (Passavant's ridge) on the nasal surface of the palate which may assist closure of the nasopharyngeal isthmus (Piggott and Makepeace, 1975; Piggott, 1977)
Palatoglossus muscles	Fibres originate in the sides of the tongue and ascend into the palate in the form of an arch (palatoglossal arch or anterior faucial arch)	Pull the soft palate down (Fritzell, 1969) Antagonistic to the levator palati muscles; assist in rapid flickering movements of the palate in connected speech
Levator palati muscles	Fibres arise in the petrous portion of the temporal bone, descend along the route of the Eustachian tube and are inserted into the palatal aponeurosis	Elevate the soft palate. Most important muscles for competent palatopharyngeal closure
Palatopharyngeus muscles	Fibres arise in the palatal aponeurosis and enter the lateral walls of the pharynx, forming the posterior faucial arch Specialised fibres form Passavant's muscle or ridge which enters the superior tube of the superior pharyngeal constrictor muscle (Fritzell, 1969)	Assist in sphincteric closure of the nasopharynx in swallowing, causing bunching of the lateral pharyngeal walls

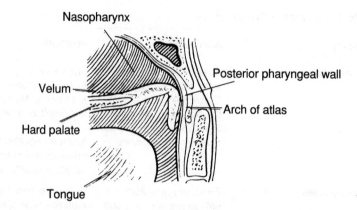

Figure 2.22 Site of contact of elevated velum.

smell, which is far less sensitive in humans than in many animals. Although the tongue distinguishes sweet, sour, bitter and salt, the subtle flavours of food are experienced by smell.

The nasal cavities affect the sound of the voice when the velopharyngeal port is open and sound energy passes into the nasal tract. Nasalised vowels are produced when sound energy passes through the nasal and oral tracts simultaneously. For the production of nasal consonants, the oral resonator is closed. Although the importance of certain supraglottic air spaces as resonators of the vocal note is generally acknowledged, there is disagreement concerning the contribution of the nasal cavity and paranasal sinuses. Proctor (1980) stated that one of the purposes of the paranasal sinuses is the provision of resonators for the voice. Bunch (1982), however, believes that 'the sinuses play little or no part in the vocal resonance that is actually perceived by the audience', although vibration will be felt by singers in the air spaces and bones of the head. The current view is that the sinuses play no role in the acoustics of the externally transmitted signal.

Summary

- This chapter describes the essential anatomy and physiology of the larynx and the structures and systems, apart from respiration, to which it is related and by which it is supported.

- Text and diagrams alone tend to convey the complexity of the larynx, but are inadequate in clarifying the three-dimensional reality and its biomechanics. Laryngeal dissection is helpful as a means of appreciating the various structures while extensive viewing of videos of the larynx during phonation is invaluable for helping to understand vocal fold movement.

3 CHAPTER

The lower respiratory tract

Speech breathing and breathing for singing are modifications of the processes of respiration that exist primarily for the metabolic gas exchange necessary to sustain life. The generation of sound in the larynx depends on the coordination of the laryngeal and respiratory systems, with appropriate levels of air pressure, air volume and airflow being fundamental to phonation and articulation. It is important to remember that, although breathing processes affect phonation during connected speech, laryngeal behaviour also affects breathing patterns because of the resistance that varying degrees of laryngeal valving provide. When this concept is extended into the area of voice disorders, it has important implications for treatment planning and the selection of intervention strategies. Disordered breathing patterns adversely affect the voice but aberrant vocal fold adduction and abduction inevitably affect breathing patterns. This chapter describes the anatomy and physiology of breathing.

The **lower respiratory tract** is protected by the larynx. It is housed in the **thorax** (chest cavity), which is bounded by the 12 **thoracic vertebrae** of the spinal column posteriorly, the **ribs** laterally and the **sternum** (breast bone) anteriorly.

Thoracic skeleton

The thoracic skeleton, or rib cage, houses the lungs and provides a movable scaffold for the attachment of the muscles of respiration. The cage consists of 12 pairs of ribs in males and females. The first pair of ribs is immobile, being attached to the vertebrae posteriorly and to the manubrium (handle) of the sternum anteriorly. The second to seventh pairs are attached to the vertebrae posteriorly and to the sternum anteriorly by synovial joints which allow smooth rotation. The eighth to tenth pairs are attached to each other anteriorly by flexible cartilage and fibrous bands. They are attached only indirectly to the sternum because the eighth pair of ribs is bound to the seventh. The eleventh and twelfth pairs are known as 'floating ribs' because the anterior attachment is not to the sternum but to the abdominal wall by fibrous membranes (fascia) (Figure 3.1 and Table 3.1).

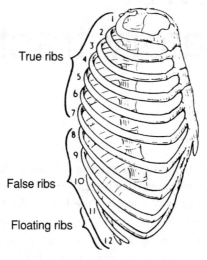

Figure 3.1 Thoracic skeleton.

Table 3.1 Rib pairs of thoracic skeleton

Rib pair	Anterior attachment	Posterior attachment	Movement
First (top)	Manubrium (handle) of sternum	Thoracic vertebrae	Immobile
Second to seventh	Sternum by synovial joints	Thoracic vertebrae	Second to sixth lift sternum to increase anteroposterior dimension
Eighth to tenth	Adjacent rib by flexible cartilage and fibrous bands (indirect attachment to sternum via attachment of eighth to seventh)	Thoracic vertebrae	Seventh to tenth widen thorax
Eleventh to twelfth 'Floating ribs'	Abdominal wall by fibrous membranes (fascia)	Thoracic vertebrae	Follow abdominal movements, backwards and forwards

The movement of the second to sixth pairs of ribs about their axes increases the anteroposterior dimensions of the chest by lifting the sternum. Cotes (1979) likened the movement to that of a farmyard pump handle. The seventh to tenth pairs of ribs act like bucket handles and, as they rotate about the anteroposterior axis, they widen the chest dimension. Expansion of the lungs is greatest in this region.

Tracheobronchial tree

The **trachea** extends from the lower border of the cricoid cartilage of the larynx at the level of the sixth cervical vertebra (C6) and is approximately 10–11 cm long and 2 cm wide. It is composed of incomplete rings of cartilage, the **tracheal rings**, which are connected by fibroelastic membranes. This structure allows flexibility during swallowing and inspiration. The trachea is lined with ciliated epithelium and mucosecretory cells. At the level of the fifth thoracic vertebra (T5), the trachea divides into the right and left **bronchi** which enter the **lungs**, a pair of sponge-like structures, where they divide further to form **bronchioles** and finally **alveoli** (**air sacs**). There are approximately 300 million alveoli, each 0.3 mm in diameter (West, 1979). The specialised epithelial cells of the alveoli manufacture **surfactant**, a liquid that lubricates the air sacs in order to facilitate their expansion and that lowers surface tension to prevent their collapse (Dikeman and Kazandjian, 1995). An air-tight sac, the **visceral pleura**, surrounds each lung.

Air is carried into the lungs via the trachea, bronchi and alveoli so that oxygen enters the venous blood stream. Carbon dioxide moves out through the capillaries wrapped about the very thin membrane that encloses the alveoli. The lung, besides the function of gas interchange, also filters out toxic particles from polluted air. These are swept out in a flow of mucus by the ciliated epithelium lining the bronchial walls. Large particles are filtered out by the nasal passages. Some particles settle in the alveoli and diminish their efficiency whereas some substances, such as coal dust and smoke, permanently damage the lungs (Cotes, 1979). Cilia can be destroyed by toxic gases and nicotine; the alveoli become blocked and lose their elasticity, with resultant emphysema. The **mediastinum**, containing the heart, great vessels and oesophagus, divides the thorax into right and left halves.

Thoracic muscles

The thoracic muscles (detailed drawings and descriptions of these muscles can be found in Netter, 1979) activate expansion and contraction of the chest and lungs and maintain the rhythmic excursions of inspiration and expiration. The thoracic muscles:

- connect adjacent ribs (**intercostal muscles**)
- span several ribs between their attachments
- connect ribs to the sternum
- connect ribs to the vertebrae.

The most important respiratory muscle is the **diaphragm** (see below). The movements of respiration consist of highly coordinated movements of the thoracic and abdominal muscles. For ease of description, these muscles are divided into 'inspiratory' and 'expiratory' ones, but this over-simplifies the real nature of their coordinated functions.

Inspiratory muscles

The muscles most active in inspiration are the **diaphragm** and the **external intercostal muscles,** with the accessory muscles (see below) also contributing to chest movements. Contraction of the inspiratory muscles provides the force to overcome the resistance of the lung and chest wall. This results in air passing along the tracheobronchial tree into the alveoli of the lung. The diaphragm is a dome-shaped muscle which divides the thoracic cavity from the abdominal cavity. The fibres of the diaphragm originate in the circumference of the thorax, the sternum, the ribs and the vertebral column. They are inserted in a trilobed central tendon which acts like a piston. The diaphragmatic aponeurosis operates much like the diaphragm of a bellows. The fall and rise of the diaphragm fill and empty air from the lungs (Figure 3.2). Its expiratory movement is passive and controlled by the abdominal and intercostal muscles. It is devoid of proprioceptive nerve endings, unlike the rest of the respiratory muscles. The breather is therefore unaware of the rise and fall of the diaphragm taking place within the chest cavity and experiences sensation from the chest wall and abdomen only (Campbell, Agostini and Davis, 1970). Although the external intercostals fill in the interstices between the ribs and elevate them on contraction to increase the dimensions of the thorax, it is the diaphragm that is the major muscle of inspiration, being responsible for two-thirds of the vital capacity (Williams et al., 1995). Three diameters of the thoracic cavity can be increased (Table 3.2). The thoracic movements for maximum inspiration and expiration are summarised in Table 3.3.

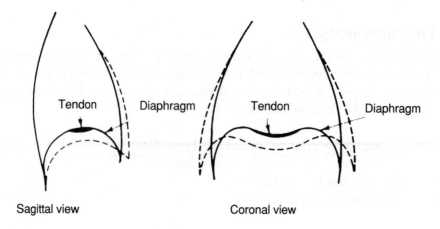

Sagittal view   Coronal view

Figure 3.2 Diaphragmatic movement.

Table 3.2 The three diameters of the thoracic cavity that can be increased on inspiration

Vertical diameter	When the diaphragm contracts, the domes are flattened and the diaphragm is lowered
Anteroposterior diameter	The ribs are drawn together and raised by the intercostal muscles, and the sternum is thrust forwards
Transverse diameter	As the ribs are raised (like bucket handles) the transverse diameter of the thoracic cavity is increased

Table 3.3 Thoracic movements for maximum inspiration and expiration

	Maximum inspiration	*Maximum expiration*
Abdominal wall	Relaxed	Contracted
Diaphragm	Descended	Raised (relaxed and stretched)
Ribs	Raised	Depressed
Spine	Fixed backwards	Flexed forwards

Expiratory muscles

The muscles of expiration are the **internal intercostal** and **abdominal muscles**. The internal intercostals are most active during expiration but are not as strong as the external intercostal muscles. They oppose the external intercostals and pull the ribs down, diminishing the size of the thoracic cavity. The ability to regulate air pressure is essential for speech breathing. Consequently, exhalation for phonation cannot depend on positive recoil forces alone but involve the speaker in active control of the expiratory process (Orlikoff, 1994) (Table 3.4).

Abdominal muscles

The abdominal muscles, the **external** and **internal oblique, rectus abdominis** and **transversus abdominis**, are chiefly active in forced expiration. The abdominal wall contracts and exerts pressure on the abdominal contents (viscera) so that the diaphragm is pushed upwards, the lungs are compressed and air is expelled. The abdominal muscles are active in speech breathing and also play an important role in singing. Coughing, defaecation and vomiting are dependent on contraction of the abdominal muscles. Non-phonatory expiration is largely passive, brought about by the elastic recoil of the chest wall components as the inspiratory muscles relax. In normal vegetative or tidal breathing, the diaphragm's height changes approximately only 1.5 cm, but in forced inspiration and expiration a total

Table 3.4 Respiratory muscles: function and innervation

Respiratory muscles	Function	Nerve supply
Thoracic muscles		
External intercostals	Elevate ribs on inspiration, enlarging thoracic cross-section	Intercostal spinal nerves T2–T11
Internal intercostals	Depress ribs on exhalation (also involved in rib elevation)	
Diaphragm	Descends on inspiration to enlarge thorax vertically	Phrenic nerves (paired C3–C5)
Abdominal muscles		
External oblique	• Supports abdominal contents • Pulls ribs downwards	Thoracic spinal nerves T6–T12
Internal oblique	• Supports abdominal contents • Pulls ribs downwards	Thoracic spinal nerves T6–T11, lumbar L1
Rectus abdominis	• Pulls ribs downwards	Thoracic spinal nerves T6–T11
Transversus abdominis	• Contracts abdominal cavity	Thoracic spinal nerves T6–T11, lumbar L1
Accessory muscles		
Sternocleidomastoid	• Supports head • Raises sternum and clavicle on inspiration	Cranial nerve XI
Scalene	• Inspiration: elevates rib cage	Spinal nerves C2–C8

After Dikeman and Kazandjian (1995).

excursion of 10 cm may occur (West, 1979). This is accompanied by increased movement of the chest wall and abdomen. Hixon, Mead and Goldman (1976) stress the fact that the diaphragm and abdomen behave as a single unit, the 'chest wall', because, as the diaphragm descends, the abdominal contents press the abdominal wall forwards. The reverse is the case on expiration. Each component of the chest wall system is independently capable of changing the lung volume. Indeed, it is possible for one part of the system to be moving in an inspiratory direction, while the other is engaged in an expiratory gesture.

Accessory muscles of respiration

The accessory muscles of respiration are those of the shoulder girdle: the scaleni and the sternocleidomastoids (see Chapter 2) (Campbell, 1974). These muscles assist in elevation of the ribs and are usually called into play only during exercise. The sternocleidomastoid becomes active only at high levels of ventilation and can be seen to contract during severe asthma, for example, elevating the sternum and slightly enlarging the anteroposterior and longitudinal dimensions of the chest. Forceful breathing occurs with maximum expansion of the rib cage in all directions to produce the ballooning of the lungs.

Lung ventilation and volume

Lung capacity varies considerably among individuals and there are measurable differences between men and women. Age, exercise, size, weight, posture, health and smoking all affect lung volumes and function (Cotes, 1979). Consequently, it is possibly more relevant to obtain information about single individuals when needed than to establish scientific statistical data concerning mean values (Hixon, 1987). A number of standard terms are used to describe lung capacity variation (Campbell, 1974; Slonim and Hamilton, 1976) (Figure 3.3 and Table 3.5).

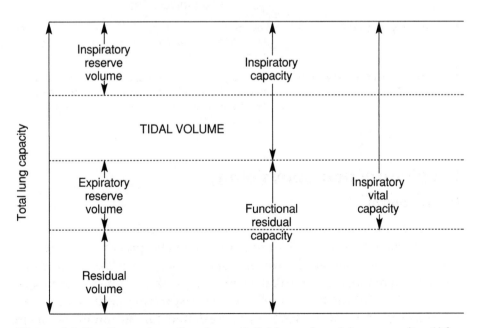

Figure 3.3 Ventilatory lung function: subdivisions of total lung capacity. (After Cotes, 1979.)

Table 3.5 Respiratory volumes

Tidal capacity (TC)	The volume of air inspired and expired in normal breathing at rest. This volume can be doubled or trebled according to the needs and activity of the individual. Average normal adult volume: 500 ml
Inspiratory reserve volume (IRV)	The volume that can be inspired beyond the end of tidal inspiration; it is the reserve that is available for increasing the tidal volume. Average normal adult volume: 2.5 litres
Expiratory reserve volume (ERV)	Maximum volume of gas that remains to be expired at the end of spontaneous expiration. Average normal adult volume: 1.5 litres
Residual volume (RV)	The volume of gas left in the lungs after maximal expiration. Average normal adult volume: 1.5 litres
Functional residual capacity (FRC)	The volume of gas in the lungs after normal expiration. Average normal adult volume: 3 litres
Vital capacity (VC)	The exhaled volume after maximal inspiration. This is also described by Cotes (1979) as the extent to which total lung capacity exceeds the residual volume. Vital capacity in healthy males is in the range 2.0–6.6 litres. The range for the healthy female is 1.4–5.6 litres. Height, weight and age all affect vital capacity. During normal conversational speech only 20–25% of the vital capacity is used (Orlikoff, 1994)
Total lung capacity (TLC)	Volume of gas in the lungs at the end of maximal inspiration, i.e. the maximum volume of gas that the lungs can contain
Total ventilation (TV) and minute volume (MV)	The volume of air inspired and exhaled in a minute. There are on average approximately 15 breaths/minute (15 × tidal volume is equal to 7500 ml/min)

Respiratory neurophysiology

Reflex control

The chief function of respiration is to oxygenate the blood and to remove excess carbon dioxide. This vegetative, automatic process is carried on continuously throughout life whether one is asleep or awake. It needs no conscious attention. The respiratory muscles work in a finely coordinated rhythmic fashion which is controlled by the **respiratory control centre** or 'central controller' (West, 1979) in the **reticular formation of the brain stem**, a collection of neurons in the **pons** and **medulla**. The level of ventilation is controlled by two types of sensor:

- **chemoreceptors,** which instantaneously feed back information to the control centre regarding the oxygen and carbon dioxide balance in the arterial blood
- **stretch receptors** in the lungs and pleurae, which respond to lung expansion.

This balance of oxygen and carbon dioxide is constantly changing with bodily activity, but is adjusted by the central control that programmes ventilation and action of the respiratory muscles. The rate of breathing is correlated with stress factors as well as physical demands (Lenneberg, 1967). Failure in coordination can occur when the inspiratory muscles operate as antagonists to the expiratory muscles. This may occur in pre-term babies when asleep. Respiration in at-risk infants needs careful monitoring because certain respiratory abnormalities are thought to be related to sudden infant death syndrome.

Sasaki and Weaver (1997) point out that, although the existence of central and peripheral chemoreceptors and thoracic stretch receptors was discovered during the nineteenth century, it was not appreciated that the larynx had a respiratory role until 1949. Sir Victor Negus observed that the glottis opens a fraction of a second before the descent of the diaphragm causes air to be inspired. Sasaki and Weaver cite the work of Suzuki as clarifying that this laryngeal activity is a direct effect of the medullary respiratory centre. Suzuki also demonstrated that the glottis widens as the result of rhythmic bursts of activity in the recurrent laryngeal nerve. It has been established that the posterior cricoarytenoid and cricothyroid muscles act together to widen and lengthen the glottic chink during inspiration, thus increasing the diameter of the glottal airway anteroposteriorly (Sasaki and Weaver, 1997). Expiration is also influenced significantly by the larynx acting as a valve, with the cricothyroid muscle again performing a major role in altering airway resistance and thus affecting the duration of expiration.

Voluntary control

Breathing is also under voluntary control and the cortex can take over control of the respiratory centres to some extent. Breath can be held, for example, or respiration slowed down or greatly accelerated causing the distressing experience of hyperventilation (hypocapnia) (see page 225). If an individual loses consciousness, the respiratory centres will usually take over control and the individual will resume normal breathing. Breathing pattern is altered at will by attention being directed to movements of the chest and abdomen. This awareness is developed to a high level during the acquisition of particular breathing methods for speech and song. Breathing for speech develops from the first cry of the neonate and the incoordinated gasps and spluttering of the infant. Control of breath for speech develops on a continuum as the child begins to produce babble sounds and as muscular and neurological control systems mature (Langlois, Baken and Wilder, 1980). Voluntary control emerges gradually and becomes automatic, almost reflex. This is important to note because it explains why individuals who have vocal strain commonly do not associate their problems with breathing or realise that breath provides the energy source for voice.

Respiratory function

The general principle underlying the processes of inspiration and expiration is that air flows from regions of higher pressure to those of lower pressure.

Inspiration

At the onset of inspiration, the diaphragm contracts and descends whereas the rib cage expands. The root of the lung descends and the level of the bifurcation of the trachea may be lowered by as much as two vertebrae (Snell, 1995). This enlargement of the thoracic cavity leads to the lungs being stretched, causing an expansion of alveolar air and a decrease in alveolar pressure. As a result of this drop in lung pressure in relation to the atmospheric pressure, air flows into the chest cavity in order to equalise the internal and external pressures. When the pressure in the alveoli equals the atmospheric air pressure, inspiration is completed. The inspiratory muscles continue to be active into the early part of expiration, however, with the force that they exert gradually decreasing. Their role during the first stages of expiration is to act as a releasing brake against the recoil forces of the lung (Hixon, 1987).

Forced breathing occurs when more air is required during physical effort. During forced inspiration, the accessory respiratory muscles may be employed in order to achieve maximum expansion of the thorax as rapidly as possible. In this situation, every muscle that can raise the ribs is brought into action, including the sternocleidomastoid (Snell, 1995).

Expiration

When alveolar pressure exceeds atmospheric pressure by an amount sufficient to overcome resistance, air flows out of the lungs. During quiet breathing, expiration is a largely **passive** process, which is brought about by the elastic recoil of the lungs, and the relaxation of the intercostal muscles and the anterior abdominal wall, which forces the relaxing diaphragm upwards. The pressure that is produced by entirely non-muscular activity of the respiratory system is known as **relaxation pressure**. More forceful expulsion of air is achieved by **active expiration**, during which the expiratory muscles are used to decrease the size of the thorax. Forced expiration occurs as the result of the forcible contraction of the anterior abdominal wall.

In normal resting subjects, expiration and inspiration times are equal (approximately 2 seconds) with a slight pause occurring at the end of expiration and the rate of the respiratory cycle at 16–20 times per minute. This rate is faster in children and slower in elderly people. In the adult, there are differences in the breathing patterns of men and women. Women tend to rely mainly on the movements of the ribs rather than on the descent of the diaphragm on inspiration. This is called the thoracic type of respiration (Snell, 1995). Men generally use both the abdominal and thoracic forms of breathing, but the abdominal pattern predominates. In the abdominal pattern, the descent of the diaphragm is the main element of increasing thoracic capacity on inspiration, resulting in marked inward/outward excursion of the anterior abdominal wall (Snell, 1995).

Speech breathing

In respiration for speech, the breathing pattern is significantly different. Air pressures, flows and resistances are constantly changing and vary considerably according to the type of phonation. The following stages occur:

- Inspiration is relatively quick so that continuous speech is interrupted as little as possible. As the nasal passages are too narrow for the rapid inspiration necessary for speech, breathing becomes oral. Most conversational speech of normal loudness requires deeper breaths than in quiet breathing, with lung volumes ranging from 35% to 60% of the vital capacity (Hixon, 1987), with women typically having higher lung and rib-cage volumes than those used by men (Stathopoulos and Sapienza, 1993). The extent of each inspiration is influenced by the type and length of the anticipated utterance.
- Immediately before phonation, the vocal folds are abducted during rapid inspiration, while the larynx is simultaneously lowered in the vocal tract. This is described by Wyke (1983) as the pre-phonatory inspiratory phase.
- This is followed by the pre-phonatory expiratory phase as the diaphragm and intercostal muscles relax.
- The vocal folds adduct and contribute to the control of the expiratory airflow. As a result of this high resistance in the vocal tract, the air leaves the lungs more slowly with the effect of lengthening the

expiratory phase. As a result, subglottal air pressure is generated and phonation is initiated as described in Chapter 2. The expiratory muscles play an important role during talking and singing, controlling and modifying relaxation pressure during expiration. Expiration can be prolonged to 10–15 seconds (Fry, 1979).

The adducted vocal folds act as a valve to control the expiratory transglottal air flow. The subtle interaction of vocal fold adduction and subglottal air pressure is the basis of establishing and maintaining the **intensity of the vocal note**. A monosyllable might require only minimal modification of the breathing pattern, but a shout or peroration necessitates significantly increased subglottal air pressure to achieve adequate intensity and length of utterance. Expiratory airflow control also has a role in the **prosodic features** of speech to mark stress, prominence, intonation and rhythm. These features are monitored by the linguistic system, which influences the action of the expiratory muscles. Stressed syllables, for example, require an increase in subglottal pressure obtained by the internal intercostal muscles (Ladefoged, 1974). In connected speech, the abdominal muscles influence expiration by controlling the rate of the ascent of the diaphragm (Hixon, Mead and Goldman, 1976). Hixon (1987) considers that the intercostals are the most important muscles in everyday speech. Their position and size mean that they have a significant influence on the volume of the rib cage and because of that they are instrumental in effecting rapid and small variations in the driving pressure supplied to the larynx and airway. A baseline pressure in the lungs is established in order to produce sequences of speech segments and is dependent on the intercostal muscles and the diaphragm interacting with the elastic recoil of the lungs. The muscles make adjustments to keep this pressure constant as the lung volume diminishes (Gould, 1981).

It is important to understand that adequate air intake for speech in a healthy individual is not dependent on forcefully taking or gasping air into the lungs. When the rib cage expands and the diaphragm lowers, negative pressure is created in the thorax. As a result, air from the exterior rushes in to equalise the pressure. It is the extent of the rib cage expansion, therefore, that largely determines the amount of pulmonic air available for phonation. This is an important concept for the individual with a voice disorder, or for a performer. Many individuals think mistakenly that effortful air intake will provide them with increased air for voice production.

Control of speech breathing

In ordinary everyday conversation, natural breathing occurs without awareness or training. Adjustments in tidal airflow take place but these are minimal. Inspiration time quickens and expiration time lengthens with fluctuations in the activity of the respiratory muscles. The variations in the degree of effort required are largely unnoticed by the normal untrained speaker, although actors and singers regard training and development of breathing patterns as an essential foundation for developing vocal skills. The role of the abdominal wall in controlling the ascent of the diaphragm during expiration has long been recognised by singers and actors. Traditional exercises included those for strengthening the abdominal muscles by lying prone and moving weights up and down on their stomachs. Control of expiratory airflow was developed by attempting to sing a vowel in front of a lighted candle, without causing it to flicker. Subsequently, aerodynamic studies (see page 456) have disproved some beliefs and verified others. Large expansions of the chest and the expulsion of high volumes of air, for example, are not necessary to produce good voice. Slight abdominal contraction is apparently essential as part of the adjustments made by the chest wall before phonation, although rib-cage movements may vary (Wilder, 1983). Reported research into airflow and pressure levels has not suggested that control of speech breathing is unimportant or that training in correct use of the respiratory muscles is not necessary in rehabilitation.

Luchsinger (1965a), having drawn attention to the changed rhythm in respiration at rest and in speaking or singing, wrote with commendable logic:

> The longer the available air lasts, the more can be said or sung on one breath. Here is the essential secret of breath control for speaking and singing: to achieve prolonged phonic expiration through proper muscular coordination.

Differing opinions exist, however, regarding the value of 'breathing exercises' as an element of voice therapy. Some voice therapists consider that, as breathing for speech is a natural activity, raising the speaker's awareness is either unnecessary or creates tension which is counterproductive. The opposing view is that individuals who have clinical voice disorders frequently do not breathe normally and naturally; the laryngeal dysfunction may lead to inappropriate breathing patterns which become habituated. It is also clear, as Gould (1981) concluded, that:

> Defects in or misuse of the pulmonary apparatus lead to laryngeal dysfunction. A clear understanding of the pulmonary laryngeal system is needed so that preventive or corrective measures may be taken during voice training more intelligently.

In addition, when speech breathing patterns are affected by anxiety and tension, the problem is compounded by the compensatory strategies that subsequently evolve in an attempt to produce useful voice. As a result, patients may need information and practice in appropriate speech breathing patterns. As Wilder (1983) stated, modification of respiratory patterns is an important issue in voice therapy.

Posture

The traditional view that posture has a significant effect on breathing was confirmed by studies conducted by Hixon (1987). In the upright position, the vital capacity is at its greatest because the abdominal contents are pulled down by gravity, allowing full descent of the diaphragm. Sitting and supine positions reduce the vital capacity. Consequently, a speaker's habitual posture is a fundamental factor to be considered in the assessment of patients with voice disorders and in treatment programmes.

Breathing variations for phonation

According to which muscle movements predominate, various types of breathing are recognised as variants of the normal breathing pattern during which costal and abdominal movements occur simultaneously and regularly. There is evidence that speech breathing varies according to body type. The normal breathing pattern of the tall, thin ectomorph may be different from that of the rotund endomorph (Hixon, 1987).

ABDOMINAL BREATHING

In this type of breathing, there is very little costal movement but movement of the abdominal wall is evident as the diaphragm moves up and down. This may follow pregnancy when the abdominal muscles are weak. It is also common in corpulent individuals with pronounced girth who take no exercise and are constantly short of breath. Excessive fat deposits impair lung function (Cotes, 1979).

CLAVICULAR BREATHING (UPPER CHEST BREATHING)

This is the reverse of abdominal breathing and is associated with anxiety and tension. It also occurs in individuals who have asthma. The external intercostal muscles and the accessory muscles elevate the shoulder girdle and the upper portion of the chest. Tension and effort radiate into the infrahyoid muscles (see page 27).

'BREATH SUPPORT' IN SINGING

This is a breathing technique used in singing and differs greatly from that used in speech because of the greater phrase length and increased vocal intensity frequently required. The technique greatly increases vocal volume and pitch range, as well as enhancing vocal quality. It is generally agreed to be essential for producing all the aesthetic features of artistic performance. There is much disagreement over how it is achieved and what exactly is the nature of the control exerted over the respiratory muscles. Luchsinger (1965a) reviewed the conflicting theories that endeavour to explain this support to the singing voice, called 'appoggio' by the Italians, 'appui' by the French, 'Stutze' by the Germans and 'rib reserve' by the British. Isshiki (1964) contributed a scientific investigation into the interrelationship of the intensity, subglottic pressure, glottal resistance and airflow rate in trained singers. However, this was related to the behaviour of the vocal folds rather than the respiratory muscles. A study of respiratory function by Gould and Okamura (1973) showed that total lung volumes are not significantly larger in the trained singer when compared with those of the untrained singer. The most obvious difference is the increase in vital capacity and decrease in residual volume in the trained singer.

The support given to the voice is felt subjectively as a great increase in the mastery of performance and power. This is accompanied by a feeling of tension in the chest. Last (1984) suggested that this is evoked by the opposing actions of the external intercostals and the diaphragmatic movement. On inspiration, as the ribs elevate, the diaphragm is pulled down by the central tendon and the internal intercostals, and a pull against the external intercostals is felt. Expiration is then controlled by the contraction of the abdominal muscles with the rib cage still held in its elevated position. Air pressure is raised below the glottis and air is used under great control very sparingly, with vocal fold vibrations adjusted for intensity and pitch by the ear. When the diaphragm has achieved its resting elevated position, the ribs can be lowered and the 'rib reserve' of air is useful for extending the phonation time for a phrase or exacting aria. The importance of abdominal muscle support in singing is clearly illustrated by Sataloff, Reinhardt and O'Connor (1984). A professional singer, unable to sing after becoming quadriplegic, was provided with a device to provide abdominal support which restored his singing ability and substantially improved respiratory function. It is interesting to note that, in order to enhance the tension of the abdominal wall and to provide support for the action of the diaphragm, some traditional Japanese singers bind the abdomen while performing (Kirikae, 1981).

Although speech–language pathologists will have ill-trained and untrained singers of all types of music referred for treatment, it is outside the province of the voice therapist (unless a trained singer) to teach the required breathing patterns. The fundamental principles of natural voice production will set the artist on the right path but the competent singing teacher is the appropriate instructor in the art of singing and its aesthetic qualities.

Summary

- Adequate speech–breathing capacity and control is fundamental to all aspects of normal phonation.
- Superior control of speech–breathing patterns is essential for increased vocal demands, such as singing and public speaking.
- Respiratory disease and conditions affecting respiratory control are reflected in vocal function.
- Voice disorders disrupt normal speech breathing patterns.

4 CHAPTER

Voice and phonation

After the previous chapters, which describe the structures of the vocal tract, this chapter is concerned with the normal voice, its features and the underlying laryngeal biomechanics. Every feature of a voice, normal or abnormal, has a biomechanical basis. There is always a physical reason for the sound of a voice; whatever the underlying aetiology of a voice disorder, therefore, the acoustic product is a manifestation of vocal tract events. The many potential variations in the voice reflect the capacity of the component parts of the larynx and vocal tract to change constantly. In addition, age-related changes occur throughout life and their effects contribute to the voice on a more long-term basis (see Chapter 5).

Voice is the acoustic signal generated by the larynx and vocal tract. The physical process of exhaling air between adducted vocal folds and so producing voice is called **phonation**. It is extremely difficult to define normal voice because each individual's voice has distinctive features and differs significantly from the voice of every other person. In addition, the same person exhibits markedly different vocal features according to factors such as mood, tiredness, illness and the perception of the communication context (Tosi, 1979; French, 1994). Although we think that we are able to recognise a familiar voice after a few words have been spoken, because of its apparently unique features, it has been shown that individuals' voices are not sufficiently consistent to distinguish them reliably. Attempts by forensic scientists to compare criminal and suspect recordings on a wide range of auditory and acoustic–phonetic dimensions cannot establish speaker identity with absolute scientific certainty (French, 1994). Instrumentation is not yet able to identify the voice unequivocally in the way that a fingerprint provides conclusive evidence (Levi, 1994).

The simplest definition of normal voice might be that it is ordinary or unremarkable, but this does not allow for the voice that is considered to be particularly beautiful. It is easier, therefore, to consider whether or not a voice falls within normal limits. Within these boundaries there are certain features to which a **normal voice** adheres:

- The vocal note has **clarity**. Generally, it is not rough or excessively breathy and it does not crack or sound 'gravelly'. It is also **consistent** and does not disappear unintentionally for parts of an utterance.
- It is **audible** within a wide range of settings and can be heard even when there are relatively high levels of ambient or background noise. It should be possible for most people with normal voices to shout loudly and to be able to maintain loud conversation in a social setting.
- A normal voice is **age** and **sex appropriate**.
- It fulfils its **linguistic** and **paralinguistic roles** to the speaker's satisfaction.
- It has **stability** and does not change unexpectedly in any of its parameters either at the onset of phonation or during continuous speech. The speaker is able to rely on the way it will perform.
- It has **flexibility** of pitch, loudness and quality.
- It has **stamina** so that it can usually be used throughout the working and social life without deteriorating.
- Normal phonation is **comfortable**. Most people are unaware of any physical sensations associated with speaking, unless they have to increase vocal loudness significantly or produce voice at the limits of their pitch range.

The sound of the voice is dependent on the physical structure and behaviour of the vocal tract. Each person's voice and the changes that are heard depend on the biomechanics of the larynx and the supra- and sub-glottic vocal tract. The size, length, tension and mass of the vocal folds affect the quality, pitch and loudness of the fundamental vocal note, which is subsequently modified by other parts of the vocal tract (Tucker, 1987c; Titze, 1995). Whatever the underlying emotional, linguistic or paralinguistic motivation, the vocal changes are directly related to the physical characteristics of the phonatory mechanism. This fact underlies the assessment and treatment of clinical voice disorders; all vocal features, whether long term or transitory, are the manifestation of events within the vocal tract.

The biomechanics of phonation

Appreciation of the normal patterns of vocal fold movement and the way in which laryngeal adjustments affect the sound of the voice is essential to evaluating laryngeal findings in cases of disordered voice. Considerable variations of structure and function can be found even in the normal larynx, and there are probably even more permutations of laryngeal behaviour. The role of the voice therapist is to modify vocal behaviour; planning successful treatment depends, with other factors, on accurate interpretation of the relationship between the laryngeal image and the vocal profile.

INITIATION OF VOICE

Immediately before phonation, the vocal folds rapidly abduct to allow the intake of air. This has been termed the 'pre-phonatory inspiratory phase' by Wyke (1983). Subsequently, the vocal folds are adducted by the lateral cricoarytenoid muscles (see page 23). Subglottic air pressure increases below the adducted vocal folds until it reaches a level that overcomes their resistance and blows them apart, thus setting in motion the vibratory cycles, which result in phonation. The vocal folds, in common with all vibrators, have a degree of inertia that has to be overcome in order for phonation to occur. The amount of air pressure required to begin voicing is known as the **phonation threshold pressure** (Farley and Barlow, 1994). The size and tension of the vocal folds in combination with the viscoelastic properties of the vocal fold cover will affect the phonation threshold pressure (Titze, 1994b).

To produce a voice within normal limits, the vocal folds have to be structurally and functionally symmetrical and on the same plane. In production of notes of middle pitch, the interarytenoid muscles adduct the cartilaginous portion of both vocal folds and hold them together, while the anterior portion of each fold is gently adducted but free to vibrate in the expiratory airflow. Although full vocal fold adduction during phonation has traditionally been regarded as the norm, clinical observation and various studies have refuted this view by showing that normal phonation can occur when there is incomplete glottal closure (Biever and Bless, 1989; Gelfer and Bultemeyer, 1990). This pattern of vocal fold adduction is more common in women than in men. In particular, incomplete glottal closure can be considered normal in high-frequency modal voice and in falsetto, when hour-glass or spindle glottal configurations can occur in normal subjects (see page 435) (Murry, Xu and Woodson, 1998). It also appears that different types of glottal configurations are associated with different age groups. Biever and Bless (1989) found that incomplete closure of the posterior part of the vocal folds (posterior glottal chink) is a common finding in young and middle-aged women (Sodersten, Hertegard and Hammarberg, 1995). Elderly women are more likely to exhibit anterior chinks. It is essential that clinicians dealing with vocal pathology recognise that incomplete vocal fold closure may be a normal glottal configuration during phonation in certain subjects and at certain frequencies. A comprehensive range of vocal tasks throughout the patient's pitch range during laryngoscopic examination (see Chapter 13) is essential, therefore, if inappropriate conclusions regarding laryngeal pathology are to be avoided.

THE VIBRATORY CYCLE

Each vibratory cycle of the vocal folds consists of three phases: **adduction**, **aerodynamic separation** and **recoil**. As the increased subglottic air pressure overcomes the resistance of the adducted vocal folds at the onset of phonation, the vocal folds peel apart from their inferior border. When they finally separate at their superior margin, a puff of air is released. The resulting negative pressure in the glottis, caused by the Bernoulli effect,* results in the vocal folds closing rapidly as they are sucked together, the inferior vocal fold margins closing first. Contact between the vocal folds increases until the subglottic air pressure is high enough to blow the vocal folds apart again, and the cycle recommences. Each cycle of adduction, separation and recoil is the manifestation of a mucosal wave travelling from the inferior to the superior surface of each vocal fold. The process by which this undulating wave of movement of the mucous membrane occurs is dependent on what is known as the **cover/body theory**, i.e. the vocalis muscle provides the firm body of the vocal fold over which the mucous membrane cover of the vocal fold is blown by the expiratory airstream. These undulations of the vocal folds' thin cover can be observed using stroboscopy (see page 432) or high-speed photography (Titze, 1994c).

The periods of vocal fold contact and lack of contact in one vibratory cycle can be divided broadly into **closed** and **open phases**, respectively, with associated **closing** and **opening phases** (Hirano and Bless, 1993). The closing phase of the vocal folds is more rapid than the opening phase. The phases of the vibratory cycle (Figure 4.1) can be classified, therefore, into four stages as shown in Table 4.1.

---

*The Bernoulli effect is a drop in pressure dependent on particle velocity. In relation to the vocal tract, Maran (1988) describes it as follows: 'When air passes from one large space to another (e.g. from lung to pharynx), through a constriction (the glottis), the velocity will be greatest and the pressure least at the site of the constriction'. As a result of the drop in pressure at the glottis, the vocal fold mucosa is drawn into the space between the vocal folds.

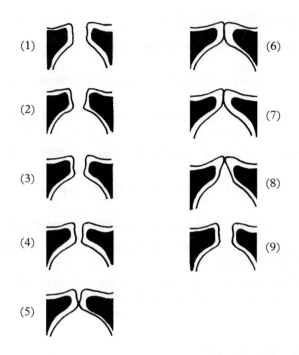

Figure 4.1 Vocal fold vibratory cycle. (coronal view)

Table 4.1 The periods of vocal fold contact and lack of contact in one vibratory cycle

Closing phase	The vocal folds begin to close rapidly from their lower margin
Closed phase	The medial edges of the vocal folds are in full contact
Opening phase	The vocal folds begin to separate from their lower margin and gradually peel apart. The superior margin remains in contact until the end of this phase
Open phase	The vocal folds are separated The longest part of a normal vibratory cycle

Insufficient approximation of the vocal folds results in air wastage and production of breathy voice. The vocal folds fail to approximate completely along their membranous portion, with a slightly increased aperture in the cartilaginous section. As a result, turbulent air escapes and is audible in the voice. The vocal folds must vibrate symmetrically, be at the same level and close rapidly in order that a clear vocal note can be initiated and maintained (Woo et al., 1991).

Some of the biomechanical principles governing the vocal folds are listed in Table 4.2. The choice of remediation strategies for treating voice-disordered patients depends, in part, on understanding these principles.

Table 4.2 Phonation: biomechanical principles

- Phonation is the result of interaction between airflow, air pressure and vocal fold biomechanics

- The size of the glottic opening and the degree of vocal fold tension affect airflow and air pressure

- Incomplete vocal fold adduction results in greater airflow and reduced subglottic air pressure

- Tight vocal fold adduction may result in reduced airflow and increased subglottic air pressure

- Increased tension of the vocal folds requires greater force to displace them and to initiate movement

- Increased vocal fold mass also requires greater force to displace the vocal folds

- Increased vocal fold mass results in lower frequency of vibration and, as a result, lower pitch (all other things being equal)

- Increased subglottic air pressure in conjunction with increased vocal fold tension results in increased loudness (and a small increase in frequency)

Acoustics of the voice

The voice heard by the listener is not the basic sound produced by the larynx alone, but the acoustic product of the entire vocal tract. Consequently, perceptual and instrument assessment of a voice problem requires identification of the various acoustic features that enable the clinician to describe the disordered voice as a foundation for treatment planning.

SOURCE-FILTER MODEL

The basis of the voice is the sound generated in the larynx. There are various terms used to refer to this sound: **glottal signal, voice signal, source signal** or **vocal note**. They all apply to the sound made at the lower end of the vocal tract by the vocal folds. The glottal signal is periodic and composed of a series of sine waves (or harmonics). It is subsequently filtered by the supralaryngeal tract with some harmonics in the source signal being resonated more than others. This explanation of the process is referred to as the source-filter model of voice. The shape of the vocal tract is the primary factor in its frequency response. The resonance peaks of the vocal tract are known as **formants**. Each formant is identified by a formant number. Vowels are distinguished by a number of formants of which $F1$ and $F2$ are recognised as being the most conspicuous in contributing to vowel differentiation. Howard (1998) points out that the fourth, fifth and sixth formants are thought to be important in operatic singing and that $F3$

might convey information that helps to identify individual speakers. As well as varying from speaker to speaker and in children, men and women, vowel formants vary in the articulation of the same speaker, according to the phonetic context in which they occur and by which they are influenced (Gimson, 1962). Although formants occur in all speech sounds, the term is usually confined to the description of vowels. Values of mean frequencies of $F1$ and $F2$ have been compiled by Fry (1979), Baken (1987) and Kent and Read (1992) (Table 4.3).

Table 4.3 Formant frequencies of some English vowels

Vowel	F1 (Hz)	F2 (Hz)
/i:/ (eel)	300	2300
/i/ (bit)	360	2100
/ae/ (hat)	750	1750
/ʌ/ (cut)	720	1240

After Fry (1979).

The varying shapes of the oral and pharyngeal cavities in articulation of vowels are shown in Figure 4.2. Note the elevation of the soft palate which alters position and is most tensed for /i:/. The diaphragm of the velum will reflect sound waves but also acts as a sounding board with sound waves passing into the nasal cavity. These are too weak to cause nasal tone but impart nasal resonance, which is missed if there is nasal obstruction, as in an upper respiratory tract infection. Note also the marked variations in

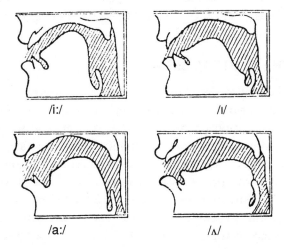

/i:/   /ɪ/

/a:/   /ʌ/

Figure 4.2 Oral and pharyngeal modifications during articulation of vowels.

tongue positions for the various vowels and, as a result, the way in which the shape and space of the oral cavity is modified.

One of the most significant modifications of the vocal note can be effected by the soft palate. The balance of oral and nasal resonance is determined to some extent by the action of the velopharyngeal sphincter. The soft palate is normally raised towards the posterior pharyngeal wall in connected speech, apart from the nasal phonemes /n/, /m/ and /ŋ/. Significant lowering of the soft palate will cause **excessive nasal resonance** or **hypernasality**. The balance of resonance is also affected by the degree of mouth opening, tongue bunching and pharyngeal tension. In extreme forms, these characteristics will be perceived as abnormal, but moderate changes fall within what are regarded as normal limits. For example, the speaker whose mouth is relatively closed and whose tongue tends to be raised and retracted will produce a voice with a more nasal quality than the individual with a relaxed, relatively open mouth and lowered tongue.

Baken and Orlikoff (2000) draw attention to the fact that, in addition to modifying the glottal signal, the supralaryngeal vocal tract has a significant role in modifying vocal fold function. They give the example of constriction at some point within the vocal tract (e.g. linguopalatal contact), which causes an increase in subglottal air pressure; this, in turn, modifies the glottal signal because of a change in air pressure within the glottis. This interaction between the source and the filter has potentially important clinical implications.

Ultimately, therefore, the acoustic signal that is heard by the listener is an amalgam of the glottal signal and the filtering effects of the supralaryngeal tract. As the glottal source is resonated and modified, the particular 'timbre' or 'colour' of the voice is produced as well as the vowel characteristics. This final output is known as the radiated or propagated acoustic signal (Kent and Read, 1992).

QUALITY OF THE GLOTTAL SIGNAL

The quality of the glottal signal depends on the competency of vocal fold adduction and the periodicity and symmetry of the mucosal waves. The sound generated is composed of periodic and aperiodic waves (random noise). Noise is a sound that is not a harmonic of the glottal signal. The percentage of periodic waves to aperiodic waves contained in the vocal signal can be calculated with appropriate software to give the **harmonics-to-noise ratio** (HNR). Any increase in the noise component of the vocal note impairs the harmonic structure of the voice and, when it is a dominant feature of the sound of the voice, it will be perceived as hoarseness and regarded as abnormal (see Chapter 6). The greater the increase in aperiodic sound (i.e. reduced HNR), the more severe the hoarseness. The terms 'breathy' or 'rough' are used to describe a voice in which there is an increased noise component. Although the HNR measurement provides information concerning noise in the vocal signal, it does not indicate the laryngeal abnormality that gives rise to the increased noise quotient (Yumoto, 1983). Normal voices exhibit varying degrees of **breathiness** and this is largely the result of air leakage via the glottis (Hirano, 1981), resulting from inefficient vocal fold closure. When this is excessive and results in functionally inefficient phonation, it will be regarded as a clinical voice disorder. **Roughness,** which can occur intermittently even in an otherwise normal voice, is the result of irregular glottal pulses (Dejonckere, 1995). The complexities of vibratory patterns occurring in rough voice are being investigated increasingly by non-linear dynamic analysis (*chaos theory*) which might explain various vocal irregularities (Baken, 1994, 1995; Berry et al., 1994; Herzel et al., 1994). HNR measurement was recognised for many years as a potential tool for quantifying hoarseness objectively (Yanagihara, 1967a; Yumoto, Sasaki and Okamura, 1984), but the evolving software remained unsatisfactory until recently (Awan and Frenkel, 1994). As a baseline measure of vocal pathology and as a monitoring measure of change during treatment, HNR is an important measure for the voice clinician.

FREQUENCY

The time taken by one vibratory cycle is called its **period**. The **frequency** is the number of periods per second, and is measured in hertz (Hz). The perceptual correlate of frequency is **pitch,** and the perceived pitch of a sound increases in proportion to the frequency of oscillation. The rate of the vibration of the vocal folds is dependent on vocal fold length, tension, elasticity and mass, and resistance to subglottic air pressure. As long as these factors remain constant the frequency does not vary. As the vocal folds increase in length and the vocalis muscles thin and stiffen them, frequency increases.

It has to be remembered that high pitch is not necessarily the result of high frequency but may be caused by the acoustic characteristics imparted to the voice by the supraglottic vocal tract. Consequently, Fo may be a poor indicator of vocal pitch.

Speaking fundamental frequency (SFo)

Speaking fundamental frequency, or habitual pitch, depends on the sex and age of the speaker as well as the type of communication and the speaker's emotional status. It can be affected by a range of variables such as speaking against background noise, reading aloud and talking on the telephone. It has been found that, when people drink alcohol, the vocal pitch is raised (McClelland, 1994), although this will probably depend on the degree of intoxication. Lowered pitch may be a feature of depression. Fundamental frequency and its variation with sex and age has been the subject of many studies. Extensive normative data on SFo and other vocal parameters have been collated by Baken (1987). The average habitual pitch levels, varying according to the individual and the circumstances, appear in Table 4.4.

Pitch and pitch changes reflect vocal fold length and tension, sub-glottic air pressure and activity of the thyroarytenoid muscles (Table 4.5). Most of the tension is taken by the epithelium of the vocal folds as they are stretched by the contraction of the cricothyroid muscles (Atkinson, 1978) (Figure 4.3). As a result, voice pitch is largely determined by tension in the vocal fold epithelium (Scherer, 1991). Scherer also points out that, when subglottic air pressure increases, there is an associated increase in frequency. The mechanical reason for this is that increased subglottic air pressure causes maximum lateral excursion of the vocal fold to increase during each vibratory cycle. Consequently, as the vocal fold is stretched more during the cycle there is greater tension, which results in faster return to the start position, resulting in increased frequency. This also accounts for the association between increased vocal loudness and increased pitch. The

Table 4.4 Average speaking fundamental frequencies

	Men	Women	Children
Average habitual pitch (Hz)	128	225	265
Median speaking Fo (Hz)	Bass 98–110 Baritone 117–133 Tenor 147–165	Contralto 220 Mezzo-soprano 226 Soprano 262	

Table 4.5 Vocal fold changes required to raise and lower fundamental vocal note frequency

	To raise Fo	To lower Fo
Subglottic air pressure	Increases	Decreases
Vocal fold length	Lengthens	Shortens
Vocal fold tension	Increases	Decreases
Vocal fold depth	Thins	Thickens

Similar principles apply when vocal folds are abnormal. For example, an increase in mass (e.g. as a result of vocal nodules) lowers the fundamental frequency of the vocal note, whereas a decrease in mass (e.g. as a result of a loss of muscle in an aged larynx) causes the fundamental frequency to rise.

(a)

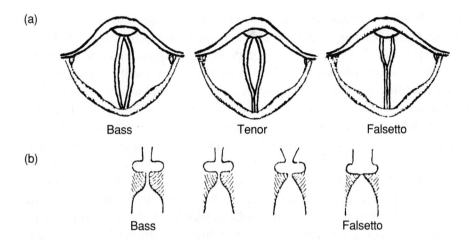

(b)

Figure 4.3 Superior and coronal diagrams of vocal folds in phonation.

highest vocal frequencies can be achieved only by maximum cricothyroid muscle activity and minimum thyroarytenoid muscle activity (Farley and Barlow, 1994). The control of pitch is highly complex because the frequency of the vocal note not only changes as a result of increased muscle tension and subglottal air pressure, but also varies with sudden transglottal pressure changes (Baken and Orlikoff, 1991).

Pitch range

In addition to the habitual vocal pitch, the pitch range of a voice is an essential aspect of vocal function for both speaking and singing. It is dependent on the vocal fold changes described above. Titze (1995) explains that low frequencies are enhanced by the entire vocal tract, whereas high frequencies are enhanced in the supraglottic laryngeal space. These high frequencies can be enhanced further by widening the posterior part of the larynx, as in an anticipated yawn. The capacity for rapid flexibility within the pitch range is as important as the potential for an extensive pitch range if the vocal requirements of speech and singing are to be fulfilled. Figure 4.6 (page 86) shows the pitch ranges for men and women.

Vocal registers

The subject of vocal registers is confusing and controversial. This is partly because the definition of what constitutes a register has been unclear but also because a number of terms are used to describe each register. Traditionally, registers have been regarded as the perceptually distinct regions of vocal quality over certain ranges of pitch and loudness

(Titze, 1994b), but listener identification of the change from one register to another is not reliable (McGlone and Brown, 1969). The terms used vary according to whether they are being employed by singers or speech scientists, but even then their use is not uniform. Singers tend to classify the registers as **head, middle** and **chest**, but these terms are regarded as unsatisfactory by voice scientists, many of whom refer to three main vocal registers: **falsetto, modal** and **vocal fry**. These classifications, however, do not relate directly to each other. Baken (1987) notes that the problems of definition and terminology have been clarified by Hollien's (1974) suggestion that registers should be defined in terms of laryngeal behaviour, rather than in acoustic terms, because registers are governed by the degree of contraction of the vocalis muscle. As a result, the terms **loft, modal** and **pulse registers** can be used with less confusion; they describe the vibratory pattern of the vocal folds and the acoustic parameters being produced (Hirano, 1981)

- **Loft register (or falsetto)** covers the highest frequencies of the voice. The vocal folds are lengthened, extremely tense and thinned so that there is minimal vibration. The knife-thin free edges are almost adducted and subglottic air pressure is high. During the production of these high frequencies, the larynx is raised by the suprahyoid muscles and the pharynx is shortened (Shipp, 1975) (Figure 4.4).
- **Modal register** encompasses the range of frequencies usually employed in speech and singing. The membranous portions of the vocal folds are adducted and make complete closure in the closed phase of each vibratory cycle. In cross-section, the vocal folds are

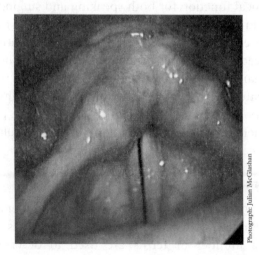

Photograph: Julian McGlashan

Figure 4.4 Normal falsetto phonation.

triangular in shape. In low notes, the intrinsic muscles relax, the folds increase in bulk and their opposing surfaces deepen from 3 mm to 5 mm. They vibrate slowly along their whole length, the lower surfaces of their 'lips' making contact and separating as the upper surfaces approximate in a rolling motion or figure of eight. In lowest notes, the infrahyoid muscles pull the larynx down (Shipp and McGlone, 1971).

- **Pulse register** (or **glottal fry** or **vocal fry** or **creaky voice**) occurs during the lowest vocal frequencies and is a feature of normal speech (Fry, 1979). This terminology reflects the pulsatile nature of the laryngeal sound generated. There is a long closed phase in each vibratory cycle.

The terminology and underlying modes of vocal fold behaviour during the production of each register are outlined in Table 4.6.

Table 4.6 Vocal registers

Register	Equivalent terms may include	Vocal folds	Fo range (Hz)
Loft register			
Highest vocal frequencies	Falsetto	Thin, tense, lengthened minimal vibration	275–1100
Modal register			
Range of fundamental frequencies most commonly used in speaking & singing	Chest, head, middle Heavy voice	Complete adduction	100–300
Pulse register			
Lowest range of vocal frequencies: laryngeal output is perceived as pulsatile	Vocal fry Glottal fry Creaky voice	Long closed phase	20–60

The terminology related to vocal registers is not consistent. Various overlapping terms are used which have different theoretical bases (see text). During classical singing voice quality should remain constant regardless of pitch and the transition from one register to another, known as the passagio, should be as smooth as possible. This is achieved by careful control of vocal fold tension in combination with an appropriate level of subglottic air pressure.

Counter-tenors are normal males with normal speaking voices who are able to sing in the falsetto register. Alfred Deller popularised counter-tenor singing in the 1930s and the English counter-tenor James Bowman has been extremely popular more recently. The voice of the male falsetto singer is rather richer in harmonics than that of the boy by reason of the larger adult resonators. These singers' voices have a range of two octaves (164–698 Hz) (Jackson, 1987).

Pitch perturbation (jitter)

When consecutive vibratory cycles of the vocal folds vary in frequency so that there is short-term frequency variation, the phenomenon is referred to as pitch perturbation or jitter. These terms are applied to frequency variability resulting from involuntary changes in the fundamental frequency. Jitter ratio measurements are higher in pathological voices and in some elderly normal voices (Hartman and Von Cramon, 1984b; Zyski et al., 1984; Dejonckere, 1995), and are important in the evaluation of voice disorders and laryngeal abnormality.

AMPLITUDE

Amplitude refers to the size of the oscillations of the vibrator – the vocal folds – and is perceived as **loudness** or **intensity**. The amplitude of the vibrations depends on the energy or force of the excitor – the airflow and pressure. The intensity of sound is measured on a logarithmic scale in units known as decibels (dB), which are measured in relation to the threshold of audibility.

Vocal loudness (Table 4.7) varies according to respiratory airflow and subglottic pressure, which affects the rate of glottal closure and the size of the excursions executed by the vocal folds. Increased loudness can be achieved only by increasing vocal fold resistance to increased airflow. Frequency and intensity modifications are closely related because of the air pressure and vocal fold tensions, which are common to both. Not only do maximum and minimum vocal intensity change with fundamental frequency, but increased intensity can also result in increased frequency.

There are wide variations in vocal loudness according to context, mood and content. Even conversational speech will be extremely loud when background noise level is high and volume will increase if the speaker is addressing an audience. Fry (1979) recorded the average intensity of conversational speech, a metre from the speaker, as 60 dB, which is similar to Vilkman's (1996) suggestion that the sound level of speech in a silent room

Table 4.7 Vocal intensity for speech and singing

Vocal loudness	dB
Quiet voice	35–40
Average intensity	60–70
Shouting: forte	80
Shouting: fortissimo	90
Singing	100

Sources: Fry (1979); Baken (1987); Hacki (1996).

is normally 50 dB at a distance of 1 metre. Vilkman also notes that the sound level of the speaking voice increases by 3 dB for each 10 dB increase in ambient noise level from 40 dB, as a result of the Lombard effect. During quiet voiced speech, the average level is approximately 35–40 dB and, during shouting, 75 dB. Data reviewed by Baken (1987) indicated that connected speech lies in the region of 70 dB. Hacki (1996) reports that an individual with a normal voice can reach a *forte* intensity of 80 dB and a *fortissimo* of approximately 90 dB with the speaking voice, while shouting and some singing reaches an average of 100 dB. Trained classical singers achieve maximum volume by shaping the mouth into a horn shape, rather like the end of a trumpet or clarinet, by lowering the jaw and widening the mouth. This produces a graduated opening of the vocal tract into free space which conveys the voice to the audience as loudly as possible (Titze, 1995).

Amplitude perturbation (shimmer)

Amplitude perturbation is a short-term instability of the intensity of the vocal signal and is conceptually comparable to pitch perturbation (see above). Shimmer measurements quantify the variability of the intensity of the fundamental vocal note. Baken (1987) cites research that demonstrates the importance of shimmer to the perception of hoarseness.

The vocal profile

The voice can be described, therefore, in terms of its parameters: vocal note quality, pitch, loudness and resonance. Subcategories of flexibility, particularly of pitch range, and stamina are also important descriptors. Each parameter can be described in isolation and one element can be changed while others remain constant. For example, vocal pitch can be raised and lowered while talking quietly. In reality, however, the various vocal features are interdependent and the alteration of one can affect another. This occurs, for instance, when increased vocal loudness is invariably accompanied by raised pitch. Together, the vocal parameters create an acoustic profile (Table 4.8).

Normal vocal variants

The potential flexibility of the vocal tract and vocal folds allows an enormous variation of vocal behaviours to be executed. Many of the resulting changes in the voice occur constantly without the speaker being aware that they are taking place. Other vocal behaviours, such as singing, are developed as vocal skills and can make great demands on the individual's ability to fulfil what is regarded as superior vocal function. In between these two extremes are the vocal behaviours that are used intentionally in order either to be

Table 4.8 Vocal profile parameters	
Vocal parameters	*Acoustic measure*
• **Vocal note quality**	Harmonics-to-noise ratio (HNR)
• **Habitual pitch**	Speaking fundamental frequency (SFo)
• **Pitch** – pitch range – pitch instability	Voice range profile Jitter (pitch perturbation)
• **Loudness** – loudness instability	Intensity Shimmer (amplitude perturbation)
• **Resonance**	Spectrum/spectral peaks
• **Flexibility** (pitch and loudness)	
• **Stamina**	

appropriate for a particular situation or to elicit a particular response in the listener. As a result of this vocal flexibility and because the voice is affected by the body's physiological requirements, the demarcation between normal and abnormal voice is inevitably poorly defined. In reality, there is a normal–disordered continuum (Mathieson, 2000); a voice that is generally regarded as normal will produce features from time to time that might be regarded as abnormal if the voice sample were heard out of context.

Example 1

After running, when the speaker is out of breath, phrases are short, the voice is breathy and it is difficult to increase vocal loudness. These vocal features are the direct result of the body's physiological need for rapid breathing in order to replace oxygen. The inevitable effect is that the speaker is unable to maintain vocal fold adduction and create adequate subglottic air pressure for normal phonation because of the overwhelming need for greater ventilation. Phonation during the recovery time is therefore grossly abnormal but is a normal vocal variant.

Example 2

After prolonged crying, there is hyponasal resonance because of increased nasal secretions and swollen nasal mucosa. The fundamental note sounds 'wet' because secretions are pooling in the area of the larynx.

Example 3

When a heavy weight is being lifted, the individual takes a deep breath and firmly adducts the vocal folds in order to build up enough subglottic air pressure to fix the shoulder girdle This provides a fixed point so that the strain of the weight can be taken. If speech is attempted while lifting the weight, the voice has a squeezed or pressed quality, which is grossly abnormal when compared with the voice at other times and which mimics the phonation of certain neurological voice disorders.

Voice-onset variants

Hard glottal attack

Hard glottal attack occurs at the onset of phonation when the vocal folds momentarily make full closure, so that the expiratory breath stream is interrupted and then released explosively. It reaches its maximum amplitude rapidly and shows greater air consumption than soft attack (Koike, Hirano and von Leden, 1967). This onset pattern is normally used for emphasis in words with an intial vowel, e.g. 'I said so', and in some English dialects, such as those in parts of London, the glottal stop replaces certain lingual plosive consonants, e.g. 'Got a lot of butter' (gδəʔδəbʌə). It is also the normal mode of articulation in German for vowels occurring initially in words. In moods of fear, anger and impatience, it occurs as the speaker's tension increases (Luchsinger and Arnold, 1965). When use of the glottal stop is linguistic, it is innocuous but, when it is a physiological symptom of laryngeal tension and abusive phonation, it can be harmful and result in damage to the vocal fold mucosa. The singer who mistakenly develops this method of initiating phonation, thinking that it will increase articulatory clarity, risks producing an unpleasant sound in addition to damaging the vocal folds (Bunch, 1982).

Soft attack (breathy onset)

When soft attack is used, the vocal folds do not fully adduct at the onset of phonation and air passes through the resulting glottic chink, without vocal fold vibration, immediately before voice onset. Such phonation can be associated with emotions of joy and pleasure. Soft attack is not appropriate for the singer who is aiming at a clear vocal note, because the breathy quality will be apparent at onset whereas volume and projection will be radically reduced. To achieve precise and clear voice onset, the classical singer has to coordinate a 'precise momentary closure of the vocal folds' (Bunch, 1982) with a gentle breath stream.

Whisper

In whisper, the glottis is narrowed and turbulent air passes through the resulting glottic chink (Figure 4.5). There is no vocal fold vibration. In quiet whisper, the vocal folds are slightly separated along their anterior two-thirds, but there is a triangular posterior glottic chink because the arytenoid cartilages do not adduct. In strong whisper, the folds are adducted firmly along the anterior two-thirds and air is forced through the posterior chink with considerable friction (Luchsinger, 1965a). Monoson and Zemlin (1984), in a quantitative study of whisper, noted that vocal fold position in whisper is variable in different speakers and that the degree of transglottic airflow is an important characteristic of whisper.

Breathy voice

During breathy voice, the vocal folds are not fully adducted but they are vibrating. Turbulent air through the glottis is heard simultaneously with the vocal note, which gives the vocal note its breathy quality. As a result of air escaping through the glottis during the production of breathy voice, phrase length will be shortened and it becomes difficult to increase vocal loudness.

Harsh voice

During the production of harsh voice, the vocal folds are more strongly adducted than in breathy voice. Perceptually, the resulting vocal quality has a hard edge but is also breathy (Howard, 1998).

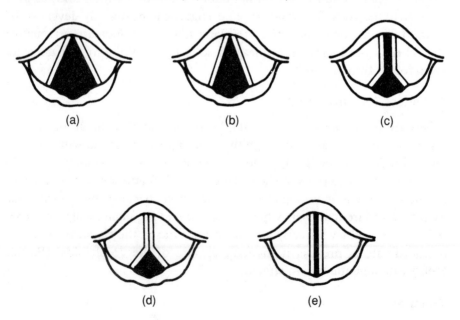

(a)　　　　　　　　(b)　　　　　　　　(c)

(d)　　　　　　　　(e)

Figure 4.5 Position of vocal folds in full abduction, gentle abduction, gentle whisper, stage whisper and phonation.

Pressed voice

This vocal quality occurs when the vocal folds are relatively firmly adducted during phonation and there is raised subglottic air pressure. Phonation is effortful and can become uncomfortable if increased loudness is attempted or the voice is used over a long period. It is usually accompanied by hard voice onset. Although a low level of pressed voice can be within normal limits, this vocal behaviour is well advanced along the normal–disordered continuum to becoming a voice disorder.

Singing voice

The singing voice employs much more extensive pitch and loudness range than speaking. There is some disparity between the measurements given by various writers arising from different assessment methods. Luchsinger and Arnold (1965) suggested a singing range of 147–349 Hz for men and 249–698 Hz for women, whereas Perkins and Kent (1986) give ranges of 80–700 Hz and 140–1000 Hz, respectively. Maximum frequency range can extend from a lowest Fo of 77 Hz to a highest Fo of 567 Hz in a young man and from 134 Hz to 895 Hz for young women (Baken, 1987). To achieve these very high notes, subglottic air pressures are much higher and in trained singers the closed quotient of each vocal fold vibratory cycle is longer (Howard, Lindsey and Allen, 1990; Akerlund and Gramming, 1994; Carroll et al., 1996). It has been suggested by Carroll et al. (1996) that, because of the differences that have been observed in trained singers from the generally used vocal parameter norms, separate normative data should be available for this group. See Figures 4.6 and 4.7 for the frequency ranges of male and female singing voices in Western culture.

Certain traditions of singing have developed characteristic vocal behaviours which are described below.

Covered voice

In the teaching of singing, the mastery of special singing techniques is essential, especially for the opera singer. In western European classical singing, the means of increasing vocal substance and a swelling tone is agreed to be the 'covered' voice. How this is actually achieved has long been a bone of contention among singing professors. The Italian school advocates the open singing technique with open mouth and smiling lips, a wide open and relaxed throat being apparently the chief aim. For dramatic singing, the 'covered' voice is advocated mainly by the German school because it gives added power and emotional tension to the voice. The technique necessitates descent of the larynx, simultaneous widening of the pharyngeal cavity and increased air pressure. Luchsinger (1965a) stated that 'covering' the voice

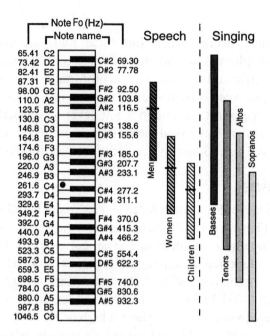

Figure 4.6 Speech and singing ranges. ©Whurr Publishers Ltd. Reprinted by permission of Professor David M. Howard.

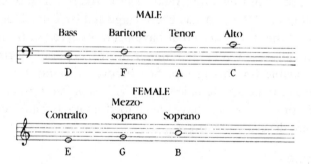

Figure 4.7 Middle notes of singing ranges.

means a slight 'darkening' of the vowels on higher pitch levels to avoid excessively bright timbre in singing. This accords with the view that lip-rounding is essential in achieving covered voice because all formant frequencies decrease uniformly with lip-rounding (and increase with lip-spreading) and with increased length of the vocal tract (Titze, 1994b). Covering is also used to facilitate changes from one register to another.

Sundberg (1974, 1977, 1995) has made important contributions to understanding the nature of vibrato and covered voice in his acoustic studies. In particular he brought attention to what he termed the 'singer's formant'. This is formed by a fusion of the third and fourth formants of the fundamental note. The combination of these peaks of resonance results in a band of maximum energy in the region of 2500–3000 Hz. The singer's formant is most likely to occur at high fundamental frequency and intensity (Hollien, 1980). This optimal frequency occurs in a bandwidth in which orchestral energy is low. As optimal use is being made of resonance, the operatic singer is able to be heard without using excessive effort, above the apparently much greater volume of the orchestra. Sundberg (1974) also provided an articulatory interpretation of the singing formant. In male singers, the envelope peak is in the region of 2.8 kHz and, in order to achieve this, three conditions of the vocal tract have to be met:

• The cross-sectional area must be at least six times wider than the laryngeal tube orifice. If mismatched an extra formant is added.
• The sinus of Morgagni (laryngeal ventricle) must be wide in relation to the larynx tube and if mismatched an extra formant may be added between the third and fourth formants of normal speech.
• The pyriform fossa must be wide, which reduces the fifth formant to about 3 kHz.

These three conditions can be fulfilled when the larynx is lowered. The two linked resonators of larynx and pharynx produce the resonance characteristics of voice. Sundberg (1974) avers that there is no case for the terms 'head', 'chest' and 'mask' resonance currently used in vocal pedagogy, but such terms can be useful in teaching students. Achievement of the singing formant is dependent, therefore, on lowering the larynx and lengthening and widening the pharynx while relaxing the tongue and mandible. It is important that the pharyngeal muscles are relaxed and the voice is produced effortlessly. This will not occur if the larynx is forced down in the vocal tract and if the supraglottic resonators are tense. Bunch (1976), in a cephalometric study of structure of head and neck during sustained phonation of covered and open singing, confirmed that enlargement of the pharyngeal cavity is a major factor in production of covered voice.

A comparative study by Burns (1986) of the singing voices of opera singers and 'country and western' singers illustrates the importance of the use of the singing formant as a protective mechanism, in addition to its aesthetic function. He hypothesised that country and western singers use a faulty singing technique that does not incorporate the singing formant and that this accounts for the vocal abuse frequently occurring in this group. Acoustic analysis of the speaking and singing voices of both groups revealed that, as expected, the opera singers used the singing formant but the country and western singers used formants almost identical to those of speech when they were singing. Unfortunately, for country and western singers, and for rock and many pop singers, attempts to use the singing formant would destroy the vocal quality that is highly popular and an integral part of a particular style of singing.

In the mountains of Mongolia and some Tibetan monasteries, the resonators are used differently to produce 'overtone chanting' or 'throat singing', during which the fundamental vocal note and its formants can each be perceived separately but concurrently. This is achieved by adopting certain mouth and tongue postures.

Vibrato

Vibrato is a skill used by singers to add emotion and beauty to the voice. It varies according to the type and culture of singing, giving Western operatic singing its warm, rich tone. A fundamental frequency modulation occurs at a rate of 5–7 Hz over a range of one semitone. There is a simultaneous intensity modulation of a few decibels; on average, the intensity increase is 9 dB. The hub frequency swing varies but is in the region of a quarter of a tone. The frequency undulations are the result of pulsating contractions of the cricothyroid muscle (Sundberg, 1995), in association with oscillations of the soft palate, the epiglottis, the lateral walls of the hypopharynx and the inferior part of the oropharynx, at certain pitch and loudness levels in most singers. In trained singers, vibrato tends to develop automatically and it is possible that this is cultivated from a 4–6 Hz physiological tremor in the cricothyroid and thyroarytenoid muscles (Titze, 1994b). Sundberg suggests that, in popular singing and in non-Western cultures, the vibrato quality appears to develop from pulsations of subglottic air pressure rather than pulsations of the cricothyroid muscle. The rate of vibration is slightly faster in females than in males and tends to accelerate under the influence of emotion. Individual frequency and pitch differences in vibrato have been recorded in different singers. Enrico Caruso produced a frequency undulation of 6.54 Hz (Dejonckere, 1995) and Maria Callas an undulation of 7.5 Hz. Lily Pons produced 'quaver' rather than vibrato of 7.5 Hz. When properly controlled, vibrato enhances the singing voice. If absent, the voice sounds metallic. An excessively high number of pulsations gives rise to the unpleasant quality known as **tremolo** while slow pulsations result in **wobble**. This decrease in vibrato rate to a 2–4 Hz range tends to occur with ageing. When the vibrato features of opera singers were compared with the vocal characteristics of patients with pathological vocal tremor in a study by Ramig and Shipp (1987), there were only minor differences between the two groups. Although the regularity of the fundamental frequency variation was somewhat greater in singers, the vibrato rate in singers was 5.5 Hz compared with the vocal tremor patients who produced a rate of 6.8 Hz.

Trill

Trill is achieved by rapid variation of pitch between a base note and a note higher by either a whole tone or a semitone (Proctor, 1980; Titze, 1994b), whereas in vibrato the singer attempts to remain on the same note. Vennard and Von Leden (1967) submitted the trills of four outstanding sopranos to spectrographic analysis. They concluded that the rate of pitch fluctuation in a trill is very little faster than that of a vibrato, but the extent of the pitch variation is increased so that the ear can perceive the two pitches involved. Rhythmic contractions of the whole laryngeal structure accompany a trill, but the visible movement of the larynx has no connection with the 'wobble' voice quality resulting from excessively slow vibrato.

Yodel

Yodelling is a particular style of singing that figures prominently, for example, in songs of the Swiss Alps and the American south-west. It is thought to have originated in imitation of the alpenhorn and the shawm, an ancient wind instrument similar to the clarinet and common to all pastoral people (Luchsinger, 1965b). The yodel consists of sudden jumps in pitch from modal to falsetto voice on vowel sounds only, not words. Good air support is necessary and this is provided by activity of the diaphragm. The yodel has great carrying power and is an effective means of calling the attention of a neighbour on another mountain top and is not, as might be expected, for rounding up lost sheep and goats.

Perfect singing technique will greatly improve a mediocre voice and enhance an excellent voice. However, perfection depends on the singer's musical talent coupled with the genetic anatomical endowment. It is this that accounts for a Caruso, Ferrier, Callas, Pavarotti, Norman, Te Kanawa or Domingo.

Determinants of phonation

This chapter has been concerned with many aspects of the generation and modification of the vocal note within the vocal tract. In reality, the acoustic signal is affected by the complex interaction of much wider factors both intrinsic to the speaker and arising in the context in which the utterance takes place. The flow diagram in Figure 4.8 illustrates that the structure of

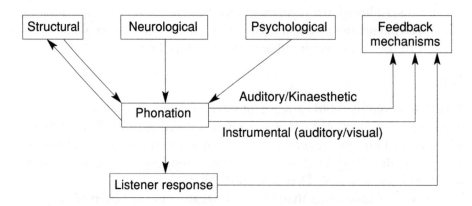

Figure 4.8 Determinants of phonation.

the vocal tract and its neurology are fundamental to normal phonation. Aberration in these areas will undoubtedly produce vocal abnormality. The speaker's psychological state also influences the voice directly as well as indirectly because of its influence on the nervous system and subsequently on muscle tone. Fry (1979) attributed the emotional colouring of the voice to changes in fundamental frequency resulting from changes in tension of the vocal folds matched to anxiety or content. These vocal fold changes also affect the quality of the glottal signal. It is also possible for the process of phonation to cause changes to the structure of the vocal fold mucosa if the use of excessive effort causes damage. These changes in structure will, in turn, feed back into the vocal behaviour as the speaker attempts to make adjustments for these abnormalities and tries to produce normal voice. The interaction with a listener can also have a significant effect on the voice. If there is a negative response, this might result in a quavering, quiet, breathy voice, for example, if the speaker is made to feel nervous. The voice can develop features that immediately reveal how the speaker is feeling and listener response is one of the important elements of feedback loops that can affect all voices. Others include the sound of the speaker's own voice and the physical sensations that accompany phonation, i.e. the auditory and kinaesthetic feedback. The speaker usually monitors these without awareness unless certain vocal features appear to be inappropriate. Patterns of phonation can also be monitored by instrumental auditory and visual feedback which are fundamental to clinical practice as well as in singing teaching, the tuition of presentation skills and other methods for modifying vocal behaviour. It is essential for the clinician, voice scientist, singing and voice teachers, and all professionals involved in analysis and pedagogy to take these factors fully into account in dealing with the individual and the voice.

Summary

■ The voice is the product of a glottal signal which is filtered by the supraglottal tract.

■ A voice can be described in terms of a vocal profile.

■ The vocal profile can comprise the following parameters: vocal note quality, pitch, loudness, resonance, flexibility (of pitch and loudness) and stamina.

■ Changes in the vocal parameters reflect the biomechanics of the vocal tract.

■ Each individual produces a wide range of vocal behaviours.

■ There is an overlap between normal and abnormal voice.

■ At any particular moment, an individual's voice reflects: the structure and function of the vocal tract; the person's neurological and psychological status; the auditory and kinaesthetic feedback that he or she is receiving; and the behaviour of the listener or audience.

Voice development: infancy to senescence

The larynx and all parts of the vocal tract are changing throughout life and the voice reflects these changes. Some vocal features are the result of gross alterations such as the size of the vocal folds and the dimensions of the vocal tract structure, but others are the result of more subtle changes, such as the changing histology of the vocal folds and the timing of the neuronal impulses that initiate and regulate phonation. The structure and the controlling mechanisms of phonation are in a process of maturation for the first 20 years of life. At certain ages, such as puberty, dramatic developments are obvious but it is not until approximately the end of the second decade that all aspects of the vocal tract are matured. From age 20 to 29 years, the third decade, the body undergoes only minor physiological changes although, even at this time of relative anatomical and physiological tranquillity, women will be experiencing menstruation and, possibly, pregnancy, both of which can affect the voice. The fourth decade brings the beginning of degenerative changes throughout the body which progress at a different rate in men and women and from person to person. From infancy to old age, therefore, the maturation and subsequent decline of the anatomy, physiology and histology of the vocal tract and its related systems result in acoustic changes in the voice. Throughout the lifespan the voice is affected by a number of internal and external factors (Table 5.1).

Infancy

UPPER RESPIRATORY TRACT

Laryngeal position

The configuration of the infant aerodigestive region is radically different from that of both the child and the adult. At birth, the larynx is high in the vocal

Table 5.1 Factors affecting the voice from infancy to senescence

- Growth, e.g. bones, muscles, cartilages
- Hormones, especially androgens and oestrogens
- Health: good, poor
- Use: occupation and leisure activities
- Lifestyle, e.g. busy, relaxed, smoking, excessive alcohol, gastric reflux
- Environment, e.g. quiet, pleasant, unpleasant, noisy, dusty, excessively dry atmosphere
- Psychological status, e.g. happiness, serenity, depression, anxiety, stress
- Cultural factors, e.g. vocally loud social/family group
- Degenerative changes, e.g. bones, muscles, cartilages, nervous system, respiratory system

tract with the lower border of the cricoid cartilage at the level of cervical vertebrae 3 and 4 (C3–C4) (Maddern, Campbell and Stool, 1991). The tip of the epiglottis is parallel with the upper portion of the body of C1 and in some cases it is in contact with the soft palate (Laitman and Reidenberg, 1997). This arrangement allows the infant to breathe and swallow almost simultaneously, as in some other mammals. The root of the tongue is in the oral cavity but, during the first 4 years of life, the larynx and the root of the tongue descend into the pharynx (most of the descent occurs in infancy). The vocal tract above the larynx is also primitive in development and restricted in resonance variability. The narrowest point of the airway in the neonate is the subglottis within the cricoid ring, whereas in the adult the narrowest point is the glottis itself (Tucker, 1987c). It is estimated that, in about 50% of infants, the epiglottis is omega or U-shaped. At this early stage of life, the hyoid bone and the thyroid cartilage are closely approximated, but they gradually separate as the larynx descends in the vocal tract throughout childhood.

Vocal fold length

There is some difference of opinion concerning the exact length of the vocal folds at birth, but the most notable feature is the minute size of the laryngeal sphincter. Negus (1949) reported that the folds are 3 mm long at 14 days, 5.5 mm at 1 year, 7.5 mm at 5 years, 8.0 mm at 6 years 6 months, and 9.5 mm at 15 years. Hirano, Kurita and Nakashima (1983), in the examination of 88 Japanese infants, calculated that the length of vocal folds in the newborn varied from 2.5 mm to 3.0 mm (Table 5.2). Von Leden (1961) and Hollien (1980) reported that the length of the vocal folds increases about 80% from birth to 12 months of age. Variance in size and weight of infants determines laryngeal size. More than 50% of the glottic opening in the infant is cartilaginous, in contrast to two-thirds of the glottis being bordered by soft tissue in the adult (Tucker, 1987c).

Table 5.2 Vocal fold length

Age	Vocal fold length (mm)	Data source
Neonate	2.5–3.0	Hirano, Kurita and Nakashima (1983)
14 days	3	Negus (1949)
1 year	5.5	Negus (1949)
5 years	7.5	Negus (1949)
6 years 6 months	8	Negus (1949)
9 years	9	Mueller (1997)
Puberty	12–15	Mueller (1997)
Women	12–17	Mueller (1997)
Men	17–23	Mueller (1997)

Vocal fold histology

The fibres of the vocalis muscle are incomplete at birth and develop along-side the thyroarytenoid muscle, which increases considerably in size from the ninth postnatal month. The mucosal cover of the vocal folds is very thick in relation to its length and there is no vocal ligament observable in early infancy. This develops between 1 and 4 years. The intermediate and deep layers of the lamina propria are not differentiated into collagenous and elastic fibres. The thick loose layer of the lamina propria is prone to develop acute oedema which is the cause of croup. Although the airway becomes constricted, total obstruction does not occur because the membranous length is almost the equivalent of the cartilaginous length of the fold (Hirano, 1981; Hirano, Kurita and Nakashima, 1983; Kahane, 1986). Hirano, Kurita and Nakashima (1983) provide an excellent set of histological pictures illustrating the differences in structure of the vocal folds at birth, in the child and in the adult.

LOWER RESPIRATORY TRACT

Structure

Before birth, the lungs are yellowish and solid, tucked away in the back of the chest. Immediately the child is delivered, 'the tissues of the lungs expand like the petals of a flower and the colour changes to rose red' (Thomson, 1976). This is because of the inrush of blood and air into the expanding lung tissues. From the dramatic moment of the birth cry, the infant is launched into automatic life-supporting respiration. The glottis is sphincteric and widens and narrows reflexly in concert with inspiration and expiration (Terracol, Guerrier and Camps, 1956). The pharynx is hypersensitive which ensures instant spasmodic closure of the glottis at the slightest excitation from saliva or milk. This is followed by immediate expulsion by coughing and spluttering accompanied by poorly coordinated inspiratory and expiratory action which, however, proves effective. The diaphragm is the chief muscle involved in respiration in infancy. The ribs are relatively perpendicular to the spine and do not contribute to thoracic movement until the child is able to sit and assume upright posture. The act of crying necessitates changes in respiratory patterns and provides essential preliminary exercise for phonic respiration.

Function

During the first year, control over vegetative respiration gradually develops. The infant acquires the ability to change from quiet breathing to the changed rhythm and volume necessary in vocalisation, in babbling and eventually in speech. Study of respiratory movements can be registered by magnetometry, which tracks the anteroposterior diameter of the rib cage and abdominal wall. Impedance pneumography measures the circumference of the same structures. Such measurements are non-intrusive but accurate, and have revealed that breathing in infants is extremely variable. At 1 month, breaths may be taken at a rate of 87/min and irregularity is not uncommon (Perkins and Kent, 1986). The rate decreases gradually to 61 breaths at 6 months and 42 at 12 months (Langlois, Wilder and Baken, 1975; Langlois, Baken and Wilder, 1980). As the infant grows and the laryngeal airway increases in size, the airflow increases and airway resistance decreases (Netsell et al., 1994).

PHONATION

Infant cries

The voice is used to signal distress and discomfort and to emit cries for help. The first cry at birth is probably the most dramatic use of voice that an individual will ever make. It signals that the infant is alive and respiration has commenced. The primitive nature of the baby's vocal apparatus means that comparison with a musical instrument at this stage is invalid. The sounds emitted encompass a considerable range of frequencies and an amazing volume of sound considering the tiny size of the instrument (Murry, 1980; Raes and Dehaen, 1998). The vocal tract of the newborn is incapable of producing the full range of speech sounds, although the formants of vowels /æ/ and /ʌ/ are apparent in sound spectrographic analysis (Ringel and Kluppel, 1964; Stark, 1978) The formants produced inevitably reflect the characteristics of a vocal tract that, at birth, resembles that of non-human primates more than that of human adults

(Lieberman, 1967). The larynx is elevated in the vocal tract during crying.

The cries of the newborn have been studied extensively with spectrographic and other acoustic analyses. Following a spectrographic and acoustic analysis study of 39 boys and 4 girls (age range 1–30 days) and 87 infants (age range 1–7 months), Wasz-Höckert et al. (1968) classified the cries into four characteristic signals (Table 5.3).

An early study was carried out by Fairbanks (1942) on his son from the age of 1 to 9 months. He recorded the fundamental frequency of hunger wails. At 1 month, the mean fundamental frequency was 373 Hz and subsequently increased to a mean of 814 Hz at 5 months, and then stabilised, to a decreased mean of 640 Hz at 9 months. He attributed the regular and rapid rise in frequency up to 5 months to increased neuromuscular development and not to increasing length of the vocal folds. The plateau was thought to result from conditioning to the speech environment. These data have been confirmed by Siegel (1969) with infants aged 3 months as well as Osgood (1953) and Lenneberg, Rebelsky and Nichols (1965), who also studied vocalisations of infants in their first year.

A study, by Sheppard and Lane (1968), of a male and female for the first 141 days of life showed that the fundamental frequency for the male baby's cry was 443 Hz with a range of 404–481 Hz. The mean for the female baby was 414 Hz with a range of 384–481 Hz. Ostwald (1963) emphasised that the fundamental frequency of a newborn infant's cry may fluctuate from 400 Hz to 600 Hz. Other studies have shown that a pitch range from 300 Hz to 800 Hz is possible. The cries of pain and hunger of the average neonate are produced within a frequency range rising to

Table 5.3 Characteristic cry signals of newborn babies

Cry	Characteristics
Birth	Tense, raucous and short duration of 1.5 seconds or less
Pain	Tense, longest signal of the four cries most reliably identified Max. mean frequency: **740 Hz** Min. mean frequency: **460 Hz** Melody: falling or flat
Hunger	Max. mean frequency: **500 Hz** Min. mean frequency: **320 Hz** Melody: rising–falling
Pleasure	Occurs from 3 months onwards, relaxed, often nasal, no glottal plosives, vocal fry or subharmonic breaks Max. mean frequency: **650 Hz** Min. mean frequency: **360 Hz**

Data source: Wasz-Höckert et al. (1968).

500 Hz (Maddern, Campbell and Stool, 1991) This accounts for the heart-rending and ear-splitting potential of the infant cry. The amplitude of these wails appears not to have engaged the interest of most researchers in the field. Langlois, Baken and Wilder (1980) comment on the fact that scant attention has been paid to the infant's development of respiratory control despite its relevance to the understanding of speech development.

It is generally believed that a mother is able to identify the cause of her baby's crying, whether hunger or pain, by its acoustic quality. However, it has been found that mothers could not identify cry samples correctly according to the cause of the cry. In a review of studies of perceptual identification of cry types, Hollien (1980) concluded that cries actually contain insufficient perceptual information to identify the reason for crying. The cry attracts the mother's attention and is subsequently categorised by environmental clues. Increases in amplitude and duration of wails provide information regarding the degree of distress. However, a mother can identify the voice of her own infant crying. Valanne et al. (1967) examined the ability of mothers to identify the hunger cry of their own newborn infants during the lying-in period. They found that mothers were successful in identifying their own babies from an audiotape recording that included various other infants. Formby (1967) and Murry (1980) reported similar findings. The baby's cry has individual and personal characteristics, as one would expect from the fact that they have different physiognomies.

Vegetative sounds

Infants produce a range of non-crying sounds described as 'vegetative'. These include coughs, burps, hiccups, lip smacking and sucking, spitting, etc., accompanied by ingressive as well as egressive breathing. The study of vegetative sounds is naturally less interesting than that of infant cries. The gradual emergence of 'comfort sounds', as Lewis (1936) described them, as distinct from discomfort cries, is the first step in the acquisition of speech. Vocal play and babbling are an important transitional stage of development leading into the prosodic features of speech.

Prelinguistic tonal development

Lewis (1936), in his classic study of infant speech, distinguished both discomfort and comfort sounds. He stressed the pleasure evinced by the baby in making and experimenting with musical vowel-like sounds, and also the pleasure shared by the mother and her response in encouraging these first elements of vocal communication. At 6 weeks an advanced baby's response to a strange face and voice is negative, but mother's face and voice evoke pleasure. The baby will respond with pleasure to the mother's voice even when she is out of sight. The first smile appears a couple of weeks later and coos, gurgles and little shrieks are produced, especially when the baby is spoken to and caressed (Weisberg, 1963; Stark, 1979; Illingworth, 1980). Mother and responsive childminders reinforce social reactions, especially by talking to the baby, all of which is crucial for normal emotional and speech development. The child therefore needs to be caressed and talked to when handled.

The comfort sounds increase steadily. A healthy sign is the variability and pitch range of the musical glides that are emitted. This tallies with maturation of the vocal folds and improved muscular coordination. Expiration is matched to phonation and control of breath groups subserve vocal expression (Lieberman, 1967). Throughout the developmental sequence cortical and neuromuscular maturation keep pace. Greene and Conway (1963), in collecting material for their audio-recording of infant speech development, evaluated recordings of dozens of infants. They were interested in the earliest appearance of musical sounds, as distinct from crying and scolding noises. The progressive development of inflectional glides in cooing and babbling was noted. The earliest appearance of an upward glide C3 to C# was in a girl aged 2 weeks, and in the same child the range increased from C3 to E3 at 7 weeks. A baby boy ranged from C# to F# in glides of a semitone on one breath at 5 weeks and achieved an inspiratory crow at G4#. This child had varied vowels and diphthongs and varied musical inflection at 16 weeks, rising and falling between C2# and E2. He produced these musical glides up and down the scale within the range of C2# and E2# and as a social response at 18 weeks when rhythmic syllables and babbling were developing rapidly. This child spoke early and was followed up until the age of 2 years. (See Table 5.4 for conversion to hertz.)

Upward glides appeared in these babies first, then rising and falling glides which increased in quantity and range progressively, covering approximately an octave at 6–7 months. The influence of heard speech, described by Piaget (1952) as 'contagion', is obviously strong in this development and is present as early as 1 month of age. The great versatility in vocal behaviour is confirmed by Murry, Hoit Dalgaad and Gracco (1983) in their study of one child's hunger, discomfort and non-distress cries from 2 to 12 weeks of age. They clearly distinguished seven melody types in each of the three categories of vocalisation. The rapid shifts and wide frequency range reflected increasing respiratory and phonatory control, exhibiting early communication behaviour. The emergence of cooing was studied by Stark (1978), and features of infant vocalisation by Stark, Rose and McLagan (1975), in the first 8 weeks of life.

Table 5.4 Fo to musical note conversion

Musical note	Frequency (in hertz) for octaves							
	C_{-3}	C_{-2}	C_{-1}	C_0	C_1	C_2	C_3	C_4
C	16.35	32.70	65.41	130.81	261.63	523.25	1046.50	2093.00
C# and Db	17.32	34.65	69.30	138.59	277.18	554.37	1108.73	2217.46
D	18.35	36.71	73.42	146.83	293.66	587.33	1174.66	2349.32
D# and Eb	19.45	38.89	77.78	155.56	311.13	622.25	1244.51	2489.02
E	20.60	41.20	82.41	164.81	329.63	659.26	1318.51	2637.02
F	21.83	43.65	87.31	174.61	349.23	698.46	1396.91	2793.83
F# and Gb	23.12	46.25	92.50	185.00	369.99	739.99	1479.98	2959.96
G# and Ab	25.96	51.91	103.83	207.65	415.30	830.61	1661.22	3322.44
A	27.50	55.00	110.00	220.00	440.00	880.00	1760.00	3520.00
A# and Bb	29.14	58.27	116.54	233.08	466.16	932.33	1864.66	3729.31
B	30.87	61.74	123.47	246.96	493.88	987.77	1975.53	3951.07

After Baken, 1987.

Pathological and diagnostic factors

An abnormal cry in the newborn is an important diagnostic sign because the crying of healthy and sick infants differs (Karelitz and Fisichelli, 1962; Michelsson, Raes and Rinne, 1984).The cry can reflect neurological, respiratory and certain structural abnormalities. Cries will also differ in full-term and pre-term infants; the differences are more marked the more pre-term the baby. In particular, the pre-term baby has a cry of much higher pitch. Early cries in infants with neurological disorders have been studied extensively because the cries of these babies are particularly different, with considerably higher pitch and a different melody type. Results of studies by Michelsson et al. (1982) have shown that infants with central nervous system disturbances have increased maximum and minimum frequencies compared with healthy babies. It is also significant that, in these babies, rising and fall–rising melody patterns are more common, as are unstable vocal signals. In babies with kernicterus, it is well known that the level of serum bilirubin does not always reflect the presence or absence of neurological damage, but acoustic analysis of the babies' cries can be a useful indicator. Down's syndrome babies have characteristic cries and the cri-du-chat of the chromosome 5 deficiency is unmistakable (Michelsson and Wasz-Höckert, 1980). The diagnosis of cri-du-chat syndrome can be made in newborn babies on the basis of a combination of low birthweight, craniofacial abnormality and the characteristic high-pitched cry, the frequency of which is one or two octaves above the cry of a normal baby. On acoustic analysis, it has some of the properties of the cry of young cats (Niebuhr, 1978; Romano et al., 1991).

There is also evidence that the cry of the baby at risk from sudden infant death syndrome (SIDS) has acoustic characteristics that could help to identify the vulnerable infant. Stark and Nathanson (1975) found that, in addition to these cries exhibiting higher fundamental frequency levels than normal, there was evidence of sudden shifts or breaks in pitch level and voiced inspiratory sounds. Their acoustic studies showed more instances of vocal tract constriction and this was thought to result from the back of the tongue touching the soft palate and therefore obstructing the airway intermittently. Laitman and Reidenberg (1997) have suggested that the occurrence of SIDS may be related to the subtle changes in laryngeal position and central and peripheral neuromotor control of the larynx during the first year of life. Studies by Steinschneider (1972) and Steinschneider and Rabuzzi (1976) concluded that SIDS infants have a high degree of respiratory instability and that the unusual features of the cry may be another sign of poor respiratory control. Pre-term infants have incoordinated muscular activity, especially during sleep. The thoracic muscles may try to inspire while abdominal muscles expire (West, 1979).

The reviews by Colton and Steinschneider (1980) and Michelsson and Wasz-Höckert (1980) of cry analysis in early infancy are recommended for further study. Michelsson, Raes and Rinne (1984) have also used a cry score as an aid in infant diagnoses.

Predictions of speech and language development

Greene and Conway (1963) also observed several male children whose vocalisations were limited in pitch range and duration, and whose speech development was delayed. Clinicians have, in these inflectional melodies, indicators of delayed or normal speech development. Absence of pre-linguistic vocalisation may, however, signify general developmental delay, socioeconomic deprivation or neglect, in which the child is not encouraged with loving speech and attention (Winitz, 1969).

Between 3 and 6 months, babbling of syllables develops. This is common to all races and is a biologically determined human trend. Wasz-Höckert et al. (1968) found no difference between Swedish and Finnish babies. Deaf babies babble in the same way as hearing children, but this soon dies away without the stimulation of heard speech. Between 6 and 12 months, vocalisation begins to assume the characteristics of communicative speech. The child is said to be 'talking scribble' or jargon, and the inflections of speech are so real and well organised by rhythm, intonation and breath group that 'pretend' conversations can be held, i.e. they are pretend for the adult but so animated that they must be real for the child, in that the intention to convey meaning is there. This is the origin of prosody

which precedes words and provides whole tonal patterns into which seg-
mented features will come to be fitted during the second year. The 'first
word' becomes stable and identifiable at 12–14 months. The linguistic, segmental and grammatical stage of speech has begun (Crystal, 1976).

Childhood

UPPER RESPIRATORY TRACT

From 4 years until puberty, the dimensions of the entire vocal tract are
increasing in conjunction with improving neuromuscular coordination.
The larynx of the 2-year-old child is at the level of the mid-portion of C5,
and it continues to descend relatively rapidly until it is at the level of C6 at
the age of 5 years. It does not reach its adult position with the lower border
of the cricoid cartilage at the level of the C6–C7 vertebral disc until the
individual is aged 15 years (Maddern, Campbell and Stool, 1991).

LOWER RESPIRATORY TRACT

Throughout childhood, there are developmental changes in the respiratory
system and breathing for speech differs significantly from adults' speech
breathing patterns. Four-year-old children, for example, exert far more
expiratory effort in speech breathing than adults, and 7 year olds use relatively higher lung volumes to initiate vocal fold vibration than older children and adults (Netsell et al., 1994). Before puberty, lung function is
almost identical in boys and girls of equal size. Boys' chests, however, grow
in lateral and longitudinal dimensions more than those of girls. It is interesting to note that a low level of activity in childhood affects the size of the
lungs. Cotes (1979) found that children living in high blocks of flats, where
the opportunity for exercise was limited, had 7% less vital capacity than
physically active children. This is a factor that must not be overlooked in
measurements of airflow and phonation time in children.

PHONATION

The fundamental frequency continues to decrease with age as the larynx
enlarges and the vocal folds increase in mass (Robb and Saxman, 1985).
By 5 years, the child's speaking voice settles at a median pitch in the region
of middle C, or maybe two or three semitones higher. The child's singing
range varies very little between boys and girls at the age of 7 years
(Tarneaud, 1961). At 8 years, the lower range is only slightly extended and
by 9 years the range extends a little further in both directions from B2 to
D4. The range of voice in both girls and boys is similar despite the vocal
folds of boys being 8% larger (Cotes, 1979). In brief, the voice range for

both sexes remains constant at about two and a half octaves between 6 and 16 years (Aronson, 1980).

Adolescence

UPPER RESPIRATORY TRACT

Laryngeal skeleton changes

At the onset of puberty and during the period from 10 to 14 years, there is a dramatic period of general growth associated with increased secretion of androgens in the male and oestrogens in the female. As the hormonal changes take place, male and female secondary sexual characteristics emerge. The mutational period may be complete at 14 years in boys, but in girls it continues on average until 15 years. The dimensions of the vocal tract reflect this period of growth and differences between males and females. Laryngeal dimensions in the male are generally larger and the thyroid cartilage changes its configuration. Until puberty, the angle of the thyroid cartilage is 120° in both males and females. During pubertal change in the male, the thyroid cartilage enlarges significantly and the angle decreases to 90°, giving rise to the marked thyroid prominence known as the Adam's apple (Figure 5.1).

Vocal fold length

The increased size of the laryngeal skeleton is reflected in the length of the vocal folds. In girls, the mean length of the vocal folds is 15 mm before puberty and this may increase to 17 mm in a contralto. During the mutational period, a boy's vocal folds double in length and may increase to a maximum

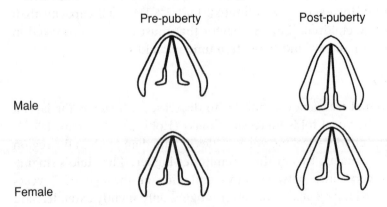

Pre-puberty   Post-puberty

Male

Female

Figure 5.1 Laryngeal changes at puberty. Transverse section of the larynx. Note the internal angle of the thyroid cartilage which changes at puberty from 120° to 90° in the male as the vocal folds double in length.

of 23 mm in the bass voice. The normal minimum vocal fold length for the male is 17 mm, so it can be seen that a tenor and a contralto may have much the same pitch range, but it is the larger resonators of the larynx, pharynx and the chest that distinguish the male from the female voice.

Vocal fold histology

The layer structure of the lamina propria of the vocal fold continues to mature in adolescence and it is not until 16 years that it resembles the structure of the adult vocal fold. Before this, the layers are less well defined. This change in the inner structure of the vocal fold mucosa is a significant factor in voice mutation, besides the increase in length of the vocal folds.

LOWER RESPIRATORY TRACT

The young adult has approximately four times the lung volume of the 5 year old. Vital capacity is at its peak during the late teens and early 20s, after which it gradually deteriorates with reduced diaphragmatic action. Breathing rate at rest is between 10 and 22 breaths/min (Perkins and Kent, 1986).

PHONATION

Speaking fundamental frequency

As the vocal folds double in length in the male, the voice drops an octave whereas girls' voices mature gradually as a result of the less dramatic enlargement of the larynx, consistent with general body growth. Voice mutation and vocal pitch are associated with the growth of the larynx and lengthening of the vocal folds (Figure 5.2). It is possible, however, that the dramatically lowered speaking fundamental frequency in the male does not result entirely from the lengthening of the vocal folds, but also reflects changes in their mass and the developing differentiation of the histological layers (Harries et al., 1998). McGlone and Hollien (1963) found that a girl's vocal pitch is at its highest at 7–8 years, drops 2.4 semitones between 11 and 15 years, and remains at much the same level throughout life. Michel, Hollien and Moore (1966) recorded the speaking fundamental pitch of 15-, 16- and 17-year-old girls and found that this was 207 Hz. This indicates that fundamental frequency is established at 15 years in girls when pubertal mutation is over, although body growth continues up to 20 years of age and beyond.

Vocal shifts and breaks

The pitch breaks that occur in children's voices over the age of 7 years have received much attention on account of the need to understand and manage

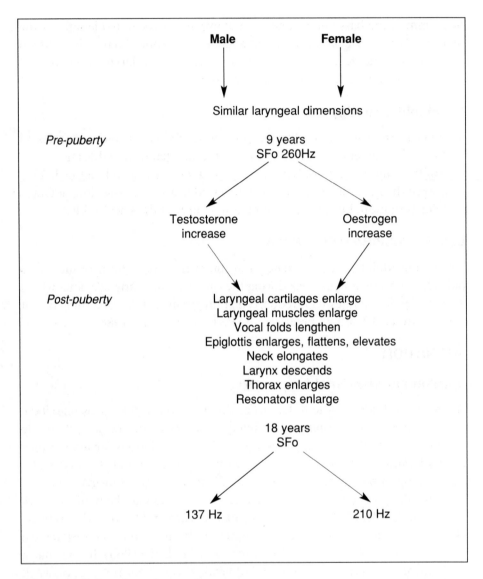

Figure 5.2 Pubertal vocal tract changes.

the voice mutation difficulties of adolescence in singing. Weiss (1950), in his comprehensive survey of the literature, cited 334 sources. We are also indebted to him for his clarification of the problems involved. Weiss defined 'break of voice' as a sudden and involuntary change in the pitch and quality. 'Voice break' should therefore be properly confined to the characteristic fluctuations in pitch and quality in adolescence during the period of voice mutation. The voice may rise or fall an octave, rising to falsetto or falling to the bass notes. The voice 'breaks' analysed in the work of American workers described below refer either to the mutational period of voice break in adolescence or to 'shifts' in pitch during childhood. These shifts consist of abrupt and uncontrolled rises and falls in vocal pitch resulting from poor coordination of the laryngeal musculature, associated with general bodily growth. In prepubertal boys, these shifts do not have the masculine quality that is so conspicuous and bizarre a feature of the real break of voice in adolescence. The young boy's resonator system naturally cannot produce the necessary resonance characteristics of the adult male voice.

Vocal shifts appear to be a normal physiological feature of juvenile laryngeal function. These shifts may also be aggravated by vocal strain imposed by vocal abuse in children who shout and scream at football matches and in the playground. Vocal shifts and subharmonic breaks were recorded in infants by Wasz-Höckert et al. (1968). Fairbanks, Wiley and Lassman (1949) studied the voice breaks in voices of 7- and 8-year-old boys and girls. They concluded that the pitch changes recorded occurred as frequently in girls as in boys and were not sex linked or confined to adolescence.

Luchsinger (1962) stated that the real voice 'break' or 'stormy' mutation occurring in male adolescence is not the general rule and is encountered in only a minority of boys as a result of vocal or psychogenic strain. Weiss (1950) suggested that the sudden drop or rise in the voice, changing momentarily from the childish treble to the adult male voice or vice versa, is so conspicuous that it has accordingly been considered the main characteristic of the pubertal voice change, whereas it is actually uncharacteristic.

Singing in adolescence

In his book *The Voice of the Boy* (1919), Dawson attributed pitch breaks to collapse of the voice caused by misuse and vocal strain. None of his pupils suffered from 'breaking' of the speaking or singing voice. The boys' voices just slid down the scale. He evaluated the pitch of their singing voices at frequent intervals and shifted them after 12.5 years from soprano to alto, and gradually to tenor or baritone by 15 years as their voices dropped with growth of the larynx. He attributed failure to sing well to vocal abuse in early childhood and advocated early training in breathing technique. Most experts stress the dangers for both boys and girls of singing in the mutation period and will not permit serious voice training to begin until 17 years with girls and 18–19 years with boys. Weiss pointed out that very few choirboys, possibly a mere 2%, ever turn into good adult singers and this he attributed to the irreparable damage that had occurred in adolescence. Some singing teachers and choirmasters have little knowledge of the anatomy and physiology of the vocal tract, do not instruct their pupils in the fundamentals of good voice production and fail to appreciate the dangers of the pubertal period.

The mutational period of the singing voice lasts much longer than that of the speaking voice and this also is not often understood and recognised. Growth in height may continue long after the voice has 'broken', and during this time the voice is vulnerable and cannot achieve its adult potential on account of physiological immaturity.

Female hormonal changes

Women are subject to variations in their levels of sex hormones from the onset of menstruation (the menarche) at puberty and during the menstrual cycle and pregnancy. The human larynx is a hormonal 'target organ' (Abitbol et al., 1989) and oestrogen target cells have been identified in the epithelium of the vocal folds (Fergusson, Hudson and McCarty, 1987). These oestrogen receptor sites on the membranes of the epithelial cells are proteins that bind with specific hormones in the fluid component of the cell. It is suggested that a decrease in oestrogen levels causes water retention, oedema and venous dilatation of vocal fold tissue, which result in increased vocal fold mass. There are indications that these variations are reflected in the voice and that finally the menopause triggers more permanent vocal changes (Figure 5.3).

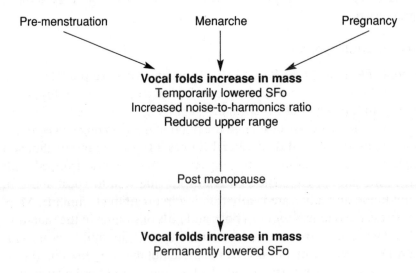

Figure 5.3 Female hormone-related voice changes.

Premenstrual changes

Most of the reports of premenstrual vocal changes are anecdotal and in many cases the hormonal fluctuations produce only subtle effects that might be noticed only by a professional voice user, such as a singer or actor. Although indications of an increase in vocal fold mass suggest that changes in pitch might be the chief problem, a study by Hirson and Roe (1993) concluded that changes in jitter and shimmer measures and harmonics-to-noise ratio were significant, although there were no significant changes in frequency throughout the menstrual cycle. Professional singers, however, report a range of vocal changes related to the premenstrual phase of the cycle. These predominantly refer to problems of pitch range, vocal note quality and more general unpredictability of vocal function (Davis and Davis, 1993).

Menopausal changes

The menopause signifies permanent cessation of the menstrual cycle as ovarian activity ceases. As production of the female hormones oestradiol and progesterone decline to imperceptible levels, the ovary starts to secrete androgens (male hormones) in addition to the androgens being produced by the adrenal glands. This relative increase in androgens in the post-menopausal woman leads to increased mass of the vocal folds and the typical lowering of speaking fundamental frequency. It is difficult to distinguish between the effects of the menopause on the voice and general age-related changes, although there is some indication that more women than men experience vocal change around the age of 50 years (Boulet and Oddens, 1996). General effects of the menopause include connective tissue changes throughout the body which result in osteoporosis, reduced skin thickness and reduced collagen content, all of which will be reflected in the laryngeal tissues. The advent and more widespread use of hormone replacement therapy (HRT) for peri- and postmenopausal women has raised the possibility of limiting some of the undesirable changes occurring at the menopause, including those apparent in the voice. Very little research has been done in this area. Although it might be logical to presume that HRT would benefit the voice (Emerich, Hoover and Sataloff, 1996), problems appear to arise in prescription of the oestrogen/progesterone ratio. It is known that oestrogen stimulation results in thickening of the superficial epithelium of the vocal folds and progesterone causes changes in the intermediate layer of the lamina propria. Voice changes appear to be associated with this hormone balance and there is anecdotal evidence that some women who are taking HRT are aware of adverse vocal symptoms as they change from the oestrogen to the progesterone element of the prescription. It should also be remembered that the menopause, apart from its physical effects, is a major change in a woman's life that frequently occurs as her children leave home. The significance of this time of her life and the associated emotions can also affect vocal behaviour.

The adult: degenerative changes

Age-related changes are exhibited throughout the body and result in change or loss of function. They are not manifestations of disease, but there is an increased susceptibility to pathological changes as a result of these normal degenerative processes. The timing and extent of these changes vary significantly from one individual to another, but as they occur they will inevitably affect the vocal tract. In most individuals the major changes occur in the sixth and seventh decades. The body systems affected by age-related changes are listed in Table 5.5. These changes inevitably affect the anatomy and physiology of phonation.

Age-related anatomical and physiological changes are reflected in the vocal tract, its supporting systems and vocal function.

UPPER RESPIRATORY TRACT

Laryngeal cartilages

The cartilages of the larynx may begin to ossify and lose their elasticity after the age of 25 years, although this is not necessarily the case. Zenker

Table 5.5 Body systems reflecting age-related changes

Body system	Age-related changes
Muscular	Muscle atrophy
Neurological	Neurons atrophy Nerve conduction slows Neurotransmitter deficiencies occur
Skeletal	Cartilages ossify so that structures that have had some flexibility may become rigid and acquire the rigidity of bone Bone is resorbed so that bone mass is reduced and skeletal shrinkage occurs
Cardiovascular	Poor circulation may result in breathlessness and a general reduction in vigour
Respiratory	Muscular, skeletal and tissue changes result in reduced expendable volume of air
Hormonal	Androgens and oestrogens affect vocal tract development, structure and function throughout the lifespan

(1964) reported that the thyroid cartilage may still be elastic at the age of 70 years, yet be rigid in much younger individuals. In Kahane's study (1983) of excised larynges, the laryngeal cartilages showed signs of ossification from the third decade in men, from 25 years onwards, and from the fourth decade in women. Pantoja (1968) examined the cartilages of 100 normal adults. He found that ossification in the thyroid cartilage begins in the inferior horns and progresses along the inferior and posterior borders, and then along the anterior border and angle. He confirmed that calcification is not constant and may be absent even in the oldest patients. It is generally agreed that female laryngeal cartilages change more slowly, and that these changes progress less far, than in males (Kahane, 1983). There is some evidence that changes in the articular surfaces of the arytenoid and cricoid cartilages interfere with smooth arytenoid movement and that the ligament of the joint capsule can loosen with advancing age (Kahane, 1987). This contributes to less efficient vocal fold approximation and reduced glottic efficiency.

Vocal fold histology

Ageing results in atrophy of the laryngeal muscles and changes in the laryngeal mucosa. Luchsinger (1962) described the false folds as narrower and the true vocal folds as more visible on laryngeal examination of the elderly larynx, so that the opening into the laryngeal ventricle appears very wide. As a result of extrinsic laryngeal muscle changes, the speed and extent of the vertical laryngeal excursions during swallowing and phonation are reduced (Sonies, 1992). The efficiency of vocal fold adduction and abduction is affected by the degeneration of the intrinsic muscles. Atrophy of the vocalis muscle not only reduces vocal fold tonicity, but also compromises its control of the shape of the vocal fold. These changes contribute to less effective vocal fold abduction and adduction, and consequently to reduced efficiency of the laryngeal valve.

The vocal folds are visibly less tense and may exhibit bowing. The mucous membrane can be reddish or show yellow or brownish pigmentation. Honjo and Isshiki (1980) studied a number of individuals, of mean age 75 years, and attributed changes in colour of the vocal folds to fat degeneration or keratosis of the mucous membrane. The age changes differed significantly between men and women. Vocal fold atrophy and glottic gap were frequently seen in aged men, whereas in women oedema of the vocal folds was a predominant characteristic. The changes in the male vocal folds were judged to be the result of senescent change of muscle and mucous membrane. It was suggested that hormonal imbalance during the menopause may account for the injected appearance of the female vocal folds. Changes in mass of the vocal folds has been described by many writers (Honjo and Isshiki, 1980; Mueller,

Sweeney and Baribeau, 1985). In women, vocal fold mass tends to increase as the tissue becomes oedematous because of the reduced oestrogens and relative increase in androgens after the menopause. In contrast, there is a tendency for vocal fold mass to be reduced in men as the result of vocalis muscle atrophy. The changes in each layer of the vocal fold mucosa inevitably affect its vibratory characteristics. In less vigorous individuals, the vocalis muscle no longer provides the firm 'body' of the vocal fold, but has a tendency to vibrate chaotically as it becomes atrophic. In addition, each layer of the 'cover' of the vocal fold is changing (Table 5.6) and vibrating differently.

Table 5.6 Vocal fold histological changes in the ageing larynx in men and women

Vocal fold	Male	Female
Membranous vocal fold	Shortens markedly	Slight shortening
Mucosa	May become pigmented	May become pigmented
Vocal fold cover	Slight thickening	Thickens
Superficial layer of lamina propria (Reinke's space)	Oedema	Oedema
Intermediate layer of lamina propria (elastic fibres)	Thins – fibres atrophy and become less dense	No significant change
Deep layer (collagen fibres)	Thickens – fibres become more dense and fibrotic	No significant change

After Hirano, Kurita and Sakaguchi (1989) see page 28 for description of vocal fold histology

Supraglottic vocal tract changes

Superficial tissue in the mouth, nose and pharynx tends to become thinner and drier with advancing age. The epithelium in the oral cavity thins and there is a reduction in water content and in collagen fibres in the mucosa lining these structures (Close and Woodson, 1989). Reduced saliva production, together with changes in the laryngeal glands that lubricate the vocal folds, lead to general dryness of the vocal tract. This is further compounded by a degree of nasal obstruction, caused by changes in the nasal cartilages, resulting in a tendency for some elderly people to mouth breathe. Vibratory function of the vocal folds is inevitably affected as tissues become drier. As the bone of the mandible undergoes resorption and shrinks, oral cavity dimensions are reduced. Skeletal changes in the cervical spine similarly affect the dimensions of the oral pharynx and hypopharynx. The head tends to be thrust into a forward position so that the size, shape and dimensions of the pharyngeal resonator are altered.

Ageing also reduces the sensitivity of both the oral and pharyngeal cavities (Caruso and Max, 1997), with laryngopharyngeal sensory reduction possibly contributing to aspiration and dysphagia in some elderly individuals (Sonies, 1992; Aviv, 1997).

LOWER RESPIRATORY TRACT

Structure

Respiratory function deteriorates with increasing age because of tissue changes. These changes are more marked in men than in women and result in gradual reduction in strength of the respiratory muscles. Reduction in the mobility of the thoracic cage also occurs due to stiffness of the costovertebral joints. In advanced age, the lungs and bronchi shrink and sink to a lower position in the thorax. The sensitivity of the airway is reduced with increasing age and coughing is less likely to occur (Slonim and Hamilton, 1976). Changes vary greatly with different individuals and their lifestyles. Physical activity will prevent noticeable deterioration in respiration whereas exposure to pollutants, especially smoking, reduces the elastic recoil of the lungs. The correlation between smoking and carcinoma of the lungs is generally acknowledged, but its effect on the airway before appearance of disease is relevant when considering phonation. Cotes (1979) notes the substances in cigarette smoke and their effects on the body. Particles in the smoke cause irritation and the tar deposit damages the bronchial epithelium and contributes ultimately to emphysema. Oxygenation of the blood is impaired by carbon monoxide whereas nicotine increases cardiac frequency and systemic blood pressure. Inhalation of tobacco smoke results in an immediate rise in airway resistance, because of the smoke particles that are being deposited, and the adverse effects last many hours. If the smoker has a frequent, forceful cough the vocal folds will be abused. Comparable effects are thought to occur in the passive smoker.

Function

By the age of 75 years, respiratory efficiency is half that of a 30 year old. The residual volume (the air remaining in the lungs after maximal expiration) increases with age so that, whereas it is 1.5 litres at 20 years of age, it is 2.2 litres at 60 years. Consequently, the older individual has less expendable volume of air for all tasks, including phonation. In his review of age-related changes in respiration, Orlikoff (1994) notes that there is a tendency for elderly men to take a greater number of between-sentence breaths and a greater breath pause time than younger adult males. Similar patterns are observed in elderly women. In addition, older women typically tend to inhale to a higher lung volume and use greater exhalatory volumes during speech than younger women. Older women also tend to lose a greater volume of egressive air before initiating phonation and during non-inhalatory pauses. This might reflect the reduced efficiency of laryngeal valving and a reduced ability to maintain rib-cage elevation.

PHONATION

The ageing voice

The physical changes associated with physiological ageing naturally contribute to changes in the acoustic characteristics of voice (Ramig and Ringel, 1983; Ringel and Chodzko-Zajko, 1987a) and in general to less efficient phonation. A vocal stereotype is exemplified by some actors in the role of elderly characters, especially in men. Shakespeare describes the sixth stage of man with the shrunken shank and the big manly voice turning towards 'childish treble', which 'pipes and whistles in his sound' (Shakespeare's *As You Like it*). Perceptual terms used to describe the elderly voice include 'shaky', 'squeaky', 'weak' and 'hoarse,' but these terms do not apply to the voices of all elderly people (Sapienza and Dutka, 1996). There is considerable variation from one person to another, but with improved health and longevity vocal deterioration is greatly delayed. Physiological age can be unrelated to chronological age, the reality being that 'you are as old as you are' and the vigour experienced in the prime of life may be extended into the 70s and even the 80s. Women, however, have the advantage over men and tend to remain younger and live longer. In most cases, only subtle vocal changes are apparent and these are most obvious when maximum vocal performance, such as singing, is attempted.

Close and Woodson (1989) conclude that vocal changes in the elderly fall into three categories:

- Some changes are caused by the ageing process alone which affects the larynx, the related structures and the controlling systems.
- Others are secondary to an increased tendency to disease. The voice of the individual in poor physical condition is perceptually and measurably 'older' than that of the fit person. In disease, dysphonia signals and contributes to underlying conditions such as pulmonary disease or neuropathology.
- Some are the result of compensatory behaviours that occur as vocal effectiveness decreases. Attempts to increase vocal loudness and maintain a former habitual pitch can result in hyperfunctional phonation which amounts to vocal misuse.

The degree of deterioration of the voice is less noticeable in people who have naturally well-produced voices, and especially in professionals with training in voice production who know how to breathe, project and resonate the voice and maintain good posture. The British actress Dame Sybil Thorndike, when over 80 years of age, still had a fine acting voice, of a rich and mature quality belying her age. Martinelli, the Italian tenor, was singing and recording at the age of 76 years at the Metropolitan Opera House and sang the part of Turandot aged 82 years. Amado (1953) reported that several other male singers have preserved their voices at concert level over the age of 70 years; he named Malfia Battistini and Leon Melchissedec, but no female singers of comparable age. More recently, one can cite the case of Salvation Army Commissioner, Catherine Bramwell-Booth, who, at the age of 100 years, had an extraordinarily youthful and delightful voice. Nevertheless, it has been found that listener judgement can detect age changes in the voice and speech of the ordinary elderly person (Ptacek et al., 1966; Shipp and Hollien, 1969; Debruyne and Decoster, 1999). Judgement is not entirely related to vocal clues but to various other features of delivery. Ptacek et al.'s study involved 72 healthy subjects, none of whom had a hearing loss greater than 35 dB. The 10 listener judges were student graduates in speech pathology. They were told only the sex of each subject and had to judge whether the recorded samples of voice and speech were from people under 35 years or over 60 years. Each subject had recorded a prolonged vowel (4 seconds) and Fairbank's 'Rainbow Passage' (played forwards and backwards). There was correct age recognition judgement at a 75% mean for the vowel, an 87% mean for the 'reverse' reading and a 99% mean for the 'forward' reading. The judges listed phrasing, speed, hesitancy, voice breaks and vitality as being the features that had indicated vocal age to them and that had influenced their judgement. This study showed that even inexperienced listeners can identify the aged voice and that correct listener judgement increases with the advancing age of the speakers. The elderly voice is recognised by the features listed in Table 5.7.

Elderly people complain of reduced control over their phonation, changes in speaking fundamental frequency, reduced pitch range and deterioration of vocal quality (Mueller, 1978), whereas studies show that loudness, resonance and timing are also affected. The term 'presbyphonia' is used to refer to a voice that shows marked deterioration of functional and acoustic properties associated with ageing, in the absence of any other pathology. Presbyphonia is the result of **presbylaryngis**, a larynx that exhibits significant signs of ageing (see Chapter 16).

Table 5.7 Perceptual acoustic characteristics of the normal elderly voice

- Altered pitch
- Roughness
- Breathiness
- Weakness
- Hoarseness
- Tremulousness/instability

Pitch changes

The literature concerning pitch changes from adult life to old age is extensive but not in total agreement (Table 5.8 and Figure 5.4). Mysak (1959b) and Mysak and Hanley (1959), in their studies of men, found that voice pitch falls in middle age from that of early adulthood but thereafter rises with increasing age. In middle age, the fundamental pitch was 110 Hz but it had risen to 124.9 Hz in the 65- to 79-year-old group and to 142.6 Hz in the 80- to 92-year-old group. In another study of pitch in men by Hollien and Shipp (1972), similar results were described. The mean frequency level was found to fall progressively to age 40 years; there was a progressive rise from 60 to 80 years. The elderly women studied by McGlone and Hollien (1963) also exhibited raised pitch with increasing age with a mean fundamental pitch of 196.6 Hz in the 65- to 79-year-old group and a mean fundamental pitch of 199.8 Hz in the 80- to 94-year-old group. The reduction of pitch range occurs in singing before speaking whereas measures of pitch perturbation (jitter) are increased. At all ages, measures of jitter are

Table 5.8 Age-related changes in speaking fundamental frequency

Age (years)	Mean SFo	
	Males	Females
20–29	120	224
30–39	112	213
40–49	107	221
50–59	118	199
60–69	112	199
70–79	132	202
80–89	146	

Data sources:
Males: Shipp and Hollien (1969); Hollien and Shipp (1972).
Females: Stoicheff (1981).

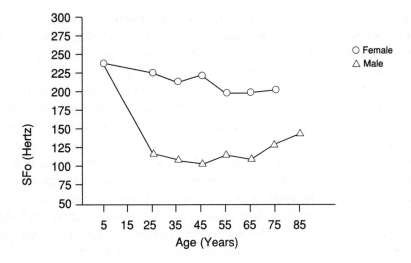

Figure 5.4 Differential trends in male and female age-related SFo changes.

higher in those who are in poor physical condition, but they are particularly increased in those of advanced age.

Honjo and Isshiki (1980) found that, as expected, the differences in vocal characteristics in elderly men and women reflect the differences that they found in the vocal folds. As a result of vocal fold atrophy, elderly men tend to have a higher fundamental frequency than younger men. In contrast, aged women frequently have a lower fundamental frequency and more restricted pitch range than young women because of vocal fold oedema.

Vocal amplitude

The reduction of expiratory volume in combination with reduced glottal efficiency adversely affect the speaker's ability to increase subglottic air pressure and so to increase vocal loudness. It has also been found that shimmer (amplitude perturbation) is significantly higher in elderly people than in younger individuals (Ringel and Chodzko-Zajko, 1987b).Vocal loudness might also appear to be reduced as resonance of the fundamental vocal note is less effective because of the changed dimensions of the oral cavity and oropharynx. On the other hand, an increase in the loudness of speech was observed by Greene (1982) and attributed to hearing loss. Ryan (1972), studying the acoustic aspects of the ageing voice, draws attention to the fact that all the sensorimotor processes slowly deteriorate and adversely affect articulation and the resonance of the voice. Hearing loss is of great significance in control of vocal volume and those who are hard of hearing need to raise the voice to hear themselves, especially against background noise. Schow and Nerbonne (1981) tested the hearing of 202 elderly residents of a nursing home with an age range 65–98 years. There was evident progressive deterioration in hearing, especially for high frequencies. This was predictable, whereas the discovery that hearing deteriorated more seriously in men than in women was rather unexpected, but is consistent with the pattern of earlier ageing in men. Deafness in old age is one of the most common threats to psychosocial communication. Wearing a hearing aid and instruction in lip-reading is often rejected but, by tactful handling from relatives and help from a speech–language pathologist, the voice can be maintained. Vision is another factor in controlling vocal volume; poor sight renders it difficult to judge the distance between speaker and listener. The voice may be deliberately reduced in intensity when not wishing a tête-à-tête to be overheard, as may be the case in hospital or residential home (Greene, 1982). Takano-Stone (1987) recommended various psychosocial remedies for the sensorially disabled.

Vocal quality

The elderly voice tends to be rougher and more breathy than that of a younger person, with a reduced harmonics-to-noise ratio. These features reflect the flaccidity of the vocal folds and incomplete glottic closure, which result in aperiodicity and turbulent air.

Timing deficiencies (Table 5.9)

Some of the changes occurring in phonation in elderly people are related to the fact that they tend to perform complex tasks more slowly than younger people (Oyer and Deal, 1985). This results partly from an increase in reaction time, but also because muscle strength declines with age. The effects of these changes are also seen in the swallowing patterns of older people (Ekberg and Feinberg, 1990). The following timing deficiencies (Table 5.9)

Table 5.9 Possible timing deficiencies in the elderly voice

- Reduced maximum phonation time (smaller lung volume; higher phonatory flow rate)
- Reduced voiceless interval/poor devoicing of voiceless phonemes (slow vocal fold abduction)
- Variable voice-onset time (VOT) (slow/poorly coordinated vocal fold adduction and expiratory airflow)
- Impaired phonation/articulation coordination (slowed diadochokinesis)

After Oyer and Deal (1985).

can occur with advancing age, but they will be most pronounced in the frail elderly individual:

- The length of time for which a vocal note can be sustained is reduced because of a smaller available volume of air and a tendency for air leakage via the glottis. Initially, this is most obvious in singing when duration of a note cannot be sustained. In advanced old age, difficulties of maintaining phonation after one air intake, and the need for more frequent breath intakes, cause reduced phrase length and can affect prosody.

- The duration of voiceless intervals, which normally occur fleetingly in spontaneous speech, tends to be reduced because of inefficient vocal fold abduction. If abduction is insufficiently extensive, rapid and well coordinated with articulation, voiceless phonemes and pauses are not effectively devoiced.

- In the frail elderly person, there is an increased latency period between beginning to initiate phonation and the actual production of the voice. This is the result of the combined effects of the various physiological changes. Similar features are seen in various physical tasks and it is interesting to note that the age differences for central processing rates appear to be less for vocal responses than for manual responses (Baron and Journey, 1989).

- With increased age, the ability to repeat an articulatory task rapidly (diadochokinetic rate) declines. Laryngeal diadochokinesis is slowed in many older individuals and can affect the ability to coordinate phonation accurately with articulation in rapid speech.

As adequate communication is of vital importance in maintaining social contacts as physical possibilities diminish, preservation of voice must not be overlooked in therapy, which principally concentrates on the linguistic failures of old age. A well-preserved voice helps maintain self-respect and self-image. At a time when so much attention is paid to hair replacement, cosmetic surgery, cosmetics and dress by both men and women in the fight against old age, preservation of the voice and its prosodic and paralinguistic features is essential. As Takano-Stone (1987) says:

> The goal of care is to assist the older person to achieve the highest level of functioning and to live the remaining years in a meaningful, satisfying manner

as defined by the individual. Families need support and advice on how to care for elderly relatives. The advice provided by Skinner and Vaughan

(1983) in their excellent practical book, *Enjoy Old Age*, is a strongly recommended guide to self-management.

Summary

■ The structure and function of the vocal tract and its support systems change throughout life.

■ Full development of the vocal tract is not established until the end of the second decade.

■ All parameters of the vocal profile can be affected by the degenerative changes of old age.

■ The effects of increasing age on the vocal tract can often be delayed and reduced by appropriate vocal hygiene and good vocal health.

Part II
Voice Pathology

Voice disorders: presentation and classification

Voice disorders range from complete absence of the voice (aphonia) to varying degrees of vocal impairment (dysphonia). Abnormalities can involve one or more of the vocal parameters: habitual pitch, pitch range, loudness, vocal note quality, resonance, flexibility and stamina. As a result, disordered voices can range from being functionally ineffective through varying degrees of inefficiency to being merely aesthetically unpleasing in their least severe form. Whatever the underlying aetiology, these vocal changes are the manifestation of disordered laryngeal, respiratory and vocal tract function, which might reflect structural, neurological, psychological and behavioural problems as well as systemic conditions. Most voice disorders can be acquired from infancy throughout the lifespan, although a small proportion are congenital because of fetal abnormalities of the vocal tract or related systems.

Acoustic features

PRIMARY PHONATORY FEATURES

The primary acoustic features of a voice disorder are those that are the direct result of the initial disordered function of the vocal tract. If the vocal folds are inadequately adducted during phonation, for example, the primary features of the voice disorder are breathiness and reduced volume. The sound of a disordered voice is frequently characterised by the abnormal quality of the fundamental vocal note, which sounds rough or breathy. Hoarseness can be mild or so severe that the voice is almost inaudible. In general, complaints regarding dysphonia concern hoarseness much more frequently than pitch or loudness (Dejonckere, 1995), although these features are usually also affected when the fundamental note is abnormal. Vocal note quality is not the only aspect of the voice that can be abnormal, as is shown in Table 6.1, which summarises the various parameters, how they can be affected and the vocal tract dysfunction that gives rise to these changes.

Table 6.1 Acoustic parameter variations and underlying laryngeal behaviours

Parameter affected	Disordered acoustic feature	Possible vocal tract dysfunction
Habitual pitch (speaking fundamental frequency/ SFo)	• Too high	• Vocal folds excessively tightened
	• Too low	• Vocal folds: – excessively short and thick – increased vocal fold mass
	• Unstable	• Vocal fold tension unstable
	• Pitch breaks	• Vocal fold tension unstable
Pitch range	• Restricted to upper or lower frequencies	• Insufficient vocal fold adjustment
	• Lowered upper and lower frequencies	• Vocal folds excessively short and thick or increased vocal fold mass
	• Raised upper and lower frequencies	• Increased vocal fold tension
	• Excessive pitch variation	• Intermittent excessive lengthening and shortening of the vocal folds
	• Insufficient pitch variation	• Minimal variation in length of the vocal folds
	• Reduced control	• Changes in vocal fold structure or in related systems, e.g. respiratory, neurological
Loudness	• Too loud	• Excessive subglottal air pressure and vocal fold tension
	• Too quiet	• Insufficient subglottal air pressure and inadequate vocal fold tension and adduction
	• Unstable volume	• Variable vocal fold adduction and tension and/or variable subglottal air pressure
Vocal note quality	• Rough	• Chaotic vocal fold vibrations or ventricular fold involvement
	• Breathy	• Turbulent air within the glottis/glottic chink
	• Creaky	• Hyperadducted vocal folds
	• Voiceless segments	• Intermittent incomplete vocal fold adduction/glottic chink

(contd)

Table 6.1 (contd)

Parameter affected	Disordered acoustic feature	Possible vocal tract dysfunction
Vocal flexibility	• Reduced flexibility/control – pitch and/or – loudness	• Limited range of vocal fold lengthening and/or shortening • Limited variation of subglottal air pressure and/or vocal fold tension/adduction
Vocal stamina	• Inability to sustain vocal function of the type and for the time required without vocal deterioration	• Impaired respiratory and/or vocal fold function • Deterioration of vocal fold mucosa status with use

The vocal tract behaviours listed as possible dysfunction can be caused by structural, functional, neurological and emotional factors.

Most of these problems might be present in some voice disorders whereas others will exhibit only one or two features. In most cases, the abnormalities are interdependent. For example, if a voice is extremely breathy it will be quiet and lacking in stamina. This is because, to produce a breathy voice, the vocal folds are not fully adducted on phonation and there is a relatively high transglottic airflow. The potential for prolonged, vigorous voice use is also reduced in these circumstances because of the relatively inefficient laryngeal valve. Another example is an extremely low-pitched, creaky voice that is inflexible. The action of firmly depressing the larynx in the vocal tract during production of very low speaking fundamental frequency inhibits the usual vertical laryngeal excursions in the neck, which are associated with effecting pitch change. Vocal flexibility is reduced as a result. It is important to remember that Table 6.1 classifies only the biomechanical aspects of vocal tract dysfunction in relation to the parameters affected. In many instances, these features reflect the underlying psychosocial or sociolinguistic context in which the voice is used. A voice that is regarded as too loud, for example, might be the result of an angry or forceful speaker, but it can also indicate hearing loss or lack of neurological control.

SECONDARY PHONATORY FEATURES

As the speaker attempts to compensate for the primary features of a voice disorder, usually by increased effort, further acoustic features can be superimposed upon the initial vocal changes. These secondary features might include changes in quality, such as roughness generated by adducted false vocal folds during phonation or an unexpectedly raised speaking fundamental frequency as vocal fold tension increases with increased hyperfunction. In all aspects of normal and abnormal voices, the interrelationship of the acoustic features is the manifestation of the biomechanics of the vocal tract.

Symptom variability

It is typical of many voice disorders that the extent and severity of the symptoms are variable. These variations can occur for both physical and psychological reasons. The most extreme presentation is consistent aphonia, but this consistency tends to be unusual. Although the variability can result in improvement as well as deterioration, it is the changeable nature of a voice disorder that can cause additional frustration and distress. Various patterns of symptom presentation are listed in Table 6.2. In many cases, the patient will be able to correlate vocal deterioration with the amount and type of voice use. This means that, although vocal problems are relatively predictable in certain situations and evasive action can be taken, the speaker is frustrated by the fact that voice problems will inevitably occur in certain settings. When the presentation of symptoms occurs episodically with entirely or almost normal voice in the intervening periods, patients sometimes have difficulty in convincing clinicians of the significance of their problem. The pattern of symptom variation in any voice disorder is an important diagnostic indicator.

Sensory symptoms

Changes in sensation in the vocal tract frequently accompany vocal changes and can be unpleasant and worrying. Clinical experience suggests that for many people the associated discomfort causes as much, if not more, concern than the changes in the sound of the voice. This is partly because the discomfort is in itself unpleasant, but also because it frequently

Table 6.2 Symptom variability

Dysphonia/aphonia	Pattern of voice
Consistent aphonia	No vocal note at any time
Episodic aphonia	Episodes of voicelessness interspersed with normal or near-normal voice
Severe dysphonia/aphonia	The voice is consistently dysphonic and deteriorates to aphonia from time to time
Consistent dysphonia	The voice is always abnormal but the severity of the problem varies
Episodic dysphonia	Normal voice degenerates to dysphonia from time to time
Vocal tract discomfort	Varying degrees of discomfort associated with phonation which can be consistent or variable and which do not necessarily correlate with the severity of the acoustic features of the voice problem

gives rise to fear of serious underlying pathology, particularly laryngeal carcinoma. A study of patients with hyperfunctional dysphonia found that
62% of the subjects experienced vocal tract discomfort (VTD) (Mathieson,
1993a). The types of discomfort most commonly felt by this patient group
were aching and soreness, with the greatest number of patients experiencing coexisting aching and soreness. Patients were given a list of terms at
their initial assessment, which included **tickling, burning, soreness,
aching, tightness, pain** and **choking**. The first three terms are associated
with inflammatory changes in the vocal tract mucosa and patients supple-
mented this category with the term 'dryness'. Aching and tightness refer to
musculoskeletal discomfort. None of the patients in the study reported pain
or choking. Patients were decisive in confirming the type of VTD that they
were experiencing and their descriptions correlated well with the clinical
findings. Those with mucosal changes complained of tickling, burning and
soreness (inflammatory changes) three times more frequently than those
with no mucosal changes. The site of soreness was generally indicated by
pointing to the larynx. Patients also distinguished decisively between
aching, in the extrinsic laryngeal muscles, and tightness which was persis-
tently used as a term to describe the sensation of constriction within the
vocal tract 'inside the throat' or 'at the back' (see 'globus' on page 218).
Aching was generally indicated by laying both hands on the sternocleidomastoid muscles simultaneously or by wrapping the palm and fingers of
one hand around the front the neck. To show where tightness was being
experienced, patients frequently opened the mouth and pointed to the posterior pharyngeal wall. These findings are constantly confirmed in clinical
practice. Patients are reassured to be told that these sensory symptoms are
a significant aspect of voice disorders in many cases and that there are specific strategies for dealing with them.

Sensory symptoms are frequently accompanied by a sensation of
laryngeal fatigue, particularly after prolonged talking or when the speaker
has been talking against high levels of background noise. The accompanying physical sensations and awareness of effort on phonation are generally
associated with changes in perceptual voice quality. The speaking fundamental frequency of connected speech may change significantly. Anterior
glottal chink (see Chapter 13) has been noted as a laryngeal feature in cases
of laryngeal fatigue (Sabol, Lee and Stemple, 1995).

Clinicians tend to be concerned primarily with features of a disorder
that can be observed and measured: the sound of the voice, the structure
and function of the larynx, and respiratory function. The vocal tract discomfort that is frequently an intrinsic component of a voice disorder can
easily be disregarded by the professional because it is assumed that it will

resolve as intervention progresses. This approach is not only insensitive to the patient's complaint but can compound the problem if the patient does not receive reasonable explanations for the discomfort.

Normal–disordered continuum

It is as difficult to clarify an abnormal voice absolutely as it is to define a normal voice (see Chapter 4). This is because each voice is variable and there is an overlap between normal and abnormal according to the reasons for the vocal features and the context in which they occur. It can be helpful to consider a normal–disordered continuum rather than a clear-cut division (Mathieson, 2000). The overlap between normal and abnormal occurs for various reasons.

Physiological demands

When physiological demands take precedence over phonation, voices that are generally regarded as normal may sound grossly abnormal. These vocal changes last for a short period of time and are not usually regarded as voice disorders because of their relatively fleeting nature and the fact that they reflect other normal bodily functions. (See examples in Chapter 4)

Different repertoires

Individuals have different repertoires of vocal behaviours.

Example 1

The most obvious differences occur between vocal athletes, such as opera singers and actors, and the rest of the population. An experienced soprano who finds that she is not able to reach a certain note in her upper range might justifiably conclude that she has a voice problem. Another female who does not have the same skills would be quite reasonably unconcerned if she could not produce this note because she would not expect to produce voice at this pitch.

Example 2

An individual who is used to being able to project her voice loudly as a street trader or actor will be concerned about vocal function when it is no longer possible to increase vocal loudness. A generally quietly spoken man, on the other hand, would not necessarily be regarded as having a voice disorder if he were unable to project his voice to the back of a large auditorium.

Variability of vocal features

Certain vocal features are regarded as normal when occurring intermittently but as abnormal if they are present consistently.

Example 1

Vocal creak occurs in connected speech, predominantly on falling intonation patterns. Excessive vocal creak sounds abnormal because of its effortful quality, and prolonged use can damage the vocal fold mucosa.

Example 2

Hard glottal attack is also a vocal behaviour which is used by most people when they are angry or making a point forcefully. It is an aspect of disordered voice only when it is constantly present or contributing to trauma of the vocal folds.

Age-related changes

The voice changes throughout the lifespan and is affected by hormonal changes.

Example 1

Age-related voice changes depend on the rate and the extent of physiological ageing rather than chronological age (see Chapter 5). The point at which these changes in the voice are considered to be a voice disorder (presbyphonia) can depend on the chronological age of the individual, as well as the demands made on the voice. The features of an elderly voice would be regarded as a voice disorder in an individual of 55 years, but are unexceptional in someone of 85 years.

Example 2

During pregnancy, professional voice users in particular are sometimes aware of adverse voice changes. These can be the result of hormonal changes affecting connective tissues and the increasing size of the fetus which restricts normal breathing patterns.

Inconsistent voice abnormality

A disordered voice is not necessarily consistent in its abnormality and at times the voice might revert to normality (see below).

Example

Physical changes within the larynx, particularly inflammation of the vocal fold mucosa, can fluctuate so that the voice is within normal limits on waking, but may be dysphonic by the end of the day. In some conditions, particularly when there is a psychological basis, dysphonic or aphonic episodes occur when the voice is otherwise normal.

Borderline of normal and disordered voice

At the borderline of normal and disordered voice, the speaker can be aware that vocal function sounds or feels abnormal, although the listener cannot detect any change. Conversely, the listener observes changes of which the speaker is unaware.

In reality, therefore, the dividing line between normal and mildly or moderately disordered voice can be ill-defined, but aphonia and severe dysphonia are usually obvious to the listener. The criteria by which a voice is rated as abnormal can, therefore, depend on social, cultural and occupational norms, as well as objective evaluation. It should be remembered that, although physical changes in the vocal tract generally result in changes in the voice, a structurally normal vocal tract is capable of producing an abnormal vocal note both intentionally and unintentionally.

Effects on the individual

Normal voice is an essential part of communication and of the individual's well-being. All voice disorders reduce the speaker's communicative effectiveness in various ways. Many people are unaware of the role of the voice until problems arise, and they are distressed and surprised by the extent to which their lives are affected by the deficiency (see Voice Handicap Index, Chapter 13, page 465). The clinician should be aware that the degree of distress does not necessarily correlate with the apparent severity of the voice disorder. It is possible to have relatively minor vocal difficulties, but to be extremely distressed because of impairment of the highly developed vocal skills normally used or because of severe vocal tract discomfort. Alternatively, severe vocal problems can be perceived as inconvenient by the affected individual, but do not cause significant emotional problems. Voice disorders have the potential to cause the following effects.

IMPAIRED INTELLIGIBILITY

The functions of the voice are to make oral communication audible and to fulfil linguistic and paralinguistic roles (see Chapter 1). Any voice problem, therefore, tends to reduce the speaker's intelligibility or ability to communicate the message efficiently. Most dramatically, the sufferer cannot be heard or has difficulty in being heard in some or all situations, particularly when talking against background noise. According to the personality of the individual and to the severity of the problem, the speaker either attempts to speak more loudly or eventually abandons the attempt to speak in the difficult situation. Impairment of the more subtle linguistic and paralinguistic aspects of vocal function means that it may be difficult or impossible to convey the nuances that are fundamental to effective communication.

SELF-IMAGE DIFFICULTIES

The voice is an important component of an individual's self-image. Many people are unaware of this fundamental feature of how they present themselves and how they are perceived by the world until they develop a voice disorder. Changes in vocal quality and speaking fundamental frequency significantly affect the way in which individuals present themselves to the world. Part of sex identity is related to masculine and feminine vocal features, whilst inferences are made from certain vocal qualities such as a clear or loud voice. It is common for patients with voice disorders to feel that they are having difficulty in conveying their 'real self' and that other people are not forming an accurate impression of what they are like. Self-confidence can be affected further because people frequently interact differently with voice-disordered speakers, who may then find that they are spoken to less frequently, are talked over or even spoken to extremely loudly to compensate for the deficit.

FATIGUE

The effort involved in trying to overcome vocal deficiencies frequently results in fatigue. In some cases of severe dysphonia and aphonia, the sheer physical effort expended on phonation and the attempt to be audible is tiring. The speaker tries to increase the amount of air available for phonation by vigorous inspiration and to expel it with great effort. This frequently leads to increased transglottic airflow and the necessity of even more air being inspired and exhaled with excessive effort. Increasingly forceful glottal closure can also be a feature of these compensatory strategies, so that vocal tract discomfort in the form of soreness and aching is the result. In addition to the effort related directly to phonation, fatigue can also reflect the energy used in trying to overcome the feelings of ineffectiveness by various attempts to improve communication. This can take the form of excessive animation, using gesture and exaggerated facial expression. Many of these inappropriate compensatory behaviours are not only tiring but can cause further vocal problems which have to be dealt with during treatment.

PSYCHOSOCIAL EFFECTS

Emotional reactions vary according to the type and severity of the voice disorder, its duration, the personality of the individual concerned, and its impact on working and social life. Negative emotions can include depression and anxiety. These feelings tend to be worse if the aetiology of the problem has serious health implications, if the prognosis is poor or the recovery time is lengthy. There is evidence that, when there are multiple voice symptoms and when the voice has particular significance, the effects on the sufferer are more complex. In a study of 74 university voice students who were studying singing, Sapir (1993) found that those who had three or more symptoms of voice disorder were significantly more likely (1) to be frustrated, worried, depressed or anxious about their voices; (2) to quit performance, forego audition, limit their repertoire or quit singing altogether; (3) to speak in an excessively low-pitched voice; and (4) to have a general tendency to worry, be depressed or anxious, or have mood swings. An unsympathetic response to the condition by family, friends and colleagues exacerbates the situation and, after an initial effort to overcome the difficulty, some individuals communicate less and reduce their social contact (Figure 6.1).

ECONOMIC CONSEQUENCES

Voice problems can be responsible for absence from the workplace, the need to be moved from a post requiring significant oral communication or for job loss. The number of people who are forced to leave a job because of vocal dysfunction is probably relatively small, but many patients are concerned that they might be dismissed if their voices are not functionally adequate within a set time. This anxiety can exacerbate the voice problem significantly.

Impairment, disability and handicap

The effects of voice disorders can be classified according to the World Health Organization's *International Classification of Impairments, Disabilities and Handicaps* (WHO, 1980), which is used as a framework to describe the consequences of a disease or a disorder. Its terms are defined in Table 6.3.

This classification can be used to describe the effect of a voice disorder on the individual. The example of glottic incompetence resulting from recurrent laryngeal nerve paralysis is used by Ramig and Verdolini (1998):

- Glottic incompetence is abnormal laryngeal function and is classified as an **impairment**.
- The inability to establish and maintain increased vocal loudness is a **disability** resulting from the glottic incompetence.
- Being unable to function as a teacher because of the inability to increase vocal loudness as the result of glottic incompetence is a **handicap**.

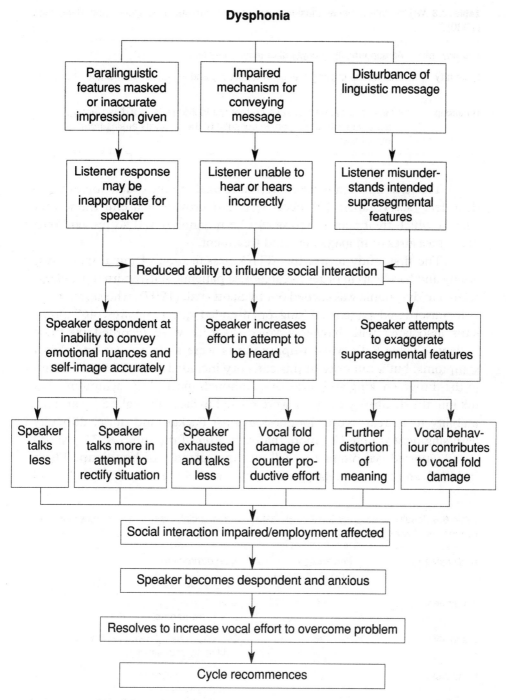

Figure 6.1 Effects of voice disorder on communication behaviour. Each individual responds differently but communication patterns inevitably change according to the speaker's personality and the type of dysphonia.

Table 6.3 WHO's International Classification of Impairments, Disabilities and Handicaps (1980)

Impairment	An abnormality in physical or mental function
Disability	A limitation in performance of an activity and in behaviour because of an impairment
Handicap	A loss of social role function so that the individual is at a disadvantage compared with other people because of the disability arising from the impairment

This classification will be referred to again in the evaluation of voice disorders (see Chapter 13) because it can provide a useful framework against which treatment progress can be monitored and so provide outcome measures of management and treatment.

The first study to use the WHO classification of impairment, disability and handicap in order to categorise patients' self-reported problems related to dysphonia was carried out by Scott et al. (1997), who studied 133 voice-disordered patients. Using open-ended questionnaires, 467 problems associated with having a voice disorder were recorded by these patients (Table 6.4). Most **impairments** were altered voice and throat symptoms, but a minority in this category included a sensation of a lump in the throat, choking and dizziness. Although most of the symptoms that fell into the **disability** category were related to lack of vocal clarity and the inability to increase vocal loudness against background noise, difficulty with singing was noted by more than a quarter of the subjects; 31 respondents reported symptoms that fell into the category of **handicap**. These included employment-related difficulties and the effects on family and

Table 6.4 Results of study by Scott et al. (1997) on the social, lifestyle and employment consequences of voice disorders

WHO category	Percentage of problems reported	Type of problem
Impairment	60	Altered voice Throat symptoms
Disability	26	Difficulty in being heard (25% noted difficulty with singing)
Handicap	14	Difficulties related to: – employment – family and social relationships – psychological and emotional issues

friends. The psychological and emotional consequences of the voice disorders were also regarded as elements of handicap.

Although the research literature related to voice disorders is extensive, this is the first study to categorise patients' self-reported symptoms related to dysphonia. Clinical awareness of patients' perceptions of their voice disorders provides an important perspective for developing symptom-specific treatment strategies and for measuring the outcome of intervention.

Voice disorders and employment

There has been increasing interest in recent years in the relationship between the voice and certain jobs or professions. Apart from the personal distress of the sufferer, the potential economic implications can be significant if voices are impaired. For example, Ramig and Verdolini (1998) cite a report by the National Center for Voice and Speech (1993) on occupation and voice data, which estimates that 24.49% (28,269,000 individuals) of the total working population of the USA have jobs for which voice use is essential. Vilkman (1996) reports that in Finland, out of a population of 5 million people, 800,000 work in professions that place considerable demands on the voice. Some types of employment become impossible if there is any vocal abnormality, whereas other jobs are relatively high risk for causing a voice disorder. If these relationships are appreciated and understood, steps can be taken to institute preventive measures and to monitor those individuals who might experience vocal problems. Voice users have been graded by Koufman and Blalock (1991) into four levels.

Level 1: élite vocal performers

This level includes, for example, professional singers and actors who depend on a consistent, special or appealing voice quality as a primary tool of the trade (Titze, Lemke and Montequin, 1997).

Members of this group require maximum vocal performance in all parameters. They are sometimes referred to as vocal athletes because of the superior quality, pitch range and loudness that they are able to achieve.

Level 2: professional voice users

This level includes, for example, lecturers, teachers, barristers, clergy and telephone operators.

The voice is an integral part of the roles of these professionals. They frequently require considerable vocal stamina over prolonged periods and, in many cases, have to make themselves heard by large groups of listeners. Titze, Lemke and Montequin (1997) define this group as those who, if afflicted with aphonia or dysphonia, would generally be discouraged in their jobs and seek alternative employment. Even low levels of vocal impairment in this group mean that it is not possible to perform the job adequately.

Level 3: non-vocal professionals

This level includes, for example, doctors, business executives and lawyers.

Members of this group would be able to carry out their roles if they were slightly to moderately dysphonic, although severe dysphonia would prevent them from fulfilling their professional commitments adequately in many cases.

Level 4: non-vocal non-professionals

Although a voice disorder might have personal consequences for members of this group, it would generally be unlikely to affect their ability to carry out their job.

Investigations into the links between job type and voice disorder have been undertaken by Titze, Lemke and Montequin in the USA (1997) and by Vilkman in Finland (1996), because of the effect they have on an individual's career and the economic implications. Vilkman notes that, in occupational health medicine, the field of voice disorders is poorly developed in comparison with other conditions such as hearing disorders. He suggests that this might be because the behavioural nature of voice use has been overemphasised. It is possible that people working in sales and sales-related occupations, who form approximately 13% of the US working population, are the largest group of professional voice users. They constituted approximately 10.5% of the voice clinic case load in the study by Titze, Lemke and Montequin (1997), which was not markedly different from their workforce percentage. More significantly, however, 19.5% of the voice clinic case load comprised teachers, who make up only 4.2% of the US workforce. Similarly, the number of singers seen in the voice clinic in this study (11.5%) was disproportionately large when the estimated number of professional singers in the USA is only 0.02% of the working population.

Relatively high figures of voice clinic attendance in relation to representation within the workforce were also seen among the groups that include clergy and telephone operators. Vilkman (1996) highlights the voice problems of teachers and quotes studies by Aaltonen and Pekkarinen, and Viljanen and Koskela, which report that 50–80% of teachers occasionally experience voice problems whereas 10% have one or more symptoms of vocal fatigue on a weekly basis. Almost 100% of kindergarten teachers were found to have voice problems. Similar vocal fatigue problems in teachers were reported in North America by Gotaas and Starr (1993) and in Europe by Calas et al. (1989), in a study of 100 teachers with dysphonia, 96 of whom complained of vocal fatigue. A 13-year study by Urbanova and Uhrova (1987) also monitored hyperfunctional voice disorders in teachers. Lejska (1967) noted similar problems in teachers 30 years ago. These difficulties result partly from the high levels of background noise encountered in teaching environments, which Vilkman reports as 75–80 dB with peak measurements of 117–120 dB. As a result, he found teachers' speech intensity to be high, varying between 58 dB and 79 dB. This increases the risk of voice problems, which are exacerbated by the dry and dusty atmosphere in many classrooms. Aerobics teachers have the additional problem of attempting to produce continuous, loud speech while performing physically demanding exercise. A study by Heidel and Torgerson (1993) concluded that aerobics instructors experience more hoarseness and episodes of voice loss during and after instructing a class, and have a significantly higher incidence of vocal nodules, than a group of individuals participating only in aerobics classes. Similar problems were noted in women army instructors by Sapir, Atias and Shahar (1990).

The chief features of professional voice use are extensive periods of talking, frequently very loudly or against high levels of background noise (Stemple, Stanley and Lee, 1995). The vocal mechanism is stressed even further during emotional speaking and singing. Vilkman (1996) refers to the additional demands made upon the voice by professional voice users as **vocal loading** which occurs in relation to:

- the amount of voice usage
- the speaking fundamental frequency being used
- vocal loudness
- phonation time
- speaking time
- vocal quality used.

Even when vocal technique is good, some individuals appear to be more at risk than others of developing voice problems as the result of vocal loading. Evidence of this is provided by the study of 30 experienced female teachers conducted by Misterek et al. (1989); 15 of the women had healthy voices and the remaining 15 had 'functional voice disturbance'. The time for which they were speaking and their vocal intensity during the teaching day were measured in conjunction with heart rate and arterial blood pressure. There were no statistical differences on these measures between the two groups. Other elements of vocal behaviour, such as phonatory effort and inappropriate speaking fundamental frequency, as well as more general factors, such as levels of stress, could account for the differences between the two groups. Although some occupations place the individual at risk because of vocal loading, it can also be the case that, when high standards of vocal function are required and expected by professional singers and speakers, there is much greater awareness of minor vocal changes than in other people.

In addition to considering the health and safety of employees, Titze, Lemke and Montequin (1997) also highlight the implications of voice disorder in people whose clear oral communication is essential to public safety. Normal voice is essential for airline pilots, air traffic controllers, firefighters and those in similar occupations if their vital instructions are to be unambiguous. The incidence of vocal problems within this group has not been established.

Classification of voice disorders

Traditionally, voice disorders have been classified as organic and non-organic, but this system does not necessarily consider the aetiology of the problem. This issue is most obvious in conditions where the vocal fold mucosa is altered as a result of the way in which the voice is being used. For example, although vocal fold nodules are undoubtedly organic they are the secondary manifestation of vocal behaviour. It is arguable that an aetiologically based classification, broadly divided into behavioural and organic aetiologies, is more logical and helps to indicate the preferred course of management. Table 6.5 classifies voice disorders according to their aetiology.

The division into organic and non-organic categories is also rejected by Titze (1994b), who prefers to classify voice disorders as 'responses of a biomechanical oscillator to environmental, systemic or traumatic conditions'. The three categories that emerge on this basis are shown in Table 6.6.

Although classifications are conveniently tidy, the clinical reality is likely to be more complex. The emotional stress involved in coping with an organically based voice disorder can introduce a psychogenic factor to the original problem. Alternatively, the physical effort required to produce a forced whisper in some conversion symptom aphonias can result in a true laryngitis. Consequently, voice disorders should not be categorised simplistically because, in reality, they can be multifactorial by the time the patient reaches the laryngologist or speech–language pathologist. As any voice pathology affects the individual's ability to communicate effectively, the problem can have far-reaching effects which, in turn, will cause vocal behaviour to change further. The presentation of many voice disorders, therefore, consists of the primary

Table 6.5 Aetiological classification of voice disorders

Behavioural	
Hyperfunctional	Muscle tension dysphonia (MTD) without observable changes in the vocal fold mucosa (also referred to as vocal strain or vocal misuse)
	MTD leading to changes in the vocal fold mucosa (also referred to as vocal abuse)
	e.g. vocal fold nodules
	oedema
	granuloma
	polyps
	vocal fold haemorrhage
	contact ulcers
	chronic laryngitis
Psychogenic	Anxiety state
	Conversion symptom aphonia/dysphonia
	Delayed pubertal voice change (puberphonia/mutational falsetto)
	Trans-sexual conflict
Organic	
Structural abnormalities	*Congenital:*
	Laryngeal web
	Nasal obstruction
	Cleft palate
	Vocal tract stenosis
	Sulcus vocalis
	Vergeture
	Acquired:
	Trauma
	Vocal tract stenosis
	Presbylarynx
Neurogenic	Recurrent laryngeal nerve paralysis/paresis
	Pseudobulbar palsy/bulbar palsy
	Cerebellar ataxia
	Benign essential tremor
	Parkinsonism
	Chorea
	Athetosis
	Dyspraxia/apraxia
	Laryngeal focal dystonia (spasmodic dysphonia)
	Post-CVA syndromes
	Multiple lesions:
	Motor neuron disease (amyotrophic lateral sclerosis)
	Multiple sclerosis
	Guillain–Barré
	Myasthenia gravis
	Wilson's disease

(contd)

Table 6.5 (contd)

Endocrinological	Thyrotoxicosis
	Myxoedema
	Male sexual retardation
	Female virilisation
	Adverse drug therapy
Laryngeal disease	Neoplasm: benign/malignant
Disease affecting the	Papillomatosis
larynx	Cysts
Inflammatory conditions	Laryngitis (acute/chronic)
	Autoimmune diseases
	Cricoarytenoid rheumatoid arthritis
	Gastric reflux
	Allergic reaction
	Syphilis
	Fungal infection
	Tuberculosis

Table 6.6 Classification of voice disorders on the basis that they are 'responses of a biomechanical oscillator to environmental, systemic or traumatic conditions' (Titze, 1994b)

Congenital (structural voice disorders)	Example
Disorders related to tissue change	
• Infection	
• Systemic changes	Dehydration, pharmacological agents, hormones
• Mechanical stress	
• Surface irritation	Smoking
• Cancer	
Disorders related to neurological or muscular change	
Vocal fatigue	

phonatory features that are the direct result of the original condition and the secondary features which develop as attempts are made to compensate.

Although the sound of a voice gives some indication of the laryngeal biomechanics involved, the underlying cause of a voice disorder must never be presumed even when there appears to be an obvious precipitating factor. Laryngeal examination is always essential in order to establish laryngeal status.

A comment is necessary here concerning the term 'functional' voice disorder, which has evolved to have significantly different meanings. Its most straightforward meaning is that a vocal tract that is normal in structure and potential function is not functioning normally and a voice disorder is the result. Functional in this usage is equivalent to behavioural in its purest sense, without necessarily implying a psychogenic component. Unfortunately, some clinicians use the term 'functional' to indicate that the voice problem is psychogenic, on the basis that, if a potentially normal vocal tract is being used abnormally, a psychological problem must be the cause. This latter use of the word functional is unsatisfactorily narrow and in some instances betrays a judgemental and pejorative view of the patient, which is neither fair nor accurate. Although some functional voice disorders are psychogenic, there are many instances where a functionally unsatisfactory pattern of phonation is the product of poor vocal skills, which have been unable to withstand excessive demands. In view of the ambiguity of the word functional in relation to voice disorders, alternative terminology is preferable whenever possible or the way in which it is being used should be clarified.

Examples of voice disorders can be heard on CDs made by Dworkin and Meleca (1977).

Incidence of voice disorders

Evidence regarding the frequency with which voice disorders occur in the population is somewhat fragmented, with more studies concerning children than adults (Ramig and Verdolini, 1998). Inevitably, data reflect those who are examined by laryngologists and exclude those who are unconcerned by their vocal abnormality or who are reluctant to seek help. In England, Enderby and Philipp (1986) suggested that the annual incidence of dysphonia could be 28 per 100,000 population but this estimate is probably low. Nearly a decade later, a review of initial contacts with patients referred to a hospital in London, England, over a representative 6-month period, produced an annual figure of 121 cases of voice disorder per 100,000 population (Mathieson, unpublished data, 1997). It is possible that the development of voice clinics and a greater public awareness of the possible significance of voice symptoms contributed to this higher figure. In the USA, voice disorders are estimated to occur in 3–9% of the total population (Wilson, 1972; Leske, 1981). It is thought that the elderly population has a much higher percentage of vocal problems, with estimates ranging from 12% (Shindo and Hanson, 1990) to 35% (Ward et al., 1989).

Among children, boys tend to present with voice problems more frequently than girls. The incidence of voice disorders in children also seems to be affected by the social environment. Multinovic (1994), in a study of 362 children aged 12 and 13 years, found that 3.92% of children who lived in a rural environment had voice problems whereas the incidence in the urban group was

43.67%. The literature on voice disorder in adults tends to conclude that voice disorders occur more frequently in females than in males, although a study of 428 individuals by Laguaite (1972) reported that only 5% of females had voice disorders in comparison with 7.2% of males. Various hypotheses are proposed to explain this difference. Although Fritzell (1996) suggests that women might have a greater need to speak than men, he also discusses the possibility that the female voice is affected more readily by the demands made on it. This latter suggestion is also proposed by Hammond et al. (1997), who concluded, from their histological study quantifying the hyaluronic acid composition of the lamina propria, that the vocal folds of men and women are morphologically distinct. It appears that the greater thickness of the lamina propria in men is the result of higher levels of hyaluronic acid in the vocal fold structure than in women, and that it acts as a shock absorber. Lifestyle also affects the level of risk for certain types of laryngeal pathology. Individuals who smoke and who have a high alcohol intake have an increased risk of malignant changes within the vocal tract (British Association of Otorhinolaryngologists, 1998). Professional voice users are more vulnerable to voice problems than others, particularly if they have no vocal training (Fritzell, 1996).

Hyperfunctional voice disorders constitute the largest group of voice disorders with presentation ranging from severe dysphonia to minimal vocal changes. The statistics collated by Ramig and Verdolini (1998) from a number of studies concerning the incidence of various types of voice disorder can be seen in Table 6.7. It should be noted that these studies list vocal fold nodules as a separate category when, in reality, they are the manifestation of hyperfunctional phonation. The figures on vocal fold nodules, and possibly on polyps, should be added to those on hyperfunctional phonation in order to appreciate the full extent of the problem of vocal misuse and abuse.

Voice disorder profile (Table 6.8)

The information concerning each type of voice disorder can be systematically compiled so that a profile of each condition emerges. Diagnostic, therapeutic and surgical decisions are made by laryngologists and speech pathologists, according to these details and to whether or not the individual's particular presentation of the problem is typical. The various categories of information are outlined below and provide the format for subsequent chapters. The procedures for acquiring the information are described in more detail in Chapter 13.

Pathology

In many cases of voice pathology there is no visible evidence of laryngeal or vocal tract pathology. The voice is abnormal as a result of abnormal function in the absence of structural changes in these cases. When organic

Table 6.7 Frequency of occurrence of various types of voice disorders

Disorder	Percentage of cases seen		
	Brodnitz (1971) 1851 cases	Cooper (1973) 1406 cases (children and adults)	Herrington-Hall et al. (1988) 1262 cases
Hyperfunction or abuse	25.8	36.6	
Polyps	19.7	4.8	11.4
Vocal fold nodules	15.3	18.1	21.6
Subtotal	**60.8**	**59.5**	**33**
Polypoid degeneration/ thickening/oedema	9.4	4.5	14.4
Contact ulcers	5.3	6.1	
Spasmodic dysphonia	4.7	3	
Neurological dysphonias		4.2	
Vocal fold paralysis			8.1
Psychogenic dysphonia	4.4		
Functional dysphonia			7.9
Mutational voice disorders	4.7		
Total	**89.3**	**77.3**	**63.4**

pathology does underlie the voice disorder, careful observation of its extent and the impact it has upon laryngeal function is fundamental to successful management (see Chapter 13). This evaluation is carried out most effectively in a multidisciplinary voice clinic with the laryngologist and speech and language therapist working as a coordinated team.

Aetiology

The aetiology of many voice disorders is multifactorial with behavioural, emotional and lifestyle factors either influencing the patient's management of the problem or being the primary cause of the problem. The outcome of intervention can be successful only if the aetiological features are accurately identified and acted upon by the clinician and patient (Stemple, Glaze and Gerdman, 1995).

Symptoms

The patient usually describes both how the voice sounds and any discomfort associated with the problem at rest and during phonation. As with all subjective accounts, the manner of the account, as well as the factual

Table 6.8 Voice disorder profile	
Pathology	
Aetiology	
Symptoms (described by patient)	Acoustic/sensory
Signs (observed by clinician)	Voice Vocal behaviour Vegetative vocal behaviour Non-vocal behaviour
Laryngoscopic findings	Structure/function
Expected vocal profile	Primary/secondary vocal behaviour
Acoustic analysis profile	Fo, intensity, jitter, shimmer, harmonics-to-noise ratio
Physiological profile	Airflow and volume measures EGG profile EMG (when appropriate)
Medicosurgical decisions	

The presentation of each voice disorder can be organised into a profile. This is compiled from information which is acquired by observation and instrumentation in addition to the patient's description of the problem. In subsequent chapters, these headings are used to present a profile of each type of voice disorder but it should be remembered that patients who have similar conditions do not necessarily have identical vocal profiles.

details, provide important information diagnostically and indicate the individual's perception of the condition.

Signs

The signs observed by the clinician fall into 3 categories: acoustic, visual and palpatory. The sound of the voice, the way in which it is produced and the individual's non-verbal behaviour provide diagnostic information and a basis for therapy.

Laryngoscopic findings

Laryngoscopic examination provides information regarding laryngeal structure and function (see page 427).

Expected vocal profile

A particular vocal profile is to be expected when the laryngeal image has been observed. Incomplete vocal fold adduction generally results in breathiness, e.g. as turbulent air passes through the glottis. When there is a mass lesion on one vocal fold, the vocal pitch is commonly lowered and there is roughness of the fundamental vocal note. Discrepancies between the vocal profile and the laryngoscopic findings require further investigation and must be considered in treatment planning.

Acoustic analysis profile

Instrumental analysis of the vocal acoustic parameters gives baseline measures in order to monitor the treatment process and assess the outcome of treatment. The results can also be compared with normative data and acoustic profiles of various voice disorders, when available, and so contribute to the diagnostic process (see page 448).

Physiological measures

Airflow and volume measures

Baseline measures concerning the respiratory potential for producing voice, subglottic air pressure and transglottal airflow provide diagnostic and progress indicators (see page 456).

Electroglottographic profile

The degree and pattern of vocal fold contact can be assessed using electroglottography (EGG), during which an electric impulse passes across the glottis between two electrodes placed on either side of the thyroid cartilage (see page 438).

Electromyography (EMG)

In cases of neurogenic voice disorders, assessment of the electrical activity of the muscles involved in phonation can be an important diagnostic and prognostic tool (see page 461). (Electromyography [EMG] is also used to monitor the administration of botulinum toxin injections in the treatment of spasmodic dysphonia, see Chapter 10.)

Medicosurgical decisions

The treatment of choice for most voice disorders is voice therapy but decisions regarding the relative merits of surgery or other types of intervention have to be carefully evaluated to ensure the most satisfactory outcome for the patient. Where surgery is essential, or a possibility, voice therapy is an integral part of the treatment plan pre- and postoperatively.

Summary

- Voice disorders affect communicative effectiveness.
- Hyperfunctional voice disorders constitute the largest category of vocal problems.
- Primary phonatory behaviours are frequently compounded by secondary vocal behaviours as the speaker attempts to overcome the initial problem.
- Vocal tract discomfort frequently accompanies a voice disorder.
- Voice disorders can present significant emotional and economic problems for the sufferer.
- The degree of distress and the extent of the economic consequences are not necessarily related to the severity of the voice problem.
- Voice disorder can be a symptom of serious disease, but
- Severe voice disorder can be present without organic pathology.

7 CHAPTER

Hyperfunctional voice disorders

Hyperfunctional dysphonia is characterised by excessive phonatory effort (Laver, 1980; Boone and McFarlane, 1988). This inappropriate vocal behaviour places undue physical stresses on the anatomy and physiology of the vocal tract, causing undesirable changes in its function and, in some cases, trauma to the vocal folds. There is excessive tension in the muscle groups involved in phonation, particularly the intrinsic laryngeal muscles. This group of voice disorders is commonly referred to as muscle tension dysphonia (MTD) and can be divided into two subgroups: **MTD without changes to the vocal fold mucosa** and **vocal fold lesions**.

Muscle tension dysphonia without changes to the vocal fold mucosa.

The voice disorder is the result of aberrant vocal tract function arising from excessive effort. This group is also referred to as vocal misuse or vocal strain. The term 'muscle tension dysphonia' (Morrison, Nichol and Rammage, 1986) has been adopted widely, whereas the terms 'habitual dysphonia' (Fawcus, 1986b) and 'mechanical dysphonia' (Gordon, Morton and Simpson, 1978) are used less frequently. Muscle tension dysphonia can exist for many years without damage to the vocal folds.

Vocal fold lesions

These include lesions, such as vocal nodules and polyps, which are the direct result of excessive effort during voice production (also referred to as **vocal abuse**). Particularly forceful adduction of the vocal folds in vocal misuse can eventually lead to damage to the surfaces of vocal folds, which penetrates the lamina propria. The acute symptoms of damage can develop

145

when vocal misuse occurs during an upper respiratory tract infection, and can persist after the infection has resolved if the hyperfunction is maintained over a prolonged period. In some cases, changes to the lamina propria are caused during isolated episodes of extremely loud and forceful singing or shouting.

Hyperfunctional patterns of phonation tend to establish a vicious circle of behaviour. Increased effort, particularly when attempting to increase voice loudness, leads to deterioration in the voice. Further effort is then employed to overcome the deterioration which subsequently leads to further vocal problems. If vocal misuse can be diagnosed early and treated appropriately, the problem can be resolved and improved patterns of phonation established with relative ease. If it is not identified and the damaging patterns of voice production, and other elements of laryngeal abuse, are allowed to continue, the situation will deteriorate. It is unlikely to remain static or to improve spontaneously.

General aetiology

The reasons for individuals using such extreme effort that hyperfunctional dysphonia occurs can be categorised, but in many cases the basis of the problem is multifactorial. It has to be remembered that the vocal manifestation of the problem is the result of the speaker's need to speak with effort and it is essential for the clinician to establish the factors involved if treatment is to be successful. The aetiological factors can be grouped under the following headings.

HIGH RISK

This category includes those who work in occupations where there is a high risk of misusing the voice, either through the demands of the job itself or because of the setting in which voice use takes place. Prolonged use of the voice alone does not usually create problems; it is the need for a very loud voice or talking against high levels of background noise that can result in abusive vocal behaviour (Vilkman, 1996). In these settings, employees do not usually receive voice training, and in some situations the demands made on the voice might not be helped by training because of the extreme volume levels required. High-risk occupations include school teaching, stock market trading and certain factory jobs where noise levels are high (see Chapter 6). Some professional voice users, such as rock singers, fall into this category and the particular problems of performers are discussed in Chapter 16. Various leisure activities, such as cheerleading and karaoke singing, can also be fairly high-risk activities for vocal abuse. The leisure group also includes the enthusiastic football supporter who shouts support as loudly as possible while driven by emotion, which results in uninhibited shouts of joy or despair at maximum physiological intensity. In this group, the speaker is intent upon making the voice as loud as possible in order to be heard, and usually is unaware of the stresses being placed on the vocal tract until vocal problems occur.

PSYCHOSOCIAL

Personality, emotional status and interpersonal relationships can be important aspects of vocal hyperfunction and frequently contribute to the way in which the voice is used. All voices are affected by changing emotions, but clinical observation suggests that certain profiles of personality type or emotional status are relevant to hyperfunctional voice disorder:

• Some very forceful and dominant individuals tend to carry out most activities with excessive effort: the 'sledgehammer to crack a nut' approach to life. They might be generally noisy and, in particular, they communicate forcefully. Phonation might be used to control and influence others. The relevance of personality to this type of voice disorder can be observed most dramatically in children. It is not the quiet, retiring child who usually develops vocal fold changes as the result of hyperfunction, but the outgoing, extremely sociable, keen player of team games who plays and observes sport with a passion that involves considerable shouting. This child does everything with great intensity: singing, arguing, discussing and relating the day's events. (Children's voice disorders are discussed in more detail in Chapter 16.) Among friends and colleagues these individuals are known for having very loud voices that can be heard above others. Very often, this loud and forceful behaviour reflects an exuberant temperament, but it can also be one aspect of a bombastic, and less pleasant, pattern of behaviour. Many are energetic, active, anxious, ambitious and self-driven, always competing and trying to excel. They may be perfectionists and find it hard to delegate responsibility and resent offers of help, which they regard as interference. The business executive, the singer and the actor may have this tension, ambition and drive, as well as individuals involved in local committees and societies. These individuals are not necessarily neurotic but may be well adjusted and successful.

• Arnold (1962) and Luchsinger and Arnold (1965) stated that vocal nodules represent the reaction of local tissue to mental strain imposed by difficulties in adjusting to the demands made by society in persons of a certain personality structure. There are patients who do not speak excessively loudly but with such tension and use of hard glottal attack that the folds have been damaged. Arnold (1962) noted that the disorder is common in pyknic and athletic types and rare in asthenic individuals. There is such a strong anxiety component in the personality structure of some individuals who suffer from vocal abuse that it appears to be akin to a psychosomatic disorder (Linford Rees, 1982). Morrison, Nichol and Rammage (1986) reported that the majority of individuals with muscular tension dysphonia seen in their voice clinic had problems coping with stress.

- Cultural patterns of communication within a family or social group vary considerably with regard to loudness, forcefulness and pitch. A pattern of hyperfunctional voice problems can be observed in certain families, for example, where family life is conducted with televisions, radios and hi-fi equipment providing high levels of background noise. Members of the family talk loudly in competition with this background and with each other, frequently from room to room or even from downstairs to upstairs. This pattern of communication becomes habitual so that even when they are talking in a quiet setting, excessive volume and force are used although inappropriate.

- Changes in emotional status can also lead to hyperfunctional phonation. Although very forceful yelling in anger or at a sports event can damage the vocal fold mucosa and the individual is instantly aware that something has happened in the larynx, in most cases it is more prolonged emotional stress that causes behavioural voice changes. As the vocal tract muscles tighten and speech-breathing patterns become shallow in reaction to the situation, phonation is more effortful as a result. A vicious circle is then steadily established during which increasing levels of effort are used in order to overcome the initial vocal inefficiency. It is important to recognise that these changes in vocal behaviour, once established, do not necessarily disappear when the causative emotional episode has passed.

SOCIOLINGUISTIC

The importance of the voice in conveying information about the speaker has been discussed in Chapter 1. Hyperfunctional voice problems can arise if attempts are made to maintain vocal features that are at the limits of physiological potential. Problems commonly occur, for example, when an impression of increased gravitas or authority is sought, either consciously or unconsciously. This phenomenon is observed more frequently in males than in females. Speaking fundamental frequency is lowered and is usually accompanied by a degree of vocal creak. Consequently, the larynx is forcefully depressed in the vocal tract so that the normal vertical excursions, particularly laryngeal elevation, become restricted. The extrinsic laryngeal muscles become increasingly tense as the speaker attempts to maintain the lowered pitch. When this phonatory pattern is accompanied by vocal creak, during which the closed phase in each vibratory cycle of the vocal folds is increased, further stresses are placed on the vocal mechanism. This example of hyperfunctional phonation demonstrates clearly that hyperfunctional voice is not necessarily loud; the essential feature is that it is effortful. Using an unduly low SFo is in itself an effort but, because it has limited carrying power, the speaker is also frequently trying to increase volume which adds a further hyperfunctional component.

POST-INFECTION

During an upper respiratory tract infection that affects the voice because of acute laryngitis, excessive secretions or respiratory difficulties, phonation can become hyperfunctional as attempts are made to normalise the voice. Coughing and throat clearing are also involved. As the infection subsides, the changes in vocal behaviour may continue, partly because they have become habituated, but also because the previous sensations (the kinaesthetic model) of voice production have been compromised. The patient describes not being able to remember how normal voice used to feel. If vigorous throat-clearing has also become a habit this becomes part of the hyperfunctional picture.

COMPENSATORY

Hyperfunctional voicing patterns can also occur as a secondary feature of laryngeal pathology or in an attempt to overcome an existing hyperfunctional voice disorder. This pattern of vocal behaviour accompanies and compounds many organic voice problems, as well as the various difficulties described above. The inevitable result is a vicious circle of increasingly counterproductive effort. Attempts are made to overcome a primary voice problem by increasing phonatory effort. These become increasingly ineffective and effort is increased still further with the same result. As the speaker becomes fixed in this circular behaviour, tense forceful phonation becomes habituated. Koufman and Blalock (1991) have remarked that it can be argued that all voice disorders have a hyperfunctional element, whether as a primary or a secondary feature.

INADEQUATE VOCAL SKILLS

The speaker is at risk of vocal strain, misuse and abuse when demands on the voice exceed vocal skills. Many professional voice users tend to fall into this category because loud voicing that reaches the limits of pitch range is often required for prolonged periods. The skilful coordination of appropriate subglottic air pressure and vocal fold tension, in combination with maximum use of the supraglottic vocal tract spaces, is essential if the vocal mechanism is to withstand these demands. Even when less athletic vocal performance is required, difficulties arise when the voice can meet only the required levels of loudness and pitch with excessive effort.

ANATOMICAL AND PHYSIOLOGICAL FACTORS

Although it is generally accepted that the anatomy of the larynx and vocal tract is symmetrical, it is evident that there are asymmetries in normal speakers. It is possible that these variations increase the likelihood of hyperfunctional phonation as the speaker unconsciously compensates. Speculation within the literature concerning the higher incidence of certain voice disorders among women includes histological differences between the vocal folds of men and those of women. It is possible that women's vocal folds are less able to cope with the demands made upon them than those in the male. The higher quantity of hyaluronic acid in men's vocal fold structure (see Chapter 2, page 29) appears to act as a shock absorber, giving the folds greater protection (Hammond et al., 1997). The relatively high number of cases of vocal fold nodules in women probably also reflects the higher speaking fundamental frequency which results in greater impact stress on the vocal folds.

MULTIFACTORIAL AETIOLOGY

Although hyperfunctional voice disorders can be categorised as above to some extent, the aetiology is frequently multifactorial. The problem might fall into one of the above categories and be compounded by additional factors. Alternatively, a number of disparate elements may coincide to cause the voice disorder. In a significant number of patients, the vocal fold mucosa is additionally irritated by gastric reflux, which has to be managed in conjunction with the abusive vocal behaviours if the voice disorder is to be successfully resolved (see Chapter 11). Even non-phonatory tasks such as playing woodwind instruments (King, Ashby and Nelson, 1987) and working with weights in a gym can cause forceful vocal fold adduction and contribute to voice problems.

Case history

AF, a 27-year-old female marketing executive, was found on laryngoscopic examination for hoarseness to have very early vocal fold nodule formation, 6 weeks after an upper respiratory tract infection (URTI). She reported that she had always been lively and sociable, and was known by her family and friends for being generally 'loud'. She reported that she had had a rather deep voice since childhood. Her voice had never concerned her until she had lost it almost completely during her recent infection. Until then, she had also been a cigarette smoker, but finally stopped as a result of this episode. During this time, however, she continued to work, giving presentations and dealing with clients. She had found that, if she increased the effort with which she spoke, it was possible to produce more voice. Throughout the acute stage of the infection, and for some weeks after it had resolved, she had been coughing forcefully. Subsequently, she continued to use her voice vigorously both at work and socially. She played hockey, which involved a great deal of shouting, and her social life was based in clubs where there was loud music and people were smoking. Although she was severely dysphonic, she did not seek medical help until phonation involved considerable effort, and talking and swallowing were painful.

This case exemplifies the multifactorial nature of many voice disorders and encompasses most of the aetiological factors listed previously. Socially, AF fell into a moderately **high-risk** category; many individuals find that they are hoarse after an evening in clubs where there are high levels of background noise. Perhaps more important were the **psychosocial** and **sociolinguistic factors**. She was a forceful and sociable individual who put maximum effort into everything she did, even **during and after the infection**. It was part of her self-image to be energetic and she perceived that her successful marketing career could be maintained only with maximum animation and impact on her clients. This involved talking loudly and rapidly at all times. Her method of dealing with her vocal problem was, therefore, to increase the effort that she put into communicating and so further traumatise vocal folds recovering from acute laryngitis. This inappropriate **compensatory** approach compounded the problem in combination with the prolonged period of coughing.

Although she had had no problems when giving presentations before this infection, it became evident that her **inadequate vocal skills** for projecting her voice contributed further to her voice problem subsequently, as she increased laryngeal effort but had no awareness of the need for adequate subglottal air pressure and resonation of the fundamental vocal note. It is also arguable that, being a woman, her vocal folds were **physiologically** less able to withstand the trauma to which they were subjected. Clinical experience suggests that it is less common for a man to produce similar vocal fold changes in this situation. AF's voice disorder was not, therefore, purely the result of having the URTI, as she thought. There were sufficient elements of her personality, previous vocal behaviour and lifestyle that predisposed her to developing the disorder when she contracted the URTI. Resolving the problem depended on identifying the contributory elements and helping AF to gain some insight into the way in which her voice problem had evolved and become established. Her general enthusiasm was also applied to cooperating with voice conservation advice and to changing her vocal behaviour. It is interesting to note that, although there were a number of contributory factors, these did not include underlying stress and emotional tensions. Clinicians become very aware of the range of emotional problems that may underpin patients' voice disorders. As a result, it is possible to overlook the fact that some individuals approach life and tackle their problems with such energy that they can develop symptoms of vocal abuse.

These aetiological factors of hyperfunctional voice disorders (Table 7.1) can occur in isolation or coexist. In many cases the aetiology is multifactorial.

Muscle tension dysphonia (vocal misuse)

SYMPTOMS

Onset

Patients frequently describe the onset of the problem in sensory terms (see Chapter 6). A tired and aching throat may have been noticed before changes in the voice were apparent. Some patients describe their voices as having been their 'weak spot' since childhood, with a history of URTIs, which includes

Table 7.1 Hyperfunctional dysphonia: aetiological factors

Contributory factors

- Vocally high-risk occupation/social life
- Psychosocial
- Sociolinguistic
- Post-infection
- Inadequate vocal skills
- Anatomical and physiological
- Multifactorial

---

relatively frequent episodes of acute laryngitis and voice loss as well as hoarseness after prolonged talking. Shouting and speaking against noise, stress at work or in the domestic situation, fatigue and poor health all aggravate the condition. The tendency of the vocal fold mucosa to be irritable means that exposure to pollutants such as dust, fumes, dry atmosphere, spirits and especially smoking causes coughing. Patients complain of both transient and persistent voice changes which generally relate to the amount and type of voice use. Transient voice changes tend to occur after specific events such as shouting at a sports event, singing or public speaking. The patient may describe the voice as usually returning to normal by the following day but at the time of seeking help these episodes of vocal deterioration are occurring more frequently or lasting longer. In cases of persistent voice change, onset can be sudden after shouting or attending a social function in a very noisy setting, for example. More commonly the voice has degenerated over a period of time, the length of which can vary from a few days or weeks to months or even years. The various symptoms complained of by this group of patients tend to fall into well-defined categories and common terms are used to describe the vocal and sensory changes associated with these voice disorders (Table 7.2). A profile of muscle tension dysphonia is given in Table 7.3.

Acoustic

Personal descriptions of the abnormal voice reflect the changes in the various vocal parameters. Common descriptions of a reduced harmonics-to-

Table 7.2a Hyperfunctional dysphonia symptoms: patient descriptors

Vocal change symptoms

Parameter	Common patient descriptors
Vocal note quality	Husky, hoarse, breathy, rough
Loudness	It's too quiet I can't control the volume I can't be heard when it's noisy
Pitch	My voice is much lower/deeper I can't reach my high/middle/low notes It cracks/breaks
Vocal note onset/continuity	My voice disappears at the end/beginning of words/ sentences I keep losing my voice
Stability	It wobbles/sounds unsteady
Stamina	The more I talk the worse it gets My voice gets tired

Table 7.2b

Vocal tract sensory symptoms

Vocal tract discomfort	Patient descriptors
Symptoms of inflammation	Sore, burning, tickling, irritable It hurts when I swallow It feels bruised
Musculoskeletal symptoms	Aching, constriction, tightness It hurts when I swallow It's an effort to speak Lump in the throat
Increased secretions	I have to clear my throat frequently I have a lot of mucus/catarrh in my throat

The terminology used by individuals who have voice disorders tends to be very similar and can provide important information about the underlying vocal tract status

noise ratio include *rough, gravelly* and *breathy*, while one patient, who had little knowledge of acoustics, accurately described his voice as: 'sounding as if it has too much noise in it. Like a radio that needs tuning in.' The inability to achieve higher notes in the normal vocal range, particularly during singing, is a common complaint. Many note that the voice appears to be considerably higher or deeper than usual. Voiceless segments are described as 'my voice cuts out' or, in one case, 'it sounds as if my voice has holes in it' whereas delayed voice onset is often described as my 'voice isn't there when I start talking'. Complaints of vocal instability, lack of stamina and reduced loudness complete the account.

Sensory

Vocal tract discomfort is a common feature of hyperfunctional dysphonia (Mathieson, 1993a; Roy, Ford and Bless, 1996) and it is an additional stress that can compound the primary problem. Not only is it an unpleasant experience in itself, but it frequently gives rise to fear of serious underlying pathology, particularly laryngeal carcinoma. The discomfort felt reflects inflammatory changes and musculoskeletal tension, and it has been shown that patients are extremely reliable in identifying the various types of discomfort even when they coexist (Mathieson, 1993a). Those with mucosal changes complain of soreness considerably more frequently than patients with muscle tension dysphonia alone who describe aching and tightness. Coexisting aching and soreness is understandably mentioned more frequently by those with mucosal changes. Table 7.2 shows the terms used by patients to describe vocal tract discomfort.

Table 7.3 Muscle tension dysphonia profile	
Pathology	• MTD (vocal misuse/vocal strain – no changes in the vocal fold mucosa)
Aetiology	• Hyperfunctional phonation occurring for various reasons (see text) but frequently multifactorial
Signs and symptoms	• Varying degrees of vocal deterioration usually of gradual onset, ranging from intermittent to constant • Vocal tract discomfort (VTD) • Laryngeal irritability • Excessive throat clearing
Laryngoscopic findings	• Normal vocal fold and laryngeal structure • Medial and/or anteroposterior constriction of the glottic and/or supraglottic tract, including false vocal fold adduction • Hyperadducted vocal folds or various glottic chink configurations (see text) • Reduced vocal fold vibration • Reduced mucosal wave • Prolonged closed phase if vocal folds hyperadducted • Prolonged open phase if pronounced glottal chink
Expected vocal profile	• Rough, breathy, harsh vocal note • Hard glottal attack • Excessively high/low habitual pitch • Extreme or reduced intonation patterns • Reduced pitch range • Excessively loud phonation or reduced loudness
Acoustic analysis	• Reduced harmonics-to-noise ratio • Speaking fundamental frequency raised or lowered
Airflow and volume measures	• High transglottal airflow if glottic chink • High subglottic air pressure if vocal folds hyperadducted
Medicosurgical decisions	• Voice therapy. Referral for psychological counselling if necessary/appropriate

Emotional

Patients' reactions vary considerably and the degree of concern or distress will not necessarily correlate with the severity of their symptoms. Fear of cancer because of the death of a family member or acquaintance from 'throat cancer' is mentioned as an important concern by some patients and their distress and anxiety can be considerable. It is more usual for patients to report the general fatigue associated with hyperfunctional voice disorders. The phonatory effort required to overcome the vocal inefficiencies affecting intelligibility can be tiring, but attempts to convey personality and paralinguistic vocal features appear to contribute to this fatigue. There is also a tendency, particularly where the primary voice disorder is related to certain vigorous personality and behavioural factors, for the speaker to use excessive force and effort to overcome the problem. This aggravates the original condition and increases still further the effort required and the tendency to general fatigue.

SIGNS

Onset

Hyperfunctional voice disorders are generally of gradual onset but they can start suddenly after acute trauma to the vocal folds. Some patients recall vividly the vocal deterioration following an upper respiratory tract infection or shouting during an argument. The majority merely recount steady deterioration of the voice to the critical point when they seek help.

Communication patterns

Effortful phonation is the common feature of all hyperfunctional voice disorders, but the presentation varies and the extent of the musculoskeletal tension is not always apparent immediately. The patterns of communication in these patients tend to fall into one of two groups:

- Loud, rapid speech is the classic pattern associated with vocal abuse and misuse. Communication is forceful and voluble, with the speaker frequently dominating the conversation and speaking over others. Loud voice in itself, however, does not give rise to vocal problems – it is the way in which that loudness is achieved (Neils and Yairi, 1987).
- Some quiet speakers use considerable effort to phonate but do not appear to be abusing their voices. This can mislead the clinician who is looking for overt signs of hyperfunction. These speakers frequently have tense oral musculature and reduced mouth opening as they speak which reduces the resonating efficiency of the oral cavity. This sometimes occurs in combination with a lowered chin, which then depresses the larynx in the vocal tract. In some cases, the relatively closed mouth is accompanied by significant oropharyngeal tension, which causes increased nasal resonance. A naturally quiet, tense speaker tends to use considerable effort when required to use a louder voice, particularly when it is necessary to speak in public.

Laryngeal irritation

- Hyperfunctional phonation tends to cause laryngeal irritation. As a result, increased sensitivity of the laryngeal mucosa can lead to paroxysmal coughing in response to minimal stimuli, such as a particularly rapid intake of air, temperature changes or certain spicy foods.

- Irritation of the vocal folds resulting from misuse causes increased laryngeal secretions. As a result, vigorous throat clearing is a common feature. This, in turn, causes further irritation of the vocal fold mucosa which leads to further secretions. Few patients are aware of this cycle and attribute the excessive laryngeal mucus to postnasal secretions or 'catarrh'. Certain conditions such as allergic rhinitis, asthma and gastric reflux do cause increased secretions in the vocal tract, but it is also apparent that many individuals without these problems resort to excessive throat-clearing, which has been caused by hyperfunctional phonation. It seems to be inevitable that people who abuse their voices with vigour also clear their throats with considerable force. In addition, the individual's conclusions as to the origin of these secretions affects the way in which they are cleared from the vocal tract. For example, some patients think that the excessive laryngeal secretions are noxious and must be removed as thoroughly as possible. It is common for these patients to cough and clear the throat vigorously or to spit out the mucus, particularly in the morning on waking, in an attempt to prevent the mucus being swallowed.

- The tense vocal tract and tendency to overuse the larynx as a sphincter causes many of these patients to vocalise for non-vocal tasks. Laryngeal valving or more obvious grunts can be heard for simple tasks such as rising from a chair, reversing a car or picking up an object that is not heavy. In the absence of organic laryngeal obstruction, inspiration and expiration may be noisy at the laryngeal level because the vocal folds are held partially adducted. The individual is usually unaware of this laryngeal behaviour, but it can be a source of irritation to family and colleagues.

- Laryngeal irritation can be aggravated, or caused, by: tobacco smoking, excessive use of alcohol and gastric reflux. (These factors are discussed in more detail in Chapter 11.)

It has been suggested by Morrison, Rammage and Emami (1999) that some patients present with a group of symptoms that can be termed 'irritable larynx syndrome' (ILS). The following are the criteria for diagnosis of ILS:

1. Symptoms that can be attributed to tension of the laryngeal muscles, i.e. dysphonia and/or laryngospasm with or without globus and/or chronic cough.
2. Visible (laryngoscopic) and palpable signs of tension of the laryngeal muscles.
3. Evidence of a sensory trigger of the above symptoms, e.g. dust, gastric reflux, odour.

Morrison, Rammage and Emami (1999) postulate that ILS is caused by a change in the central nervous system, which results in hyperexcitability of the sensorimotor pathways. Conditions such as emotional distress, postviral illness, gastric reflux and habitual postural muscle misuse are cited as possible causative factors. These may cause the neuronal networks in the brain stem, which control the larynx, to be held in a constantly hyperexcitable state. As a result, they react inappropriately to sensory stimulation.

Excessive extralaryngeal muscle tension

Excessive tension of the sternocleidomastoid muscles may be obvious visually. This is seen most easily in those individuals with relatively thin necks. The larynx may be seen to rise dramatically at the onset of phonation and to stay in a raised position or to be held in a lowered position. In both cases, its normal vertical excursions during phonation tend to be restricted. On palpation, the extrinsic laryngeal muscles are frequently tense and can be extremely tender to gentle digital pressure. Tenderness is most pronounced either in the belly of the sternocleidomastoid or at the points of attachment. The distal sections of the hyoid bone are also points of tenderness, which can cause the patient to flinch involuntarily when touched, referred to by Roy, Ford and Bless (1996) as the 'jump' sign. The supralaryngeal area, the floor of the oral cavity, may be firm to the touch. The marked tension of the various muscles can also alter the relationships of the laryngeal cartilages, so that the distance between the hyoid bone and the superior edge of the thyroid cartilage is reduced.

A similar reduction may also be found in the space between the inferior edge of the thyroid cartilage and the cricoid cartilage, referred to by Harris (1998) as a closed cricothyroid visor. As a result of the excessive tension in the surrounding muscles, the larynx is frequently highly resistant to lateral digital pressure. In an averagely relaxed neck, the larynx can be moved from side to side easily, although some crepitus (quiet clicks as the larynx is moved laterally) can be felt in many individuals. When the laryngeal muscles are excessively tense, however, the larynx is either resistant to lateral digital pressure or the crepitus is very marked and an unpleasant sensation for the patient. A common additional feature of the presentation can be obvious jaw clenching and a history of teeth grinding or temporo-mandibular joint problems. It is unsurprising, therefore, that the voice rapidly fatigues when laryngeal function is required to take place under such constraints. Patients find the analogy of attempting to drive a car using the accelerator and brake simultaneously helpful in trying to understand this process. The discomfort and sensation of strain rapidly resolve if the voice is rested but return when used again. This appears to be because an inappropriate vocal tract posture has become established, and the more it is used the more the kinaesthetic image for this posture is reinforced. Consequently, although the way in which the voice is being produced feels abnormal, it is difficult for the speaker to change the muscle adjustments without help. The inability to raise the speaking fundamental frequency when the larynx is held in a particularly lowered position or to lower the pitch when the larynx is held high in the vocal tract is inevitable, even when the speaker is aware of the need for such a change.

Inefficient speech–breathing patterns

Air intake is often shallow with increased upper chest movement as the speaker attempts to increase loudness. Rapid, relatively noisy air intake is a common feature of hyperfunctional voice disorders. Phonation on residual air is also frequently observed as the speaker attempts to maintain voice, although the available air has been used. The increase in phonatory effort as the subglottic air pressure diminishes is easily observed. There appear to be various reasons for this behaviour. Some individuals with MTD are rapid, 'driven', communicators who ignore and attempt to override the basic physiological necessity of taking a breath. It is only when they are compelled to pause for breath, having been speaking on residual air, that they inspire again. In cases where the larynx is forcefully depressed in the vocal tract, speaking on residual air is also a common feature accompanying the 'pressed' voice production. When the reasons for attempting to speak as long as possible on one air intake are discussed with patients, it frequently emerges that there is conscious or unconscious concern that other people might intervene in the conversation before the point has been made. This is a common factor for business executives or professional and academic staff who attend numerous meetings. The need to express their views on certain issues is important to them and the need to perform well in front of a challenging peer group, while trying to manage with an inadequate voice, compounds the problem.

LARYNGOSCOPIC FINDINGS

In cases of MTD alone, no pathology is evident and there are no structural abnormalities. Occasionally, slight inflammation of the vocal folds at the free edge is apparent. The dysphonia is a reflection of disordered vocal tract function at the glottic and supraglottic levels. Where hyperfunctional phonation has culminated in organic secondary changes such as nodules and polyps, these secondary changes contribute to further vocal tract behaviour, which is described in the relevant sections below. Morrison and Rammage (1994) and Koufman and Blalock (1991) have described the effects of excessive tension in relation to lateral and anteroposterior constriction of the vocal tract. In simple vocal misuse, the vocal folds frequently reflect medial constriction (also referred to as medial compression or contraction). They adduct forcefully and are then maintained in a hyperadducted posture during phonation. Stroboscopic examination reveals a prolonged closed phase in each vibratory cycle with mucosal waves being reduced in amplitude and possibly asymmetrical. In some cases, together with over-adduction of the vocal folds in the anterior section, there is a wide posterior glottic chink as the result of excessive tension in the posterior cricoarytenoid muscles. Morrison and Rammage (1994) have named this condition laryngeal isometric disorder. In some cases, the laryngeal muscles contributing to the vocal fold hyperfunction appear to fatigue so that the vocal folds cease to be over-adducted and exhibit, in contrast, insufficient approximation. In the past, this laryngeal presentation was referred to as myasthenia laryngis.

When medial constriction occurs in the supraglottic structures, the false vocal folds approximate during phonation and can completely obscure the true vocal folds. This is known as false vocal fold voice or plica ventricularis voice. There is frequently a strong psychogenic background to this disorder. Anteroposterior constriction in the supraglottis also tends to obscure the vocal folds to varying degrees. During the production of very low-pitched voice, described by Koufman as the 'Bogart–Bacall syndrome', the posterior half or two-thirds of the vocal folds are obscured by partial anteroposterior contraction as the arytenoid cartilages are pulled anteriorly. The vocal folds are completely obscured by extreme anteroposterior contraction of the supraglottis when the laryngeal posture is sphincteric during phonation. Table 7.4 summarises these laryngoscopic features.

EXPECTED VOCAL PROFILE

Hoarseness is the chief symptom in hyperfunctional dysphonia. The predominant vocal features are likely to be breathiness when there is glottal insufficiency and, more variably, harshness (Morrison, Nichol and

Table 7.4 Muscle tension dysphonia: patterns of vocal tract contraction

Region of tension	Vocal tract appearance during phonation	Comments
Glottic		
Sustained posterior cricoarytenoid muscle contraction	Wide posterior glottic chink	
Medial contraction	Hyperadducted vocal folds Prolonged closed phase Mucosal waves – reduced amplitude – asymmetrical	High-impact approximation at the onset of phonation
Supraglottic		
Medial contraction	Approximation of false vocal folds	Known as false vocal fold voice or plica ventricularis voice
Partial anteroposterior contraction	Posterior half or two-thirds of vocal folds obscured because arytenoids are pulled anteriorly	Excessively low pitched voice (Bogart–Bacall syndrome)
Extreme anteroposterior contraction	Vocal folds completely obscured	Sphincteric vocal tract posture

Excessive tension in the larynx and related structures can lead to dysfunction of the glottis and supra-glottis. Contraction can occur anteroposteriorly and medially.
After Koufman and Blalock (1991); Morrison and Rammage (1994).

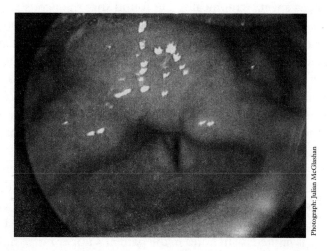

Photograph: Julian McGlashan

Figure 7.1 False vocal fold adduction during hyperfunctional phonation.

Rammage, 1986). Frequent hard glottal attack is a common feature with the majority of vowels that occur initially in words being produced with forced onset, even when the speaker is attempting to speak quietly or gently. In some cases, excessive vocal creak is a noticeable feature, which is particularly marked on falling intonation patterns. The quality of the voice reflects the degree of constriction of the glottis and supraglottis. A strongly sphincteric posture with a long closed phase in each vibratory cycle of the vocal folds produces a squeezed, effortful voice, but glottal insufficiency results in a weak voice that lacks loudness. A voice that is low in pitch and has a rather muffled 'throaty' quality reflects false vocal fold approximation, partly because the voice has been lowered by the speaker initially, but also because the bulk of the false vocal folds vibrate at a lower frequency and overlie the true folds. In contrast, when the vocal folds are tense and relatively hyperadducted, with the larynx held high in the vocal tract, vocal pitch rises and tone is harsh. Pitch breaks occur in MTD, particularly when the speaker attempts to increase vocal loudness, as the result of excessive vocal fold tension. Voiceless segments may also be present, particularly when higher vocal notes occur in speech or singing. These features may be accompanied by delayed voice-onset time (VOT) at the initiation of phonation if vocal fold approximation is inadequate. Tension also results in fatigue so that vocal stamina is reduced and the vocal note tends to be unstable.

ACOUSTIC ANALYSIS PROFILE

The hoarseness associated with MTD represents an increased noise component of the vocal note. Yanagihara (1967b) analysed the formants in hoarse voices spectrographically. He found that the acoustic properties of hoarseness in the cardinal vowels analysed were noise components occurring in the main formants, especially the second formant, and loss of energy in high-frequency harmonic components. On this basis he postulated that confusions in subjective evaluation might be eradicated and a classification of hoarseness on a basis of noise components and loss of harmonics might be achieved. However, the extreme irregularity of the glottal waves, and the fact that the spectrographic results showed wide variance from production to production, made such classification impossible.

As the quality of the vocal note is abnormal in most disordered voices, the harmonics-to-noise ratio is an important baseline measure for monitoring progress and outcome. Speaking fundamental frequency can be within normal limits but too high or low for the particular speaker. In most cases pitch range is limited, with notes in the patient's upper range no longer being achieved.

ELECTROGLOTTOGRAPHY

Electroglottographic (EGG) findings do not produce a standard picture in cases of MTD, but will vary according to the particular laryngeal presentation of the excessive laryngeal tension. In cases of vocal fold hyperadduction, the trace rises rapidly as the vocal folds approximate and retains a prolonged peak, indicating a prolonged closed phase of the vocal folds in each vibratory cycle. This will be seen even when there is a posterior glottic chink, because the waveform reflects any vocal fold contact. In cases of false vocal fold approximation, their contact cannot be distinguished from that of the true vocal folds. Glottal insufficiency in MTD produces a trace with a prolonged trough, indicating an increased open quotient. (See Chapter 13 for details of EGG.)

AIRFLOW AND VOLUME MEASURES

Transglottic airflow is raised if there is a glottic chink and maximum phonation time is reduced because of the consequent loss of air via the glottis. The speaker may feel breathless if prolonged conversation is attempted and, as a result, may take more frequent inhalations than usual. Alternatively, when the vocal folds are hyperadducted, there may be a tendency to continue to speak on residual air in an attempt to maintain phonation for as long as possible on a single air intake. In this case, the transglottic airflow is significantly reduced. It is to be expected that speakers with relatively inefficient, premorbid, speech–breathing patterns are more susceptible to vocal strain. This was confirmed in a study of two groups of female cheerleaders by Reich and McHenry (1987). Group 1 consisted of cheerleaders who reported acute cheer-related dysphonic episodes whereas group 2 reported only minimal or no history of voice problems. Vital capacity, inspiratory capacity, inspiratory reserve volume and tidal volume were measured. It was found that group 2 exhibited significantly greater vital capacity and inspiratory reserve volume than group 1. Respiratory efficiency appeared to have contributed to protecting the second group from voice problems, although the vocal loading required was similar for both groups.

MEDICOSURGICAL DECISIONS

Voice therapy consisting of voice conservation and vocal hygiene advice, followed by a programme of vocal re-education, is the appropriate treatment route for MTD when there are no secondary lesions of the vocal fold mucosa. Appropriate psychological counselling may constitute part of this therapy when anxiety, depression and stress-related factors underlie the voice problem.

Laryngeal pathology in hyperfunctional dysphonia (vocal abuse)

Many hyperfunctional voice disorders are not associated with lesions of the vocal fold mucosa. Minor inflammatory changes can be seen after prolonged or demanding vocalisation in some patients, but these changes are transitory and disappear with voice rest. Vocal abuse usually has to be persistent to produce lasting changes in the epithelium and the lamina propria. The epithelium tends to thicken as it undergoes various modifications in response to irritation and trauma, whereas the lamina propria exhibits oedema, fibrosis or inflammatory reaction in conjunction with extracellular deposits of fibrin and vascular neoproliferation (Remacle, 1996).

An isolated traumatic episode such as shouting, a scream or an exacting singing performance may produce a tiny submucous haemorrhage, but this will be absorbed and disappear after a day or two if there is no repeat of the performance. Continuous misuse, however, can perpetuate and aggravate the damage. As Titze (1994a) explains, various types of mechanical stress involving the vocal folds – tensile, shear, inertial and aerodynamic – are an inevitable part of phonation. Titze views tensile stress as the greatest stress applied to vocal fold tissue involving primarily the stretching of the vocal ligament by the cricothyroid muscle, with maximum tensile stress occurring during the production of high notes. Any of these routine stresses, however, can result in damage to the vocal fold tissue if effort is used to increase loudness or high pitch. It should be remembered, however, that excessive demands on the voice do not necessarily result in vocal attrition, but that a number of the coexisting aetiological factors described above can precipitate vocal changes.

The aetiology, symptomatology and vocal tract behaviour described above with regard to MTD is relevant also to the conditions described below. These organic manifestations of hyperfunctional phonation are more advanced presentations on the same continuum. Specific features described must be considered in the context of the effects of hyperfunctional phonation and MTD.

VOCAL NODULES (SINGERS'/SCREAMERS' NODULES)

Appearance and site

Vocal nodules are non-malignant minute neoplasms seldom exceeding 1.5 mm in diameter (Table 7.5 and Figure 7.2). They are comparable to callouses and formed by trauma arising from contact between the opposing surfaces of the vocal folds. They are symmetrical, bilateral lesions

Table 7.5 Vocal fold nodule profile	
Pathology	• Vocal fold nodules (singers'/screamers' nodules)
Aetiology	• Trauma to the vocal fold mucosa resulting from hyperfunctional phonation
Signs and symptoms	• Gradual onset of hoarseness, initially episodic but eventually constant • Effortful phonation • Vocal tract discomfort
Laryngoscopic findings	• Bilateral mass lesions at the junction of the anterior third and posterior two-thirds of the vocal folds • Soft or fibrosed: soft nodules may range from minute to large; fibrosed nodules are small, hard, white and horn-shaped • Typical hour-glass glottic chink • Reduced vocal fold vibration • Mucosal wave may travel across soft nodules • Mucosal wave absent in region of fibrosed nodules • Supraglottic activity
Expected vocal profile	• Breathy/rough vocal note • Voiceless segments • Low pitch and reduced pitch range • Voice deteriorates with use
Acoustic analysis	• Reduced speaking fundamental frequency • Reduced harmonics-to-noise ratio • Reduced intensity when nodules well established
Airflow and volume measures	• Usually, high transglottal airflow • In some cases of soft nodules the vocal folds are hyperadducted so that subglottal air pressure is high
Medicosurgical decisions	• Voice therapy is the treatment of choice in most cases • Phonosurgery may be required in cases of fibrosed nodules, but voice therapy is essential in order to change vocal behaviour and prevent recurrence

usually occurring at the junction of the anterior and middle thirds of the vocal folds, the midpoint of the membranous vocal folds. Vocal fold nodules occur, therefore, at the site of greatest vibratory amplitude and maximum impact. Occasionally, the diagnosis of a unilateral nodule is made, and in these cases some reddening or slight swelling will commonly be apparent on the contralateral vocal fold, caused by the irritative action of the node. (Clinicians tend to disagree on whether or not it is possible to have a unilateral nodule and some suggest that this unilateral lesion is, in fact, a form of polyp. The histology in such cases is not always conclusive [Remacle, Degols and Delos, 1996]).

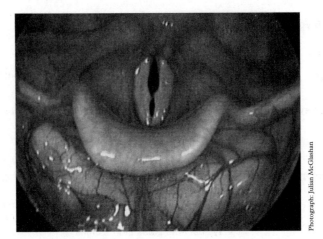

Photograph: Julian McGlashan

Figure 7.2 Vocal fold nodules.

Specific aetiology

Titze (1994a) uses the analogy of hands clapping to illustrate the impact of the vocal fold surfaces across the glottis: the force of the impact is greater when the free edges of the vocal folds are far apart at the onset of closure. Trauma appears to arise, however, not only from the collision of the vocal folds. Jiang and Titze (1994) report that, after the impact phase of vocal fold adduction, there is a pre-open phase during which intraglottal pressure increases as the result of subglottal pressure being applied to the tissue, starting from the inferior surface and ending at the top lip of the vocal fold. In addition to the amplitude of the vibration being relevant to mucosal changes, the frequency of the vocal fold collision probably also has a part to play. Vocal nodules, therefore, tend to occur more frequently when voices are loud and high pitched. There is also evidence that structural abnormalities of the vocal tract, such as a laryngeal web or an incompetent palatopharyngeal sphincter, can predispose the speaker to nodules (see Chapter 9).

Initially, beading of mucus occurs on the vocal folds at the predestined sites of the nodules. Starting with local inflammation and oedema, the nodules appear initially as soft red swellings on the free edges of the fold. At this stage the nodules are either oedematous or telangiectatic, if the trauma has been sufficiently violent to injure microvessels (Remacle, Degols and Delos, 1996). It is possible to reverse the changes at this stage with voice therapy. If there is no intervention, the swellings gradually fibrose and harden as connective tissue proliferates and chronic nodules, white in colour and conical in shape, become established. The tissue surrounding the nodule may be oedematous.

Incidence

Vocal fold nodules are the most commonly occurring vocal fold lesions caused by hyperfunction. They occur most commonly in children and more frequently in boys than girls under the age of 20 years (Heaver, 1958; Kleinsasser, 1968). After adolescence, the incidence decreases in males and increases in females when the highest incidence appears to be in young to middle-aged women. It has been postulated by Fritzell (1996) that perhaps women have a greater need to speak than men, but he also suggests that the female voice is less able to cope with the demands made upon it. This latter suggestion appears to derive some support from the findings of Hammond et al. (1997) (see page 140).

Specific sensory features

Before vocal nodules become fibrosed, the patient may complain of episodes of marked laryngeal soreness after vigorous voice use, in addition to the sensory features associated generally with MTD. With increasing fibrosis of the nodules, soreness usually disappears.

Laryngoscopic findings

Bilateral nodules in the classic position at the midpoint of each membranous vocal fold (i.e. at the junction of the anterior third and posterior two-thirds of each vocal fold) create an hour-glass-shaped glottic chink (see Figure 7.2). The area surrounding the nodules might be inflamed and oedematous. On stroboscopy, the mucosal waves will be reduced throughout the fold and absent in the area of each nodule when the nodules are fibrosed and hard, but can be seen to travel over soft, oedematous nodules. Early organic changes are evident in the form of incipient nodules, where pooling of mucus and a minimal amount of organised tissue can be seen at the site of potential nodules. While nodules remain soft, it is possible for relatively good vocal fold approximation to be achieved by increasing phonatory effort. This obviously undesirable manoeuvre literally squeezes the nodules out of the way, but the mucosal wave continues to be affected. Advanced, white, fibrosed nodules obstruct vocal fold approximation.

Differential diagnoses

A submucosal cyst and the traumatised area on the contralateral vocal fold have a similar superficial appearance to bilateral vocal fold nodules in some cases. The mistaken diagnosis of vocal fold nodules is easily made in children where a hoarse voice and vigorous vocal use are seen so frequently. An abnormal voice since birth is a common feature of the history of a cyst, although careful laryngoscopic examination frequently reveals that the lesions are not in the classic position and that they are of significantly different sizes. On stroboscopy, the cyst might be distinguished from the traumatised area on the opposing fold by differences in the mucosal wave. Trial voice therapy can assist the diagnosis where laryngeal examination is inconclusive.

Expected vocal profile

The voice is hoarse with elements of roughness and breathiness. These vocal features arise in part from the glottal insufficiency that occurs as the nodules meet and so prevent approximation of the full length of the free edges of the vocal folds. Impaired mucosal waves contribute further to the rough vocal quality. In addition, as a result of the increased mass of the vocal folds, which then vibrate at a lower frequency than normal, vocal pitch is lowered. For

(a)

(b)

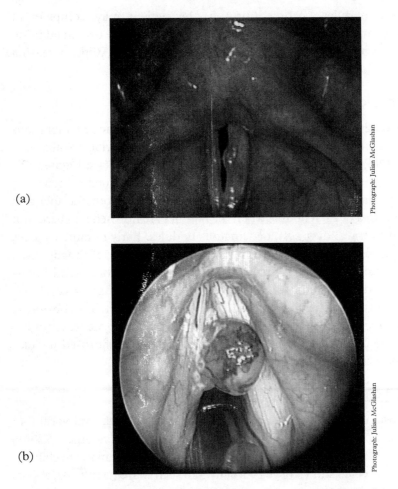

Figure 7.3 Vocal fold polyps (a) sessile polyp (b) pedunculated polyp.

similar reasons, pitch range is lowered at its upper and lower limits. Although the severity of the dysphonia tends to reflect the size of the nodules, this is not always the case. When vocal nodules are soft, the clarity of the vocal note can be considerably improved by increased hyperadduction (see above), a manoeuvre that must be discouraged. In contrast, small vocal nodules can be associated with more severe dysphonia than expected if certain inappropriate supraglottic postures are employed (see above), either as a compensatory measure or as part of the primary hyperfunctional vocal behaviour.

Acoustic analysis profile

For an acoustic analysis profile, see Table 7.5 (page 165).

Medicosurgical decisions

Voice therapy is the preferred course of treatment for nodules, however large, while they are soft and while fibrosis is absent or minimal. Surgical intervention should be avoided if at all possible, in order to minimise the risk of damage to the layers of the lamina propria. It is salutary to note that, on occasion, when nodules are removed by laser and although the vocal folds look normal on indirect laryngoscopy, stroboscopic examination reveals reduced or absent mucosal waves at the site of the excised lesions as a result of tethering of the lamina propria. This situation can only partly be redeemed by voice therapy. If there are doubts concerning the appropriate intervention route, a trial programme of voice therapy should be instigated initially. Fibrosed nodules require surgical removal but surgery should be preceded by voice therapy in order to reduce inflammation and surrounding oedema, and to give the patient insight into prevailing vocal behaviours. Microsurgery should always be preceded by advice from a speech–language pathologist and followed by voice therapy as soon as possible, so that the damaging vocal behaviours can be replaced by more efficient vocalisation. Postoperatively, the voice should not be used at least until re-epithelialisation of the vocal folds has taken place, usually a period of approximately 3 days. During this period, forced whispering can cause damage; to produce a forced whisper, the anterior two-thirds of the vocal folds are tightly adducted and air passes through the triangular posterior glottic chink under pressure.

POLYPS

Appearance and site

Vocal fold polyps are either pedunculated or sessile. A pedunculated polyp is attached to the vocal fold by a stalk, but a sessile polyp is attached at its base and has no stalk. The typical site is 3 mm behind the anterior commissure on the free edge or the subglottic surface of the vocal fold (Figure 7.3 and Table 7.6).

Specific aetiology

Polyps tend to be the result of acute trauma to the vocal fold mucosa, in combination with infection, allergy, pollution or endocrine disorders (Remacle, Degols and Delos, 1996). Histologically, there are several types of polyp; the most common is the oedematous polyp which appears as a soft, translucent structure. If small blood vessels have been affected by the vocal trauma, submucosal bleeding in combination with connective tissue

Table 7.6 Vocal fold polyp profile	
Pathology	• Vocal fold polyps (sessile or pedunculated) • Usually occur singly
Aetiology	• Acute trauma to the vocal fold mucosa, often in combination with other factors (see text)
Signs and symptoms	• Hoarseness • Vocal tract discomfort as in other hyperfunctional voice disorders • Reported sensation of 'something' in the throat which cannot be cleared
Laryngoscopic findings	• Small or extremely large mass on or attached to vocal fold • Pedunculated polyp may hang into subglottis and be visible only on phonation • Glottic chink anterior and posterior to polyp • Asymmetrical vocal fold vibration • Polyp inhibits vibration of the affected fold and the contralateral vocal fold • Polyp may vibrate separately and slightly after the vocal fold on each cycle
Expected vocal profile	• Breathy/rough vocal note • Lowered pitch and reduced pitch range • Voice deteriorates with use
Acoustic analysis	• Reduced speaking fundamental frequency • Reduced harmonics-to-noise ratio • Increased measures of jitter and shimmer • Reduced intensity
Airflow and volume measures	• Slightly increased transglottal airflow • Subglottal air pressure almost normal
Medicosurgical decisions	• Trial voice therapy initially for small sessile polyps, before considering phonosurgery • Large sessile and pedunculated polyps require surgical intervention, preceded and followed by voice therapy

forms a haemorrhagic polyp. The majority of polyps occur singly. In a series of 100 operated cases Kleinsasser found that 79% were single and 21% presented with two or more polyps. It is generally accepted that hyperfunctional vocal fold adduction is the chief cause of vocal fold polyps (Luchsinger and Arnold, 1965; Morrison, Nichol and Rammage, 1986).

Incidence

Vocal fold polyps are the second or third most frequently occurring lesions resulting from vocal abuse, depending on the studies cited (see Chapter 6, Table 6.7).

Specific sensory features

In addition to the various elements of vocal tract discomfort experienced by many with hyperfunctional dysphonia, patients with polyps, particularly when the polyp is large, frequently report a sensation of 'something in my throat'. They discriminate this sensation from a lump in the throat, but it is likened to stubborn mucus that they have difficulty in clearing from the larynx. As a result, throat clearing is vigorous and frequent.

Laryngoscopic findings

Polyps range in size from the equivalent of a small 'blood blister' to a large pedunculated mass. When the polyp is on the free edge of the vocal fold, it is easily visualised, but some large polyps that hang into the subglottis are only fully visualised as they are blown superiorly into the glottis during phonation. All polyps affect glottic competency on vocal fold adduction; the size and shape of the glottic chink depend on the size and position of the polyp. On stroboscopy, the polyp inhibits mucosal waves on both the vocal fold site of the lesion and the contralateral vocal fold.

Differential diagnosis

Small sessile polyps can present as unilateral vocal fold nodules and, as Remacle, Degols and Delos (1996) point out, if the clinician relies on histopathology to establish or confirm the laryngoscopic diagnosis: 'he is very often disappointed. In most cases, the pathologist's protocol is descriptive and concludes that there is compatibility between the microscopic image and the diagnosis suggested by the surgeon, but without removing doubt.'

Expected vocal profile

The vocal features are similar to those associated with vocal fold nodules, although polyps generally occur singly. The increase in mass of one vocal fold tends to lower vocal pitch and to restrict pitch range. The vocal note is rough and breathy, partly because vocal fold approximation is incomplete as a result of obstruction by the polyp and also because vocal fold vibratory patterns are asymmetrical. The severity of the voice disorder generally reflects the extent of the lesion.

Acoustic analysis profile

Speaking fundamental frequency is reduced. This reduction tends to correlate with the size of the lesion. Frequency range is reduced because frequencies in the upper part of the normal vocal range cannot be achieved. This is because of the increase in vocal fold mass and the reduced ability to thin the vocal fold. Jitter and shimmer measures may be increased because the polyp tends to lag behind the vocal fold vibration and has its own vibratory pattern, the successive vibrations of which are often aperiodic (Hirano and Bless, 1993; Remacle, 1996). The incompetent vocal fold adduction allows air to leak, causing an increase in noise in the vocal note, which is reflected in a reduced harmonics-to-noise ratio. Poor vocal fold closure may also result in reduced intensity as the potential to increase subglottal air pressure is reduced.

Airflow and volume measures

Transglottic airflow measures are raised according to the size of the lesion and the extent to which it prevents competent vocal fold approximation.

Medicosurgical decisions

Voice therapy is a possible course of intervention when a sessile polyp is small, but in most instances microsurgery is required to remove the lesion. The patient should be seen by the voice therapist preoperatively for voice conservation and vocal hygiene advice. In some cases a short course of preoperative voice therapy is helpful in order to reduce inflammatory changes. Unless polyps are small, however, they interfere with phonation so significantly that changes in vocal behaviour are difficult to achieve. Surgery should be followed by voice therapy in order to reduce the possibility of recurrence.

CONTACT ULCERS

Appearance and site

Contact ulcers occur on the posterior part of the vocal fold which overlies the vocal process of the arytenoid cartilage (Figure 7.4 and Table 7.7). They consist of crater-like forms with highly thickened squamous epithelium piled up

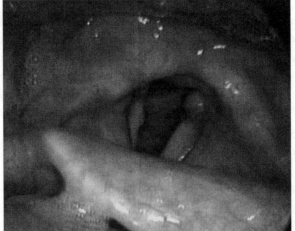

Photograph: Julian McGlashan

Figure 7.4 Contact ulcer/granuloma.

Table 7.7 Contact ulcers profile	
Pathology	• Contact ulcers
Aetiology	• Hyperfunctional phonation: forced, effortful, low-pitched voice • Possibly associated with gastric reflux
Signs and symptoms	• Hoarseness of gradual onset • Marked vocal tract discomfort: soreness and aching • Speaker tends to depress chin when phonating
Laryngoscopic findings	• Inflamed, bulky posterior vocal folds and tissue overlying arytenoid cartilages • Medial and anteroposterior contraction of glottis and supraglottis • Reduced vocal fold vibration
Expected vocal profile	• Rough vocal note • Low pitch with 'pressed' quality • Restricted pitch range
Acoustic analysis	• Low speaking fundamental frequency • Reduced harmonics-to-noise ratio
Airflow and volume measures	• High subglottal air pressure
Medicosurgical decisions	• Voice therapy for early lesions • Surgical intervention for advanced contact ulcers in combination with voice therapy

over connective tissue, with some oedema. The classic description of a raised granuloma on one side and a crater on the other, which fit together on contact like a ball and socket, applies only in very advanced cases. In the early stages, the arytenoid (cartilaginous) portions of the folds may simply appear oedematous and reddened. The anterior two-thirds of the folds may not appear healthy and may exhibit some thickening of the epithelial cover. A glottic chink between the vocal folds anteriorly is often observable. The ulcer may be confined to one arytenoid region or both may be involved.

Specific aetiology

Contact ulcers are the result of an extreme form of vocal abuse typified by the speaker's excessively low speaking fundamental frequency, high levels of vocal creak and effortful phonation. The voice is characteristically very deep and hoarse, and has a forced or 'pressed' quality. The aetiology of ulceration of the folds in the arytenoid region was first related to vocal abuse by Jackson and Jackson (1935). They gave the condition its now accepted name of 'contact ulcer', on account of the trauma of 'hammer and anvil' with which the arytenoids strike each other in the forced type of phonation employed by these individuals (Jackson and Jackson, 1935). The mechanism of the arytenoid joint was also studied by Von Leden (1961) during vocal fry phonation. The arytenoids perform a rocking movement in two planes, making a wide excursion in low frequencies. In the deep throaty voice, prolonged approximation of the arytenoid surfaces occurs in the region of the vocal processes which exposes the folds to excessive stress and is the cause of the contact ulcer. This action causes inflammation, and eventually ulceration and granuloma or neoplasm formation on the mucous membrane covering the arytenoid region of the fold. Arnold (1962) distinguished between contact ulcers, which consist of granuloma of the cartilaginous portion of the folds, and pachydermia of the posterior commissure. This is the area between the arytenoids over the cricoid elevation where no hammer and anvil or crater appearance is present. This interarytenoid pachydermia is caused by chronic infections and pollutants, especially smoking, and is not caused by vocal abuse. Kleinsasser (1968) defined contact ulcers as contact pachydermia, the two names being synonymous for the one condition. He stated that the lesions are not true ulcers or granulomas.

In addition to certain phonatory patterns, gastric reflux (see Chapter 12) also appears to contribute to the problem in many cases. Cherry and Margulies (1968) described three patients with contact ulcers that failed to heal when treated by conventional voice rest and voice therapy. These patients were found to have pharyngo-oesophagitis caused by peptic acid reflux. Peptic reflux while the patient is asleep can seep into the posterior larynx and cause inflammation and ulceration. (Cherry and Delahunty [1968] experimentally painted the vocal folds of dogs with gastric juice and found this produced inflammation and then ulceration.) The sequence of aetiological factors is difficult to determine. It is unclear whether certain patterns of vocal abuse, in which there is strong medial compression of the arytenoid cartilages, render the speaker more susceptible to the effects of gastric reflux or whether reflux irritation of the arytenoids changes vocal behaviour because of the discomfort arising from the inflammatory changes. Contact ulcers do not usually occur until middle age, and it is arguable that patterns of vocal abuse would be expected to give rise to the problem earlier in life. It is possible, therefore, that gastric reflux is the pre-cipitating factor. It is also evident, however, that the typical vocal quality tends to be the vocal behaviour of the older male who is attempting to add gravitas to what he is saying, which suggests that vocal behaviour might be the primary cause. In most cases of contact ulcers, the two factors become interdependent and successful treatment depends on managing both areas.

The equivalent of contact ulcer can be produced by anaesthetic intu-bation traumatising the vocal folds. In this case, vocal abuse is not a con-sideration and voice conservation measures to promote healing is the necessary course. This condition is described further under laryngeal trauma (page 256).

Incidence

Contact ulcers are almost exclusively a male complaint. Vibration of the arytenoids occurs naturally in the pulse register (vocal fry) and contact ulcers develop in people with deep voices. Women do not employ similar methods of voice production and do not develop contact ulcers. This con-dition is far more common in America, it seems, than in Europe where the condition is very rare (Brodnitz, 1961). Landes (1977) draws attention to the proclivity of American men to cultivate bass voices and comments: 'Somehow our culture seems to dictate that a bass voice is a mark of mas-culinity.' The high incidence of contact ulcers in the USA would appear to be a social phenomenon, with many American men using a lower part of the pitch range than British men (Giles and Powesland, 1975).

Specific sensory features

The attempt to phonate may be very painful, with a burning sensation in the larynx or shooting pain in the ear. This is understandable when the action of the arytenoids is seen in the high-speed cinematographic film by Von Leden and Moore (1960). The arytenoids are seen to approximate forcefully in phonation and the pars respiratus is closed, providing a 'posterior air shunt' (Proctor, 1974).

Laryngoscopic findings

The inflamed, bulky, posterior part of the vocal folds is immediately obvious. The vocal folds approximate forcefully and are hyperadducted, particularly in the area of the arytenoid cartilages, so that there is a prolonged closed phase in each vibratory cycle. Extreme inflammation in the posterior larynx suggests the effects of gastric reflux.

Differential diagnosis

Bulky, inflamed tissue on the arytenoid cartilages is a classic presentation of contact ulcers that is easily recognised. Pachydermia laryngis, which appears within the interarytenoid space, differs in its formation and site. It is important to consider the relative contribution of coexisting contributory factors to the formation of the contact ulcers in each.

Expected vocal profile

Habitual pitch is low and pitch range is restricted to the lower part of the speaker's range. The voice is hoarse and harsh, with high levels of vocal creak and a rough vocal note. The speaker finds that, in order to increase vocal loudness, even greater effort is required, but attempts to project the voice are relatively ineffectual and quickly cause further discomfort or even pain. Many patients with contact ulcers describe that they are aware of speaking 'in the basement' but are unable to initiate a high pitch.

Acoustic analysis

The harmonics-to-noise ratio is reduced and jitter is increased. Speaking fundamental frequency is low and pitch range is limited.

Airflow and volume measures

As a result of the firm vocal fold adduction, the transglottal airflow is reduced.

Medicosurgical decisions

Newly formed contact ulcers should not be operated upon, but treated with voice conservation and vocal hygiene measures followed by a programme of vocal re-education. Gastric reflux medication may be prescribed concurrently (see page 325). Myerson (1952) claimed that removal of specific irritants could result in immediate alleviation of symptoms, if at a mildly oedematous stage. He reported that heavy smokers had lost their ulcers within 24 hours of ceasing to smoke. With established contact ulcers, surgery is necessary. The hypertrophic epithelium, which develops through the effort to approximate the vocal folds as the separation of the arytenoids increases with development of the ulcers, may be removed from the anterior sections of the folds. Absolute voice rest is advisable after surgery until healing is complete. Voice therapy is essential and smoking should be abandoned if possible. Although the adverse effects of smoking are not substantiated by Peacher (1961) or Brodnitz (1961) (see below), it must be remembered that smoking is generally considered to be a prime cause of acute oedema and laryngitis in vocal misuse (Kleinsasser, 1968).

Contact ulcers are comparatively unusual in Europe, but there are valuable accounts available concerning quite large groups of patients in America. It is evident from these studies (Table 7.8) that severe cases of contact ulcers require surgery, sometimes several times, and that treatment is frequently long and difficult. Voice therapy is an essential part of treatment.

Table 7.8 Contact ulcer studies

New and Devine (1949)	• 53 subjects (9 of these had ulceration resulting from endotracheal intubation – 6 females, 3 males) • 39 received surgery; of these, the contact ulcers eventually resolved in 32 cases (total of 73 operations, some patients undergoing 5 operations) • All patients had vocally demanding jobs • No voice therapy given
Peacher and Holinger (1947)	• 16 subjects • 6 received weekly voice therapy/control group of 10 treated surgically, by voice rest or both but no voice therapy • Results: – contact ulcers in both groups only healed if subjects changed vocal behaviour – voice therapy group: complete or almost complete resolution of ulcer over 1–4 months – control group: recovery time of 7 months to 3 years
Peacher (1961)	• 70 subjects monitored following voice therapy • 36 no surgery 34 subjects underwent 80 operations before and during voice therapy (not a control group; subjects had advanced pachydermia and required surgery pre-voice therapy) • Results: – non-surgery group; average healing time 10.05 weeks – surgical group; average healing time 26.52 weeks – no correlation between healing time and smoking, drinking, voice rest or duration of hoarseness before treatment

(contd)

Table 7.8 (contd)

	• Conclusion: chief contributory factors – vocal abuse and emotional tension (Vocal abuse = hard glottal attack, low pitch, poor breath control, excessive coughing and throat clearing)
Brodnitz (1961)	• 26 subjects • High correlation between contact ulcers and emotional stress • No correlation between contact ulcers and drinking alcohol and smoking • Common features: constant throat-clearing, characteristic pain radiating to ear
Cooper and Nahum (1967)	• 16 subjects • Authors described three stages of contact ulcer development: (1) vocal fatigue and hoarseness by end of day + arytenoid oedema which may improve with rest (2) continual hoarseness and fatigue + occasional pain on swallowing + severe arytenoid inflammation (3) constant severe hoarseness and fatigue + pain on swallowing and talking + arytenoid ulceration • Treatment: voice therapy and reflux medication and management • Results: ulcers resolved within 3–6 months

Case notes

Contact ulcers were diagnosed in a young man of 23 years who, after achieving a university degree, was employed by a firm of merchant bankers in the City of London. He was extremely ambitious and determined to achieve rapid promotion. In an unconscious attempt to sound as mature and substantial as possible, particularly on the telephone, he had lowered his vocal pitch dramatically; this was accompanied by a posture of tucking his chin in towards his neck, which maintained the larynx in an uncomfortably low position in the vocal tract. A therapeutic programme of establishing awareness of this behaviour and the reasons behind it, combined with improved voice production, eventually resolved the problem.

REINKE'S OEDEMA

(Synonymous terminology: polypoidal degeneration, polypoid corditis, polypoid laryngitis, chronic hypertrophic laryngitis, polypoid fringe.)

Appearance and site

Reinke's oedema involves the superficial layer of the lamina propria (Reinke's space), which fills with fluid and becomes oedematous and distended, primarily on the superior surface of the vocal fold (Figure 7.5 and Table 7.9). The oedematous swelling is usually bilateral and symmetrical, but in some cases there is a marked difference in the size of the oedematous folds. Occasionally, the swelling is unilateral. Zeitels et al. (1997) have proposed a grading system for this condition based on the severity and extent of the vocal fold abnormality on inspiration, with normal tidal volume and abducted arytenoids:

- Grade I: vocal fold contact is confined to the anterior third of the musculomembranous vocal folds.
- Grade II: contact is confined to the anterior two-thirds.
- Grade III: contact is extended to the full length of the vocal fold.

Although the term 'polypoid' occurs in a number of the synonymous terms, Reinke's oedema is regarded as a separate entity from vocal fold polyps (Bennet, Bishop and Lumpkin, 1987).

Specific aetiology

Prolonged smoking is accepted as the primary cause of Reinke's oedema (Kleinsasser, 1968; Bennet, Bishop and Lumpkin, 1987; Remacle, Degols

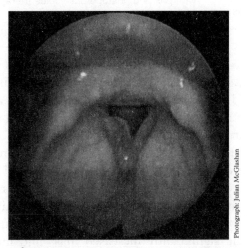

Photograph: Julian McGlashan

Figure 7.5 Reinke's oedema.

Table 7.9 Reinke's oedema profile (polypoid degeneration, polypoid corditis, chronic hypertrophic laryngitis, polypoid fringe)

Pathology	• Reinke's oedema (oedematous enlargement of the superficial layer of the lamina propria)
Aetiology	• Prolonged smoking • Vocal abuse
Signs and symptoms	• Low-pitched, effortful phonation • In advanced cases, sensation of some airway obstruction on exertion
Laryngoscopic findings	• Bilateral swelling of both vocal folds, sometimes involving the entire length • Injected blood vessels on surfaces of vocal folds • Complete glottal contact during phonation • Amplitude of mucosal waves is increased and may be asymmetrical. (Mucosal waves are absent in advanced cases as the cover of the vocal fold increases in stiffness)
Expected vocal profile	• Very low pitch • Upper and lower limits of pitch range are lowered • Speaker unable to increase vocal loudness effectively
Acoustic analysis	• Speaking fundamental frequency lower than normal measures and those of other vocal pathologies
Airflow and volume measures	• Subglottal air pressure is relatively high when there is complete contact of the vocal folds during phonation. • Considerable air pressure is required to overcome the increased mass of the vocal folds
Medicosurgical decisions	• Phonosurgery is the primary treatment route, in combination with pre- and postoperative voice therapy. Voice therapy alone is ineffective

---

and Delos, 1996). The resulting chronic glottal mucositis may then be further compounded by gastric reflux (see page 325). Although opinions regarding the contribution of vocal abuse vary, Zeitels et al. (1997) suggest that the primary irritants render the vocal folds more susceptible to trauma, which finally results in the lesion. They conclude that most patients with this condition are vocal abusers, but Bennet, Bishop and Lumpkin (1987), although agreeing that smoking was the major factor, reported that only 25% of patients with Reinke's oedema in their study exhibited vocal abuse. Clinical observation suggests that, even when vocal abuse has not been a primary cause, the significantly increased mass and inertia of the vocal folds necessitate much greater phonatory effort than normal. Consequently, vocal abuse is an inevitable secondary feature that exacerbates the initial changes in Reinke's space.

Incidence

Women over the age of 40 years are the most common group presenting with Reinke's oedema (Kleinsasser, 1968; Bennet, Bishop and Lumpkin, 1987; Zeitels et al., 1997). Although the condition is also seen in men of a similar age, it is unclear whether women seek help more frequently because they find the very low speaking fundamental frequency associated with the increased vocal fold mass more unacceptable than men, who are less concerned by the lowered pitch. It is possible that other factors, such as hormonal effects, predispose women to the condition.

Specific sensory features

Sensations of effort during phonation and of a reduced airway on exertion are commonly reported by patients with Reinke's oedema. These symptoms are the result of the greatly increased mass of the vocal folds. Greater aerodynamic effort than usual is required to overcome the inertia of the distended vocal folds, in order to produce voice, and their bulk impinges on the airway even when the vocal folds are fully abducted. Complaints of soreness are unusual.

Laryngoscopic findings

The laryngeal appearance of bilateral distension of the vocal folds is classic, although unilateral Reinke's oedema does occur. The degree of oedema of each fold can differ significantly. Injected blood vessels can be seen on the surface of the vocal folds. On stroboscopy, the glottis is completely closed during phonation and the amplitude of the mucosal waves is generally increased as the mucosal cover of the vocal fold is less stiff. The extent of the waves varies from patient to patient, depending on the viscosity of the oedema and the increased depth of the free edge of the vocal fold. The mucosal waves may be asymmetrical when the extent of oedema on each vocal fold is asymmetrical. On phonation, the false vocal folds are sometimes medially compressed as the speaker exerts excessive effort. In advanced cases, the range of movement of the vocal folds on adduction and abduction appears to be greatly reduced because of their increased mass.

Differential diagnosis

Well-established, bilateral cases of Reinke's oedema are distinctive, but early, unilateral presentations bear some resemblance to a sessile polyp.

Expected vocal profile

As a result of the greatly increased mass of the vocal folds, pitch is extremely low and correlates with the severity of the condition. In their study of the vocal characteristics associated with Reinke's oedema, Bennet, Bishop and Lumpkin (1987) found that not only was the speaking fundamental frequency much lower than normal, but it was even lower than in cases of laryngeal carcinoma. For this reason, they regarded it as a diagnostic indicator. The extremes of the pitch range are affected, with both the upper and the lower limits significantly lowered. Loudness is also reduced because, although the glottis is completely closed, the relative flaccidity of the vocal folds on account of the oedema reduces the potential for increasing vocal fold tension.

Acoustic analysis

Speaking fundamental frequency is significantly lower than normal and pitch range is reduced. Harmonics-to-noise ratio is reduced. Jitter and shimmer measures are raised. Intensity is low.

Airflow and volume measures

Airflow measures correlate with the extent of the oedema. When there is complete vocal fold contact throughout the length of the vocal folds, subglottal air pressure may be high in order to overcome the increased inertia of the vocal folds.

Medicosurgical decisions

Microsurgery is the primary treatment route, together with a programme of voice therapy. Voice therapy alone does not resolve the oedema. Preoperative advice and assessment by a speech–language pathologist should be arranged and postoperative voice therapy should be carried out routinely, in order to reduce the habituated hyperfunctional patterns of voice production. Fritzell, Sundberg and Strange-Ebbesen (1982) describe a patient who did not receive voice therapy postoperatively and who subsequently developed vocal fold nodules. It is important that laryngeal irritants, particularly smoking, are eliminated or significantly reduced.

The aim of surgery is to reduce the volume of the superficial layer of the lamina propria while preserving its characteristics, and to ensure that the deeper layers of the mucosa remain intact. To achieve this, an incision is made in the superior surface of the vocal fold, an epithelial flap is raised and the excess contents of the superficial space are aspirated. It may be necessary to take a biopsy so that the possibility of malignant disease in a persistent inflammatory condition can be excluded.

In cases where gastric reflux is a contributory factor, anti-reflux advice and medication should be given.

SUBMUCOSAL VOCAL FOLD HAEMORRHAGE

Appearance and site

Haemorrhages on the surface of the vocal folds can range from isolated minute blood vessels to involvement of the surface of an entire vocal fold (Figure 7.6 and Table 7.10).

Specific aetiology

Vocal fold haemorrhages are frequently the result of the rupture of a varicose vein on the superior surface of the vocal fold. Sataloff (1991) notes that this condition in professional voice users is commonly seen in premenstrual women who are using aspirin products. Any type of trauma involving forceful vocal fold adduction, particularly when there is a coexisting upper respiratory tract infection or acute laryngitis, exacerbates these vascular events.

Incidence

Vocal fold haemorrhages can occur in isolation or coexist with other laryngeal pathology. As a result, figures do not appear to be available.

Specific sensory features

Patients do not generally experience any discomfort from the haemorrhage.

Laryngoscopic findings

Small telangiectatic blood vessels can be seen on the superior surface of the vocal fold, although in cases of the most extensive haemorrhage the entire vocal

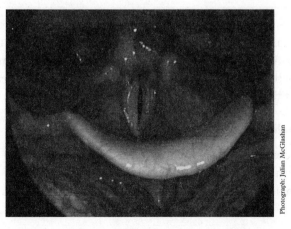

Photograph: Julian McGlashan

Figure 7.6 Resolving left vocal fold submucosal haemorrhage.

Table 7.10 Submucosal vocal fold haemorrhage profile	
Pathology	• Submucosal haemorrhage
Aetiology	• Rupture of a varicose vein on the superior surface of the vocal fold. • May be associated with forceful vocal fold adduction during phonation or coughing, often in conjunction with upper respiratory tract infection • May be associated in premenstrual women with the use of aspirin
Signs and symptoms	• Sudden onset vocal changes, possibly masked by an acute infective laryngitis
Laryngoscopic findings	• Vascular changes in the vocal fold mucosa, ranging from small ruptured blood vessel to entire vocal fold appearing dark red • Reduced mucosal wave in area of haemorrhage • Asymmetrical mucosal waves
Expected vocal profile	• In some cases the speaking voice is perceptually well within normal limits and the pathology is apparent only during singing • The vocal note is rough but this feature may be apparent only at certain pitches or with changes in subglottal air pressure • Roughness may only be minimal, even when the entire vocal fold mucosa is affected by the haemorrhage
Acoustic analysis	• Reduced harmonics-to-noise ratio; may be apparent only at certain pitches
Airflow and volume measures	• Usually within normal limits
Medicosurgical decisions	• Voice therapy • Phonosurgery in some cases of repeated haemorrhages and if benign mass lesions of the vocal fold are associated with the haemorrhage

fold appears dark red. Although vocal fold adduction is usually unaffected, the movement of the mucosal wave can be impaired by the haemorrhagic area. Underlying pathology, such as a submucosal cyst, might be revealed as the primary cause of the haemorrhage on stroboscopic examination.

Differential diagnosis

It may be necessary to clarify whether the haemorrhage is an isolated event or whether other factors have increased the susceptibility of the vocal fold mucosa to this damage. Stroboscopy is an important tool in making these judgements.

Expected vocal profile

In most cases the vocal note is slightly rough because of the altered oscillation of the vocal folds. Pitch breaks may also occur for this reason, but may also be caused by increased tension as a result of compensatory behaviours.

Acoustic analysis profile

Speaking fundamental frequency can be relatively unaffected, although notes in the upper part of the range might be impaired. The harmonic-to-noise ratio is reduced and jitter and shimmer measures tend to be increased.

Medicosurgical decisions

In cases of simple trauma, even when the haemorrhage is extensive, voice therapy facilitates the spontaneous resolution of the vascular damage. Surgery might be necessary when vocal fold structural abnormalities, such as cysts, nodules or polyps, have been the basis of the glottic trauma. Postoperative voice therapy should be arranged. Sataloff (1991) also advises that, when recurrent vocal fold haemorrhage is clearly related to the menstrual cycle, hormonal adjustments should be considered in discussion with an endocrinologist.

Summary

- The predominant feature of hyperfunctional voice disorders is excessive effort on phonation.
- In some cases, there is no evidence of any change to the vocal fold mucosa, whereas in others there are obvious mucosal changes.
- The aetiology of this category of voice disorders is frequently multi-factorial.
- Hyperfunctional phonation may be a primary cause of a voice disorder, but it is frequently evident as a secondary feature of many types of voice disorder.
- Modification of vocal behaviour is essential to resolve voice disorders of this type.

8 CHAPTER

Psychogenic voice disorders

The normal voice and vocal tract reflect the changing emotional state of the individual. The previous chapter on hyperfunctional voice disorders has described the contribution of the patient's psychological status to muscle tension voice disorders. Stresses and anxieties that are reflected in the voice and the way in which it is used fall within the normal range of human experience. Psychogenic voice disorders, although being part of the same continuum of experience, can be discussed as a distinct category because, in many instances, the aetiology and presentation have distinct features. This chapter is concerned with the description of psychological states associated with disturbances of the autonomic system and of the personality that result in voice disorders. Some understanding of these psychopathological states by the laryngologist and speech–language pathologist is essential, although mental illness is the domain of the psychiatrist and patients must be referred to the appropriate professional for treatment as necessary. It is not always easy to distinguish patients who are severely disturbed and neurotic at first interview and, in some instances, voice therapy may be inappropriately prescribed when referral to a psychiatrist is essential. Many psychogenic voice disorders are, however, successfully treated by voice therapy with or without the support of suitable counselling from other professionals. A carefully compiled case history may clearly indicate psychiatric illness. The content of the patient's speech is highly significant and the clinician should not become so involved with observation of the patient's vocal behaviour that the content is ignored.

Classification of mental and behavioural disorders

Classification of psychiatric illness changes with each revision of the *International Classification of Diseases* (ICD) by the World Health

Organization. The most recent revision – *ICD-10: The Classification of Mental and Behavioural Disorders* – was produced in 1992 and consists of a group of documents related to the various categories, which are intended for international use. A significant departure from previous classifications is the avoidance of the terms 'neurosis' and 'psychosis', although these terms are used descriptively (Murray, Hill and McGuffin, 1997). The terms 'psychogenic' and 'psychosomatic' have also been omitted from the classification, but continue to be used by professionals in the field. The categories are listed in Table 8.1.

Table 8.1 WHO ICD-10: the classification of mental and behavioural disorders (WHO, 1992)

- Organic, including symptomatic mental disorders
- Mental and behavioural disorders due to psychoactive substance abuse
- Schizophrenia, schizotypal states and delusional disorders
- Mood (affective) disorders
- Neurotic, stress-related and somatoform disorders
- Behavioural syndromes and mental disorders associated with physiological dysfunction and hormonal change
- Abnormalities of adult personality and behaviour
- Mental retardation[a]
- Developmental disorders
- Behavioural and emotional disorders with onset usually occurring in childhood or adolescence

[a]The current terminology is learning disability.

When a voice disorder is only one manifestation of serious mental illness, a speech–language pathologist is usually unlikely to be involved in the patient's treatment. (There are occasions, however, when a comprehensive assessment of such patients' speech, language and voice is part of the evaluation procedure and where symptomatic voice therapy might be arranged.) It has been estimated that only 7% of all those with psychiatric disorders in the UK are seen by psychiatrists (Lewis and Wessely, 1997). This suggests that there is potentially a large population of people who might seek medical help through other routes because of symptoms arising from psychological problems. Patients with mental and behavioural disorders can present with voice disorders and clinical experience suggests that the most frequently represented category is: ICD-10: Neurotic, stress-related and somatoform disorders. The primary features of neurotic disorders are listed in Table 8.2.

Table 8.2 Features of neurotic disorders (after Lewis and Wessely, 1997)

- Anxiety, characterised by somatic, cognitive and emotional symptoms, or depression, characterised by feelings of hopelessness

- No overall loss in perception of external reality (unlike psychotic disorders)

- Neurotic disorders include:
  Generalised anxiety disorder (GAD)
  Phobias
  Obsessive–compulsive disorder
  Panic
  Stress disorder
  Post-traumatic stress disorder

- Impaired insight

NEUROTIC, STRESS-RELATED AND SOMATOFORM DISORDERS

Neurotic disorders are typified by anxiety and depression which are caused by both childhood experiences and adult life events. Lewis and Wessely (1997) suggest that anxiety occurring in the absence of depression is linked to problems in childhood rather than those in adult life. The persisting anxiety that affects efficiency and health, becoming an anxiety state (Linford Rees, 1982), is caused by experiences such as parental loss and separation, and by parental attitudes and child-rearing practices. Skynner (1976) emphasises that parental behaviour reflects the behaviour of their own parents, because they treat their children in the same way as they themselves were brought up. Anxiety is in part genetic and is handed down from generation to generation. The case for a genetic component lies in the fact that babies demonstrate, from birth, very different temperaments before falling prey to the family atmosphere and, later, the psychological structure of the family unit. Some children ride the storms better than others: some are equable and happy, others are the reverse. Neurotic individuals tend to be attracted to each other and fall in love, have children and perpetuate their problems (Skynner and Cleese, 1983). There is a distinction between worry and anxiety, although in experiencing these states they tend to overlap. Worry can be defined as an 'unpleasant process involving recurrent thoughts about a problem or concern' (Lewis and Wessely, 1997). Every normal individual experiences worry and anxiety when confronted by certain events – illness in a child, visiting a doctor or dentist, addressing a meeting, taking examinations or a driving test. Certain situations, such as unemployment, are associated with higher rates of all forms of psychiatric disorder (Murray, Hill and McGuffin, 1997), but normal anxiety is not crippling and it does not last. It disappears when the feared event is over.

It is a necessary emotion, alerting the individual for 'fight or flight' and releasing energy and drive that are essential in all competitive activity. A chronic anxiety state is characterised by somatic and emotional symptoms that are the result of underlying anxiety, although the individual might not be conscious of worrying.

In adulthood, the *anticipation of losing* something extremely important, such as a loved person, status at work or in the community, or a home, appears to lead to anxiety. Depression tends to be the result of *actual loss* or *humiliation*. Individuals who have undergone such loss may also experience anxiety as they contemplate what can go wrong next. It is significant that studies of neurotic disorder show an association with poor social support, although the causal relationship is unclear. Anxiety is characterised by three groups of symptoms: **somatic**, **cognitive** and **emotional**. The somatic symptoms have considerable relevance to psychogenic voice disorders and can be divided into three groups as shown in Table 8.3.

Individuals in a state of anxiety find it extremely difficult to remove the sense of fear and foreboding. The sense of confused uncertainty also means that it is difficult for them to make and take decisions. Consequently, they become trapped in a circle of fear that is exacerbated by their inability to change their experience without treatment.

Table 8.3 Symptoms associated with anxiety

Somatic symptoms	Autonomic arousal causes sweating, abdominal discomfort, palpitations, muscular tremor
	Muscular tension gives rise to muscle pain and tenderness, leading to muscular fatigue in addition to the motor problems associated with muscle tension (there is no evidence that all dysphonic individuals with muscle tension have a neurotic disorder, but patients with generalised anxiety state are vulnerable to muscle tension dysphonia)
	Hyperventilation: can lead to a number of unpleasant symptoms such as paraesthesia, chest pain, headache, dizziness and faintness because of a drop in the CO_2 level in arterial blood (see below)
Cognitive symptoms	In these patients, the anxiety is directed towards concern that some dreadful incident will occur such as dying, losing control in public or being humiliated
Emotional symptoms	In addition to any of the above symptoms, the patient feels anxious. This can affect the whole pattern of communication significantly and vocal behaviour will reflect these emotions

PERSONALITY DISORDER

Individuals with personality disorders also experience anxieties and tensions that can affect the voice. There are various categories of personality disorder.

Obsessional

These personalities are obsessional about order, routines and how things are done. Meticulous attention to detail and over-conscientiousness interfere with accomplishing tasks, and drive colleagues and family to desperation. The individual's rigid behaviour cannot be altered easily and changes are fiercely resented because they threaten the security of the routines in which the individual is entrenched. Compulsive actions arise from obsessional thoughts, the basis of which is usually a fear or a phobia. A common example is compulsive hand-washing, where the fear of contamination leads to increasingly lengthy rituals for cleaning the hands. Compulsive neuroses can produce laryngeal spasms, vowel prolongations and constantly repeated rhythmic patterns in a form of compulsive stammering.

Histrionic

Everyday incidents and encounters are exaggerated and embellished so that nothing is ordinary. Individuals' anxieties, fears and concerns are reinforced by their own dramatic accounts.

Paranoid

There is a fear that others are always critical and judgemental. As a result, offence is taken when none is intended, injustices and imagined insults are brooded over and, subsequently, the individual withdraws.

Schizoid

These personalities show emotional coldness and detachment. Few activities give pleasure.

Anxious

This is the worrier who anticipates problems and is constantly tense, apprehensive and fearful. Some people are timid, insufficiently assertive, rather humble and apologetic, while suppressing normal feelings of anger and hostility which, on occasion, explode.

Dependent

These personalities are loathe to take full responsibility and rely on others. Feelings of anxiety surface if the relationships on which the individual depends are unsatisfactory.

Emotionally unstable

This category might take the form of impulsiveness and unpredictability. The case history will reveal difficulties and anxieties at home, at work and in social contacts as a result of the personality of the individual. There may be a recital of difficulties at school, a succession of jobs or marriages, and general signs of instability. Anxiety, therefore, takes many forms and when a traumatic event or long accumulation of worries explodes into a voice problem it can indicate that the patient has reached breaking point and that this is caused by a breakdown in personal relationships. These anxious individuals are difficult to get on with and their sensitivity, prejudices, intolerances and criticisms of others create disagreements, ill-feeling and lack of cooperation. They become immersed in their own miseries and have a distorted perception of events, unable to see both sides of the question. Unable to cope, the voice disorder is a cry for help that is not necessarily recognised and, in any case, could not be admitted overtly, because this would be an admission of failure and inadequacy, and recognition of suppressed fear.

AFFECTIVE (MOOD) DISORDERS

Affective disorders typically involve depression. The term 'bipolar disorder' is now used to refer to manic–depression. Depression is graded as mild, moderate or severe, with the patient appearing depressed and uninterested by usual activities. Feelings of guilt, worthlessness and fatigue predominate and are compounded by anxiety. The uniformity of intonation and a limited pitch range are characteristic of depression (Moses, 1954), whereas excessively wide pitch variation, high pitch and fast tempo are typical of manic states.

Somatisation and psychosomatic symptoms

Somatisation is a feature of a number of categories of psychological disturbance. It is the tendency to produce symptoms that either appear to be physical or are attributed to physical illness by the sufferer in the absence of organic or neurological aetiology. There is frequently a long history of physical complaints with negative findings on investigation. Despite a lack of pathological evidence followed by detailed reassurance, many patients continue to request further clinical investigations. These symptoms tend to occur at times of particular stress, but the underlying cause is frequently genuinely denied by the patient as being related to the symptoms. Somatisation does not necessarily occur in isolation. The clinical picture can be complicated when it coexists with and contributes to physical illness. Anxiety upsets the homoeostasis of the whole organism, including the regulatory mechanisms of the body that are controlled by the autonomic and sympathetic nervous system, thus influencing the endocrine mechanism and release of hormones (Linford Rees, 1982). In this way, psychogenic disorder produces physical symptoms known as psychosomatic symptoms because the mental and physical states are interdependent. When in harmony or homoeostasis, health endures. When out of tune, illnesses of every sort can appear. Psychosomatic symptoms assume many forms and only careful medical examination can determine whether or not such symptoms are organically based. The following conditions frequently have a psychosomatic component and many of the symptoms of these conditions can be mimicked by psychosomatic symptoms.

- Respiratory: vasomotor rhinitis, hay fever, asthma, hyperventilation.
- Dermatological: eczema, urticaria, psoriasis.
- Endocrinological: hyperthyroidism, diabetes mellitus.
- Cardiovascular: hypertension, cardiac symptoms, palpitations, headache.
- Hormonal: premenstrual tension, menopausal disturbances.
- Gastrointestinal: ulcer, indigestion, anorexia nervosa, dry mouth, urgency.
- Excessive sweating: particularly on forehead, upper lip, palms of hands.
- Sleep disturbance: insomnia and fatigue.
- Thought disturbance: forgetfulness, confusion, disorganisation, phobias.
- Musculoskeletal tension: joint pains and muscle pains (myalgia).

A thorough medical examination is necessary to ascertain the validity of the patient's complaints and to prescribe appropriate treatment. Such symptoms as peptic ulcer and high blood pressure are not difficult to diagnose. It is in less well-defined areas, such as asthma, migraine and rheumatic pains, that the degree of psychological involvement is difficult to ascertain, particularly as it is known that there is a threefold increase in psychological disorder in patients with medical illness (Murray, Hill and McGuffin, 1997).

Differential diagnosis

There are a number of organically based symptoms of ill-health that can be mistaken for emotional disturbance. For example, thyrotoxicosis and hypoglycaemia can present with complaints of anxiety, and complaints of breathlessness could be confused with asthma and pulmonary embolus. If the patient is not incapacitated by the symptoms, it is frequently expected by the doctor that they must be endured although, in fact, they may be helped by medication. The attribution of symptoms to psychological factors should be a diagnosis of exclusion; possible organic causes must always be investigated fully in order to ensure that serious organic aetiology is not overlooked (see case history on page 194). This tenet applies to voice disorders as well as the conditions below, which might also coexist with psychogenic or organic dysphonia.

MENSTRUAL DISORDERS

Hormonal disturbance in women, associated with menstrual and reproductive functions, affects mood and energy. Premenstrual syndrome, postnatal depression and the menopause can produce excessive fatigue, irritability and anxiety. Suitable hormonal treatment is available in many instances. Progesterone may be prescribed for premenstrual syndrome and hormone replacement therapy (HRT) is being used increasingly to relieve the unpleasant symptoms of the menopause. Such treatments can restore the patient's energy and feeling of well-being.

CHRONIC FATIGUE SYNDROME

Chronic fatigue syndrome (CFS) is also known as postviral fatigue syndrome, myalgic encephalomyelitis (ME) or neurasthenia. CFS may follow an acute attack of 'flu and the patient feels tired and depressed for many months and years. The aetiology of this condition has been the subject of much debate, but increasingly it is thought to be multifactorial. A possible course is fatigue after a viral infection from which most individuals gradually recover. In the case of the CFS sufferer, recovery might be delayed by other factors such as stress or depression, and is then further compounded by prolonged inactivity and the belief that the continuing problem is likely to be exacerbated by too much activity. These patients may be regarded unsympathetically as neurotic and hyperchondriacal, or told that their condition is entirely physical. Persisting fatigue and lethargy can be purely psychological, as in the case of John Cleese (Skynner and Cleese, 1983) who appeared to suffer from 'low grade flu symptoms' for 2 years before embarking on a successful course of family therapy to treat his depression (Skynner, 1976), but syndromes such as CFS continue to be the subject of debate between doctors regarding the contributions of organic and psychogenic factors.

ALLERGY AND HYPERSENSITIVITY

Reactions to specific substances can produce results that resemble psychogenic symptoms. An interesting case is described by Freeman et al. (1987). The episodic dysphonia of a young professional woman was initially diagnosed as 'hysterical and/or spasmodic dysphonia'. Although there was no evidence of earlier allergic reactions, careful stroboscopic investigation by the research team revealed a hypersensitive reaction to a particular loft insulation material. This reaction occurred only in the larynx and consisted of oedema and stiffness of the vocal folds. There was complete absence of the closed phase of vocal fold vibration. Freeman et al. (1987) concluded that reaction to specific environmental agents should always be considered in cases of psychogenic dysphonia.

NEUROPATHOLOGY

The differentiation of psychogenic and neurogenic dysphonia can be complex, particularly in the early stages or when the condition is subject to remissions and relapses. The early stages of neurological disease can mimic psychogenic dysphonia. Aronson (1971) describes a case of early motor neuron disease masquerading as psychogenic breathy dysphonia. The situation is even more complex if the dysphonia is accompanied by a neurological condition that might potentially affect the voice, but that is not necessarily giving rise to a voice disorder. The diagnostic problem is compounded by the fact that some diseases of the central nervous system can affect the voice, although no abnormality is visible on laryngoscopy (Sapir and Aronson, 1987). As a result, neurological dysphonias can be misdiagnosed as psychogenic. The case below also illustrates the importance of careful clinical investigation particularly when the context of the onset of symptoms and ambiguous signs lead the clinician to an initial diagnosis of a psychogenic condition.

Case histories

Neuropathology presenting as possibly psychogenic

A 34-year-old male patient was admitted to the ENT ward with swallowing difficulties the day after a low-impact road traffic accident (RTA). During the previous afternoon, he was sitting in his car in a line of traffic when the car behind hit the rear of his stationary vehicle at an estimated 15 mph. Although he was shaken by the incident, he was not injured. During the night, he reported, he had woken aware that he was having difficulty swallowing his saliva and was coughing after attempted swallows. During the first day of the patient's admission, the results of various examinations were negative; the only hard sign continued to be his dysphagia, including his inability to swallow his own secretions. The patient was calm and cooperative. In the light of the negative findings, over the next 24 hours members of the clinical team began to suggest that the presentation was possibly psychogenic. It is well known that symptoms can be produced or exacerbated by litigation and, in this case, there was the possibility that the patient might initiate legal proceedings against the driver who had crashed into his car. Meanwhile, the speech–language pathologist was asked to see the patient regarding his swallowing difficulties. It was noted that there was mild hoarseness but the voice quality was probably on the borderline of normality.

Careful attention to the patient's speech patterns revealed minimal hypernasality and barely audible nasal emission of air, most obvious on the articulation of bilateral plosives. Simple oromotor examination was almost unremarkable, but on second and third repetition of the examination there was slight deviation of the tongue to the left on protrusion and minimal deviation of the soft palate to the left on elevation. When each task was repeated, the deviation became more pronounced. On being asked if he had noticed any other problems, the patient reported that the only rather odd thing that he had noticed was that, when he had used his deodorant that morning, he could feel the spray under one armpit but not under the other. At the ward round early on the third morning of the patient's admission, palatal movement appeared normal but the dysphagia was unchanged. Although the psychogenic possibility was again discussed, it was felt that a neurological opinion should be sought. The neurologist concluded that the patient was presenting with lateral medullary syndrome, a condition affecting the nucleus ambiguus and resulting in palatal and pharyngeal involvement, with vocal fold paralysis a common presenting feature. It is possible that this patient had sustained this damage during the collision. The lack of positive findings initially, in conjunction with the patient's calm acceptance of the fact that he was having severe swallowing difficulties, led the clinical team to consider that his dysphagia might be psychogenic. Repeated, careful testing of oromotor movements provided enough evidence to merit a neurologist's opinion.

Psychogenic aetiology presenting as possibly organic

A 32-year-old woman was referred for voice therapy because of her intermittent dysphonia. She complained that her throat felt extremely constricted and that she was finding it difficult to swallow. She was very thin, looked unwell and reported that she was losing weight rapidly. Laryngeal examination was normal and videofluoroscopic examination of her swallowing was within normal limits. The results of a range of blood tests and other examinations were unremarkable. When it was explained to her that no abnormality had been found, the possibility of stress-related factors was introduced carefully. Her response was very aggressive and she was not prepared to consider this possibility. As she was dysphonic and as she looked so ill, voice therapy was started with the aim of getting to know her while working on relaxation and other techniques No strategy or technique produced any lasting benefit. When some improvement could be achieved in the controlled clinical situation, her voice rapidly deteriorated after a few minutes. She continued to describe her swallowing problems, although there was no demonstrable abnormality. Eventually, she was referred to a psychiatrist. This patient appeared to have a physical condition causing her dysphagia and, possibly, her voice disorder. The fact that she looked so unwell seemed to indicate an underlying physical condition and, as psychogenic aetiology is a diagnosis of exclusion, rigorous investigations were carried out. Finally, it was concluded that there was a psychological basis for her problems that she was not prepared or able to confront.

Multiple psychogenic symptoms

Mrs E (Aged 47 years)

The laryngologist referred this patient with a normal larynx for speech therapy because her voice grew tired during long conversations. Mrs E spoke rapidly with few pauses in a light, girlish voice and used frequent hard glottal attack. Sentences were frequently incomplete and she changed subjects rapidly and bewilderingly. She asked questions and either answered them herself, or apparently did not listen to the answers because she would ask the same question again a few minutes later. Her first appointment with the speech–language pathologist was delayed because she confused the date for the first visit and, as she lost her way on the next visit, it began late. She reported that, although her voice was troublesome, her chief concern was the discomfort in her throat and she admitted that she was terrified that this was cancer that the laryngologist had overlooked. Her father had died of laryngeal cancer as had a much-loved uncle.

This patient needed reassurance and sympathetic understanding combined with a matter-of-fact pragmatic approach to establish more relaxed and effective phonation. Throughout her visits over several months, in addition to her throat symptoms, she was also experiencing stomach pains that were found not to have an organic basis. Gradually, she was able to acknowledge when her anxiety was peaking and that it was unfounded. She was the long-awaited only child of over-protective parents upon whom she had been dependent. She married a man much older than herself and retained her dependent role. Much of her anxiety seemed to arise from the fact that she did not feel that she could competently control and organise her own life. These feelings were discussed during treatment. When her throat symptoms were marked, she was seen by the laryngologist for indirect laryngoscopy to provide additional reassurance and to confirm that there was no organic basis for her symptoms. As time progressed, it was possible to discontinue clinical appointments and the patient was able to deal with her anxiety by telephoning the speech–language pathologist from time to time, and the throat symptoms abated. The voice remained 'girlish' but improved breath support, reduction of hard glottal attack and tempo ensured that it was no longer a problem.

These cases highlight the fact that psychogenic dysphonia or aphonia is a diagnosis of exclusion. While there is the possibility that any aspect of the presenting problem might be organic, even if the patient is excessively anxious or distressed and leads the clinician to the intuitive diagnosis of a psychogenic disorder, it is obligatory to pursue full investigations. Similarly, while the patient does not respond to a psychogenic treatment approach, the possibility of an organic condition or neuropathology must be borne in mind.

Symptoms of psychogenic voice disorders

Many of the symptoms of psychogenic voice disorders are similar to those described by patients with muscle tension dysphonias (see Chapter 7). The voice is frequently effortful to produce and the patient describes vocal fatigue and, in many instances, vocal tract discomfort. It is the way in which patients recount the history and their perception of the vocal symptoms that is significant for the clinician. The reaction might be excessive for the severity of the presenting problem or remarkably understated where far greater concern and distress would be more realistic in the light of significant impairment.

Signs of psychogenic voice disorders

Psychogenic voice disorders can present with a wide range of features, but there are certain common factors. They are not all necessarily found in each patient:

- The signs and symptoms are inconsistent with the clinical examination. The laryngeal findings show that there is the potential for normal phonation, i.e. the vocal folds are capable of adduction and there is no structural abnormality, but the voice is abnormal. In cases where there is coexisting laryngeal pathology, the voice may be much worse than the appearance suggests.

- The presentation is not always consistent. A normal vocal note might be heard on vegetative behaviours such as coughing, throat clearing, yawning or laughing, but not when the voice is being used for communication. During conversation the voice varies according to social context, subject matter and the mood of the patient.
- The history and presentation might be inconsistent with any known condition.
- Various therapeutic approaches can produce normal voice, however fleeting, almost immediately.
- The voice disorder might be episodic. Abnormal voice or aphonia is interspersed with periods of normal voice.
- The patient describes, or the history reveals, related stressful events or prolonged stress.

Aetiology

Psychogenic voice disorders are frequently multifactorial, and it is accepted that they are the result of psychosocial stress and triggered by emotional conflicts (Andersson and Schlalen, 1998). Depending on the duration of the problem when the patient attends for treatment, the voice reflects not only the current psychological status of the individual but also vocal habit. In some instances, the precipitating stressful event or circumstances have passed and the patient is no longer unduly stressed or distressed, but the kinaesthetic model for normal phonation cannot be retrieved and so the problem persists Other patients are overtly distressed, apparently because of their vocal problems, but it becomes clear that the voice is a focus for more widespread difficulties. Inability or reluctance to express emotion is a common feature in psychogenic voice disorders and, as a result, the individual retains a tense, stoic countenance.

A study of patients with psychogenic voice disorders by Butcher et al. (1987) supports the impression that certain life events are frequently implicated in psychogenic voice disorders. Family and interpersonal relationships are the dominant feature in most cases. Butcher et al. (1987) found that the stressful situations for these patients could be classified into three groups.

• Family and interpersonal relationship difficulties

The dominant features were marital conflicts and disturbed relationships with children in their teens and 20s. The children appeared to be immature while the parent was dominated and controlled by the child and had little independence. These patients frequently had difficulty expressing their feelings, particularly negative feelings, and feared losing complete control if they expressed their true emotions. Individuals with personality disorder also fall within this category. The most common psychological/behavioural factor in this group was excessive anxiety and musculoskeletal tension.

• Burden of responsibility

These patients were overwhelmed by family responsibilities, such as the care of an elderly parent, and had little support emotionally or practically.

• Stressful factors associated with work

When individuals work very long hours or under difficult conditions it can be extremely stressful and affects relationships at home, which adds to the stress.

Andersson and Schlalen (1998), in their study of the aetiology of psychogenic voice disorders, confirmed the importance of family and work stresses as major contributory factors. Rather than a specific life event acting as a trigger, their subjects revealed that the long-term effects of conflicts and frustrations finally gave rise to the problem. They concluded that psychogenic voice disorders indicate a disturbed capacity for emotional expression.

Psychogenic aphonia

Total loss of voice in the absence of organic pathology is a dramatic symptom and patients presenting with psychogenic aphonia can be divided into two groups. The majority of patients become aphonic because of prolonged stress and so produce a stress-related aphonia. A smaller number develop a true conversion symptom aphonia.

STRESS-RELATED APHONIA

Most of these patients are women who usually present as tense, anxious and distressed by their aphonia. Some suspect that the loss of voice is related to life events, whereas others are extremely upset that they have produced a psychogenic symptom. It is a common feature of this group that, during detailed case history taking, as information concerning family and work is discussed, the patient is either near to tears or begins to weep. Some patients describe that they have not cried throughout a long period while they have been under stress. In some instances, the precipitating feature is a major life event such as a bereavement, whereas in others there is a much longer history of either a sequence of stressful events or a prolonged period of stress.

A significant number of cases appear to be extremely competent individuals who regard themselves as being able to deal with most difficult situations. They are relied on by others because they are known for their coping abilities and as a result they become over-burdened. The onset of the aphonia can be associated with an upper respiratory tract infection, although not necessarily. Prognosis is good in patients who are able to develop insight into the psychosomatic basis of the aphonia (Harris and Thompson, 1999). Although this group has the symptom of non-organic aphonia in common with conversion symptom aphonia (see below), stress-related aphonia is not necessarily a symptom of underlying psychiatric illness. It is an indication that stress has become intolerable.

CONVERSION SYMPTOM APHONIA

A conversion symptom is a physical symptom that occurs in the presence of normal physical structure and potentially normal function of the body part involved. It is essentially a psychogenic illness with a characteristic motive of gain of which the individual is unaware. It differs from psychosomatic symptoms that are the reaction of the autonomic system to stress. In the individual suffering from a conversion symptom, the physical symptom concerns the somatic nervous system, although it appears to be involuntary and is outside the patient's control. The conversion symptom conforms to the patient's concept of the disability and will therefore exhibit various anomalies. Someone with writer's cramp, with the hand and arm going into painful spastic spasm, has the symptom in writing only and in no other movement. A conversion symptom anaesthesia may be found to involve the lower part of a limb, following a 'glove and stocking' distribution and therefore not neurologically viable. No voice is produced in conversion symptom aphonia, although the vocal folds adduct and behave normally during other functions. The conversion symptom is not evidence of malingering because it is not produced consciously or for intentional advantage or avoidance. Aronson (1990) lists the criteria for conversion reactions:

- They produce specific physical symptoms or syndromes that cannot be traced to any anatomical or physiological disease.
- They are unconscious simulations of illness that the patient is convinced are organically based.
- They serve the psychological purpose of enabling the patient to avoid awareness of emotional conflict, stress or personal failure that would be intolerable if faced directly.

- They can occur in any sensory or voluntary motor system.

In the past, conversion symptoms were known as 'hysterical' conditions, which derives from the Greek for womb or uterus, *husterikos*. As these conditions occur more commonly in women than in men, they were thought to result from disturbance of uterine function (Thomson, 1976).

Specific symptoms

The patient reports complete loss of voice of sudden onset, sometimes after an upper respiratory tract infection. Some patients describe a history of aphonic episodes of increasing frequency and duration, whereas others find that they have no voice on waking one morning. The lack of voice may be accompanied by globus sensations (see page 218). Typically, the patient does not associate the problem with emotional issues.

Specific signs

- On examination there is no vocal tract structural abnormality or any neuropathology.
- Conversion symptom aphonia is unusual in its dramatic presentation. There are relatively few organic conditions that result in such total lack of voice. Occasionally, squeaks of voice are heard during conversation but a normal vocal note might be heard on vegetative behaviours. It is significant that the patient does not appear to recognise these manifestations of the normal voice as potentially useful for speech. Some patients are almost silent as they speak and, although some over-articulate in an attempt to make themselves understood, a small number use minimal articulation or write down whatever they want to communicate.
- Onset is frequently sudden and in some cases there is a history of episodes of aphonia interspersed with periods of normal voice.
- Symptom incongruity can result from the tendency of the condition to conform to the patient's conception of the disorder. For example, some patients resort to writing because they feel that they are unable to talk. They do not consider the possibility of articulating without voice, although they are capable of doing so.
- A pronounced feature of the disorder is the detached attitude sufferers exhibit towards their afflictions, described by Janet (1920) as 'la belle indifference'. Organically based paralysis of the leg or hand normally produces acute concern about the cause and the future economic consequences of the inability to work. However, the 'hysteric' exhibits indifference and real lack of concern, conveyed positively in

the paralinguistic behaviour, although the inconveniences may be expressed verbally. A long-suffering attitude is attenuated by a certain stoicism and the patient obtains sympathy and commendation for being so courageous in the face of such adversity.

- Voice can be elicited almost immediately by appropriate strategies in many cases.

Aetiology

The conversion symptom personality

This personality differs from that of someone with an anxiety state. Someone with a conversion symptom personality craves attention and seeks the limelight, with a proclivity for histrionics and a tendency to exaggerate and dramatise. The craving for love and attention is so acute and the individual can be so demanding that people are driven away. At the same time there may be considerable manipulation of family members, friends, colleagues and even strangers. When things are going well, a conversion symptom is not necessary. The conversion symptom is assumed without conscious awareness of any connection between its appearance and the reason for it and the advantage that it represents. The exact nature of the mental process that happens 'when the mysterious leap from the mental to the physical' is made (Freud, 1943) is not fully understood. Freud thought that the imaginary symptom symbolised conflict and reflected the conversion of mental torture into acceptable physical discomfort.

Precipitating factors

The onset of a conversion symptom may be precipitated by an emotional shock such as a disaster in the family or at work. In many instances, however, it appears that the gradual accumulation of stress eventually results in the conversion symptom when the individual can no longer cope and suffers the proverbial straw that breaks the camel's back. In such cases it may be precipitated by illness, particularly an upper respiratory tract infection and a viral laryngitis. In unusual circumstances, previously stable and well-integrated individuals produce conversion symptoms when life is intolerable. Smurthwaite (1919) and Sokolowsky and Junkermann (1944) reported hysterical voice disorders in soldiers returning from the battle front in World War I.

Disassociation

Under intolerable stress, the individual evades it by disassociating thoughts from the stressful situation and directs them into imagined disability which effectively provides a means of escape. For example, loss of voice in a teacher solves the horror of trying to control an unruly class.

Primary and secondary gains

Although the patient does not produce the symptom consciously, it inevitably brings certain advantages. The primary gain of a conversion symptom aphonia is that the lack of voice prevents the patient from communicating effectively in an intolerable situation. The attention and sympathy that accrue from the obvious disability comprise the secondary gain.

> ### Case history
>
> Mrs C (36 years) was referred for speech therapy with aphonia which started with an upper respiratory tract infection. On indirect laryngoscopy there was no laryngeal abnormality. She had been aphonic for 16 months, during which time she had visited her general practitioner repeatedly for advice and medication without improvement. Eventually she was referred to a laryngologist.
>
> During the interview with the speech–language pathologist, she was vivacious and verbose, all conversation being conducted in a forced whisper. She was not unduly concerned by her lack of voice. Having reassured her that there was no reason why the voice should not recover completely, the therapist gently massaged her extrinsic laryngeal muscles so that the larynx could be moved freely. She was encouraged to cough and then to give a cough immediately followed by various vowels. Within 5 minutes she was counting, saying the days of the week, etc. and after 10 minutes was phonating throughout conversation. The patient was tearful and amazed that her voice had returned so quickly after its long absence. As a result of the explanations given to her about the reasons for such symptoms, she was soon able to identify the precipitating factor. She had two children, a girl of 14 years and a boy of 10 years. She felt that there had been constant conflict with her daughter over everything from homework to the time that she should come home and the suitability of her clothes. The arguments between mother and daughter were disrupting the whole family, with her husband blaming her for not being able to control their daughter. It was significant that the family had been more cooperative since the mother had been voiceless, and that the father fulfilled a more positive role in relation to his daughter since his wife had been unable to shout. Two further appointments directed at establishing a secure voice through traditional voice therapy in combination with counselling ensured the stable return of her voice.

Incidence

Conversion symptom aphonia is more common in women than in men, occurring in a ratio of 7:1. Its greatest incidence is between the ages of 18 and 34 years. The reaction is rare in childhood, although cases do occur. It appears that aphonia as a conversion symptom is on the decrease as a result of a better informed and more sophisticated public. During the past 30 years, we have observed that the conversion aphonias seen in our clinics have become less naive in type and pattern. We no longer see cases where the voice disappears on Monday morning as the unpleasant working week starts, only to return on Friday evening and then continue the pattern as the week begins again. We have the impression that increased knowledge does not allow the individual to produce a symptom of such transparency.

Laryngoscopic findings

The vocal folds abduct satisfactorily but do not adduct fully during phonation. Complete adduction is seen for other tasks such as coughing but not necessarily if the patient is requested to perform the manoeuvre. Occasionally, in the absence of the atrophy of the elderly larynx, the vocal folds in the case of conversion symptom aphonia are bowed or elliptical (Morrison and Rammage, 1994). Morrison, Nichol and Rammage (1986) also note that conversion symptom dysphonia may present as hyperadducted ventricular band aphonia as well as the more classic glottic chink. Their studies reveal no direct correlation in psychogenic dysphonias between laryngoscopic appearance and the various psychiatric diagnoses. The indirect laryngological examination may be easily accomplished as a result of reduced sensation of the throat and palate. This is a distinguishing difference from anxiety state where patients can be very apprehensive and resistant to laryngeal examination and apparently hypersensitive to any contact by the laryngoscope, resulting in gagging.

Case note

Two young women patients, each in their 20s, attended the combined voice clinic on separate occasions with conversion symptom aphonia. The similarities in the way they presented were striking. In both cases the symptom they produced was not the forced, loud whisper more commonly heard but an almost silent aphonia. Their demeanour was poised and restrained. On examination, in each case, it was possible to touch the soft palate, the faucial arches and the posterior wall of the pharynx without causing gagging. Both women started to shed tears silently during the examination while continuing to cooperate and without resisting. The clinical team subsequently discussed the similarity of these cases and the unusual features. In sessions with the speech–language pathologist, it was discovered, as the voice returned in each case, that these women had both been sexually abused in childhood and during their teens. Now in their 20s, the memories of these experiences were becoming increasingly difficult to deal with. Following discussion, they were both relieved to be referred to a psychiatrist.

Expected vocal profile

Most patients with a conversion symptom voice disorder are aphonic and the aphonia can range from silent mouthing of words to a forced, loud, 'stage whisper'. Some patients present with a **conversion symptom dysphonia**. The dysphonic variant can present very differently within the same patient so that the vocal profile differs according to the context and content of the conversation. Conversion symptom dysphonias represent the diversity of all possible phonation types. Forced, creaky, diplophonic voice produced by a 'sphincteric' larynx occurs as well as voice that is weak, breathy and lacking in power.

Acoustic analysis profile

It is neither appropriate nor relevant in clinical practice to subject these patients to instrumental assessment of vocal function, which might only compound and reinforce the conversion symptom. The case history, laryngoscopic examination and perceptual evaluation should indicate the diagnosis of conversion symptom aphonia. It is incumbent upon the speech–language pathologist at this point to implement the strategies for restoring the voice with minimal delay (see Chapter 15).

Medicosurgical decisions

Following laryngoscopy, management decisions should be taken and implemented without delay. Most cases should be seen by the speech–language pathologist as soon as possible, preferably immediately, with the aim of restoring voice in the first treatment session. Subsequent treatment sessions stabilise the voice and provide support and counselling. It will become apparent gradually that the emotional difficulties of some patients, even when the voice has been restored, will require the help of a trained counsellor or psychotherapist. Patients with a history of psychiatric disturbance whose behaviour gives cause for concern or patients who exhibit signs of marked mental or behavioural illness should be referred to a psychiatrist. Voice therapy is successful with patients in whom conversion is not too deeply entrenched. Indicators for early recovery are an acute onset, short duration, stable relationships and permanence of occupation. In favourable circumstances, the speech–language pathologist may be more successful than a psychiatrist. If the patient's voice does not recover after a few sessions, referral for a psychiatric opinion should be considered. Lengthy unsuccessful treatment not only reinforces a conversion symptom but might also ignore an alternative aetiology.

Psychogenic spasmodic dysphonia

It is now accepted that spasmodic dysphonia (SD) is a focal laryngeal dystonia of neurological origin (see Chapter 10), although there are a number of patients who present with the signs of SD whose difficulties are psychogenic. In both manifestations, the spasmodic adduction or abduction of the vocal folds during phonation dramatically interferes with phonation. The adductor form, resulting in effortful laryngeal spasms, is more common than the involuntary voiceless segments of the abductor type. Emotional elements are significant in both conditions. Aronson (1980) established that 40% of the patients he examined had experienced emotional trauma before onset of the condition. The bizarre phonatory spasms of laryngeal dystonia inevitably affect communication and attract unwanted attention, leading to feelings of depression and anxiety (see page 292). In psychogenic SD, the psychodynamics appear to be similar to those of conversion symptoms. The individual seeks help because of the inconvenient problem, but is not necessarily particularly distressed. A history of episodic SD combined with evidence in the case history will indicate a psychogenic condition. Trial voice therapy that resolves the condition confirms the tentative diagnosis (Damsté, 1983).

Case histories

Mr F

Mr F (38 years), a married man with two young children, was referred for voice therapy with the diagnosis 'hoarse voice; vocal cords normal'. As he spoke, there was frequent laryngospasm and speech required considerable effort. The symptoms were those of spasmodic dysphonia. His manner was incongruously cheerful in the light of his obvious difficulty in phonating; his laughter was normal.

The case history revealed that a 'catch' in his voice had become noticeable shortly after he had been told that he was to be made redundant from his job as an accountant. Phonation had become increasingly effortful in the 5 weeks before seeing the laryngologist. He was now in the process of applying for another job. Although he found it difficult to believe that there was any connection between losing his job and his dysphonia, he was highly motivated to comply with therapy because of forthcoming interviews. Relaxation and breathing strategies, followed by work on voiced sighs and the elimination of hard glottal attack in order to avoid inducing laryngospasm, proved to be the most effective method of treatment. Cheerfully and politely, he rejected all attempts at discussion of the underlying aspects of his problem. As he became able to produce vowel strings with normal voice and his confidence increased in applying these principles to normal speech, carryover was apparent. Although the voice was not entirely normal, he dealt with the job interviews successfully and started his new job. Eventually, he telephoned to report that he was too busy to have further treatment and that his voice was fine, which did indeed seem to be the case. There was no evidence of the spasmodic dysphonia which must have been psychogenic.

Mrs L

Mrs L, a middle-aged woman who worked in a hospital, was referred for voice therapy for her aphonia. She was devoted to her husband who was retired. (They had no children.) He had not been well recently and had 'passed out' several times and been admitted to hospital for tests. While she was talking over her concerns about her husband, and the thought of having to leave him at home alone while she was at work, her voice returned. It was discovered that her husband had diabetes and he soon returned home with a strict diet to observe. Some weeks later the patient returned. This time she was not aphonic, but her voice 'sounded terrible' and she was having difficulty speaking. She had a typical adductor spasmodic dysphonia. The precipitating problem was that her husband's diet was expensive and she was having financial difficulties. Once she had exposed her anxiety and fears, symptomatic treatment restored the voice to normal. She was then referred to the dietitian for advice about her husband's diet and to the medical social worker for help with financial problems. This case of conversion symptom aphonia initially and subsequent spasmodic dysphonia that responded rapidly to treatment was unquestionably a psychogenic disorder.

Mrs D

Mrs D was referred for voice therapy with a diagnosis of spasmodic dysphonia. The presentation was classic, apart from the fact that the history was of dysphonic episodes with normal voice in the intervening periods. Mrs D was adamant that there were no obvious correlating events and that she was not under any stress. All was well with her three children and her marriage was happy. Working on the basis that there was almost certainly a common factor to these episodes, the speech–language pathologist explored Mrs D's lifestyle during conversation, and also explained that it is possible to have trigger factors that are not obvious. The cause of the problem gradually emerged. Although Mrs D was happily married and very fond of her husband, she had a lover of whom her husband was unaware. She also had a second lover, unknown to either of the other men. As her husband was very good to her, she asserted that she did not want to hurt him and that it was essential that he should not find out about her lovers. During the conversation, she realised that each episode of spasmodic dysphonia occurred at a time when her illicit relationships were almost discovered. Within the next 20 minutes, after some simple voice exercises, her voice returned to normal. She was reviewed from time to time during the following year and her voice remained normal throughout.

Table 8.4 Psychogenic spasmodic dysphonia (SD)	
Symptoms	Patient complains of 'catch' in the voice initially which progresses to effortful, 'strangled' voice
Signs	'Strangled' phonation Episodes of SD interspersed with normal voice Vegetative laryngeal functions, e.g. coughing, laughing, may be normal Sung notes may be normal
Aetiology	Psychogenic; resembles a conversion symptom
Laryngoscopic findings	Vocal folds – normal structure and function except on phonation Uncontrolled, sphincteric, vocal fold adduction on phonation
Expected vocal profile	Normal apart from laryngeal spasm on phonation
Acoustic analysis profile	As with conversion symptom aphonia, instrumental analysis of vocal function is inappropriate
Medicosurgical decisions	Management depends on the differential diagnosis between SD (laryngeal dystonia) and psychogenic SD. It might be possible to determine the correct aetiology only by trial voice therapy Psychogenic SD: refer for voice therapy

Puberphonia (mutational falsetto)

During adolescence, the boy's larynx achieves adult dimensions, the vocal folds double in length and the voice 'breaks' and drops an octave into the male register. Occasionally, despite normal growth and the development of secondary sexual characteristics the adolescent retains his prepubertal voice. This is known as puberphonia, but is also referred to as failure in voice mutation or mutational falsetto. There are a number of physical conditions that may render normal voice mutation impossible and these are described in Chapter 11.

SYMPTOMS

Acoustic symptoms

The patient complains that the pitch of his voice is too high or that it has never 'broken' and that it does not have sufficient power. In some cases, he reports that he produces a deeper voice when he coughs or laughs, but that these occasions are fleeting. He may also explain that he is able to produce a deeper voice but that it feels so unnatural he is unable to sustain it in everyday life.

Sensory symptoms

Phonation can be effortful and the voice tires easily when excessive loudness is required. Some patients experience supralaryngeal pain as a result of the larynx being maintained abnormally high in the vocal tract (Hartman and Aronson, 1983). However, excessive tension does not necessarily always exist in association with falsetto voices and, when an individual produces this voice quite easily, vocal strain does not necessarily occur.

Emotional status

Distress at the failure to develop a mature voice is commonly expressed because of the social consequences. Boys in their teens are frequently subjected to taunts and ridicule based on the victim's perceived lack of manliness.

SIGNS

- A postpubertal male patient with normal secondary sexual characteristics presents with an unbroken or falsetto voice. Pitch breaks into the mature male voice may or may not be heard during spontaneous conversation or during vegetative behaviours such as coughing, laughing or shouting.
- The larynx is held high in the vocal tract.
- The patient is generally very concerned about his symptoms and highly motivated to learn about and reverse the condition. A small number of patients are unconcerned by the problem and have been persuaded to attend for treatment by friends and family. The prognosis for this group is poor.

AETIOLOGY

Various explanations for the retention of the child's voice have been suggested, and it is possible that a number of factors contribute to the disorder:

- Unusually early 'breaking' of the voice which renders the boy self-conscious among his contemporaries leading him to favour the boy's voice. The tension adjustments required to retain a prepubertal voice in a maturing vocal tract become habitual and the speaker finds that he is unable to achieve normal voice voluntarily (West, Ansbury and Carr, 1957).
- Late development of sexual maturity may cause similar problems.
- A desire to retain an outstanding treble voice that has brought distinction when it is known that loss of this singing voice will mean loss

of attention. During the period immediately before puberty, the boy might have singing obligations to fulfil in his treble voice, although his larynx is beginning to undergo changes. This can again create a habitual problem.

- Fear of assuming a full share of adult responsibility or of losing maternal protection. There is unconscious assertion of immaturity by prolongation of a childish voice, especially when the boy is an only child and there is a strong bond with the mother, although the father is unsympathetic because excluded. Most of our patients have been only children or, where there are more children, the only male child. We prefer this explanation of mutational dysphonia to the complicated tale of the Oedipus complex. According to Freudian psychology, puberphonia is explained by the Oedipus complex. The boy's love for his mother reaches full strength and fantasies of incest which are unacceptable terrify him. Denial of sexual maturity and adulthood requires rejection of masculinity and use of the mature male voice. It seems evident that, whatever the fundamental origin and the relationships with his parents, there is in most cases a strong bond between mother and son. Over-protection in childhood leads to overdependence and fear of assuming adult responsibilities. Frequently, the father is seen by the boy as threatening or, at least, as a peripheral member of the family.

- If the pubertal voice change has been delayed for any reason, embarrassment at switching over to a new and more appropriate voice may ensure the perpetuation of an undesirable vocal habit. Sometimes a deeper pitch can be produced quite easily, but the patient just lacks the confidence to use this in public knowing that it will cause comment and possible ridicule.

- Hero worship of an older boy or man by a boy with a strong feminine inclination, if encouraged, may also result in rejection of the masculine voice.

- The possession of a natural tenor voice or small larynx with short vocal folds would appear to be a predisposing factor in puberphonia, although any of the above factors may help to crystallise the condition. A tenor register seems to occur more frequently than a baritone or bass in the adjusted voices of puberphonic patients, but in this Greene's (1961) observations conflict with those of Weiss (1950), whose experience with many more cases was the exact opposite.

- Severe deafness, and the inability to hear his own voice and appreciate adult male voices, may result in retention of the prepubertal voice (Greene, 1961, 1962; Wirz, 1986).

- Homosexual tendencies may be at the root of the failure to obtain vocal maturity if there is a rejection of those qualities that are associated with masculinity. Many adolescent boys pass through a pseudo-homosexual phase, which is regarded as a normal phase of development and is apparent in the 'hero worship' of an older boy or a teacher. The majority outgrow this phase and form heterosexual relationships in which male voice is an attribute.

Many cases of puberphonia resemble hyperfunctional phonation and do not appear to have an unusual or complex psychogenic aetiology. For boys whose voices steadily deepen, adjustment is relatively uncomplicated, but for others a sudden growth spurt results in a rapidly enlarging larynx and a poorly coordinated phonatory mechanism that tends to emit an erratic voice. It is understandable that, in this situation, a boy might increase laryngeal muscle tension in an attempt to stabilise the vocal note with which he is familiar. As this vocal behaviour becomes established, it becomes increasingly difficult to produce a mature voice. Van Riper and Irwin (1958) stressed the force of vocal habits in dysphonia; even if the voice symptoms start as a psychogenic symptom and the expression of emotional conflicts, they may become purely reflex and habitual.

LARYNGOSCOPIC FINDINGS

The dimensions of the larynx are within normal limits for a postpubertal male, the structure of the vocal folds are normal and they are fully mobile. On phonation, the vocal folds adduct normally but they are tense and thin with minimal mucosal waves.

DIFFERENTIAL DIAGNOSIS

The diagnostic criteria for puberphonia are a normal larynx and evidence of secondary sexual characteristics. A voice can also sound puberphonic if secondary sexual characteristics have failed to develop because of a deficiency of testosterone (see page 357). A laryngeal web (see page 239) can produce a similar effect.

EXPECTED VOCAL PROFILE

Although the predominant characteristic of the puberphonic voice is its unnaturally high pitch, there are many variations in the voices of these patients. Sometimes, the voice is a true falsetto, high and thin and exhibiting no abrupt vacillation in pitch. Most commonly, the pitch of the voice is inconsistent and breaks occur inadvertently. The voice reverts to falsetto as the deep pitch is rejected. The fundamental vocal note is clear; there is no roughness or breathiness because the vocal folds are tightened, lengthened and approximated, without air turbulence at the glottis or chaotic vocal fold vibration. It is also possible, but less common, for the voice to be perceived as particularly high pitched, although the frequency of the glottal source is within normal limits. In these cases, the supraglottal vocal tract is tense and affects the resonance of the vocal note. It is clinically important, therefore, to distinguish between the factors that underlie the puberphonic voice.

ACOUSTIC ANALYSIS PROFILE

Speaking fundamental frequency falls within the female range. Intensity and harmonics-to-noise ratio are within normal limits.

AIRFLOW AND VOLUME MEASURES

A long open phase and a short closed phase is confirmed by electroglottography (Carlson, 1995a).

MEDICOSURGICAL DECISIONS

• Voice therapy is the treatment of choice. Despite the possible psychogenic reasons for puberphonia, the results of voice therapy are excellent. The majority of patients will be highly motivated to achieve an appropriate postpubertal voice, because they have been made painfully aware of the social and career disadvantages of the 'unbroken' voice. Treatment is unlikely to be successful if the individual has no real desire to change the voice, but has responded to the pressure of others who think that treatment should be sought. Normal laryngeal growth and length of vocal folds ensure that male voice can be produced as long as the patient is cooperative. Individuals who can produce mature male voice momentarily are much easier to treat successfully than those who can produce only falsetto. Younger patients are generally easier to treat because their vocal behaviours are less entrenched and more easily modified. If treatment is given during the mutational period before years of habit have established the abnormal voice, acquisition of male voice should not be difficult.

• In the relatively few cases where voice therapy is unsuccessful, it has been suggested by Woodson and Murry (1994) that an injection of botulinum toxin (see page 298) into each cricothyroid muscle can be helpful. They hypothesise that mutational falsetto is a habitual vocal dysfunction with inappropriate activation of the cricothyroid muscles, which results in lack of use of the vocal fold adductor muscles. By temporarily deactivating the cricothyroid muscle, the remaining laryngeal musculature functions more normally. Unlike surgery, the effects of botulinum toxin are reversible.

It would be logical to assume that individuals consistently using a raised pitch so foreign to their natural pitch range might produce vocal nodules, This, however, proves to be the exception rather than the rule, and we have encountered only two patients with vocal nodules – one aged 26 years and the other 69 years.

Case histories

Case A

Aged 18 years, case A was apprenticed to a jeweller. He presented with a voice that cracked from falsetto to baritone with great ease and he was able to speak in a mature male voice at the first interview when merely asked to do so. His larynx was normal but his posture was stooping and breathing was clavicular. He had mild learning difficulties. When asked if he was 'tied to his mother's apron strings', he was astonished and replied, 'That's what my father is always saying'. He had a clever younger brother who was the father's favourite child and who 'picked on' the patient. His mother was kind and protected him from his father. However, he resented the fact that at times she was over-protective and prevented him from doing things he wanted to, such as going abroad with his friends. Both his father and mother came to the clinic separately because trouble had arisen when the patient reported to his parents that the speech–language pathologist had suggested that he should be developing his independence. Father was delighted, saying 'At last I have an expert agreeing with me'. Mother was upset. It transpired that mother would never accept that her elder son was a poor scholar and had insisted that he should stay at school until he was 18 in order to pass examinations with special tuition. He had failed to do so and, with great difficulty, his father had been allowed to find him a job that was acceptable to the mother. Father was a successful self-made man and denied that he favoured the younger son and 'picked on' the patient. He only wanted the boy to be tough.

Although A switched to a mature voice when asked to use it in the clinic, he continued to use the creaky falsetto outside. As pressure increased to use the normal voice, he ceased to attend, his mother telephoning on his behalf with a succession of excuses. She refused to let her son be referred to a psychiatrist, which was necessary, and voice therapy was terminated.

Case B

Case B was aged 16 years. The patient sought treatment because his application to become a member of a dramatic society had recently been rejected on the grounds that his voice was unsuitable, and he felt that it was not 'strong' enough for dramatic work. He was the youngest of a not very prosperous family. His speech was fast and accompanied by fidgeting movements of the head, arms and legs. His manner and dress were effeminate. He had a friend some 10 years older whom he admired greatly and with whom he spent most of his spare time. The friend had suffered from a similar disorder and had been cured by voice therapy, and had suggested similar treatment for B.

The patient was able to laugh on a normal pitch and to sing falsetto, tenor or baritone with facility and had been able to do so since the age of 13 years. He said he could not speak in a deeper voice because it made him feel silly. When a recording of his speaking voice was played, he could hardly bear to listen to it, however, because it sounded to him 'so girlish' – a healthy admission.

A tenor voice was established in exercises but great difficulty was encountered with speech. The matter was decided when the good and bad voices were recorded and contrasted, but even then prolonged discussion was necessary before he could be persuaded to speak normally outside the clinic. He first practised at work by talking to a female secretary who was fortunately profoundly and favourably impressed. Eventually he was able to use his deep voice with the men with whom he worked who had previously ridiculed his voice.

Immature voice in women

Vocal immaturity in women is less conspicuous than in males because, during adolescence, the female voice drops only 3 or 4 semitones compared with an octave in young men. However, if the woman's voice does not mature and remains that of a girl, it is an indication of an immature personality. Women who shun acceptance of adult responsibility and desire to cling to the shelter and security of childhood may cling unconsciously to the vocal pitch of childhood as a symbolic expression of their unconscious desires (Moses, 1958, 1959). The immature voice may be accompanied by immature articulation, a lisped /s/ or defective /r/. Father's or mother's little girl never grows up and this, of course, may be very appealing to the protective male, in which case it has its advantages, especially in marriage. We have treated several women with conversion symptom aphonia and dysphonia whose habitual voices were inappropriately girlish and immature. In some cases referred with vocal strain and laryngitis, the pitch disorder was obviously psychogenic. In working to produce a lower pitch and improve quality, it was also necessary to explore the immature emotional attitudes to people and problems at work and in the home. A common feature was the feeling expressed by these patients of being 'put upon' and being asked to do too much, whereas in reality they were often avoiding full responsibility. They capitalised on the kindness and helpfulness of long-suffering colleagues or indulgent relations, using voice to gain protection by emphasising their helplessness.

Trans-sexual voice

During the past 20 years, since surgical sex change procedures have been more readily available, an increasing number of trans-sexuals have been referred to speech and language therapists. A trans-sexual is an individual who is convinced that he or she is of the opposite sex to that of his or her body; this conviction frequently establishes itself early in childhood and usually before puberty. The majority of trans-sexuals seeking medical help are male (Gelder, Gath and Mayou, 1983). Female trans-sexuals can take androgens which have the effect of increasing the mass of the vocal folds with a resulting drop in vocal pitch. For this reason the female trans-sexual is less likely to be referred for voice therapy than the male whose vocal folds are not significantly affected by the oestrogen that is administered. This section therefore deals with male trans-sexuals.

AETIOLOGY

There is a feeling of estrangement from the body and a desire to alter the body to resemble that of the opposite sex. Throughout childhood and into the teens, the trans-sexual is increasingly motivated to live as a member of the opposite sex although social pressures frequently prevent the realisation of this goal. Initially, dressing as a female enables the individual to feel like a woman, although this may be possible only when alone. The condition is different from that of the transvestite where the man enjoys dressing as a woman for the purpose of sexual arousal, but continues to perceive himself as a man and does not wish to cross-dress permanently or to lose his male characteristics. It is probable that there is an overlap area in relation to trans-sexualism and transvestism. In this respect trans-sexuals are also unlike homosexuals who may dress as women in order to attract other homosexuals. The trans-sexual's sex drive is typically low (Gelder, Gath and Mayou, 1983).

The aetiology of trans-sexualism is not fully understood. Although there does not appear to be a well-defined organic basis for the condition, some researchers have suggested that little understood hormonal abnormalities during intrauterine development may be a contributory factor (Gelder, Gath and Mayou, 1983). Others propose psychological and environmental causes, although the precise mechanisms involved are unclear (Oates and Dacakis, 1983). A combination of physical and psychological factors may be the reality.

MANAGEMENT PLAN

The male trans-sexual frequently decides to seek medical help during the late teens or early 20s. The most logical treatment would appear to be directed at changing the individual's conviction that he is a man in a woman's body. However, psychotherapy is unsuccessful and the professional approach is increasingly to approach the problem with a multidisciplinary team (Bralley et al., 1978; Oates and Dacakis, 1983). The team is composed of psychiatrists, surgeons, medical social workers, speech therapists and others because of the complexity of the medical, psychological and surgical issues that must be considered in each case. Treatment is conducted on the basis of attempting to satisfy the individual's aims of taking on a woman's appearance, living as a woman and changing the body to resemble that of a woman.

GENDER REASSIGNMENT SURGERY

Presurgical phase

The individual's involvement with the team will be long term. Surgical sex change will be undertaken only when it has been established that the man is able to adjust to living daily as a member of the opposite sex. It is also essential that the man fully appreciates the problems that accompany such surgery. Sim (1981) stresses the importance of thorough psychiatric examination because of the mutilating nature of the operation which leaves the individual sterile and incapable of orgasm. In Britain, even after surgery, the male trans-sexual is still legally regarded as male. This presurgical period usually lasts for about 2 years and during this time hormones of the desired gender are prescribed.

For medical, psychological and social reasons, it is important that the change should be gradual. In response to the female hormones, breasts and female distribution of body fat develop. Hormones may produce unpleasant side effects such as nausea and dizziness or more serious risks, including thrombosis and malignant breast tumours (Gelder, Gath and Mayou, 1983). The lengthy process of electrolysis for the removal of facial hair is started and breast enlargement may be further enhanced by mammoplasty.

It is during this transition period that the speech–language pathologist usually begins to advise and treat the patient.

Postsurgical adjustment

Although there is a compelling desire to become a woman, the onset of femininity brings enormous problems. There is fear that family, friends and strangers will discover the situation if attempts are made to conceal what is happening, but complete honesty may result in rejection and isolation. In some instances the unwanted attention of curious males has to be dealt with. The individual needs encouragement for a considerable time and depression is a common feature. When gender reassignment surgery, which involves castration, penectomy and the creation of an artificial vagina (Oates and Dacakis, 1983), is eventually performed, the postoperative period may produce severe depression (Sim, 1981). Moreover, it is extremely expensive and time-consuming for the professionals involved, and the person, after much suffering, may not be satisfied with the outcome. Having undergone this prolonged pursuit of femininity and assuming female dress, hair-style and make-up, the visual result is frequently convincingly female, but the mature masculine voice is a major factor in not being accepted as a woman.

COSMETIC SURGERY AND PHONOSURGERY

Treatment procedures have as their basis a vocal tract that is anatomically and physiologically normal for a male, but not for a female. In addition, established patterns of verbal and non-verbal communication are essentially masculine. Possible treatment for these communication problems can be divided into surgery and voice therapy.

Cosmetic surgery

Surgical reduction of the thyroid cartilage (Adam's apple), also known as laryngeal shaving, is performed in order to give the much flatter appearance of the female larynx.

This is a cosmetic operation which allows the neck to resemble the female neck more closely. It does not affect the quality of the voice (Isshiki, 1980).

Phonosurgery

Phonosurgery (surgery involving the vocal folds) for trans-sexuals is still relatively experimental and does not always produce satisfactory results. Various procedures are advocated to raise vocal pitch by changing the mass, length and tension (or stiffness) of the vocal folds. Isshiki (1980) notes that stiffness is the most important factor. Bralley et al. (1978) describe restriction of the anterior third of the vibrating segment of the vocal folds. These authors also note the work of Donald (1982) who describes a procedure in which a laryngeal web is created in order to obtain raised vocal pitch. A procedure that involves removing the anterior third of the vocal folds, and then stretching them and reattaching them to the thyroid cartilage, is described by Oates and Dacakis (1983). This has the effect of increasing vocal fold tension and decreasing vocal fold mass so that higher fundamental frequency is produced.

Isshiki (1980) regards three types of intervention as possible in these cases:

1. Increasing vocal fold tension by cricothyroid approximation.
2. A longitudinal incision of the vocal folds.
3. Steroid injection into the vocal folds in order to reduce mass. The rationale of the steroid injection is that steroids cause local atrophy but the authors report that the results are unsatisfactory.

Surgical intervention in these cases is still experimental and maintaining an unobstructed airway and avoiding marked deterioration in voice quality are major considerations.

Voice therapy

Voice therapy is only one aspect of a speech therapy programme concerned with many aspects of verbal and non-verbal communication, including a careful analysis of the individual's communicative behaviour (see Chapter 15).

Other psychogenic vocal tract disorders

GLOBUS PHARYNGEUS (GLOBUS SYMPTOM; GLOBUS SYNDROME)

Globus pharyngeus refers to the sensation of a lump in the throat in the absence of true dysphagia. It may accompany aphonia or dysphonia. It was previously known as 'globus hystericus', but this terminology is now regarded as outdated as evidence regarding a multiplicity of factors that give rise to the symptom has been amassed. Many individuals experience the sensation of a lump in the throat at times of strong emotion either when they are unable to express their feelings or when it would be considered inappropriate to give vent to these feelings. This sensation is relatively transitory but the globus symptom is persistent and may recur constantly. It is either relieved

or not affected by swallowing although in true dysphagia swallowing is difficult and pain, or a sensation of obstruction, develops within 15 seconds of the
pharyngeal stage of the swallow (Bradley and Narula, 1987). These authors
found that approximately 1–4% of new patients seen in an ENT clinic were
referred for treatment of globus symptoms and that, in women aged 50 years
or younger, the incidence is three times more frequent than in men. After 50
years of age, the incidence is comparable to men (Moloy and Charter, 1982).
(See Table 8.5 for profile of globus pharyngeus.)

Physical aetiology

It is essential that the possibility of a true dysphagia is excluded in cases of
globus pharyngeus. Full investigation includes a barium swallow, diagnostic oesophagoscopy and, in cases where there is reason to suspect undiag-
nosed problems, videofluoroscopy. Thorough visualisation of the
oropharynx and supraglottis is carried out to exclude the presence of disease, particularly malignant tumour. Various physical conditions can cause
a sensation of a lump in the throat in the absence of dysphagia (Table 8.6).

    The studies listed in Table 8.7 show the correlation between gastric
reflux and other disorders of the gastrointestinal tract.

Table 8.5 Globus pharyngeus	
Symptom	Persistent feeling of a lump in the throat relieved or not affected by swallowing
Signs	Negative findings on diagnostic oesophagoscopy and barium swallow Evidence of gastric reflux in many patients
Aetiology	Psychogenic Depressed and/or stoic and controlled individuals who do not express emotion easily Associated with gastric reflux
Laryngoscopic findings	Normal structure and function (globus can also coexist with benign mass lesions and hyperfunctional voice disorders when excessive effort is used to phonate)
Expected vocal profile	Voice unaffected by globus pharyngeus but effortful phonation can be associated with globus symptoms
Management	Full investigation must exclude organic aetiology Trial antacid reflux medication Reassurance Speech/language therapy when associated with voice changes

Table 8.6 Possible causes of globus pharyngeus ('a lump in the throat' sensation)

- Anxiety/depression: pharyngeal tension
- Gastric reflux: reflex cricopharyngeal spasm
- Hiatus hernia
- Gastrointestinal tract lesions
- Cervical osteophytes: bony outgrowth on vertebrae of the cervical spine creates pressure on pharynx
- Upper respiratory tract infection
- Enlarged lingual tonsil
- Osteoarthritis of cervical spine: referred pain to pharynx
- Enlarged thyroid gland: pressure symptoms
- Tense extrinsic and intrinsic laryngeal muscles

Table 8.7 Globus pharyngeus studies

Author(s)	Subjects with globus pharyngeus	Findings
Malcolmson (1968)	307: 217 females: 90 males	38% had miscellaneous local lesions 62% had distal lesions (most common distal lesion [69%]: hiatus hernia)
Delahunty and Ardran (1970)	25	22 patients had reflux oesophagitis resulting in acid-induced motility disturbance Globus pharyngeus eliminated by acid-free regimen
Moloy and Charter (1982)	103	Incidence of gastric reflux 38% compared with 36% in general adult population Globus symptom not eliminated even when gastric reflux treated successfully
Nishijima, Takoda and Hasegawa (1984)	290	76% had gastrointestinal tract lesions As a result of their findings, the authors recommend gastrointestinal tract roentgenography for all globus patients

Psychogenic aetiology

In those patients where physical causes have been excluded, it appears that a true conversion symptom (see page 200) is uncommon. Studies suggest that depression is the most common psychological feature related to the globus syndrome. Clinical experience shows that patients with voice disorders who also describe a sensation of a lump in the throat usually appear to have their emotions under careful control and are reluctant to express their feelings. In many instances the approach to life is stoic and they continue to carry out their family and work commitments in spite of real emotional and practical difficulties. They regard the need for support from family and friends as a sign of weakness and yet there is pride in providing support for others even if, at times, it is accompanied by resentment and feelings of being 'put upon'.

Case history

Mrs A (48 years) was referred for voice therapy because of intermittent dysphonia. The laryngoscopic examination was normal although the laryngologist noted that she was 'rather tense'. Mrs A was extremely thin and her posture was upright and rigid. She had minimal facial expression; this lack of affect was disconcerting for the listener because of the limited feedback from the patient during conversation. Phonation required visible effort and yet the voice was only just loud enough to be heard in normal conversation. She complained that her throat felt constricted and that there was a sensation of a lump in the throat almost continually, to the extent that she felt unable to eat at times and that swallowing was uncomfortable. All investigations were normal.

A story gradually emerged of divorce proceedings 5 years previously which had been followed by a very happy relationship with a married man. Unfortunately, without warning, he ended the relationship by letter. The patient was devastated when this happened 3 months before her referral to the ENT department. She was quite unaware of the link between these events and her present problems. During a lengthy interview, she revealed that she had felt unable to show her feelings at the break-up of this relationship because her teenage children would have been upset by their mother's distress. She had not been able to express her grief and anger at the termination of the relationship and the way it was ended. As she gave this account, she began to sob uncontrollably and she expressed the fear that she would not be able to stop crying. When she did stop weeping, she put her hand to her neck as she realised that the 'feeling of a lump in the throat' had gone.

This interview was followed by weekly sessions with the speech–language pathologist which provided emotional support and traditional voice therapy. As her self-respect increased and as she talked about her feelings of loss, the globus symptom reduced in intensity and eventually disappeared. Her voice returned to normal and her facial expression, which had indicated depression, became increasingly animated and responsive.

FUNCTIONAL AIRWAY OBSTRUCTION (PARADOXICAL VOCAL FOLD MOTION)

Functional airway obstruction (FAO) is a non-organic respiratory condition that can occur in isolation or in conjunction with asthma or other respiratory conditions (Imam and Halpern, 1995; Mobeireek et al., 1995; Shiels, Hayes and Fitzgerald, 1995; Elshami and Tino, 1996; Poirier, Pancioli and DiGiulio, 1996). It imitates asthmatic attacks and usually occurs paroxysmally. Occasionally, it can present in a chronic form with relatively stable signs and symptoms (Warburton et al., 1996). It is characterised by inspiratory and early expiratory vocal fold adduction with resulting airflow restriction at the laryngeal level. In some cases airflow restriction occurs on either inspiration or expiration alone. Stridor may or may not be a feature of the disorder.

The inappropriate vocal fold adduction is referred to as paradoxical vocal fold motion or vocal fold dysfunction (Newman, Mason and Schmaling, 1995). Attacks are not under the patient's conscious control and when they occur they are very frightening for the patient and observers. FAO can be extremely dramatic in its presentation because of the airway restriction, and it is often the cause of frequent attendance at hospital accident and emergency departments. It has been recognised increasingly over the past decade as an unconscious vocal tract behaviour that mimics organic respiratory conditions such as bronchial asthma, organic airway obstruction and anaphylaxis. Misdiagnosis, particularly of asthma, can lead to high levels of medication and, in some cases, unnecessary intubation. FAO, therefore, is increasingly considered as a differential diagnosis in cases of respiratory distress. Poirier, Pancioli and DiGiulio (1996) suggest that FAO should be considered if the patient does not have a typical history and physical findings associated with reactive airway disease. It is also significant, in cases where asthma is suspected or exists, that the patient with FAO tends to have difficulty on inspiration rather than expiration. Spirometry and flow–volume loop tests are considered to be the most important clinical diagnostic tools (Mobeireek et al., 1995).

This condition can occur in children and adults, particularly after an emotional event, but it occurs most commonly in young women. In a study of 95 patients with vocal fold dysfunction conducted by Newman, Mason and Schmaling (1995):

- 53 (of the 95) also had asthma
- the patients without asthma were predominantly young women
- the patients who were eventually found not to have asthma had lived with an incorrect diagnosis for an average of 4.8 years; their medications were identical to those of a control group with severe asthma
- 28% of the patients with FAO had been intubated during an 'attack'.

Clinical experience suggests that speech–language pathologists can make a useful contribution to the successful treatment of FAO and that some patients with the condition are predisposed to hyperfunctional voice disorders, which respond to explanations, reassurance and a programme of treatment to reduce vocal tract hyperfunction. The main features of the condition are summarised in Table 8.8.

Table 8.8 Functional airway obstruction (FAO)	
Symptoms	Patient feels airway is restricted at the laryngeal level
	Sensation of throat being closed
Signs	Dramatic episodes of breathing difficulty
	Stridor – inspiratory and expiratory
	Patient struggles to inspire
	Shortness of breath
	'Wheezing'
	Frequent emergency hospital attendances
	Extrinsic laryngeal muscle tension
	Fixed larynx
	Can mimic bronchial asthma, organic airway obstruction and anaphylaxis
Aetiology	Can be precipitated by emotional events
	Coexists with asthma in some patients
	Occurs with and without organic conditions
Laryngoscopic findings	Normal structure
	Vocal fold dysfunction (paradoxical motion) at rest and can occur on phonation
Management	Correct diagnosis is essential in order to avoid high levels of medication and unnecessary intubation
	Voice therapy
	Counselling / psychological or psychiatric intervention

Case history

Mr P (58 years) had suffered from asthma for most of his adult life but it was generally well controlled by bronchodilators and corticosteroids. Asthma attacks occurred infrequently. He kept a meticulous record of his medication and his peak flow measures. Approximately 1 year before he was referred to the speech and language therapist, he had an extremely severe asthma attack while travelling on a hot, crowded, London underground train. He was taken to hospital by ambulance from the next station. During the following year, he had nine more attacks and was eventually admitted to hospital by the respiratory physician for a full assessment and adjustment of his medication. The dosage of his corticosteroids was increased. Within 2 weeks of being discharged, another attack occurred and he was referred to another respiratory physician who concluded after further observation that, although the patient had asthma, these distressing episodes were possibly chiefly the result of functional airway obstruction. His decision was based partly on the relatively normal peak-flow measures at the time of the attacks.

Mr P was somewhat mystified by his referral to a speech and language therapist, but was so concerned about his condition that he was keen to explore any avenue that might improve the situation. It was noted that there was considerable vocal tract tension. As he spoke, his chin was markedly depressed and the larynx forced downwards so that its vertical excursions were restricted. There was moderate vocal creak and he tended to talk on residual air. He talked a great deal and his accounts of the attacks were detailed and histrionic. Careful questioning confirmed that the breathing obstruction was at the laryngeal level during these episodes rather than his chest. On palpation, the extrinsic laryngeal muscles were very tense and moderately tender. The larynx was highly resistant to lateral digital pressure. After explanations concerning the anatomy of the vocal tract and the process of paradoxical vocal fold movement, his sternocleidomastoid muscles were massaged and the supralaryngeal area was 'kneaded' (see page 500). He was reassured and pleased that his throat felt 'better', lighter and more open than usual. This changed kinaesthetic model was reinforced by various vocal strategies which encouraged easy voice onset, reduced creak and effortless phonation (see page 477). During two further treatment sessions, he was also shown how to recognise and alter degrees of vocal fold closure so that he could feel a certain amount of control over his laryngeal behaviour and the consequent translaryngeal airflow. He reported that this strategy, in combination with his understanding of the process, had been the most reassuring and helpful aspect of treatment. After these three treatment sessions, he was reviewed at monthly intervals for 4 months, chiefly for reassurance. During this period he had no further 'asthma' attacks and no further appointments were arranged. He made contact 6 months after his first appointment to report that he had started to experience the onset of an attack, but had managed to abort it by thinking through the laryngeal processes involved and then modifying vocal fold approximation together with relaxed breathing patterns. A year after the first appointment he had not had any 'asthma attacks'.

HYPERVENTILATION SYNDROME

Hyperventilation and panic attacks (Table 8.9)

Hyperventilation is a serious disturbance of breathing in individuals suffering from anxiety state. As a result of over-breathing the lungs are ventilated in excess of metabolic needs causing arterial hypocapnia, a persistent drop in the CO_2 level in arterial blood and expired alveolar air. Breathing irregularity is well known to be associated with anxiety and emotional disturbances and over-breathing occurs in people who have an anxiety state when they are undergoing a panic attack. A frightening situation triggers an attack which will subside gradually, but individuals may become conditioned and react in this way in similar circumstances or even at the memory of an attack (Lum, 1976). Breathing is not only rapid but irregular and may be accompanied by sighing (Innocenti, 1983). A sudden acute panic attack is accompanied by excessive panting and upper chest, clavicular breathing with heaving shoulders. It may be seen in aircraft passengers when going through a period of turbulence or landing in thick fog. Although an acute attack is very alarming to witness, it is not fatal. However, it is necessary to be aware that hyperventilation may be provoked, for example, when a patient is given a breathing exercise or if a sensitive topic is touched upon

Table 8.9 Hyperventilation syndrome: profile	
Symptoms	Patient has episodes of anxiety and breathing difficulties
Signs	Breathing rapid and irregular Increased heart rate Sweating Muscle tension Arterial hypocapnia
Aetiology	Anxiety and emotional disturbance
Management	Counselling Re-education of breathing patterns Beta-blockers

in taking a case history. The clinician should remain calm and assume a reassuring and quietly authoritative manner, exhorting the patient to breathe slowly and from the 'stomach' (Greene, 1984).

Medication

Situational anxiety, stage fright, examination nerves and the fear of flying can best be alleviated by beta-blocking drugs, i.e. beta-adrenergic receptor-blocking drugs such as oxprenolol (Gates and Montalbo, 1987). Administered half an hour before a dreaded ordeal, concomitant anxiety is dispersed without affecting concentration, clarity of thought or reaction time. Tranquillisers may be prescribed by the physician, but these are addictive, have side effects and do not solve the patient's emotional problems. Patients treated by Greene (1984) said that the tranquillisers did not help to allay the panic.

Over-breathing in anxiety states

There can be marked over-breathing in anxiety states without any dramatic episodes of hyperventilation. Patients suffer from a wide spectrum of psychosomatic disorders simulating diseases and listed previously. They are described by Lewis (1959) and Magarian (1983), who gives an excellent account of hyperventilation syndrome in discussing 'infrequently recognised expressions of anxiety and stress'. There is a wide range in the severity of symptoms in hyperventilation. Borderline cases of hypocapnia and chronic anxiety may have only occasional stressful situations. Psychosomatic symptoms may be so severe and the patient's complaints so persistent that they frequently result in extensive medical examinations in one hospital department after another. The patient's case notes will provide evidence of many investigations of heart, lung, gastric and endocrine function all proving negative (Greene, Timmons and Glover, 1983, 1984).

Measurement of hypocapnia

Precise measurement of CO_2 levels in each expiration can be obtained by passing expired air through a capnograph, which also indicates the number of respirations per minute. Normal breathing rate is approximately 12/minute and rates in excess of this indicate the presence of hyperventilation. The capnograph is difficult to operate and testing requires an experienced technician and medical assistant. A 'provocation' test of panting rapidly for 3 minutes is required, after which the CO_2 readings are monitored for a recovery period of 3 minutes. The level should return to that of the testing level and, if it fails to do so, hyperventilation is diagnosed

(Greene, 1984). The respiratory rate can be timed and irregularities and sighing noted, especially in relaxation therapy. Confirmation of diagnosis is reinforced by the case history and indicates the need for emphasis in treatment of respiratory training.

Greene, Timmons and Glover (1983, 1984) subjected a number of dysphonic patients attending a speech clinic to capnograph assessment. Two patients who were failing to progress proved to be hyperventilators with hypocapnia. They had typical case histories and suffered from anxiety state and a series of unconfirmed physical disorders. Two cases with spasmodic adductor dysphonia were not hyperventilators. Two newly referred patients were tested before being given speech therapy and diagnosed as hyperventilators, and then given a course of breathing therapy and counselling. They responded well to treatment. Individuals who have chronic anxiety cannot be so easily cured, but their condition can be alleviated and sympathetic support helps them to carry on without breakdown or resort to drug therapy.

Summary

- The voice and vocal tract are affected by the individual's psychological status.
- Psychological factors are the primary cause of psychogenic dysphonia or aphonia, but emotional factors can contribute to or be a secondary feature of all voice disorders.
- 'Psychogenic voice disorder' is a diagnosis of exclusion. The possibility of organic pathology must be fully explored and eliminated before this diagnosis is made.
- Psychogenic voice disorders are precipitated by emotional factors, which disturb vocal behaviour in the absence of organic or neurological factors, although they can coexist with these conditions.
- In many cases of psychogenic voice disorder, the symptoms are inconsistent with the history and findings.
- Successful resolution depends on addressing the underlying psychopathology as well as suitable symptomatic voice therapy.

Structural abnormalities of the vocal tract

The voice can be affected adversely by structural abnormalities anywhere in the vocal tract. Laryngeal anomalies compromise the vocal note whereas resonance is altered by abnormalities of the supraglottic vocal tract. When the lower respiratory tract is involved, subglottic air pressure can be inadequate for phonation or it might be necessary to re-route the airstream surgically, in cases of laryngeal obstruction, so that air does not pass between the vocal folds, but leaves the airway via a stoma in the neck. The various structural abnormalities can be congenital or acquired (Table 9.1).

Nasal abnormalities

PATHOLOGY

Deflected (deviated) septum

This common structural abnormality of the nasal septum involves either the bony or the cartilaginous portions, or both. It can be congenital and often occurs in association with cleft palate. An acquired deflected septum may occur if a broken nose is not surgically repaired successfully before healing takes place.

Hypertrophy of the nasopharyngeal adenoid

This condition occurs most frequently between the ages of 3 and 7 years. The tonsils are generally also enlarged. Inflammation of the nasal mucosa (rhinitis) accompanied by constant nasal discharge (rhinorrhoea) is a common and troublesome cause of insufficient nasality. Mouth-breathing results from the nasal obstruction and the child may present with the typical adenoid facies of pinched nostrils and prominent incisors in the later stages (Ballantyne and Groves, 1982). Inflammation may involve the

Table 9.1 Structural abnormalities of the vocal tract

Vocal tract locus	Structural abnormality		Effect
	CONGENITAL	ACQUIRED	
NOSE	deflected (deviated) septum	• enlarged adenoid pad • neoplasm • deflected/deviated septum • vasomotor rhinitis • allergic rhinitis • rhinitis medicamentosa • polyps • foreign body • trauma • pharyngoplasty	• nasal obstruction causes hyponasality
PALATE	• cleft palate • submucous cleft • short soft palate (with or without associated deep and wide pharynx)	palatal paresis see neurogenic voice disorders (Chap 10)	• velopharyngeal incompetency causes hypernasality and, possibly, audible nasal escape
LARYNX	• webs • laryngomalacia • laryngocele • sulcus • laryngotracheal stenosis • syndromes: cri-du-chat Down's Arnold–Chiari	• laryngeal skeleton and mucosal trauma • subglottic stenosis • sulcus • webs	• abnormalities of the vocal note • airway restriction with or without stridor
TRACHEA	tracheo-oesophageal fistula tracheomalacia stenosis	tracheostomy laryngotracheal stenosis	• airway narrowing adversely affects translaryngeal airflow for phonation • tracheostomy: no pulmonic air for phonation

laryngeal and pharyngeal membranes and produce chronic hoarseness. Adenoids alone do not cause complete nasal obstruction and mouth-breathing. Rhinitis and sinusitis may persist after adenoidectomy unless appropriate medical attention is given to any infection remaining after the operation. Even when nasal obstruction has been removed, hyponasality can sometimes persist through force of habit until speech therapy is initiated.

Neoplasms

Nasal and nasopharyngeal tumours in adults are rare and require immediate investigation and treatment by surgery and/or radiotherapy if malignant.

Polyps in the nasal passages may be related to conditions of chronic allergic rhinitis or have no obvious aetiology. Polyps may be removed surgically in order to facilitate nasal breathing and improve nasal resonance. They tend to recur and may also occur in the larynx (page 169).

Pharyngoplasty

Nasal obstruction can occur after pharyngoplasty and pharyngeal flap operations in connection with surgical correction of velopharyngeal incompetence.

Note that **vasomotor rhinitis, allergic rhinitis** and **rhinitis medicamentosa** are conditions in which the nasal mucosa is swollen, resulting in nasal obstruction (see Chapter 12).

SIGNS AND SYMPTOMS

Nasal obstruction causes the sufferer to feel as if the nose is blocked and to mouth-breathe. The resulting denasalised resonance of the voice is typical.

EXPECTED VOCAL PROFILE

When there is an obstruction of the nasal airways that renders nasal breathing difficult or impossible, the voice lacks sufficient nasal resonance (Table 9.2). Lack of adequate nasal resonance destroys the bright ringing quality that is characteristic of head resonance. Vowel sounds are denasalised and the voice is dull and muffled, but lack of nasality is most evident in the articulation of the nasal consonants /m/, /n/ and /ŋ/. These continuants may not be adequately maintained but may resemble their plosive counterparts /b/, /d/ and /g/ on account of the precipitate release of the articulators. As the nasal consonants are frequent in the English language, their denasalisation renders speech distinctly abnormal and even unpleasant to the listener, who rightly associates the lack of nasality with nasal obstruction. Severely denasalised speech is rare and a certain degree of nasality is possible for most speakers, even when there is considerable obstruction of the nasal airway, provided that the airway is not entirely closed. An individual is frequently able to compensate for lack of nasal resonance by increased pharyngeal constriction and deliberate prolongation of the nasal continuants.

Hyponasality is not entirely related to the degree of nasal blockage. Although nasal obstruction always causes the voice to be deficient in nasal resonance, it may not result in a voice that is perceived as markedly hyponasal. Insufficient nasality may persist by force of habit after removal of nasal obstruction.

Case notes

- A male patient (18 years) continued to be hyponasal after the complete removal of a large tumour which extended from the nasopharynx into the nasal cavity. Normal resonance did not return until he underwent a short course of voice therapy.
- It is noticeable that many children with cleft palate, who are hyponasal as a result of nasal obstruction and malformation of the septum, still continue to speak in the same way when the septum has been straightened and the airway obstruction cleared.
- A child who had severe audible nasal escape after adenoidectomy gradually reverted to her habitual hyponasality as movement of the palate developed, although she could now breathe through her nose without difficulty.

Table 9.2 Causes of disorders of nasal resonance

Hypernasality (excessive nasal resonance)		Hyponasality (insufficient nasal resonance)	
Congenital	Acquired	Congenital	Acquired
cleft palate	post-adenoidectomy	deflected (deviated) septum	deflected (deviated) septum
submucous cleft	psychogenic		upper respiratory tract infection (URTI)
short soft palate	palatal paresis		
deep and wide pharynx	palatal trauma		enlarged adenoids
			neoplasm
palatal paresis			nasal polyps
			allergic rhinitis
			vasomotor rhinitis
			rhinitis medicamentosa
			pharyngoplasty
			psychogenic

Excessive nasal resonance is usually caused by structural and functional inadequacies of the hard and/or soft palate and the pharynx. Hyponasality arises from conditions that obstruct the upper respiratory tract

In these instances of habit, the individual continues to apply the same auditory and kinaesthetic patterns to speech production after removal of the cause of the hyponasality and obstruction in the nasal resonator. The habitual sounds are produced, probably unconsciously and at a reflex level, but articulation and resonance are adjusted to compensate for the lack of nasal obstruction. This pattern will continue unless the individual is re-educated.

MEDICOSURGICAL DECISIONS

Surgery is required to remove the nasal obstruction, when appropriate. Voice therapy cannot overcome the effects on the voice of a nasal obstruction, but it can be an important element of postoperative treatment.

Palatal abnormalities

Palatal abnormalities are associated with inadequacy of the velopharyngeal sphincter and, as a result, hypernasal vocal resonance (see Table 9.2). In some cases, there is audible nasal emission of turbulent air via the nose, known as nasal escape, during articulation of consonants. Hypernasality is also referred to in the literature as excessive nasality, hyperrhinolalia, rhinolalia aperta and, more simply, nasalised speech. It has to be remembered that, in normal speech, degrees of nasality vary according to culture and for sociolinguistic reasons. Resonance that is considered normal in one setting can sound excessively nasal to outsiders. Speakers of standard English are considered to have nasal speech by the Dutch and, to the English, some American accents have a marked nasal twang. Vowels associated with the nasal consonants /m/, /n/ and /ŋ/ assimilate slight nasality which tends to be more marked in American English. Nasalised vowels are phonemic in French but not in English. In normal speech, increased nasality is the result of a tense oropharynx and elevation of the back of the tongue, not an incompetent velopharyngeal sphincter. When the sphincter is inadequate, however, the resulting hypernasality will be exacerbated by excessive pharyngeal tension and tongue elevation. Perceived nasality can also result from inappropriately timed movements of a perfectly competent soft palate.

CLEFT PALATE

The lip, hard and soft palate normally fuse during the first 3 months of fetal life. Fusion can fail entirely or in part. Unilateral or bilateral cleft of the lip can occur in isolation or involve the alveolus and part of the hard palate. The uvula can be bifid, and the cleft of the soft palate isolated or extend into the whole or part of the soft palate. A complete cleft runs right through from the lip to the uvula. It is the posterior cleft of the palate that engages us in the study of hypernasality.

Cleft lip and palate are the most common congenital deformities in the craniofacial region and have been reported throughout history world wide, and were discovered in Egyptian mummies. There is some difficulty in ascertaining the incidence because of incomplete records, but a central system of registration has existed in Denmark for the past 50 years. Incidence was estimated at 1.3 per 1000 live births during the first 5 years, but there has been a steady increase, rising to about 2 cases per 1000 (Fogh-Andersen, 1980). More recent figures suggest that cleft lip and/or palatal malformation occurs in 1 in 700 births (Murray, 1998). Cleft lip and palate are more common in males but cleft palate alone is more frequent in females.

The causes of clefting are thought to fall into three groups. Direct causes include certain drugs taken in pregnancy, including phenytoin and corticosteroids. Maternal hypoxia is also thought to be a direct cause. In some families there appears to be a genetic predisposition to these malformations. It is also thought that certain unidentified environmental factors are the cause in some cases.

Aetiology of speech problems

The communication problems associated with cleft palate are multifactorial. In addition to abnormalities of nasal resonance resulting from velopharyngeal dysfunction, speech can also be affected by dental problems and problems of occlusion, oronasal fistulae and hearing problems. Other factors that can influence speech adversely are syndromes associated with cleft palate, social, neurological, cognitive, developmental, environmental and emotional influences (McWilliams, Morris and Shelton, 1990). The main features of speech problems in this group are hypernasality, audible nasal emission, abnormal consonant production, nasal grimace and delayed language development (Sell, Harding and Grunwell, 1994).

Expected vocal profile

Abnormal voice in patients with velopharyngeal dysfunction can arise from two sources: the quality of the glottal source and abnormal resonance of the vocal note.

- Dysphonia arising from **vocal misuse** and **abuse** can result from the excessive effort used by some speakers for a number of reasons (McWilliams, Lavorato and Bluestone, 1973; Leder and

Lerman, 1985). In some cases of velopharyngeal incompetence, it appears that attempts to increase vocal loudness because of the relative lack of volume of a hypernasal voice contribute to glottic hyperfunction. Reduced intelligibility can also contribute to the desire to speak more loudly in order to be understood. Vocal abuse also results from the glottis being used inappropriately as an articulator, with certain phonemes being produced inappropriately as glottal sounds instead of in the normal oral placement (Stengelhofen, 1993).

- Resonance disorders: hypernasality, hyponasality and cul-de-sac resonance. **Hypernasality** is generally associated with velopharyngeal dysfunction. In any speaker, the degree of hypernasality will vary according to which vowels are being produced because different vowels require varying degrees of velopharyngeal closure (Stengelhofen, 1993). Low vowels, such as /a:/, are affected by hypernasality far less than high vowels, such as /i:/, because the resonators are more balanced when the oral cavity is more open. **Hyponasality** can also occur if there is significant nasal obstruction as a result of a severely deflected nasal septum or collapse of the nasal airway. **Cul-de-sac resonance** results from an occluded or obstructed nasal airway in conjunction with significant pharyngeal tension. This is the quality that occurs when speaking while the nose is being pinched.

Medicosurgical decisions

It is essential that patients with cleft palate malformations are treated by a multidisciplinary team where each member can provide high-quality specialist care. Teams in specialist centres see a high volume of patients and the delivery of care is constantly being reviewed and refined. Surgical repair of the cleft lip takes place when the baby is 6–12 weeks old, although in some centres this may be earlier. Subsequently, between 3 and 18 months of age, the palate is repaired in order to achieve normal palatal activity as early as possible. This reduces nasal regurgitation and speech development is facilitated. Some surgeons consider that such early palatal repair inhibits facial growth and do not operate until the child is 5–8 years old. There is evidence that this can affect speech development adversely (Murray, 1998). The quality of the primary procedure to repair the palate has a significant effect on whether or not further surgery will be necessary to improve speech, and the amount of speech and language therapy that will be required. Normal speech develops spontaneously in 50% of children after repair of the cleft palate. Secondary velopharyngeal surgery will be required by 25% of cases and 25% need speech and language therapy (Murray, 1998).

The following conditions also cause hypernasality.

SUBMUCOUS CLEFT

Rarely, the mucosal cover of the soft palate is entire, concealing a cleft of the muscular segments of the palate beneath. This is known as a submucous cleft. As the cleft is invisible and suckling and swallowing can function adequately, the submucous cleft may be unsuspected until hypernasal speech develops in the child. A translucent line may be detected running down the centre of the palate and a notch may be felt in the posterior edge of the hard palate. These are easily performed clinical tests carried out by a speech–language pathologist in assessing nasal dysphonia. The incidence of submucous cleft palate is about 1:1200, but only 5–10% have palatopharyngeal incompetence. Those children who have submucous cleft frequently have other associated abnormalities, according to Bumsted (1982), deafness and learning disability (mental handicap) being the most frequent.

CONGENITAL PALATAL PARESIS

This condition also occurs rarely and may be confused with submucous cleft until thorough investigations eradicate this possibility. Surgical treatment is not successful but a palatal prosthesis can help.

ACQUIRED PALATAL PARESIS

Palatal paralysis and paresis caused by neuropathology result in an inadequate palatopharyngeal sphincter. These conditions are described in Chapter 10.

CONGENITAL SHORT PALATE, WIDE PHARYNX

Incompetent palatopharyngeal closure and hypernasal speech may also be caused by a congenital short palate with the associated deformity of an unusually deep and wide nasopharynx. This may become evident only after removal of adenoids that have hitherto reduced the dimensions of the nasopharyngeal cavity, and made closure by the palate possible. Damsté (1962) stated that the condition, although rare, is twice as common as submucous cleft. Pharyngoplasty as for cleft palate is the usual curative surgical procedure.

POST-ADENOIDECTOMY HYPERNASALITY

Removal of a grossly enlarged adenoidal pad may result in a temporary velopharyngeal incompetence and hypernasality. There has to be a mechanical compensation for lack of the adenoidal pad against which the soft palate made contact. Nasal escape may last for only a few days and then a satisfactory adjustment is made (Greene, 1957). Occasionally, removal of the enlarged adenoids reveals a true abnormality of the palatopharyngeal sphincter, which has been masked preoperatively by the mass in the nasopharynx.

PSYCHOGENIC HYPERNASALITY

Hypernasality may result exclusively from emotional disturbance in the presence of a competent speech mechanism. Speech in these cases is generally variable and characterised by hypernasality rather than audible nasal emission. It can be a conversion symptom (see Chapter 8) or it may persist for psychological reasons after adenoidectomy as a means of gaining and prolonging the attention of an anxious parent.

A full nasopharyngeal assessment will need to be carried out if hypernasal speech persists for several months. A congenital short palate is a possibility, but functional use of the palate can be misleading. The differential diagnosis between congenital short palate and psychogenic hypernasality should never be made hastily. Diagnostic speech therapy in doubtful cases should be given while the child's emotional status is explored and the possible need for such a symptom is investigated. A period of 9 months to a year should elapse before pharyngoplasty is seriously considered.

CASE HISTORIES

The following case histories illustrate the complexities of differential diagnosis in cases of hypernasality, where the aetiology is not immediately apparent.

Case 1

A girl aged 14 years had a pleasant singing voice and was in demand at local charity concerts. She had developed excessive nasal escape after a recent adenoidectomy. After 6 months' duration of the symptom, clinical and lateral radiographic assessment revealed a short palate in relation to a deep pharynx. The surgeon in charge decided to postpone carrying out a pharyngoplasty. Three months later speech and singing suddenly reverted to normal. It appears that either there had been a particularly long period of adjustment to the changed dimensions of the palatopharyngeal isthmus or that there had been a psychogenic reason for long-lasting nasal escape.

Case 2

A girl aged 7 years 9 months with normal speech underwent adenoidectomy and tonsillectomy. Postoperatively, there was gross nasal escape and grimace which had not improved 3 months later. Her soft palate appeared to be paralysed and did not elevate when touched or in articulation of the vowel /aː/. After a few weeks of speech therapy, the palate showed slight elevation on vowels. It was noticeable that hypernasality and nasal grimace, although always present, varied considerably. She was uncooperative and wilful in the clinic and unruly at home. She was the only child of elderly parents whose relationship was far from harmonious and whose business commitments provided constant anxiety and overwork. They had little time or patience for a troublesome, though much loved and indulged, daughter.

Seven months postoperatively, lateral radiographs showed that, although her palate failed to elevate in blowing and articulating vowels, there was excellent elevation and complete occlusion of the velopharyngeal isthmus on crying. During treatment sessions at this stage, she would sometimes speak without hypernasality or nasal grimace, although both returned when she was with either parent. It began to appear that her hypernasality, although originally caused by post-adenoidectomy palatal weakness, might now be a psychogenic symptom.

This hypothesis was confirmed subsequently. When she changed school aged 8 years 5 months her speech returned to normal, even at home. Subsequently, however, she developed a non-inflammatory earache followed by abdominal pains for which no organic cause could be found. Simultaneously, her speech deteriorated. After 3 weeks she returned to school and gradually settled down happily. Speech 6 months later was normal. Some years later, she was attending the child guidance clinic on account of 'night terrors'. The resemblance of these nasal symptoms to conversion symptoms is an interesting feature of the case (see Chapter 8).

Case 3

AC (9 years) had always stammered and had been diagnosed by various doctors and surgeons as having 'breathing difficulty' on account of clonic expiratory spasms. He also exhibited variable degrees of hypernasality 'according to how he felt', as his mother accurately described it. His mother had twice been admitted for inpatient psychiatric care for treatment of depression and she alternately abused and beat the boy for his naughtiness, or insisted that something should be done about his speech.

Lateral radiographs revealed incomplete nasopharyngeal closure. The speech–language pathologist did not agree in this case that the velopharyngeal mechanism was incapable of competent closure. She considered that the symptom was psychogenic, although palatal function was incompetent. Pharyngoplasty was, however, performed. The boy was very upset by his hospital stay and his speech was even more hypernasal postoperatively. The

(contd)

palate appeared to be paralysed, but this proved to be a conversion symptom and it recovered normal function during his first speech therapy session as an outpatient. Six months later, after speech therapy, his speech was no longer hypernasal on the whole and his stammer improved. Hypernasality and stammer both returned whenever he was upset at either home or school.

Case 4

Miss B (22 years) had spoken normally until she was 7 years old when her tonsils and adenoids had been removed on account of infection and hearing loss. After this her speech was hypernasal and intelligibility was poor. She had various ear, nose and throat examinations, and it was concluded that there was no abnormality and that her speech problems would resolve spontaneously. There was no improvement and at age 15 years she had more speech therapy and, after lateral radiographic investigation, her mother was told that she had 'a lazy palate', but no further intervention was arranged.

Finally, at 22 years, she now sought further help to resolve her speech problems, which were adversely affecting all aspects of her life. Examination revealed that, although her soft palate elevated well, it did not approximate to the posterior pharyngeal wall. A pharyngoplasty was performed and, immediately afterwards, as is usually the case, speech was hyponasal and there was some nasal obstruction. After 3 months speech was normal. This patient's problem was straightforward to solve. The fact that it had not been diagnosed and treated appropriately at a much earlier stage had resulted in prolonged and unnecessary distress for this young woman.

Congenital laryngeal abnormalities

Congenital abnormalities causing stenosis (narrowing) of the larynx either result in the death of the neonate or are corrected by surgery in infancy or early childhood (Holinger, 1979). Arnold (1958) described various abnormalities found in adult larynges that may be familial and associated with hoarseness in childhood. Laryngeal anomalies also occur in conjunction with other physical abnormalities. Asymmetries of the larynx include:

- one ventricle larger than the other
- one vocal fold broader than the other
- the vocal folds on different planes.

LARYNGOMALACIA

Laryngomalacia is a self-limiting congenital anomaly causing inspiratory stridor. The supraglottic laryngeal structures are soft, and the usual omega shape of the infantile epiglottis is exaggerated so that its lateral walls almost approximate. On each inspiration, the epiglottis is pulled towards the glottis, causing inspiratory stridor which is always present but becomes much more severe during exertion and crying. The vocal folds are normal. There is no serious cyanosis, although dyspnoea may be present, and the child remains comparatively healthy. Although the laryngeal stridor is usually present at birth, in 3% of cases it does not appear until 1 or 2 weeks later (Birrell, 1986). The condition gradually improves as the epiglottis becomes more rigid and resolves by the third year.

LARYNGEAL WEB

A congenital laryngeal web of mucous membrane that traverses the glottis can occur, and the extent to which the airway is compromised will vary from one baby to another. There is some indication that there is a familial tendency to laryngeal webs. Baker and Savetsky (1966) reported congenital laryngeal webs occurring in four members of the same family. Micro-webs involve only the anterior commissure, but in some cases the web extends from the anterior commissure so that the airway is almost completely occluded. In mild cases, the web may not be suspected until puberty when boys' voices fail to break and girls' voices remain childish because of the diminished length of the vocal folds capable of vibration. Asymptomatic webs are sometimes observed on laryngoscopy, and it has been suggested that micro-webs dispose the patient to vocal nodules because additional effort is required to compensate for the shortened membranous portion of each vocal fold. Inspiratory stridor needing urgent surgery occurs when there is a large web, but hoarseness since birth can signal a less extensive web. If the web is small, it may be decided that surgical intervention is inadvisable because hoarseness will not necessarily be resolved and there is the possibility of fibrosis which can cause further deterioration.

CONGENITAL VOCAL FOLD PARALYSIS

Congenital vocal fold paralysis is the third most common cause of congenital stridor and is often associated with other defects involving the central and peripheral nervous systems, heart defects and other problems. (See acquired vocal fold paralysis, Chapter 10.)

CONGENITAL SYNDROMES INVOLVING THE LARYNX

Cri-du-chat

This syndrome is caused by a chromosomal abnormality and is typified by a high-pitched, wailing cry resembling a cat's mew. Inspiratory stridor is present from birth as a result of the flaccid epiglottis. The larynx is narrow with a diamond-shaped glottis on inspiration and an open triangle on adduction, resulting from paralysis of the interarytenoid muscle (Birrell, 1986). Other congenital abnormalities include microcephaly, learning disability, hypotonia, low-set ears and visceral anomalies.

Down's syndrome

The cry of the Down's syndrome baby tends to be harsh and of a lower pitch than normal. The low pitch is usually present throughout life and the quality of the vocal note is typically rough.

Arnold–Chiari syndrome

This is also known as the Arnold–Chiari deformity or malformation, and is a congenital anomaly in which the cerebellum and medulla oblongata, which is elongated and flattened, protrude down into the spinal canal through the foramen magnum. It may be associated with many other defects, including spina bifida occulta. Vocal fold paralysis may also be a presenting feature of this condition.

VOCAL FOLD SULCUS

A sulcus is a furrow, groove or indentation in the covering epithelium of the vocal fold which can occur unilaterally or bilaterally. With the development of sophisticated instrumentation for laryngeal examination, clinicians have become increasingly aware of this vocal fold abnormality as a cause of dysphonia. Before the introduction of videolaryngostroboscopy, sulcus was a recognised deformity of the vocal fold (Arnold, 1958) but it was probably under-diagnosed.

Aetiology

There are differing views as to whether sulci are congenital or acquired. Bouchayer et al. (1985) consider that there is convincing evidence for congenital aetiology of sulci and the associated conditions of epidermoid cysts and mucosal bridges (Table 9.3). Evidence for acquired aetiology also exists. It is probable that these vocal fold anomalies are multifactorial as a result of both congenital and acquired pathology (Lee and Niimi, 1990).

Pathology

Ford et al. (1996) have classified the various presentations of sulci into three types: **physiological sulcus, sulcus vergeture** and **sulcus vocalis** (Table 9.4 and Figure 9.1). The physiological sulcus can occur in asymp-

Table 9.3 Aetiology of sulci

Factors supporting congenital aetiology	Factors supporting acquired aetiology
Dysphonia starts in childhood in a large number of cases	Onset of hoarseness after third or fourth decade
A significant number of cases in some studies have associated epidermoid cysts (Sulci are possibly the result of ruptured congenital cysts)	Significant numbers of adults report onset of symptoms
	Possible causes arise in case histories: laryngitis, vocal abuse, allergy, gastric reflux
Can be found in patients with no history of vocal abuse or laryngitis	Sulcus might be an aberrant healing response
Sulci found in children in large number of cases	
Cases of sulci and cysts occur in several members of one family	Nearly half of the laryngectomy specimens (laryngeal carcinoma) in study by Ford et al. (1996) had adjacent sulci

This table summarises the features of this vocal fold anomaly which support either a congenital or an acquired aetiology. It is possible that vocal fold sulci originate via a number of routes. (Sources: Bouchayer et al, 1985; Ford et al., 1996.)

tomatic subjects and it is thought that it might be secondary to age-related changes and vocal fold paresis. In these cases, when the thyroarytenoid muscle is relatively atrophic, the upper and lower lips of the free edge of the vocal fold appear to allow a furrow to form between them. This is not a truly pathological sulcus as in the case of sulcus vergeture, which is a linear groove along the free edge of the vocal fold, and sulcus vocalis, a pit in the vocal fold epithelium.

Laryngoscopic findings

Sulcus is rarely evident on routine indirect laryngoscopy. As a result patients with this condition can be referred for voice therapy with an apparently normal larynx and treatment cannot be soundly based. In some instances, patients undergo surgery for incorrectly diagnosed vocal fold lesions such as nodules or polyps. Stroboscopy is essential for a definitive diagnosis of sulcus. The literature is in agreement regarding the laryngeal findings, which are summarised in Table 9.5. As a result of the groove or pit in the vocal fold mucosa, the lamina propria is tethered. This has the effect of reducing the bulk of the mucosa at the site of the sulcus, so that the mucosal wave is obstructed and the vocal folds cannot fully approximate. The glottic insufficiency in turn gives rise to supraglottic hyperfunction as a compensatory manoeuvre.

Table 9.4 Sulcus types

Type 1 physiological sulcus	Type 2 sulcus vergeture (pathological)	Type 3 sulcus vocalis (pathological)
Non-pathological depression or furrow of the vocal fold	Linear furrow of the membranous portion of vocal fold causing: (1) reduction in vocal fold cover (2) bowing of affected vocal fold (3) reduction in amplitude of mucosal wave	Epithelial-lined pit or contiguous cyst causing disturbance of mucosal wave
Can be secondary to atrophic changes of the vocal fold, e.g. ageing or paresis		
Vocal fold vibratory activity preserved on videostroboscopy		
Adequate functional separation of vocal fold body and cover	Disturbance of free edge of vocal fold with loss of cover-body separation	
Intact superficial lamina propria and layers of lamina propria intact	Loss of superficial lamina propria and fixation of thinned epithelium to underlying vocal ligament	
	Linear attachment	Pit extended into or through vocal ligament, causing inflammatory reaction

Source: Ford et al. (1996). Original information tabulated with permission of Professor Charles N Ford.

Table 9.5 Sulcus: laryngeal findings

laryngeal feature	cause
spindle-shaped, bowed vocal folds	sulcus invagination and tethering of lamina propria resulting in reduced bulk of mucosa at site of deformity
vocal folds fail to approximate on phonation	as above
medial furrows can be seen on inhalation	
impaired mucosal waves	furrow or pit impedes and distorts mucosal waves travelling from subglottic to supraglottic surface of vocal folds
supraglottic hyperfunction	compensatory manoeuvre occurring as a result of attempts to achieve competent vocal fold adduction

Source: Ford et al. (1996). Original material tabulated with permission of Professor Charles N Ford.

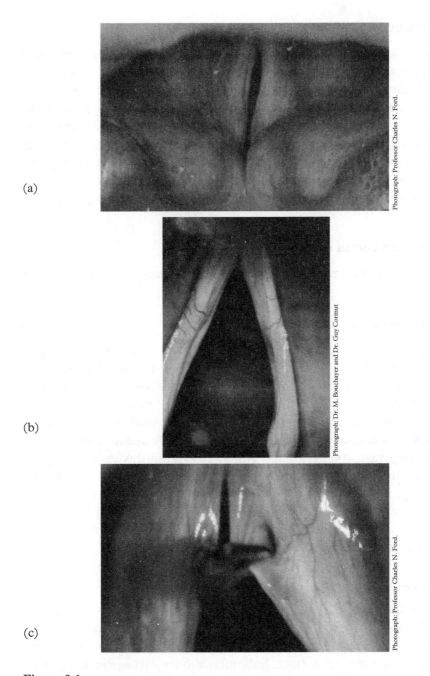

(a)

(b)

(c)

Figure 9.1
Sulcus types: (a) physiological sulcus in patient with vocal fold paralysis
(b) Sulcus vergeture
(c) Sulcus vocalis

© Annals of Otology, Rhinology and Laryngology. Reprinted by permission.

Expected vocal profile

The asthenic voice quality and hoarseness reflect the incompetent vocal fold approximation and disturbed, reduced amplitude, vocal fold mucosal waves. It is difficult for the speaker to increase loudness and, as a result, considerable effort is involved in any attempt to project the voice. Vocal fatigue, therefore, is a common feature of phonation in these patients. Supraglottic hyperfunction is the only feature of the laryngeal findings listed above that is a secondary feature and that occurs because of the effort involved in trying to increase vocal loudness. The other laryngeal findings give rise to the primary features of this type of voice disorder.

Airflow and volume measures

Glottal insufficiency results in higher levels of transglottal airflow than normal.

Medicosurgical decisions

Pathological sulci can be eliminated only with appropriate surgery. Bouchayer et al. (1985) and Ford et al. (1996) have written in detail about the surgical approaches that they have found successful. Microsurgery involves removing the affected tissue and freeing the mucosa, so that it can be functionally separate from the body of the vocal fold. Alternative approaches include injections of Teflon into the affected area to compensate for the invagination (Lee and Niimi, 1990), but this approach, while addressing the issue of glottic closure, does not deal effectively with the inadequacy of the mucosal wave. Voice therapy is essential pre- and post-operatively but it effects only minimal improvement alone. Its goal is to eliminate or reduce hyperfunctional patterns of phonation that become established in an attempt to increase loudness.

Acquired laryngeal abnormalities

Acquired laryngeal abnormalities are usually the result of trauma. Fractures and dislocations of the laryngeal framework and soft tissue damage can be caused by a variety of external injuries and by events occurring within the vocal tract. Submucosal haemorrhage in any part of the larynx as well as infection are common sequelae of laryngeal trauma. The damage affecting phonation can occur in the supraglottis and sub-glottis, as well as directly to the vocal folds. In some cases the recurrent laryngeal nerves will also be involved. Trauma to the larynx acutely compromises the airway and the management of this takes priority over phonation at all stages of recovery. The types of possible laryngeal trauma are listed in Table 9.6.

Table 9.6 Laryngeal trauma: causes

Type	Causes	Injuries
Compression (blunt injury)	Road traffic accidents Attempted strangulation Blows Sports injuries 'Clothes line' injuries	Laryngeal skeleton fractures: (1) high anteroposterior blows cause midline vertical fractures of the thyroid and cricoid cartilages (2) low anteroposterior blows cause cricoid fractures and laryngotracheal separation Soft tissue damage: haematomas, oedema, tears
Penetrating	Knives Bullets Glass	
Burns	Inhaled smoke Corrosive substances	Thermal chemical damage resulting in scarring and adhesions of the vocal folds Supraglottic stenosis
Intubation damage	Sustained during intubation for anaesthetic	Damage to free edges of vocal folds Arytenoid cartilage displacement
	Ventilator-dependent patients	Subglottic stenosis

The following are the chief effects of laryngeal injury:

- laryngeal stenosis
- pain
- dysphagia
- voice disorder.

DIRECT INJURIES

Direct trauma to the larynx falls into two groups.

Compression injuries

These occur as the result of blows or excessive pressure on the larynx. They commonly occur in road traffic accidents (RTAs) and during attempted strangulation. Blunt trauma tends to result in more severe injury to the airway and voice than penetrating trauma, probably because of the greater force needed to damage a larynx by a blow or compression (Cantrell, 1983).

Penetration injuries

These are caused by incidents such as stabbing and gunshot wounds. A penetrating laryngeal wound that is clean and localised may heal without damage to the vocal folds, but it is also much more likely to be fatal than a blunt injury.

Blows to the larynx occur most commonly in RTAs, but are not the only reason for survivors of such accidents to develop vocal problems. The multifactorial nature of post-RTA dysphonia is discussed below.

VOICE DISORDERS AFTER ROAD TRAFFIC ACCIDENTS

Road traffic accidents result not only in dramatic structural changes to the vocal tract but also in damage to the controlling and support systems of voice. The various ways in which RTAs can affect the voice are considered in this section. Comparatively few patients present with voice disorders after RTAs. This is probably because laryngotracheal injuries of any type are relatively rare and, when they do occur, the mortality rate is fairly high (Hosny, Bhendwal and Hosni, 1995). Post-RTA dysphonia cannot be viewed in terms of laryngeal damage alone, because the extensive damage that frequently ensues can give rise to a wide range of aetiologies that account for voice problems. They can be classified into three groups:

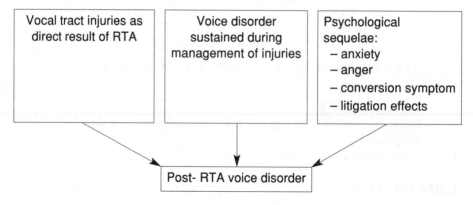

Figure 9.2 Voice disorders following road traffic accidents.

- problems affecting laryngeal structure and function
- supra- and subglottic vocal tract involvement
- concomitant problems, such as speech-breathing difficulties.

It has to be remembered that voice disorders in these circumstances are associated with severe and potentially life-threatening conditions. The effects of trauma to the vocal tract include airway stenosis, dysphagia and pain, which will have priority over the voice disorder in the management plan. Although some of the injuries causing voice disorders are sustained as the direct result of impact damage during the accident, others are the result of subsequent management during intensive care. Psychological trauma can also contribute to or cause voice disorders, whereas the needs and effects of on-going litigation frequently exacerbate residual symptoms. (Figure 9.2.)

Impact injuries

Injuries that occur at the time of the accident can cause voice problems at four main sites (Table 9.7).

Laryngeal trauma

This occurs when the body is thrown forward during sudden braking or on impact with another vehicle. Wearing a seat belt does not always provide protection but saves life and, paradoxically, increases the number of victims with laryngeal trauma (Cohn and Peppard, 1979). The usual protection of the larynx by the overhanging mandible and the forward contour of

Table 9.7 Road traffic accident injuries causing voice disorders

Site	Injuries
Front neck and laryngeal trauma	Midline fracture of thyroid cartilage Mucosal lacerations, haematomas, tears, separation, oedema Cricoid fractures, laryngotracheal separation Thermal damage
Damage to the peripheral nervous system	Unilateral or bilateral recurrent or superior laryngeal nerve damage
Head injury	Central nervous system: frontal lobe, brain-stem and upper motor neuron damage
Spinal injury	Respiratory function impairment

the chest is lost as the chin is forced upwards. As the neck extends and the larynx becomes fixed, its normal lateral and anteroposterior mobility is reduced (Casiano and Goodwin, 1991). Consequently, if contact is made with any part of the vehicle or another passenger, the larynx is subjected to maximum force. Severe laryngeal fractures occur when the larynx hits the steering wheel and the soft internal structures may be torn and the arytenoid cartilages dislocated (Harris and Ainsworth, 1965). The laryngeal injuries incurred reflect the point of impact of the blow.

High anteroposterior blows to the larynx, during which the thyroid and cricoid cartilages are crushed against the cervical vertebrae, can cause midline vertical fractures. The splaying of the thyroid lamina can cause mucosal lacerations, haematomas, tears, vocal fold injury, cricoarytenoid separation and oedema (Yen et al., 1994). The disturbed internal structures do not necessarily return to their original positions.

Low anteroposterior blows can lead to cricoid fractures and laryngotracheal separation (Roh and Fazzalaro, 1993). Fractures of the cricoid cartilage are commonly fatal because of the severe subglottal swelling. In some cases, the laryngeal skeleton is fractured so extensively that, even when the vocal folds are undamaged and mobile, they cannot be realigned to the same plane. The most severe fractures of the laryngeal cartilages can result in such marked laryngeal stenosis that laryngectomy has to be carried out in order to preserve a patent airway.

Laryngeal trauma can also take the form of **thermal damage** to the upper airway if there has been a vehicle fire after the impact. Even when gross vocal fold movements are preserved, laryngeal burns from smoke inhalation can result in stiff, red, vocal fold mucosa and minimal mucosal waves. (See laryngeal burns below.)

Peripheral nervous system damage

This occurs because of the proximity of the recurrent laryngeal nerve to the cricothyroid articulation, rendering damage to the nerve and vocal fold paralysis likely. A bilateral abductor vocal fold paralysis might not become apparent until extubation, when the patient will exhibit increasingly severe respiratory distress on removal of the endotracheal tube. Unilateral recurrent laryngeal nerve paralysis will present with typical breathy voice quality, inefficient cough and, possibly, aspiration (see Chapter 10).

Head injury

This injury acquired in high-impact RTAs can result in central nervous system damage which affects vocal fold adduction and muscle tone. Dysphonia in this instance is frequently a feature of dysarthria (see Chapter 10) with hyper- or hypoadduction of the vocal folds on phonation, according to the site of the damage. Frontal lobe damage resulting in poor affect and motivation can impair the ability to initiate phonation (Sapir and Aronson, 1985a, 1987) and oromotor apraxia might result in a patient being aphonic for volitional attempts at speech, although able to phonate involuntarily.

Spinal injury

Such injury resulting in impaired respiratory function reduces the individual's capacity for establishing adequate subglottal air pressure for the production of voice and for increasing vocal loudness.

Medical and surgical injuries

In addition to injuries acquired at the time of the accident, vocal tract changes also occur as the result of medical and surgical intervention directed at managing the recovery. Although establishing and maintaining the airway is the principal concern after the RTA, endotracheal intubation can cause a number of vocal tract changes, many of which are not revealed until extubation. These can include ulceration, oedema, granuloma, loss of vocal fold substance in the posterior vocal folds, and arytenoid dislocation followed by scar formation (Gallivan, Dawson and Robbins, 1989). Vocal fold contraction, arytenoid approximation and ankylosis of the cricoarytenoid joints continue to develop as a result of these changes. Prolonged endotracheal intubation causes granulomatous changes in the subglottis in response to friction or excessive cuff pressure in some patients, and tracheal stenosis can become so severe that a tracheostomy is necessary.

Psychological sequelae

Survivors of RTAs experience a range of psychological symptoms, which vary in type and extent according to the severity of their physical injuries, the fatalities involved, the circumstances of the crash and many other factors. These reactions can cause voice disorders such as conversion symptom aphonia or stress-related hyperfunctional dysphonia in some individuals, although there is no organic basis for their vocal symptoms. Intense emotions will also compound voice disorders as a result of physical injury, sometimes masking the true vocal profile. In cases of head injury, even when laryngoscopic examination is normal, the diagnosis of conversion symptom aphonia should be made only after neurological causes have been considered. Frontal lobe damage can result in poor affect and poor motivation, which impair the ability to initiate phonation (Sapir and Aronson, 1985a, 1987). Similar diagnostic dilemmas are caused by oromotor apraxia where the patient uses voice involuntarily but is otherwise aphonic. The emotional effects of the accident can last for many months with fluctuating levels of anxiety, anger, grief and depression. In the case of injury to others, guilt may exacerbate the psychological disturbance, giving rise to vocal symptoms such as intermittent voice loss or dysphonia. Globus symptoms are commonly associated with these emotions.

When dealing with patients whose voice problems are precipitated or appear to be maintained by emotional factors, the clinician should not overlook the effect of prolonged litigation in pursuit of claims for damages. The compensation awarded will be dependent in part on the loss of voice and damage to career prospects. In some instances, full potential recovery may be deliberately delayed until compensation is settled. Even when individuals are highly motivated to recover from the effects of the RTA, they frequently have difficulty putting the event behind them until the legal action is concluded. As the resolution of these cases can take many years, a number of factors arise in association with protracted voice disorders. The continuing stress of making statements and attending interviews with lawyers who revisit the traumatic event causes further distress. Many individuals also express concerns that, as they recover, the severity of the condition that they have suffered will be trivialised and undervalued. Although patients rarely appear to be malingering or exaggerating their voice disorders, some have to be persuaded that they can 'let go' of their symptoms and be convinced that it is possible for them to phonate normally or much more effectively.

Laryngoscopic findings

The state of the larynx is assessed by endoscopy after major trauma and regular review of laryngeal status takes place as recovery progresses. When healing is complete and inflammation and oedema have resolved, more detailed laryngoscopic examination using rigid stroboscopy helps to clarify the extent of scar tissue and laryngeal potential for phonation. Multiple laryngeal abnormalities of structure and function will be observed in many cases, as described above. The relative contributions of these abnormalities and their potential for change should be evaluated jointly by the laryngologist and speech and language therapist (Mathieson, 1997).

Expected acoustic profile

The voice will reflect the traumatic modifications of the larynx, but may also reflect respiratory and nervous system injuries as well as emotional reactions. Problems can range from aphonia through varying degrees and types of dysphonia to mild intermittent voice problems and globus symptoms. Increased vocal fold mass and any glottal insufficiency are revealed in the lowered pitch and roughness of the fundamental vocal note. It is important to identify the source of these acoustic changes during laryngoscopic evaluation, because there is much greater potential in the traumatised larynx for bizarre dimensions and approximations of laryngeal parts than in other voice disorders. For example, distorted cartilages can result in a true vocal fold approximating to a false fold, or the vocal folds each approximating to the midline appropriately but on different planes. Compression and bruising of the recurrent laryngeal nerve will give rise to the typically breathy and weak voice of vocal fold paralysis, unless there is bilateral abductor paralysis, in which case the voice is relatively normal and breathing is compromised (see Chapter 10). Electromyographic (EMG) evaluation will help in assessing the recovery potential of the recurrent laryngeal nerve in these cases (Hirano, Shigejiro and Terasawa, 1985). There is evidence to suggest that initial vocal fold paralysis indicates a poorer voice and airway result than when the folds are mobile in the early stages of recovery (Leopold, 1983).

After severe vocal tract injury, vocal recovery may take many months. The patient remains hoarse and the voice fatigues easily in conjunction with considerable laryngeal discomfort from the injured muscle tissue, ligaments and synovial joints. Inappropriate compensatory strategies can develop in an attempt to overcome organically based dysphonia, unless the patient is given guidance on the most suitable ways in which to deal with the vocal deficiencies. Some patients try to 'protect' the larynx by lowering vocal pitch and thereby unintentionally causing vocal strain. Others increase phonatory effort so that it becomes hyperfunctional as they attempt to achieve loudness. Conversion symptom aphonia can usually be overcome (see Chapter 8), but the return of voice does not resolve the emotional effects of the accident.

Medicosurgical decisions

The immediate need is to assess the extent of the laryngotracheal injury and to maintain and protect the airway by intubation or tracheostomy. If there are multiple injuries, orthopaedic, neurological and other specialists will be involved in the patient's care. Under such intensive intervention, treatment of the fractures and contused larynx may be delayed, but it is essential that the laryngologist assesses the larynx so that immediate steps can be taken to reconstruct the laryngeal cartilages and soft tissues in order to provide adequate airway protection and improve phonation. Indwelling stenting to prevent the formation of a web and stabilisation of the cartilages should be carried out as soon as practicable in order to ensure the best result for future voice (Duff, 1968; Dhillon and East, 1994).

The complexity and frequently multifactorial nature of voice disorders after RTAs necessitates a coordinated team approach by the laryngologist and speech–language pathologist. Clinical experience suggests that these patients are best served when the voice disorder is recognised and investigated at an early stage (Mathieson, 1997). The timing of a comprehensive evaluation will be determined by the patient's other injuries. A hoarse voice persisting after 24 hours following extubation should be investigated by thorough laryngoscopic examination in an attempt to mitigate future problems. Before decisions are made regarding phonosurgery and voice therapy, it is essential to obtain the best laryngeal image possible. The surgical aim is to provide a suitable airway and to repair laryngeal damage in order to establish the most efficient phonatory structure and function. Maximum functional efficiency of the damaged larynx, in the light of its biomechanical limitations, is facilitated by voice therapy. In the case of associated head injury, therapy directed at restoration of vocal function is frequently only one aspect of treatment which also concerns aphasia, dysarthria, dyspraxia and cognitive deficits.

Case histories

BC (17 years)

BC was in a collision with a car when he was riding his motorbike. His laryngeal framework was fractured when his crash helmet was pushed forward as he fell onto the road and the jaw protector crushed his larynx. An emergency tracheotomy was performed because his airway was seriously stenosed. After laryngeal reconstruction, closure of the tracheostomy and the resolution of oedema and inflammation within the larynx, his voice remained abnormal. On examination with rigid endoscopy and stroboscopy, there were obvious structural abnormalities for which he was compensating. The left vocal fold, with its irregular free edge, could be seen clearly at rest. Bulky tissue in the supraglottis completely obscured the right vocal fold.

On phonation, the true vocal folds could not be seen because of the strong approximation of the bulky false vocal folds. Consequently, it could not be established whether or not they were mobile. It was interesting to note that, on stroboscopy, there were symmetrical mucosal waves of considerable amplitude travelling across the surface of the approximated hypertrophic false vocal folds. The supraglottic activity seemed to be a compensatory function because of inadequate approximation of the true vocal folds. It is a matter of conjecture whether the glottal insufficiency was the result of vocal fold immobility or of the vocal folds not being on the same plane. The vocal profile reflected the structural and functional changes within the larynx. Vocal pitch was low because of the relatively large mass of the hypertrophic false vocal folds, and possibly because of the increased mass of the vocal folds. Roughness of the vocal note probably reflected the approximation and vibration of a number of surfaces in this abnormal larynx. As vocal fatigue set in, the voice became breathy, when it was not possible to maintain approximation of the false vocal folds and probably the true folds.

Although vocal loudness was adequate for quiet conversation, BC found it particularly frustrating that he could not be heard easily in a social setting. As a result, in the early stages of recovery, phonation was hyperfunctional and involved considerable effort. Voice therapy was aimed initially at reducing hyperfunction. This approach rapidly improved the quality of the vocal note and increased vocal loudness as a result of reducing the sphincteric laryngeal behaviour. Treatment was also directed at improving subglottal air pressure, partly through ensuring that he understood the need for adequate breath support, but also by introducing him to various strategies to ensure efficient speech-breathing patterns. Throughout treatment, which was administered in blocks over a period of 9 months, BC needed considerable emotional support from time to time. As frequently happens in such cases, the initial euphoria at surviving the trauma was followed by periods of depression, anxiety and frustration at the residual problems of communication. Regular treatment ended when he went to university. By then his voice was functionally adequate in most situations. When he was reviewed in the voice clinic over the next 2 years it transpired not only that his voice was continuing to be satisfactory, but that it had become an asset when seeking girlfriends. They found the deep pitch and a degree of vocal roughness appealing and he felt that his attractiveness was increased in their eyes.

DN (19 years)

DN was driving on the freeway when she collided at speed with a stationary truck that was at the end of a tailback of traffic. She sustained head injuries on impact and lost consciousness. The emergency services inserted an endotracheal tube at the site of the accident and she was admitted to intensive care. When she eventually recovered consciousness, there were certain cognitive deficits, related to memory and attention, but language was intact. Extubation rapidly led to respiratory distress and on laryngoscopic examination the vocal folds were observed to be approximated tightly in the midline. A diagnosis of bilateral abductor paralysis was made; it appeared that bilateral recurrent laryngeal nerve damage had been sustained at the time of the accident. A tracheotomy was performed. On occlusion of the stoma, voice was relatively normal, although there was significant vocal creak intermittently. This occurred particularly when she was anxious or distressed and reflected general vocal tract and body tension. At other times, her voice became breathy when she was tired. A Rusch valve (speaking valve) was introduced at the stoma site. Initially, her reaction to this was extremely fearful and she could tolerate the valve for only 1 or 2 minutes at a time.

Through explanations, reassurance and strategies such as easy onset phonation, she was able gradually to tolerate the valve for increasing lengths of time and to reduce the hyperadduction of the vocal folds on phonation and at rest. A narrow glottal chink became apparent over the first 3 months after the accident and a therapy programme of capping the tracheostomy tube for short periods was begun. Initially, she was able to achieve this for approximately 10 seconds only, but during the following months this time was gradually prolonged until the stoma could be capped for several hours at a time for gentle activities. She was in control of capping the stoma and could remove the cap herself at any time, for example, if she wanted to run up a flight of stairs. Vocal quality was well within normal limits and deteriorated only when she was distressed. On videostroboscopy, the vocal folds remained in the paramedian position at rest and moved to the midline on phonation. They did not abduct. Regular treatment sessions ceased when DN was managing her life well and had returned to college. She was capping the tracheostomy tube for all social situations and was very keen to have the stoma closed surgically. It was explained to her that her airway was inadequate for vigorous exercise and that an acute laryngitis could be life threatening. In addition, although surgical procedures to abduct one vocal fold would improve the airway, her normal voice would deteriorate. After 4 years her requests for stoma closure became increasingly insistent and she sought a second surgical opinion. This laryngologist excised granulomatous tissue in the subglottis and closed the stoma. DN was delighted with the result and was advised on her return to the original team to ensure that she contacted the hospital if she developed acute laryngitis at any time.

HK (24 years)

HK sustained head injuries when the car that he was driving left the road on a bend and hit a tree. He was unconscious when he was admitted to hospital and remained on a ventilator with an endotracheal tube for 3 weeks. When he resumed consciousness and the endotracheal tube was removed, his chief problems were his cognitive deficits. There were no acquired neurological speech and language problems, and his voice was normal. Over a period of days, it was reported, his breathing became increasingly laboured until he had severe difficulties and a tracheotomy was performed. He was referred to the voice clinic. He was aphonic when the stoma was occluded and it was evident that there was no transglottal airflow. On examination, the vocal folds were normal and mobile but a large granulomatous mass in the subglottis completely occluded the airway. This was the result of prolonged intubation and friction of the tube on the lining of the tracheal wall. HK was depressed and angry at his lack of voice and by the need for the tracheostomy. During long conversations with the speech–language pathologist he expressed suicidal thoughts. It was decided to remove the mass by laser. After the surgery, the vocal folds were initially oedematous and inflamed because the granulomatous tissue had encroached onto the subglottal aspect of the vocal folds. Voice therapy ensured appropriate voice conservation and vocal hygiene during the postoperative period minimised his tendency to hyperfunctional phonation as a response to being able to phonate again and helped him to adjust to normal phonation.

LB (25 years)

LB was a passenger in a car that was involved in a high-impact road traffic accident. Subsequently, she was tetraplegic and had a flaccid dysarthria. On examination, her vocal folds did not adduct fully and there was an anteroposterior glottal chink. She was unable to achieve glottal closure even on effort. Although her vocal folds were flaccid, the mucosal waves were reduced in amplitude as a result of her very limited ability to generate adequate airflow and volume of air. Her vocal profile was as expected. The vocal note was breathy because of glottal insufficiency. Quiet voice was the result of not being able to increase subglottal air pressure, because of the combined effects of limited breath support, glottal insufficiency and the flaccidity of the vocal folds. Voice therapy was based on maximising respiratory function and improving glottal closure via laryngeal valving exercises.

BD (47 years)

This patient complained of dysphonia that had been occurring intermittently since he had been hit by a car 6 months earlier. He had been digging at roadworks, at the side of the road, when he realised that another workman was in the path of a rapidly approaching car that showed no signs of slowing. He dashed to push his colleague to safety and was hit by the car himself. His leg had been broken and subsequently he had developed back problems. After the accident, he was aphonic for a short period but, although his voice had returned to normal, it was unpredictable and, at times, obviously dysphonic. He reported that his throat felt constricted and he felt that there was a lump in his throat intermittently. After laryngoscopy and having been reassured that there was no abnormality, he was referred for voice therapy. He related the voice problem to the accident and, as he explained what had happened, and how he had been unable to work subsequently, his anger was obvious. He was near to tears as he berated the stupidity of the driver who had injured him and described the endless interviews with solicitors which did not seem to accelerate the process of receiving damages.

Although he was so distressed, he listened with interest to explanations concerning the basic anatomy of the vocal tract and its response to stress. He was reassured that it was possible to experience marked voice problems and vocal tract discomfort, although there was no organic pathology, and that there was no physical reason why his voice should not return to normal. His response was positive. Understanding that the voice and vocal tract symptoms were only reflecting his anger and distress simplified the situation. He had thought that his voice had been another casualty of the accident and might signify further physical problems that might need prolonged treatment. He left the initial meeting with the speech–language pathologist saying that he felt much happier. At his next appointment, a week later, he reported that, apart from occasional tightening in his throat, he had had no problems. He felt that he was managing well and did not need further appointments, but asked if he could make further appointments if he experienced voice problems in the future. There was no further contact from this patient.

LARYNGEAL BURNS

Burns to the laryngeal mucosa may be **thermal**, as the result of a fire or explosion, or **chemical**, caused by swallowing acids or other corrosive materials, or inhaling caustic fumes. Cohn and Peppard (1979) review the possible sites of damage and the medical treatment for surface burns. Sloughing of the mucosal lining of the larynx and adhesion in healing, forming webs, may develop but this is rare with careful medical treatment. Oedema can cause difficulty in breathing and intense irritation causes coughing. Even when gross vocal fold movements are relatively normal, smoke inhalation can result in stiff, red vocal folds with markedly reduced mucosal waves. The voice will be hoarse until healing is complete and complete vocal rest must be observed during this period.

INTUBATION INJURIES

Intubation damage to the larynx has been described above in connection with contact ulcers and road traffic accident victims. Intubation damage can be sustained by two processes:

- Patients in **intensive care** are particularly susceptible to laryngeal trauma because of the long period during which the ventilator tube may be lying between the vocal folds.
- Laryngeal damage can occur **during the process of intubation** for routine general anaesthetic or for more prolonged intubation for the following reasons:
  - if the procedure is particularly difficult because of the configuration of the individual patient's oral cavity and airway
  - if intubation has been carried out with excessive force or roughness
  - if an excessively large tube is used.

Laryngoscopic findings

Intubation damage falls into two groups: **dislocation** and **abrasion**.

Dislocation

The arytenoid cartilages can be dislocated during the process of intubation. The intubation damage is not necessarily readily apparent on extubation and in some cases it is not until approximately 3 days later that inflammation and oedema of the arytenoids can be seen in association with reduced vocal fold mobility and incomplete adduction of the posterior portion (Whited, 1985).

Abrasion

Intubation can also cause superficial abrasions and granulomatous formation on the vocal processes of the arytenoid cartilages. Round, fleshy intubation granulomas form at the site of trauma to the laryngeal mucosa, frequently where an ulcer has been caused by the endotracheal tube. They vary in size and may be unilateral or bilateral (see Figure 9.3).

Expected acoustic profile

Arytenoid dislocation

This has a similar effect to vocal fold paralysis because the affected vocal fold is immobile or mobility is significantly reduced and the vocal folds do not approximate to the midline (see page 312). In some cases, the dislocation allows the vocal fold to fall to a slightly lower plane than the unaffected vocal fold. Glottal insufficiency results in a breathy vocal note and reduced loudness.

Abrasions

Abrasions to the free edges of the vocal folds cause inflammation and oedema which increases vocal fold mass and also affects the amplitude

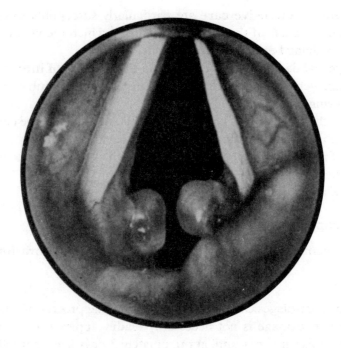

Figure 9.3 Intubation granulomas.

and symmetry of the mucosal waves. Hoarseness will vary according to the severity of the trauma and whether or not the patient abuses the voice in an attempt to compensate for the problem. Speaking fundamental frequency is lowered. **Intubation granuloma** also causes marked hoarseness.

Medicosurgical decisions

Intervention depends on the severity of the laryngeal injury. Voice conservation and good vocal hygiene followed, if necessary, by a programme of vocal re-education is the preferred course for dealing with laryngeal abrasions. It is essential to ensure that the patient does not cause further damage by using hyperfunctional phonation in an attempt to overcome the primary problem. A trial course of voice therapy can also be the first treatment route in dealing with intubation granulomas, particularly if they are small, but where both the voice and airway are affected laser removal of the lesions without damaging the underlying mucosa can be carried out (Gussak, Jurovich and Laterman, 1986).

Congenital tracheal abnormalities

The speech–language pathologist may become involved in the care of children with the following conditions in order to encourage acceptable phonation as part of the overall development of speech and language.

TRACHEO-OESOPHAGEAL FISTULA

A fistula of the tracheo-oesophageal wall is a congenital malformation that causes serious respiratory and swallowing problems in the neonate. The defect in the tracheo-oesophageal wall allows gastric contents to drain from the oesophagus into the trachea, resulting in aspiration, and air from the trachea to pass into the gut. Surgical repair or, in some cases, laryngectomy is required to ensure that the oesophagus and trachea are each patent.

TRACHEOMALACIA

This condition is similar to laryngomalacia. The walls of the trachea collapse inwards on inspiration resulting in stridor. As the infant matures the condition resolves.

TRACHEAL STENOSIS

Varying degrees of congenital tracheal stenosis (i.e. narrowing or constriction of the trachea) result in obstruction of the airway.

Acquired tracheal abnormalities

LARYNGOTRACHEAL STENOSIS

The subglottis is the most common site of narrowing in the airway (Dhillon and East, 1994). It can be the result of acute laryngeal trauma, an incorrectly sited tracheostomy or long-term intubation. The incidence of stenosis is increased after tracheostomy (Richard et al., 1996). Surgery, or in some cases dilatation of the trachea, is required to improve the airway for respiration and phonation.

TRACHEOTOMY

Tracheotomy may be performed in conditions in which the patient is unable to breathe normally through the nose and mouth. (Table 9.8) A surgically created stoma (tracheostomy) between the cricoid cartilage and the suprasternal notch allows the patient to breathe when there is upper

Table 9.8 Reasons for creating a tracheostomy

Bypass of upper airway obstruction	eg. Laryngeal carcinoma, laryngeal trauma
Artificial ventilation	eg. Neuromuscular diseases affecting respiratory musculature
Tracheal suction	eg. Chronic obstructive airway disease (COAD) when the patient's cough is ineffective

Endotracheal intubation presents fewer problems in its execution and maintenance than tracheostomy and is therefore the preferred procedure whenever possible.

airway obstruction caused by infection, a foreign body, trauma or a tumour. In these cases, it may be carried out as an emergency, life-saving procedure. In others, such as certain neurological conditions or severe respiratory disease, a decision is made after considered evaluation of the patient's problems in order to reduce respiratory difficulties or to avoid an

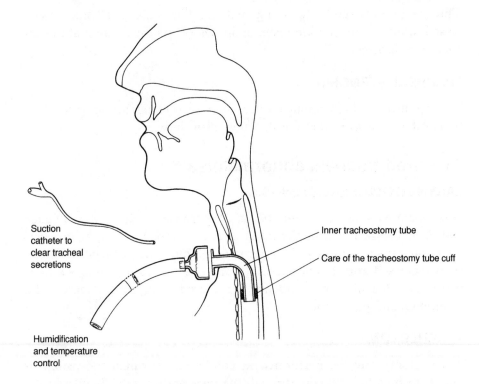

Suction
catheter to
clear tracheal
secretions

Inner tracheostomy tube

Care of the tracheostomy tube cuff

Humidification
and temperature
control

Figure 9.4 Diagram of tracheostomy tube in situ. Reproduced from 'Ear, Nose and Throat', Dhillon R.S., East CA., page 68, 1994, by permission of the publisher Churchill Livingstone.

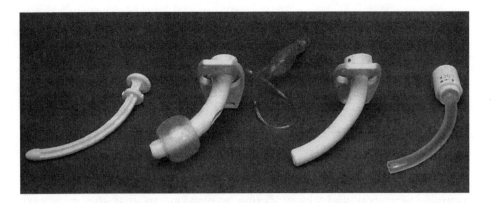

Figure 9.5 Tracheostomy tubes. From left to right: introducer; cuffed fenestrated outer tube; uncuffed non-fenestrated outer tube; inner tube. Reproduced from 'Ear, Nose and Throat', Dhillon R.S., East CA., page 68, 1994, by permission of the publisher Churchill Livingstone.

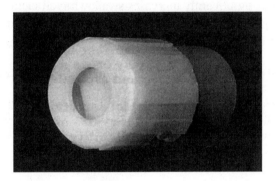

Figure 9.6 Rusch speaking valve can be attached to the tracheostomy tube. The valve opens on inspiration and closes on expiration so that air flows through the glottis to allow vocalisation. Reproduced from 'Ear, Nose and Throat', Dhillon R.S., East CA., page 68, 1994, by permission of the publisher Churchill Livingstone.

acute episode of respiratory difficulty. Whenever possible, intubation is preferred to tracheotomy because the complications of endotracheal intubation are rarer and less severe than those of tracheotomy (Dhillon and East, 1994). After tracheostomy, the patient is aphonic because pulmonic air no longer leaves the body via the larynx, but through the stoma. This lack of voice can be overcome by re-directing air through the larynx (see below). The stoma can be closed surgically if the underlying condition that makes it necessary can be resolved.

Tracheostomy tubes consist of an inner and outer tube (Figures 9.4 and 9.5). The outer tube can remain in place when the inner tube is removed for cleaning. Tubes are available with inflated cuffs, which prevent the aspiration of secretions into the lungs, and with fenestrations that allow pulmonic air to be directed through the larynx (when the stoma is occluded). When the cuff is inflated, and there is no fenestration, the patient cannot produce voice because there is no available airstream. Uncuffed tubes or tubes with cuffs that can be deflated allow the patient to produce voice when a speaking valve, such as a Rusch valve (Figure 9.6) or a Passy–Muir Speaking Tracheostomy valve, is used. The speaking valve is attached to the tracheostomy tube and opens during inspiration and closes during expiration, so that the expiratory airstream is directed to the larynx and allows the patient to phonate. An additional benefit for tracheostomised patients using a speaking valve appears to be a reduction in aspiration, which is a well-recognised tendency in patients with open tracheostomy tubes. A study by Eibling and Gross (1996) suggests that the maintenance of a closed subglottic system, which permits a rise in subglottic air pressure, significantly increases swallowing efficiency.

Table 9.9 provides a summary of the various types of tracheostomy tubes and their potential effect on phonation and swallowing.

Expected vocal profile in acquired tracheal abnormalities

Narrowing of the airway, as in tracheal stenosis, and conditions requiring a tracheostomy, inevitably affect airflow and volume for phonation adversely. Even when the larynx is normal, vocal note quality, loudness and phrase length are all reduced.

Medicosurgical decisions

Surgical intervention is required to improve or reverse tracheal stenosis. The role of the speech–language pathologist is to enable the patient to phonate as effectively as possible or to provide adequate means of communication if voicing cannot be achieved. In cases where the need for tracheostomy is the result of neurological conditions, the speech–language pathologist will also be involved in the management of coexisting dysarthria, dysphasia and dysphagia. The speech–language pathologist should also be alert to the fact that, after endotracheal intubation or tracheotomy, patients may experience swallowing dysfunction, which may be caused by weakness of the muscles involved in swallowing and incoordination of the swallow response (DeVita and Spierer-Rundback, 1990). As a result, there is risk of aspiration in these patients, even though they have been extubated or the tracheostomy has been closed.

Table 9.9 Types of tracheostomy tube

Tracheostomy tube	Reason for choice of tube	Potential for voice	Effects on swallowing
Cuffed, unfenestrated tube	Prevents aspiration of secretions. Used in ventilator-dependent patients	Pulmonic air can only leave the trachea via the stoma, therefore the patient cannot produce voice	Patient is unable to swallow
Cuffed, unfenestrated tube with deflatable cuff	Prevents aspiration of secretions but allows phonation and oral intake of food when deflated	Phonation can be achieved when cuff is deflated by occluding stoma with finger or speaking valve. Air passes up the trachea to the larynx around the tube	Patient can swallow normally when cuff is deflated and the stoma is occluded
Fenestrated tube without cuff	Allows suction of tracheal secretions and pulmonary airflow available for phonation	Phonation easily achieved when stoma is occluded by finger or speaking valve	Normal swallow when stoma is occluded
Uncuffed, unfenestrated tube	Allows suction of tracheal secretions and pulmonary airflow available for phonation	Pulmonic air passes up trachea around tube so that voice is achieved with stoma occlusion with finger or speaking valve	Normal swallow when stoma is occluded

In addition to providing a patent airway, tracheostomy tubes are chosen according to their potential to avoid aspiration of secretions into the lungs, which can result in pneumonia. When these two needs are met, the potential for allowing oral intake of food and enabling the patient to produce voice is also taken into account. The speaking valves, which are attached to the tracheostomy tube as described in this table, are entirely different from the prostheses used with laryngectomy patients (see Chapter 17). Rusch and Passy-Muir valves are used in cases where the patient has a larynx and where the airstream has to be re-routed, from exiting to the exterior via the stoma, to the vocal folds.

Summary

- ■ Structural abnormalities of the vocal tract are congenital and/or acquired.
- ■ The expected vocal profile is related to the site, type and severity of the abnormality.
- ■ But it is also influenced by any compensatory strategies that are employed in an attempt to overcome the primary deficiency.

■ Vocal potential and function can also be affected by the patient's emotional status and, in acquired conditions, by the patient's pre-morbid vocal behaviour.

■ Treatment in most cases should be a multidisciplinary approach with the laryngologist and speech–language pathologist working closely together.

■ Normal voice might not be a realistic treatment goal in every case but the patient should be helped to achieve the best voice possible, given the biomechanical limitations.

10 CHAPTER

Neurogenic voice disorders

Neurological voice disorders can occur as the result of lesions in either the central or peripheral nervous systems. When the peripheral nervous system (PNS) alone is involved, only the laryngeal and palatal muscles are affected. Central nervous system (CNS) lesions usually produce more extensive signs throughout the vocal tract, which interact to give rise to the final voice problem. Within the category of neurological dysphonias, disorders of the myoneural junction and muscles also give rise to voice disorders. Voice disorders arising from neuropathology represent a relatively small percentage of disordered voices (see Chapter 6). Many neurological conditions present with abnormal voice, however, because of their extensive effects on muscle movement and tone, as well as the timing and coordination of movements, all of which can affect the vocal tract and speech–breathing patterns. Table 10.1 summarises neurological dysphonias according to the site of the lesion, its effect on muscles (myopathy) and the possible causes. These individual conditions are described in this chapter but first the types of laryngeal dysfunction that arise from neuropathology are discussed.

Types of laryngeal dysfunction

Traditionally, the neurological dysphonias have been classified according to the site of the lesion but, in addition, classification according to the type of laryngeal dysfunction has important advantages for the speech pathologist as a basis for the goal and type of therapy which are eventually decided upon. Ramig and Scherer (1992) categorise the main features of laryngeal behaviour in neurological voice disorders as:

Table 10.1 Classification of neurogenic dysphonias

Site of lesion	Symptoms	Possible aetiology	Examples of neurological condition
Pyramidal and extrapyramidal lesions (upper motor neuron)	*Pyramidal:* • Spasticity – with associated weakness • Movements slow and reduced in range	Cerebrovascular accident (CVA) Cerebral trauma Cerebral tumour Multiple sclerosis Idiopathic	*Pyramidal:* Pseudobulbar palsy
	Extrapyramidal: • Hypokinetic • Hyperkinetic • Tremor	Arteriosclerotic Postencephalitic Infection Hereditary condition Congenital Age-related Toxic chemicals	*Extrapyramidal:* Parkinsonism Chorea (dyskinesia) Benign essential tremor Athetosis (dystonia)
Lower motor neuron[a]	Flaccidity	Viral infection Tumour Trauma Toxic chemicals Poliomyelitis Myasthenia gravis	Bulbar palsy Vocal fold paralysis and paresis
Cerebellum	Ataxia	Tumours Trauma Excessive alcohol Hereditary conditions	Cerebellar ataxia Friedreich's ataxia Legionnaires' disease[b]
Mixed lesions	Mixed symptoms	Unknown Familial	Motor neuron disease Multiple sclerosis Wilson's disease

[a]LMN lesions may involve individual cranial nerves, and therefore individual muscles, or be extensive with widespread dysarthric symptoms.
[b]Cerebellar signs are also evident in some victims of Legionnaires' disease but, although there is disruption of respiratory, laryngeal and swallowing mechanisms, the overall pattern of dysarthria is unlike the typical ataxic dysarthria (Mackenzie, 1987).
After Darley, Aronson and Brown (1975).

- problems of vocal fold adduction (hypoadduction/hyperadduction)
- phonatory instability
- phonatory incoordination.

PROBLEMS OF VOCAL FOLD ADDUCTION

Hypoadduction

The inadequate adduction of the vocal folds results in a breathy vocal note in all cases. When there is no vocal fold adduction, or when adduction is minimal, the patient is aphonic. Vocal loudness is also reduced because of inefficient glottal closure. In some cases, the flaccidity and chaotic behaviour of the vocal folds will cause diplophonia. Voiced/voiceless contrasts, e.g. bike/pike, will be affected as voiced phonemes become devoiced. Hypoadduction typically occurs in lower motor neuron (LMN) and brainstem lesions.

Hyperadduction

Uncontrolled, forceful adduction of the vocal folds gives rise to a strained, pressed voice quality. The sphincteric behaviour of the glottis in severe cases causes excessive phonatory effort and, at times, difficulties in initiating phonation because of laryngospasm, with voiceless phonemes tending to be voiced. The false vocal folds may also be involved in phonation. In milder cases, the voice is harsh, pitch breaks occur and vocal pitch is low. Upper motor neuron (UMN) lesions, in which muscles are spastic and hypertonic, can give rise to vocal fold hyperadduction.

PHONATORY INSTABILITY

In most cases of neurological dysphonia, the voice is unstable and exhibits features such as tremor and unstable pitch and loudness. The instability of laryngeal behaviour will be exacerbated by poorly coordinated speech–breathing patterns in some patients.

PHONATORY INCOORDINATION

Intelligibility is affected if phonation is not timed to match articulation. Delayed voice–onset timing (VOT) can result in voiceless segments in continuous speech and in impaired voiced/voiceless contrasts. The subtle features of normal prosody are significantly eroded when the speaker is unable to adjust the necessary intonation and stress patterns, speech rate, pitch and loudness.

Table 10.2 summarises the perceptual vocal features associated with the three categories of laryngeal behaviour found in neurological voice disorders, and the features that are observed on acoustic and EGG evaluation. In clinical practice, the patient's phonatory problems cannot be discretely categorised but vocal features will overlap, as in the patient with parkinsonism who exhibits both phonatory incoordination and hypoadduction. Each patient's vocal profile will emerge as the results of laryngoscopic, perceptual and acoustic evaluations are integrated within the context of the neuropathology.

SPEECH–BREATHING IN NEUROGENIC DYSPHONIAS

Neuromuscular disorders that affect the movements of the chest wall will inevitably affect phonation significantly due to impaired respiratory support. As a result of wasting, weakness or rigidity of the respiratory muscles, vital capacity can be reduced markedly so that, in combination with abnormal vocal fold movements, the speaking rate is slowed and fewer syllables

Table 10.2 Vocal features in neurogenic dysphonias

Vocal fold adduction abnormality:	Perceptual vocal features:	Acoustic/EGG analysis:
Hypoadduction (associated with LMN and brain-stem lesions)	Breathiness Reduced loudness Diplophonia in some cases Voiced/voiceless contrasts inadequate	Low signal-to-noise ratio Short maximum phonation time Reduced intensity range Reduced SFo Reduced/absent closed phase
Hyperadduction (associated with UMN lesions)	Pressed Strained Harsh Low pitch Voiced/voiceless contrasts impaired	Decreased airflow Short maximum phonation time Increased/decreased intensity Reduced SFo Reduced pitch range Prolonged closed phase
Phonatory instability (associated with most neurological dysphonias)	Pitch/loudness variations Vocal tremor	Increased jitter measures Increased shimmer measures
Phonatory incoordination (associated with many neurological dysphonias)	Voice-onset timing problems Dysprosody Paradoxical (inspiratory) phonation	Inappropriate voice-onset time (VOT) Abnormal Fo contours

LMN, lower motor neuron; UMN, upper motor neuron.
After Ramig and Scherer (1992)

are produced per breath. In addition to reduced mobility of the chest wall, some patients appear to have difficulty in coordinating the action of the rib cage and abdomen for speech (Murdoch et al., 1993).

In cases of neurological disorder, as in all voice pathology, the resulting voice reflects the biomechanics of the vocal folds and vocal tract, whatever the particular diagnosis of the underlying neurological condition. Regard for this essential principle ensures that the speech–language pathologist evaluates the vocal pathology of each patient without being misled by presupposition. Consequently, vocal features resulting from inappropriate compensatory strategies and the possibilities of coexisting pathologies are less likely to be overlooked.

Central nervous system lesions

Dysphonia resulting from a CNS lesion is usually only one aspect of dysarthria, a disorder of articulation as a result of CNS lesions causing paralysis and paresis of the muscles of articulation and deglutition (McNeil, Rosenbek and Aronson, 1984). CNS lesions may be acquired or congenital, as in the case of cerebral palsy. Dysarthria affects articulatory, phonatory, respiratory and phonological aspects of speech. Peacher (1949) suggested the term 'dysarthrophonia' to denote neurological dysphonia that presents as one aspect of dysarthria. Dysarthrophonia was proposed to distinguish this condition from nuclear and peripheral lesions in the LMN pathway, which do not include dysarthria but are confined to palatal and laryngeal paralysis. The term is not in general use and **neurological dysphonia** is in current use in the literature. The dysarthrias are commonly described in accordance with the Mayo Clinic classification, based on the research of Darley, Aronson and Brown (1975). No part of the nervous system is self-contained, however, and as a result discrete symptoms do not exist but may predominate in a complex of dysfunctions. In some conditions, the site of the lesion may be obscure, as in the case of tremor or dyspraxia.

The neuroanatomy underlying these neurological disorders is described in Chapter 2.

UPPER MOTOR NEURON (CORTICAL AND PYRAMIDAL) LESIONS

Pseudobulbar (spastic dysphonia)

It is important to stress that the spastic dysphonia associated with pseudobulbar palsy has to be distinguished from psychogenic spastic dysphonia and spasmodic adductor dysphonia (also sometimes referred to as spastic dysphonia) which are described elsewhere.

In pseudobulbar palsy the effects of the UMN lesion are apparent in the tongue, face, larynx and palatopharyngeal sphincter, with the result that, in addition to speech production difficulties, the face may be expressionless. Swallowing is always affected. There is emotional lability, as a result of the lack of cortical inhibition of laughing and crying, which produces emotional outbursts or excessive reactions that are not indicative of the true emotional state. This lack of control in itself causes the individual very real distress.

As a result of the bulbar nuclei receiving innervation from both hemispheres, lesions of the UMN pathway must be bilateral in order to produce vocal fold paralyses. A unilateral UMN lesion produces a spastic hemiplegia which affects the contralateral side. Impairment of the bulbar-sited cranial nerves is not severe. Although there may be facial and lingual weakness on the affected side, with the further complication of aphasia in the case of a left cortical lesion, there is no unilateral vocal fold paralysis.

The bilateral lesions resulting in pseudobulbar dysarthria cause severe speech problems. Excessive effort is used in an attempt to counteract the resistance of the hypertonic speech musculature and articulation is slow and laboured. Phonation has a distinctive 'strained–strangled' quality (Darley, Aronson and Brown, 1975) as air is forced between the hyperadducted vocal folds. Hypertonicity of the vocal tract and respiratory musculature restricts the range of movements required for pitch adjustments and, as a result, pitch is monotonous (monopitch). It might be expected that vocal pitch would be raised as a result of hypertonicity, but a classic feature of pseudobulbar palsy is excessively low pitch (Aronson, 1990). This appears to be caused by the extreme effort involved in phonation, with hyperadduction of the vocal folds resulting in the speaker phonating as if attempting a Valsalva manoeuvre while talking. Loudness is generally reduced and lacks variation because of the weakness of the hypertonic musculature. At times, however, there may be excessive loudness over short phrases.

Although there may be reflex elevation of the soft palate and symmetrical elevation on articulation of an isolated vowel, the excursion of the velum to the posterior pharyngeal wall is incomplete and slow. Consequently, hypernasality is a prominent feature of pseudobulbar palsy because the palate moves too slowly and inefficiently to coordinate with articulatory patterns.

Respiratory difficulties are apparent with breathing often out of phase with phonation, resulting in paradoxical (inspiratory) phonation and only one word, or short phrase, being uttered at a time. Breathing is shallow and there is a decrease in airflow rate. To some extent, these problems of breathing for speech arise as a result of loss of air because of the inability to form appropriate and coordinated closures in the larynx, oral cavity and velopharyngeal sphincter. Similarly, maximum phonation time is greatly reduced from normal as a result of the inability to coordinate diaphragmatic and intercostal motion with closure of the laryngeal valve. Normal prosodic features are absent and, in combination with severely distorted articulation, speech becomes unintelligible.

The characteristics of pseudobulbar palsy are summarised in Table 10.3.

Table 10.3 Pseudobulbar palsy dysphonia profile	
Pathology	UMN lesions causing spastic dysarthria and associated dysphonia
Aetiology	*Bilateral* lesions of corticobulbar tract (i.e. supranuclear lesions, above nerve X nucleus)
Signs	Spasticity of tongue, face, larynx, velopharyngeal sphincter resulting in: • motor speech disorder (dysarthria) • dysphonia: effortful phonation • dysphagia
Laryngoscopic findings	Vocal folds normal at rest Hyperadduction of true vocal folds and, possibly, false vocal folds Long closed phase
Expected vocal profile	Strained–strangled vocal quality: harsh or hoarse Excessively low pitch Reduced pitch range Reduced loudness Hypernasality Maximum phonation time reduced
Acoustic analysis profile	Reduced harmonics-to-noise ratio Lowered SFo Increased jitter and shimmer
Airflow and volume measures	Decreased airflow rate Reduced vital capacity

LOWER MOTOR NEURON LESIONS ASSOCIATED WITH DYSARTHRIA AND DYSPHONIA

Myasthenia gravis

Myasthenia gravis is a condition characterised by progressive failure to sustain a maintained or repeated contraction of striated muscle. This autoimmune disease causes the reception of acetylcholine at the neuromuscular junction to be blocked and, as a result, there is generalised muscular flaccidity (Edwards et al., 1995). It usually appears between the ages of 15 and 50 years, with a higher incidence in females than in males. General bodily weakness and extreme fatigue occur on repeated effort. The palatopharyngeal and laryngeal valves may be affected at an early stage of the disease and, as a result, hypernasality and breathy, weak voice are frequently the first diagnostic symptoms. Initially, the symptoms can be misdiagnosed as psychogenic, particularly if the voice symptoms occur in isolation. It is diagnostically significant, however, that the vocal deterioration and increased hypernasality correlate with the length of time the individual has been speaking. Reversal of the condition can be obtained by regular injections of neostigmine compounds. It is essential for the patient to avoid exertion and to rest in order to conserve energy. Voice therapy is contraindicated as the voice is normal following appropriate medical management. The characteristics of dysphonia associated with myasthenia gravis are summarised in Table 10.4.

Table 10.4 Myasthenia gravis dysphonia profile

Pathology	Generalised muscular flaccidity and weakness
Aetiology	Autoimmune disease causing reception of acetylcholine at the neuromuscular junction to be blocked
Signs	Early hypernasality and breathy voice Relatively normal speech rapidly deteriorates during prolonged speaking, becoming increasingly hypernasal and weaker
Laryngoscopic findings	Incomplete adduction and abduction In early stages, vocal fold movement can appear normal Movement may deteriorate with task repetition Long open phase
Expected vocal profile	Breathy weak voice Hypernasality Voice symptoms can occur in isolation
Acoustic analysis profile	Reduced harmonics-to-noise ratio Reduced intensity Reduced pitch range Increased jitter and shimmer
Airflow and volume measures	Increased transglottal airflow
Medicosurgical decisions	Immunological treatment: • thymectomy • corticosteroids • immunosuppressant treatment

Table 10.5 Cranial nerves involved in bulbar palsy dysarthria/dysphonia

Cranial nerve lesion	Muscle groups affected
Trigeminal (V)	Face
Facial (VII)	Face and lips
Glossopharyngeal (IX)	Tongue, pharynx, palate
Vagus (X)	Larynx, respiratory muscles, pharynx, soft palate
Hypoglossal (XII)	Tongue

Bulbar palsy dysphonia

Brain-stem lesions produce a flaccid paralysis with reduced muscle tone (hypotonia). There is atrophy (muscle wasting) and fasciculation (twitching). If a lesion occurs at a point where sensory fibres are associated with the lower motor neurons, sensation will also be affected. Table 10.5 lists the cranial nerves involved in bulbar palsy.

Typically, when the lesion is bilateral, the phonatory characteristics of bulbar palsy include breathiness, possibly with stridor, as a result of the vocal folds only partially adducting and abducting. Pitch is lowered because the flaccid vocal folds cannot be vibrated sufficiently rapidly by the expiratory airstream to achieve the speaker's normal pitch. Lack of muscle tone and the inability of the vocalis muscle to be lengthened and tightened significantly result in minimal pitch variation. Loudness is also not varied because weak vocal fold adduction of the relatively flaccid vocal folds allows air to leak at the glottis. Additional common features of bulbar palsy are hypernasality with audible nasal emission, resulting from inadequate velopharyngeal closure. The inability to produce competent closure of laryngeal, palatopharyngeal and articulatory valves also exacerbates the underlying respiratory difficulties because the expiratory airflow is uncontrolled and frequent intake of air becomes necessary, in compensation for reduced vital capacity. Consequently, clavicular breathing develops in an attempt to enlarge the thoracic movements and capacity. As a result, short phrases are used because of the reduced vital capacity and the inability to control exhalation as a result of glottal insufficiency. Attempts to phonate on residual air occur frequently. The inadequacy of vocal fold movement, combined with poor respiratory function, also make it extremely difficult for the speaker to increase subglottal air pressure for coughing, with the result that the voice frequently has a 'wet', bubbly quality arising from the collection of secretions in the larynx.

Articulation associated with bilateral lesions is affected by poor lip seal and limited tongue tip elevation arising from the hypotonic and wasting musculature. Tongue protrusion may not be possible. In some severe cases, there is great difficulty in raising the mandible to the closed position (Darley, Aronson and Brown, 1975) and therefore in producing labial and lingual consonants. Unilateral lesions are apparent in the drooping of the lips on the affected side. The tongue may fasciculate and be atrophic on the paralysed side, deviating to the affected side on protrusion. Intelligibility is poor as a result of the involvement of all parameters and the subsequent effect on prosody. The characteristics of dysphonia associated with bulbar palsy are summarised in Table 10.6.

Table 10.6 Bulbar palsy dysphonia profile

Pathology	Brain-stem lesions causing flaccid dysarthria and associated dysphonia
Aetiology	Lesions involving cranial nerves V, VII, IX, X and XII
Signs	Hypotonia, atrophy (muscle wasting) and fasciculation (twitching) of articulatory muscles Loss of sensation
Laryngoscopic findings	Incomplete vocal fold adduction and abduction Reduced vocal fold tonicity Long open phase or no closed phase
Expected vocal profile	Breathy vocal note Monopitch Monoloudness Hypernasality Reduced maximum phonation time 'Wet' vocal quality
Acoustic analysis profile	SFo decreased Pitch range reduced Harmonics-to-noise ratio reduced Jitter and shimmer increased
Airflow and volume measures	Increased airflow rate Reduced lung capacity

CEREBELLAR LESIONS

The cerebellum has an integrating and controlling role over movements that arise in other parts of the motor system. It regulates the force, speed, range, timing and direction of movements so that excesses are inhibited, and also contributes to equilibrium, posture and gait (see Chapter 2). It seems that it does not control patterns of movement but acts as a processing centre for motor activity (Darley, Aronson and Brown, 1975). A conspicuous feature of cerebellar damage is inaccuracy in targeting movements, as when a patient is asked to stretch out the arm and touch the nose with the forefinger. The basic movement pattern is intact, but the target is over- or under-shot. Intention tremor appears at the end of movements and static tremor may be present if attempts are made to maintain a limb in a steady position. For speech to be affected, the cerebellar damage must be bilateral and widespread. Patients with cerebellar ataxia are frequently thought to be drunk on account of slurred speech, wide gait, impaired balance and general incoordination.

The speech musculature is hypotonic and movements are slow and inaccurate. Unpredictable movements of articulation, phonation and respiration occur. Articulation is jerky and inaccurate with exaggerated excursions of lips, jaw and tongue. There is obvious incoordination of all speech parameters. In addition to the slowed speech rate, syllables may be produced individually with equal stress, which results in the characteristic scanning speech of ataxia. Grewel (1957a), in his classifications of dysarthria, described this as bradylalia or bradyarthria.

Table 10.7 Cerebellar dysphonia profile	
Pathology	Ataxic dysarthria with associated dysphonia
Aetiology	Cerebellar lesions
Signs and symptoms	Inaccurately targeted movements Hypotonia Intention tremor Static tremor Wide gait Impaired balance General incoordination
Laryngoscopic findings	Normal structure Intermittent hyperadduction
Expected vocal profile	Pitch variable/pitch breaks Vocal quality variable: harsh, breathy, strained-strangled Scanning speed Loud/explosive at times
Acoustic analysis profile	Unstable SFo Wide/uncontrolled pitch range Harmonics-to-noise ratio reduced and variable Intermittent increased intensity
Airflow and volume measures	Maximum phonation time reduced

Phonation is explosive and staccato at times, but hoarse, harsh and breathy at others. The lack of coordination between respiration and phonation results in reduced maximum phonation time and pitch breaks. Control of pitch and loudness is impaired and the ataxic speaker frequently speaks loudly. The presence of severe dysrhythmia disrupts normal prosody but speech, although bizarre, usually remains intelligible. The characteristics of cerebellar dysphonia are summarised in Table 10.7.

EXTRAPYRAMIDAL LESIONS

Lesions of the extrapyramidal system (see Chapter 2) result in hyperkinesia (excessive movement) or hypokinesia (reduction of movement). Hyperkinetic movements can be rapid, as in chorea, or slow as in dystonia (Aronson, 1990). The term 'striatum' is used to describe the caudate nucleus and putamen together, hence the cover term 'striatal lesions' (Brain, 1969). The nervous system acts as a whole and, although distinct features of muscular disorder are attributed to localised parts, there is uncertainty about the discrete functions of the basal ganglia. As Brain (1969) remarked, many theories concerning functions of the corpus striatum (caudate and lenticular nuclei) are debatable and do not explain all the symptoms in extrapyramidal syndromes. Damage to one cluster of cells is not discrete and any pathological damage has diffuse effects.

Hyperkinesia: chorea

Chorea is characterised by rapid jerky movements. Along with other parts of the body, the muscles of the face, lips, tongue, palate and larynx are involved, producing a quick hyperkinetic dysarthria. Sydenham's chorea (St Vitus's dance) is caused by acute rheumatic fever in children. It can occur, but rarely, in pregnancy. Huntington's disease is a hereditary form developing at about 40 years of age with choreiform movements, ataxia and progressive mental deterioration. There are irregularities in the respiratory and laryngeal movements, which produce irregular pitch and volume changes and speech arrests. These interruptions and repetitions may resemble cluttering or stammering. The characteristics of hyperkinetic choreic dysphonia are summarised in Table 10.8.

Hyperkinetic dystonic dysphonia

This condition presents as an element of slow hyperkinetic dysarthria. There are involuntary random and writhing movements of the body and orofacial grimacing. Rounding and pursing of the lips, involuntary tongue

Table 10.8 Hyperkinetic choreic dysphonia profile	
Pathology	Dysphonia associated with hyperkinetic dysarthria and generalised disturbance of body movements
Aetiology	Lesions in the basal ganglia
Signs and symptoms	Choreiform movements Ataxia Mental deterioration in some types
Laryngoscopic findings	Normal structure Intermittent hyperadduction
Expected vocal profile	Unstable pitch Unstable volume Harsh Intermittent breathiness Inappropriate inspiration/expiration
Acoustic analysis profile	SFo variable Reduced harmonics-to-noise ratio
Airflow and volume measures	Inconsistent

movements and laryngeal and respiratory spasms occur which can render speech unintelligible. Athetosis occurring in children with cerebral palsy is a type of hyperkinetic dystonia. The voice may be overloud at times and then fade to a whisper as a result of spasmodic movement of the respiratory and laryngeal muscles. Difficulty is experienced in sustaining phonation and the habitual pitch may be high and strained but drops to a groaning quality (Mecham, 1987). At rest, the patient may make disturbing grunting sounds. The characteristics of hyperkinetic dystonic dysphonia are summarised in Table 10.9.

Tremors

Healthy individuals have a small-amplitude physiological tremor. A fine tremor of 8–12 vacillations per second (Hz) is continuous both at rest and in movement. It is imperceptible but contributes to the vibrato distinguishable in the singing voice. Tremor is also associated with neurological disease and pathological tremors are manifestations of a number of underlying conditions, including bulbar and pseudobulbar palsy, and parkinsonism. Hyperthyroidism is also often accompanied by a fine rapid tremor. The tremor can cause rhythmic alterations of pitch and loudness whereas voice arrests occur in some cases, particularly when vowel prolongation is attempted.

Table 10.9 Hyperkinetic dystonic dysphonia profile	
Pathology	One aspect of slow hyperkinetic dysarthria, for example, as in cerebral palsy
Aetiology	Lesions in the basal ganglia
Signs and symptoms	Involuntary, random, writhing body movements Orofacial grimacing
Laryngoscopic findings	Normal structure Intermittent hyperadduction
Expected vocal profile	Variable in all parameters Excessively loud/whisper Unable to sustain steady vocal note Pitch ranges from excessively high to deep, groaning quality

Familial tremor (essential tremor)

Familial tremor occurs in childhood and before 25 years of age. It may occur in more than one member of a family and in successive generations (Critchley, 1949). The tremor of 4–8 Hz is generalised but most conspicuous in the hands, tongue and lips. It is not progressive but is aggravated in voluntary movement and by emotion. It must be distinguished from functional (conversion) tremor. The distinction is based on the history which will confirm the familial origin. Patients may be referred with diagnosis of functional dysphonia, in which case the tremor is audible in the voice and is of long standing. This cannot be cured, but the reason for the individual's sudden concern over the voice must be dealt with. The ways in which tremor affects phonation are summarised in Table 10.10.

Case notes

A woman employed at a hospital as a cleaner was referred complaining of voice tremor which she said had been the cause of her losing her job after being absent from work with 'flu. When the reason for being sacked was investigated and a request for reinstatement was made by the speech therapist, a different interpretation of the situation had to be made. The woman had been sacked for stealing from elderly patients' lockers. The vocal tremor was a congenital neurological disorder that had never worried her until she thought she could use it to her advantage.

Table 10.10 Vocal tremor profile	
Pathology	Isolated vocal fold tremor or associated with tremor of hands, arms, neck and mandible
Aetiology	No specific site of lesion identified
Signs and symptoms	Voice tremor which affects speech rate, articulation and rhythm
Laryngoscopic findings	Normal structure Regular hyperadduction in sympathy with tremor
Expected vocal profile	Rhythmic alterations of pitch and loudness Voice arrests Effortful phonation Dysprosody Rhythmic tremor on prolonged vowel Deteriorates with stress and fatigue

Senile tremor

Tremor that starts in old age is not present at rest but is most marked in the hands and head on the initiation of movement, and can be heard in the voice. At the onset of phonation, tremor of the extrinsic laryngeal muscles can be observed in combination with tremor of the mandibular and labial muscles. The normal, smoothly executed, vertical excursions of the larynx in the vocal tract during phonation can be inhibited or exaggerated by the tremor. Synchronous rhythmic contractions of the cricothyroid and rectus abdominis muscles have also been observed (Tomoda et al., 1987). The effect of the severe tremor is to disrupt the continuity of all aspects of phonation completely, so that conversation becomes a conspicuous struggle for the speaker. It is this aspect of voice tremor that can lead to confusion with spasmodic dysphonia (Aronson and Hartman, 1981) (see below). The differential diagnosis is based on the observation of the regularity of the tremor during phonation, in contrast with the irregularity of the laryngospasm of spasmodic dysphonia. The distinction between the two conditions can be complex, however, partly because tremor occurs in some cases of spasmodic dysphonia. In addition, the presentation can be complicated by the individual with vocal tremor who attempts to stabilise the vocal note by inhibiting the tremor. This manoeuvre can resemble spasmodic dysphonia by disrupting the regularity of the perceived tremor, and by increasing the strength of the hyperadduction of the vocal folds to resemble the laryngospasm of spasmodic dysphonia.

Toxic tremor

Toxic agents, especially alcohol, barbiturates, cocaine and mercury, can cause fine tremor.

Hypokinesia (parkinsonism)

Parkinson's disease is the epitome of hypokinesia. The disease is caused by a deficiency of dopamine-producing neurons in the substantia nigra and brain stem. Normally, the neurotransmitter dopamine has an inhibitory or monitoring effect on the release of acetylcholine, which excites muscle activity at the normal synapses. The essential maintenance of muscle tone is impaired by dopamine deficiency, so that regulation of all movement including posture, locomotion and changing from one position to another is affected. The smooth, automatic coordination and flow of movement are disrupted by hypokinesia, so that movement is slow, rigid and markedly limited in range as if a brake had been imposed on the muscles. There is a general loss of vigour. Muscles relax in jerks which can be felt if the wrist or elbow is manually flexed by the examiner. This is known as cog-wheel rigidity or rachet joint. Accompanying the rigidity is a regular coarse resting tremor of between 4 and 7 vacillations per second. This tends to subside in voluntary movement and ceases during sleep.

Although the aetiology is still not fully understood, various forms of parkinsonism are recognised. The illness usually starts after the age of 40 years. The idiopathic form (paralysis agitans) has a familial basis; otherwise, the cause is unknown. There is also an arteriosclerotic form which is associated with degeneration of cells in the basal ganglia. A postencephalitic parkinsonism can follow encephalitis lethargica (sleeping sickness) as long as 20 years after the illness. An epidemic of sleeping sickness after World War I resulted in many cases of Parkinson's disease in the 1930s and later. The incidence of sleeping sickness has decreased in the Western World and is now rare. Psychopharmacology can also induce parkinsonian symptoms: reserpine and phenothiazine have these side effects if doses are excessive or taken for prolonged periods. Damage may be irreversible but, if drugs are withdrawn in time, the parkinsonian symptoms will disperse, although this period of recovery may take up to 2 years (Williamson, 1984; Scott, Caird and Williams, 1985).

General symptoms

The disabling effect of rigidity, tremor, lack of range of movement and arrests in movement produces clear diagnostic perceptual characteristics. There is great difficulty in rising from a chair or bed and in turning in the horizontal position. Walking is greatly impaired; the patient loses balance and can fall as a result of steps becoming smaller because rigidity impedes the range of movement. Unaided, the patient totters forward with increasing speed (festinating gait) until the support of a wall or chair is reached. When changing direction, turning or attempting to start walking, the patient may become transfixed on the spot and involuntarily beat a tattoo with the feet. Manual skills are impaired. Tremor often produces a 'pill-rolling' movement between the thumb and forefinger at rest, and tasks such as fastening buttons are severely affected. Writing is also handicapped by the tremor and reduced range of movement, so that letter formation becomes increasingly small and illegible. The cog-wheel rigidity affecting smooth rotation of the wrist gives rise to further problems. Posture is typical with head, neck, trunk, hips and knees slightly flexed.

In some cases, there is intellectual decline and confusion and, more rarely, dementia. There is great variability in progression of the disease and in some fortunate patients parkinsonism is arrested (Hildick-Smith, 1980). Finally, death frequently occurs as a result of respiratory infection.

Pharmacology

A suitable drug regimen reduces the symptoms of Parkinson's disease. The aim of treatment is to compensate for the absence of dopamine with the drug levodopa. This reduces the unleashed effect of acetylcholine with anticholinergic drugs (Hildick-Smith, 1980). Initially, most patients respond to levodopa with a reduction in their motor disability, but there are side effects and a reduction in treatment effectiveness over time. Approximately 10% of patients fail to benefit from this treatment. Patients who are helped by drug therapy enjoy a marked reduction in symptoms and a great improvement in the quality of life for about 7 years. There is evidence that the drug pergolide is a useful adjunct to levodopa and can help to counteract its adverse effects (Hughes and Lees, 1991). Brain cell transplants of healthy dopamine-producing cells from aborted fetuses have been attempted but, although they have an immediate beneficial effect on the symptoms of Parkinson's disease, the long-term result is debatable.

An interesting, if barely relevant, item of information pertaining to the disease is that a lower incidence of parkinsonism has been recorded in heavy cigarette smokers (Scott, Caird and Williams, 1985).

Speech symptoms

Speech and voice are eventually involved in the progressive decline in general motor activity. It is estimated that about 50% of parkinsonian patients have speech and voice problems. Weismer (1984) suggests that phonatory characteristics are similar to the vocal behaviour of much older people, with a relatively high fundamental frequency and some vocal roughness. A further similarity to the vocal behaviour of elderly people is the reduction of the voiceless interval in parkinsonism; excessive rigidity reduces the efficiency of vocal fold abduction and this affects the ability to devoice appropriately.

There is considerable individual variability in severity of voice and speech symptoms and these have little, if any, correlation with the severity of general physical symptoms. Speech deterioration may be the first symptom of disease, particularly in unilateral cases, whereas patients with severe bodily involvement may have minimal dysarthria. The severity of speech symptoms does not necessarily correlate with the degree of tremor and rigidity. The reasons for the variation in speech deterioration from patient to patient, when degree of tremor and rigidity appear similar, remain obscure. Of course, in advanced stages all movement is severely impaired, which includes chewing and swallowing as well as speech.

Speech and voice characteristics correlate with the features of hypokinesia. There is reduced loudness, bradylalia, tremor and monopitch as a result of rigidity and reduced range of movement. Speech can be clear if one or two words at a time are uttered but festination occurs in connected speech. There are accelerations and repetitions and speech deteriorates into an unintelligible, almost inaudible, mumble. Alternatively, the body can 'freeze' and speech propulsion is arrested (akinetic mutism).

The voice lacks volume and pitch variation in addition to being breathy or, at times, rasping (Aronson, 1980). Breathy voice occurs in severely hypokinetic patients because of a marked glottal chink. When there is less rigidity, better closure may be achieved (Ludlow and Bassich, 1984). Respiratory movement is reduced in range and regularity. Phrases are short and there are frequent aphonic episodes as respiratory support ends and attempts at re-starting voice are made. Articulation is imprecise and phonemes may be repeated. The most prominent impairment is that of prosody with pitch, volume and temporal rhythmic features being disorganised. The characteristic features of dysphonia in Parkinson's disease are summarised in Table 10.11.

Paralinguistic communication

Paralinguistic communication is inevitably severely affected. The person with Parkinson's disease is liable to be misunderstood and become increasingly isolated because facial expression is absent or markedly reduced, with a resulting mask-like expression because of muscle rigidity. This will appear unfriendly and make the listener withdraw from the individual with Parkinson's disease. It has to be understood that the refined muscular control of expression is not possible but that, internally, emotions are viable. The social handicap is further compounded by the fact that laughter and gesture are not initiated spontaneously. Inability to smile, laugh and use hand and head gestures is a real social handicap.

Table 10.11 Profile of dysphonia in Parkinson's disease	
Pathology	One aspect of Parkinson's disease and related conditions
Aetiology	Damage to the substantia nigra Dopamine deficiency Various types: idiopathic, arteriosclerotic, postencephalitic
Signs and symptoms	Slow, rigid movements, which are limited in range Cog-wheel rigidity Tremor Reduced/lack of facial expression Intellectual deterioration
Laryngoscopic findings	Normal structure Incomplete vocal fold adduction/abduction Weak vocal fold movements Appearance of presbylaryngis Prolonged open phase or no closed phase
Expected vocal profile	Weak, breathy voice Raised pitch Reduced maximum phonation time Rough vocal note Reduced loudness Monopitch Delayed voice onset Dysprosody
Acoustic analysis profile	SFo increased Reduced harmonics-to-noise ratio Increased jitter and shimmer
Airflow and volume measures	Increased transglottal airflow Reduced air volume and pressure
Medicosurgical decisions	Voice therapy – intensive In coordination with patient's drug regimen

MIXED LESIONS

Mixed dysarthrias are the result of multiple lesions throughout the CNS and occur in conditions such as motor neuron disease (amyotrophic lateral sclerosis), multiple sclerosis and Wilson's disease. The speech deficits exhibit the characteristics of the different types of dysarthria.

Motor neuron disease

(Synonyms: amyotrophic lateral sclerosis (ALS); progressive muscular atrophy; progressive bulbar palsy)

Motor neuron disease (MND) is a progressive condition resulting from degeneration of spinal and cranial motor neurons and pyramidal neurons in the motor cortex, causing wasting and fasciculation of muscles (Edwards et al., 1995). Its cause is unknown, although 5% of cases are familial and the condition is irreversible. The age of onset is usually after 50 years, although occasionally it occurs in those aged 30–50 years. There is a higher incidence in men than in women. There are three main patterns of involvement.

- Progressive muscular atrophy
  In this, the spinal motor neurons are affected predominantly. Initially, there is weakness and wasting of the distal limb muscles,
- Progressive bulbar palsy
  There is early involvement of the tongue, palate and pharyngeal muscles, resulting in dysarthria and dysphagia.
- Amyotrophic lateral sclerosis
  In this there is a combination of distal and proximal muscle wasting, weakness, fasciculation and spasticity initially, followed by bulbar and pseudobulbar palsy.

In the initial stages of the disease, the predominant symptoms may be bulbar, limb or a combination of limb and bulbar, but as it progresses there is general involvement. Flaccid or spastic features may predominate at different stages of the disease. The patient remains intellectually and linguistically normal and can communicate by writing, until generalised weakness eventually makes an alternative method of communication and non-oral feeding essential. Death usually occurs within 3–5 years of the onset of the disease as a result of respiratory failure, although in some patients progression of the condition is more delayed.

A genetic abnormality was long suspected on account of the highest incidence in the world (57%) occurring in the Pacific islands of Guam among the Chamorro people. Although MND usually occurs throughout the world between the fifth and seventh decades of life, among the Chamorro it occurs in a younger population of 20–30 years of age. Life expectancy of Chamorro victims is longer and the disease is associated with parkinsonism and dementia (Spencer et al., 1987). The Third World Medical Research Foundation, led by Dr Peter Nunn, linked the disease to diet. The Mariana chain of islands used to grow cycad plantations, but these were replaced by sugar cane in all but the island of Guam. During the Japanese occupation, the Chamorro existed mainly on sago produced by the cycad plant, giving rise to the suspicion that sago contains a neurotoxic chemical. It is normally processed before being sold commercially in the West.

The mixed dysarthria of MND is a combination of bulbar and pseudobulbar palsy that impairs all parameters of motor speech production and eventually results in unintelligibility. The speech musculature is usually markedly spastic, resulting in effortful phonation with a harsh, strained–strangled quality and hypernasality. Typically the voice is low pitched and limited in range. In the early stages of the disease, however, some patients complain of raised pitch, which is apparently the result of hypertonic supralaryngeal muscles elevating the larynx and increased tension of the vocal folds. Speaking fundamental frequency changes are, therefore, a common feature, although the direction of these changes is not always consistent (Strand et al., 1994). The vocal changes result not only from the relative degree of spasticity or flaccidity in the laryngeal musculature, but also from involvement of the respiratory muscles and from compensatory strategies. Vocal characteristics in MND are summarised in Table 10.12.

Table 10.12 Profile for motor neuron disease dysphonia	
Pathology	Degenerative condition of bilateral corticobulbar tracts and lower motor neuron nuclei
Aetiology	Unknown
Signs	Brainstem and limb signs Flaccid or spastic features predominate at various stages Increasingly severe motor speech and voice problems Dysphagia
Laryngoscopic findings	Normal structure Tendency to vocal fold hyperadduction if spasticity predominates Tendency to vocal fold hypoadduction if flaccidity predominates
Expected vocal profile	Affected by predominance of flaccidity or spasticity Strained–strangled quality, sometimes sounds wet Monopitch Reduced loudness
Medicosurgical decisions	Speech therapy to maximise voice/speech effectiveness in early stages Alternative communication aids

Multiple or disseminated sclerosis (MS or DS)

MS is another disease of unknown origin, although current evidence seems to indicate a combination of immunogenic and infective influences. Demyelination of the nerve sheaths occurs randomly in the cerebral hemispheres, spinal cord and cerebellum, and peripherally, so that the affected fibres are unable to conduct impulses. It occurs in youth, rarely after the age of 40, and is progressive, although there are remissions frequently lasting for years. Early symptoms may include impaired vision. Subsequently, ataxia, nystagmus, intention tremor, dysarthria and dysphonia develop. Speech is slow and hesitant with impaired articulation and hypernasality. Respiration is adversely affected in a minority of patients.

Wilson's disease

A similar picture is seen in Wilson's disease in which there is a progressive hepatolenticular degeneration, often familial, starting early in life. The illness starts in adolescence and is a genetic metabolic disorder preventing processing of copper in food, resulting in copper deposits in the liver, brain and kidneys. Treatment is by introducing a diet low in copper and by medication such as penicillamine. Speech and voice are affected on account of muscular rigidity, tremor and ataxia; dysphagia may be a concomitant problem.

APRAXIA AND DYSPROSODY

Apraxia of speech presents an interesting neurological problem. The most prominent feature is impairment of the voluntary ability to organise the correct positions of the articulators in production of phonemes and phoneme sequences, in the absence of paralysis, sensory deficits or lack of understanding of the required movement. Controversy concerning the site of the lesion is continuously argued in the literature and is well reviewed by Buckingham (1979) and Edwards (1984). The focus of contention is whether verbal dyspraxia involving speech and phonation is a disorder of motor programming solely, or whether it is always associated with language disorder, i.e. dysphasia. The Mayo Clinic team (Darley, Aronson and Brown, 1975) were unequivocal in their view that apraxia of speech is the result of a left cerebral hemisphere injury. These authors believed that there is no impairment of muscle function (paresis or paralysis) and no disorder of comprehension or language formulation. The central language processor, they argued, is intact but the motor programming centre, possibly at the vestibular and reticular level, is impaired. The dysprosody that accompanies the disorder was considered by Darley, Aronson and Brown to be secondary to apraxia of speech and to arise as the result of impaired sequential organisation. It is, however, widely observed by many experienced speech pathologists that dyspraxic dysprosody is a linguistic suprasegmental manifestation. This view regards the dysprosody as a primary feature and considers apraxia of speech to be a disorder involving the breakdown of the inextricably linked motor and linguistic processes (Kertesz, 1983). Clinical experience suggests that most apraxic patients have dysphasic deficits of varying degree. It is considered to be an impairment of higher level planning and not only a neuromuscular disorder. The dyspraxic errors are regarded as similar to, or indistinguishable from, paraphasic errors of aphasia. Occasionally, speech may give the impression of a broad dialect or a foreign language. The famous case reported by Monrad-Krohn (1947a) is often quoted. More recently, a case is described of a patient with a 'Bronx' accent before a subcortical infarction of the left hemisphere, who subsequently spoke with an Irish accent (Seliger, Abrams and Horton, 1992). These authors suggest that suppressed prosodic patterns, to which the patient has been exposed as a child, may re-emerge after a brain injury.

Although the most obvious symptoms of apraxia are the difficulties in sequencing articulatory gestures correctly so that phonemic errors (substitutions, omissions and additions) occur, phonation is also affected in some instances. In cases of apraxic dysphonia and aphonia, laryngeal structure and function are normal but initiation and timing of voice are affected. Aronson (1990) describes three types of apraxia of phonation and respiration:

- No articulatory movement or laryngeal sound
- Whispered speech
- Articulatory movements without an exhaled airstream. The patient is unable to perform movements such as breathing in and out or coughing, either voluntarily or on command, although understanding the request and being able to perform these movements involuntarily.

In less severe cases, voice quality remains normal but anomalies of voice-onset time result in inappropriate voicing and devoicing, so that, for example, 'pan' becomes 'ban' and 'din' becomes 'tin'. Intonation patterns are also abnormal. Edwards (1984) suggested that hypernasality caused by unexplained fluctuations in soft palate elevation during speech may be the result of dyspraxia. The characteristics of apraxic speech are summarised in Table 10.13.

Table 10.13 General characteristics of apraxic speech

- Slow speaking rates; prolongation of phonologic transitions, lengthening of steady states and intersyllabic pauses (syllable segregation)

- Reduced intensity variation across syllables; slow, inaccurate articulatory gestures, inconsistent errors

- Incoordination of voicing in both vowels and consonants and difficulties in initiation

- Errors in selection of sequencing segments

- Overall difficulty in motor control of spatiotemporal schema

---

After Kent and Rosenbek (1983)

Developmental dyspraxia can occur in childhood and is associated with severely delayed speech and language development. Dysprosody becomes apparent as speech develops. As in apraxia in adults, phonation is not always accurately coordinated with articulation and intonation patterns may be abnormal, although the quality of the vocal note is normal.

The term 'dyspraxia' is not confined to speech and movements throughout the body may be affected. There is evidence that the various apraxias are associated with different areas of the brain (Bhatnagar and Andy, 1995).

APHONIA AFTER CLOSED HEAD INJURY

In some cases of severe closed head trauma, patients are mute during the early stages of recovery, and remain aphonic or dysphonic even when articulatory movements recover and laryngoscopy reveals normal vocal fold movement. Hartman and Von Cramon (1984a) in their acoustic analysis study of these patients found that recovery of phonation falls into two subgroups. The first presented with voice quality with breathy and tense components, which gradually became more normal during the follow-up period. The second group initially had normal or lax, breathy voice which became more tense.

The differential diagnosis of aphonia after closed head injury in the absence of laryngological signs can be complex. Sapir and Aronson (1985b) suggest three possible causes. The frontal lobes and limbic system are important in the regulation of affect, emotion and the vocal expression of emotion. Damage to these areas may reduce the drive and controlling mechanisms of phonation. The resulting disorder of affect is characterised by the 'flatness' of facial expression and general lack of drive, which is reflected in the aphonia or quiet voice with reduced intonation patterns. However, the symptom may also have a psychogenic basis and be part of the emotional response to brain injury. Recovery is frequently accompanied by depression and feelings of hopelessness, so that the neurological problems give rise to psychological symptoms (Sapir and Aronson, 1987). Finally, as discussed in the previous section, apraxia of phonation should also be considered as a possible cause.

SPASMODIC DYSPHONIA (ADDUCTOR LARYNGEAL DYSTONIA)

This condition is also known as spastic dysphonia but must not be confused with the voice problems associated with spastic dysarthria, which result from UMN lesions. There has been an upsurge of interest in spasmodic dysphonia (SD) with the advent of developments in treating the distressing phonatory symptoms. It remains the case, however, that misdiagnosis frequently occurs in the routine ENT clinic, with patients being told that their vocal symptoms are the result of stress, anxiety or some other psychogenic explanation (Friedman et al., 1987; Ginsberg et al., 1988). As a result, patients can be caused unnecessary further distress as prolonged, inappropriate therapeutic programmes are embarked on unsuccessfully.

Historical background

> Traube, in 1871, first described a spastic type of hoarseness characterised by a choking or strangulated dysphonia. Critchley (1939a) attributed spastic dysphonia to a neurological disorder having cranial nerve symptoms with a resemblance to facial tics and spasmodic torticollis. Thomson, Negus and Bateman (1955) compared spastic dysphonia with writer's cramp. Others compared the vocal symptoms with those occurring in severe stammering. These early neurological explanations of the condition were forgotten, however, and the disorder of spasmodic dysphonia was attributed to hysterical conversion symptom for many years (Luchsinger, 1965c). In 1960, however, Robe, Moore and Brumlik published a study of 10 patients with 'spastic dysphonia' whose encephalograms revealed CNS damage with abnormal paroxysmal discharges in the right temporoparietal region. Although these findings have not been duplicated, according to Schaeffer (1983), the possibility that a condition previously thought to be psychogenic might be neurological created great interest. Aronson et al. (1968a, 1968b) also concluded that the disorder was neurogenic. Gradually, research transferred to location of the neurological lesion and to more appropriate forms of treatment. Dedo, Townsend and Izdebski (1977) reported that histological examination of segments of the recurrent laryngeal nerve

removed from patients with SD revealed myelin abnormalities in 30% of the nerves examined. The relevance of this finding has been disputed by other investigators (Ravits et al., 1979) who argued that a peripheral nerve lesion would probably produce flaccidity rather than spasm and that such a lesion would not allow normal phonation at any time. Dedo, Townsend and Izdebski (1977) also reported, however, that neurological examination indicated brain-stem or basal ganglia disturbance in some patients with no apparent nerve disease. This line of research was also explored by Schaeffer et al. (1983a, 1983b).

Neuropathology

It is now generally accepted that adductor spasmodic dysphonia is a focal dystonia (Blitzer et al., 1985; Miller and Woodson, 1991; Blitzer and Brin, 1991). *Primary* dystonia is a syndrome of sustained muscle contractions which gives rise to abnormal movements and resulting postures (Marsden and Quinn, 1990). Typically, the abnormal muscle movement and posture are induced by the initiation of movement. The affected body part appears normal at rest, but the abnormality is revealed when it is used. In addition, many patients with dystonias exhibit rhythmic tremors. It has been suggested that dystonia is one of the most frequently misdiagnosed neurological conditions (Blitzer and Brin, 1991). *Focal* dystonia symptoms involve a specific group of muscles, e.g. eyelids (blepharospasm), oromandibular dystonia (Meige's syndrome), torticollis and writer's cramp. It is to this group that spasmodic dysphonia belongs.

The site of the neurological lesion causing the bizarre adductor action of the vocal folds seems to originate in the extrapyramidal system, probably as a result of abnormality of neurotransmitters in the basal ganglia (Swenson et al., 1992). Izdebski (1992) suggests that SD is caused by faulty processing of afferent information from the larynx and inappropriate efferent discharges from the basal ganglia, in response to the afferent discharges. The result is involuntary hyperadduction of the vocal folds (laryngospasm).

The neurological basis of the disorder has been supported by studies reporting other neurological symptoms that coexist with laryngeal dystonia. A study by Cohen et al. (1989), for example, noted that patients with SD have increased excitability of reflexes, suggesting that the dystonia involves anatomical structures in addition to the larynx. They reported earlier studies that also concluded that these patients show abnormalities, such as reduced stomach acid responses to sham feeding, reduced fluctuation in heart rate during the Valsalva manoeuvre (see page 41) and abnormal brainstem auditory responses. They concluded that these abnormalities suggested enhanced excitability of brain-stem interneurons.

It has also been proposed, however, that SD is a symptom complex associated with several neurological diseases (Hanson, Logemann and Hain, 1992).

Studies of familial patterns of dystonia reveal a significant incidence of dystonia in the families of patients with laryngeal dystonia. Blitzer and Brin (1991) report that, in a study of 260 patients with laryngeal dystonia as the primary site of onset, 27 (10.4%) had evidence of spread to another body part and 17% of their subjects had a family history of dystonia. Studies have shown that the gene responsible for idiopathic torsion dystonia has been located on chromosome 9q, and work continues to map the genes for various forms of hereditary dystonia (Sakoda, 1993)

Incidence

Spasmodic dystonia has been regarded historically as a rare condition. It is now thought, however, that its prevalence might be rather higher than previously thought, because it has not been recognised fully in the past. Marsden and Quinn (1990) reported the study of Nutt et al. (1988) on the incidence of focal and generalised dystonia in Rochester, Minnesota, USA, which recorded that there were 52 cases of SD per million. They extrapolated these figures to suggest that there might be 2000–3000 individuals in the UK with SD. Certainly, since the establishment of specialist treatment centres for SD in the UK, large numbers of patients have come forward, many of whom have been seeking a diagnosis and treatment of their voice problems over a long period.

Age of onset

The onset of adductor spasmodic dysphonia is usually in middle age with a greater incidence in women. There is some disagreement concerning the sex ratio, with Dedo and Shipp (1980) recording two women for every man and Aronson (1980) noting a male:female ratio ranging from 1:1 to 1:18. In a study by Blitzer and Brin (1991), the average age of onset was 38 years.

Wilson (1987) also refers to the condition in teenagers, in whom he notes early symptoms including moderate stridency, harshness, breathiness and slight vocal tremor. There is no sudden aphonia but hoarseness, sometimes accompanied by visible tightening of the external laryngeal muscles and elevation of the larynx during phonation. Wilson records some therapeutic success when the disorder is in the incipient stage, but confirms the general opinion of poor prognosis at the advanced stage. We have no experience of such cases in childhood.

Psychological status

Psychological disturbance, such as anxiety and depression, is to be expected from an incapacitating social and occupational handicap, which may have serious socioeconomic consequences. A marked feature of the dysphonia is lack of conversion symptoms or evidence of evading voice recovery. There is usually considerable determination to overcome the handicap, to seek treatment and to lead a normal life. This aspect induced Dedo (Dedo, Urrea and Lawson, 1973) to operate on his first patient, Mrs Mildred Younger. Although SD is not a somatoform disorder, stress can play a part in its expression causing an obvious increase in the severity of the symptoms (Ginsberg et al., 1988). For many patients, the distress resulting from the condition itself is compounded by a prolonged pursuit of a correct diagnosis and delay in receiving effective treatment.

Laryngoscopic findings

Laryngeal and supraglottic behaviour in SD can be observed most effectively using nasendoscopy. On laryngoscopic examination, the vocal folds are seen to hyperadduct when phonation is initiated. This is sometimes accompanied by increased laryngeal depression during speaking, but laryngeal elevation resulting from hypercontraction of the extrinsic laryngeal musculature also occurs (Aronson and De Santo, 1983). In addition to the involuntary vocal fold movements that interfere with the maintenance of phonation, movements of the supraglottic structures towards the midline can be observed. Anteroposterior laryngeal squeezing is also seen in some cases. Ludlow and Connor (1987) thought that only the muscles involved in vocal fold adduction are affected in these patients and it is possible, of course, that the hyperactivity of the supraglottic constrictors is a subsidiary manifestation of the effort that is required to phonate on the occurrence of the laryngospasm. A videofluoroscopic study undertaken by McCall, Skolnick and Brewer (1971) demonstrated that SD might be symptomatic of isolated laryngospasms related to phonation only, or can appear in association with a more general problem that affects the behaviour of the laryngeal and pharyngeal musculature during quiet respiration, as well as in speech. These findings were confirmed by Ludlow et al. (1987) whose study concluded that there were significantly high levels of laryngeal muscle activity in SD patients, compared with normal subjects, in both quiet respiration and phonation. They also concluded that resting muscle tone was abnormally high in this condition.

It should be remembered that laryngeal behaviour on laryngoscopy varies considerably from patient to patient, according to the severity of the condition. In many cases, laryngeal appearance is unremarkable (Hirano and Bless, 1993). This does not mean that the problem is inconsequential, as the laryngospasm during connected speech reveals. (See Table 10.14 for a profile of spasmodic dysphonia.)

Vocal characteristics

Terms to describe the vocal features of SD have proliferated as increasing numbers of laryngologists and speech pathologists have contributed to the literature. The characteristic 'strangulated' vocal quality that results from the spasmodic adduction of the vocal folds during phonation (laryngospasm) was described by Dedo and Shipp (1980) 'as though the individual is speaking while trying to lift an immovable object'. Following a review of the literature, Blitzer and Brin (1991) reported that the vocal characteristics of SD were described as:

Table 10.14 Spasmodic (adductor and abductor) dysphonia profile

Pathology	Focal dystonia
Aetiology	Extrapyramidal lesion possibly associated with abnormality of neurotransmitters in the basal ganglia Possible genetic/familial basis for dystonias
Signs and symptoms	Involuntary disruption of phonation by laryngospasms
Laryngoscopic findings	Normal laryngeal structure May be signs of minimal tremor at rest On phonation, according to severity: • normal vocal fold movements • hyperadduction at voice onset • intermittent hyperadduction • severe laryngospasm • supraglottic compression
Expected vocal profile	Effortful initiation of phonation ranging from a 'catch' in the voice to severe obstruction, as if trying to speak while performing the Valsalva manoeuvre Strained–strangled vocal quality Vegetative vocal behaviours and singing may be normal
Acoustic analysis profile	Variable according to task May be within normal limits on steady-state vowel
Airflow and volume measures	High subglottal air pressure
Medicosurgical decisions	Current symptomatic treatment: injections of botulinum toxin in conjunction with voice therapy

> ... staccato, jerky, squeezed, laboured, hoarse or groaning voice with
> voice arrests (from hyperadduction of the true and false vocal folds),
> intermittent phonation, segmented vowels, difficulty with loudness
> control, deviated pitch, vocal tension, intermittent aphonia, strangled
> voice, breathiness, glottal fry, glottal spasms, syllable repetitions,
> vowel prolongations, whispered speech, choked vocal attacks and
> hard glottal initiation.

It has been observed by Izdebski (1992), however, that the only universally accepted symptom of adductor SD is the strained–strangled, or over-pressured, voice quality and that other vocal features are the result of compensatory behaviours. There is intermittent laryngeal constriction of varying degrees during phonation and initiation is frequently effortful as the vocal folds are triggered into spasm.

The typical pattern of development is that initially the patient notices the occasional 'catch' in the voice, which gradually becomes hoarse and develops pitch breaks. The onset of the disorder is slow with progressive deterioration, stabilising after 3–5 years' duration. Respiratory viral infection, emotional trauma and injury to the head or neck have been reported to precede the onset (Finitzo et al., 1987) or there may be no obvious related factors. As the struggle to phonate progresses, facial grimaces, including eye blinking (blepharospasm) and eyebrow twitching, can become established. Voiceless sounds become voiced if the vocal folds remain adducted during the voiceless segment (Dedo and Shipp, 1980) and prosody is disturbed. Speech–breathing patterns are disrupted and exaggerated in some patients as they try to overcome the strongly adducted vocal folds. Laryngospasm is particularly marked if phonation on residual air is attempted. The musculoskeletal effort involved in phonation can result in chest and throat pain. All symptoms of the disorder tend to become more severe as the day progresses and in certain contexts, such as using the telephone (Dedo and Shipp, 1980).

Vegetative functions such as coughing, throat clearing and laughing are frequently normal. The patient might be able also to produce isolated vowels, sing, whisper and sing falsetto without spasm. Significantly, phonation on a high-pitched /i/ as required during laryngoscopy can be symptom free. Laryngospasm is reduced in some patients when there is a reduction in the communicative significance of the utterance, when the patient alters the normal mode of phonation and during whispering. Improvement is seen in some individuals when auditory feedback is eliminated. The severity of the symptoms varies so that, under stress, symptoms are exacerbated. As a result of these features and the conspicuously unusual voice and speech patterns in many cases, it is easy to see why the condition was judged to be psychogenic in the past.

The compensatory vocal features of the disorder are the result of endeavours to maintain uninterrupted speech, with the sufferer attempting to adjust any voice parameter that appears to bring relief. The patient's experience of SD is of exhausting effort in an attempt to overcome the laryngospasm and, in many cases, this aspect is as much a handicap as the voice disorder itself.

Abductor spasmodic dysphonia

Abductor SD is another, much rarer, manifestation of laryngeal dystonia (Zwitman, 1979). Studies suggest that it is not distinct from adductor SD, but that both result from the relative predominance of muscle tone between adductor and abductor muscle fibres (Hanson, Logemann and Hain, 1992). In this form, spasm of the posterior cricoarytenoid muscles results in breathy, effortful voice with abrupt terminations of voicing as the vocal folds are abducted during phonation. This laryngeal behaviour results in aphonic, whispered segments of speech, with reduced loudness overall (Aronson, 1990). As in adductor SD, vocal tremor is frequently apparent. Only a small percentage of patients present with this condition and the clinician must be aware that even some of these cases might be adductor SD sufferers who are using compensatory abductor dysphonia as a method of reducing the intensity of the adductor spasm. There is some evidence that in a proportion of these patients the vocal symptoms are psychogenic. Treatment will depend on whether it is decided that the aetiology is thought to be neurogenic or psychogenic in a particular case. Botulinum toxin injections into the posterior cricoarytenoid muscle have been beneficial in some neurogenic cases of abductor laryngeal dystonia (Blitzer and Brin, 1991; Jankovic and Brin, 1991).

Differential diagnosis

The differential diagnosis of SD depends to some extent on the diagnostician's awareness of the condition and acknowledgement that the condition might exist in the presenting patient. In some instances, it is apparent that, away from specialist centres, where few cases of SD are encountered, the diagnosis of SD has not been considered during the evaluation of the patient's symptoms.

Other conditions that appear similar to or emulate SD are **benign essential tremor** and some manifestations of **conversion symptom aphonia** (Aronson et al., 1968b). Benign essential tremor involving the larynx and musculature of the upper body occurs with intention, as the patient begins to move the affected body part. A regular tremor is clearly seen which differs from the irregular tremor occurring as part of the focal dystonia in the case of laryngeal dystonia. Marsden and Quinn (1990) note, however, that many patients with dystonias of various types show true rhythmic tremors either slower than (about 3 Hz) or at approximately the same rate as in benign essential tremor. An irregular tremor of 4–8 Hz has been described in SD patients studied by Blitzer et al. (1988), some of whom exhibited synchronous involvement of the pharynx, face and masticatory muscles.

Conversion symptom aphonia with the vocal characteristics of SD tends to exhibit certain differences from true SD. The history of the neurogenically based SD generally features a gradual onset and an uninterrupted course over many years. The onset of the conversion symptom form, in contrast, frequently starts suddenly and can occur episodically, with symptom-free periods in between. Aronson (1980) established that 45% of the patients he examined with laryngeal focal dystonia symptoms had experienced emotional trauma before the onset of the condition. Trial voice therapy, possibly with psychotherapy, helps to identify patients with psychogenic spastic dysphonia amenable to such therapy (Aronson and DeSanto, 1983). In addition, in most cases of true SD there is a determination on the part of the sufferer to seek and cooperate with any intervention that might help to resolve the problem; it is very difficult to identify any secondary gains that they might obtain from their condition. In contrast, in some instances where the SD-like vocal symptoms arise as a conversion symptom or have a psychogenic basis of another sort, secondary gains can be identified and the patient fails to cooperate with treatment procedures. Evidence in the case history and remissions in the symptoms will point to a psychogenic SD. We have seen male and female patients whose symptoms were cured by therapy and where the aetiology was obviously psychogenic. There are various reports in the literature of SD being cured by speech therapy, and these cases must have been conversion symptom disorder.

Medicosurgical decisions

There is no cure for SD, or for any of the dystonias, but a number of symptomatic treatments are used with various degrees of effectiveness. In most patients with focal laryngeal dystonia, voice therapy, psychotherapy and drug therapy alone do not significantly improve phonation in the long term (Blitzer et al., 1988; Marsden and Quinn, 1990), although they can make a significant contribution to improving patients' communication and quality of life when combined in a programme with botulinum toxin injections (see below). Trials of primodone injections, which have been reported as effective in reducing benign essential tremor, have been conducted without success (Hartman and Vishwanat, 1984). The resistance of this condition to treatment is notorious and entirely normal voice is not usually a realistic aim. Intervention is directed at reducing the severity of the laryngospasm so that the individual can communicate more easily and without the socially unacceptable struggle to speak.

Two techniques for physically reducing vocal fold adductor spasm have been evolved over the past 20 years, with injections of botulinum toxin in current use.

Recurrent laryngeal nerve section

The advent of the recurrent laryngeal nerve (RLN) section procedure initially appeared to provide a successful method of dealing with laryngospasm symptomatically, by reducing vocal fold hyperadduction, but it has been abandoned. Dedo first reported his procedure in 1976. Before surgery, an injection of lidocaine (lignocaine) into the RLN immobilises the fold temporarily, so that patient and laryngologist can assess the effect that the surgery will have (Izdebski, Shipp and Dedo, 1979). Unilateral section of the RLN paralyses the vocal fold in the paramedian position. The healthy fold, although continuing to exhibit adductor spasm, is unable to make closure of the same force with the paralysed fold across the midline. Unfortunately, the good results obtained by RLN section do not last indefinitely and the return of SD symptoms in patients who had undergone the procedure revealed the limitations of this approach (Sapir, Aronson and Thomas, 1986). Izdebski, Dedo and Shipp (1981) reported 15 cases who had benefited and retained significant reduction of symptoms over a period of 3 years. Dedo and Izdebski (1983a) reported intermediate results of 306 RLN sections for spastic dysphonia. Although, 4 years postoperatively, 90% of the patients judged their voices to be 'easier' than preoperatively, some voices lacked volume as a result of atrophy and shrinking of the paralysed fold. This was treated with Teflon injection. Another problem occurred with adduction of the paralysed fold to the midline and the return of spasticity. Spasmodic dysphonia returned in 10–15% of Dedo and Shipp's patients (1980) from as early as 1 month after surgery up to 2 years later. In cases of recurrence, Dedo and Shipp advocated debulking the paralysed vocal fold by cup forceps or CO_2 laser to produce an air leak, along a 2-mm wide strip, after a period of 1 year or more. Similar procedures were advocated by Forder (1983) and Isshiki (1980).

Aronson and De Santo (1983) reported disappointing results in follow-up of 38 patients after surgery. They found that, in 64% of the cases, the subjects' voices were worse 3 years postoperatively than they had been preoperatively. Failure among women was considerably higher than among men. In the whole group, only one patient whose voice improved had normal voice. Improved voices were breathy, hoarse, falsetto or diplophonic. Pitch breaks occurred and tremor was evident on prolonged vowels. These authors confirmed that surgery had long-term limitations.

Fritzell et al. (1982) described their experience with four subjects (three women and one man) who had RLN section for spasmodic dysphonia. Two patients who had voice therapy did not relapse, but two who did not receive therapy had a return of SD after 3 months. Electromyography indicated reinnervation of the vocal fold on the paralysed side. One patient's voice recovered with a lidocaine injection and was, as a result, operated on again to good effect. The other patient also underwent surgery, but it was impossible to locate the nerve and the voice was no better after surgery. Wilson, Olding and Mueller (1980) reported a case of return of spastic dysphonia 6 months after RLN section. Nerve section was performed again and, during this operation, the nerve was tested and found to be intact. Subsequently, botulinum toxin injection treatment directed at alleviating the symptoms has become the preferred treatment.

Botulinum toxin injection

During the last decade RLN section has been superseded by botulinum toxin injections into the vocal fold adductor muscles, in order to overcome their dystonic contractions. Botulinum toxin causes muscle paralysis (flaccidity) by acting at the peripheral nerve endings to inhibit the release of acetylcholine, thus weakening the laryngospasm. The effect of the electromyographically guided injections of the sterile substance is that of chemical denervation. This effect lasts for about 4 months. Immediately after the injection, phonation is less effortful but the voice is frequently breathy. Vocal quality continues to improve during the next 2 or 3 months with optimal improvement at about 6–10 weeks after the injection. On average, this level of phonation lasts just over a month (Aronson et al., 1993; Sapir, 1994). Subsequently, phonatory effort increases and vocal quality deteriorates as terminal sprouting restores the muscle endplate transmission.

Injections are administered unilaterally or bilaterally, usually into the thyroarytenoid muscle, but they can also be directed to the cricoarytenoid and cricothyroid muscles. There is evidence that injections at multiple sites in a single muscle are more effective than a single injection into one site (Ludlow et al., 1988). Miller (1992) reports that, in women, the beneficial effects of unilateral injections last longer than bilateral injections, whereas men have a longer period of breathiness than women, even with lower dosages. He concludes, therefore, that the treatment for women can be more aggressive. He also notes that the duration of benefit from the injection was reduced with bilateral injections, but that this did not occur with unilateral injections. Other authorities regard bilateral injections as preferable. Ludlow et al. reported that improvement occurs only with reduction in thyroarytenoid muscle activity. Hyperactivity of both thyroarytenoid and cricothyroid muscles has been found during respiration and phonation in SD.

Injection of botulinum toxin is currently recommended as the primary treatment for laryngeal dystonia (Jankovic and Brin, 1991).

Effects of laryngeal botulinum toxin injections

During the last decade, botulinum injections have brought great relief to many individuals with SD, enabling them to lead more normal lives. It is also arguable that, as an increasing number of specialist centres have emerged to provide this treatment, the condition has started to gain greater recognition, so that patients are diagnosed and directed towards appropriate intervention more frequently. There are certain disadvantages associated with this procedure, however, which must be discussed with the patient if an informed choice is to be made. Some patients experience considerable anxiety in relation to Botox injections and the possible outcome of treatment (Epstein, Stygall and Newman, 1996). If patients decide that they do not to wish to receive the injections, the clinical team must ensure that appropriate voice therapy is provided to enable them to deal with their symptoms as effectively as possible. A summary of the advantages and disadvantages is shown in Table 10.15.

Botulinum toxin injections frequently result in breathy phonation in the days after the injection and a significant number of patients experience episodes of choking on fluids in this initial period (Blitzer and Brin, 1991) with associated reduced swallowing speed (Ludlow et al., 1988). There is considerable debate as to whether these symptoms are more severe after unilateral or bilateral injections, and about which method gives the most successful result (Kobayashi et al., 1993). Ludlow et al. (1992) argue that the immediate complications of the injection are avoided by giving them unilaterally. Blitzer and Brin (1991), however, maintain that weakening or paralysing one vocal fold stresses the remaining vocal fold and exaggerates the dystonic symptoms.

It has also been reported that botulinum toxin injections can affect neuromuscular transmission in muscles distant from the site of the

Table 10.15 Advantages and disadvantages of botulinum toxin injections in the treatment of spasmodic dysphonia

Advantages	Disadvantages
Reduction of intensity of laryngospasm	Repeated injections at approximately 4-monthly intervals
Reduced phonatory effort	Breathy voice in days immediately following injection
Office procedure, no general anaesthetic	Aspiration and coughing in days immediately following injection in some cases
Improved vocal quality	Symptomatic treatment only; does not treat the underlying focal dystonia
Improved prosody	Voice symptoms gradually return as effect of injection reduces over a period of approximately 4 months
Many patients experience improved quality of life as they communicate more easily and no longer attract unwelcome attention	Some patients experience anxiety in anticipation of each injection
	Injections may affect neuromuscular transmission in muscles distant from the site of the injection
	Unknown long-term effects

injection (Ludlow et al., 1988; Comella et al., 1992). Consequently, if diffusion into the bloodstream occurs, it would be possible for patients to have systemic effects and develop antibodies. As a result they would not benefit from further treatment. In addition, the motor activity of other muscle groups may be affected. For these effects to be avoided, Ludlow et al. (1988) stress the importance of using a small dosage.

Relative effects of RLN section and botulinum toxin injections

Although RLN section and botulinum toxin injections both appear to achieve vocal improvement in SD patients by similar means, there are important differences in the effects of these procedures. Botulinum toxin partially denervates the thyroarytenoid muscle, whereas RLN section causes a complete flaccid paralysis of all the muscles innervated by that nerve. As a result, the physiological basis for phonation is markedly different in the SD speaker after intervention. This is clearly demonstrated in the study conducted by Woo et al. (1992) who compared the findings in SD patients before treatment, after unilateral recurrent laryngeal block by lidocaine (thus mimicking RLN section), after bilateral injections of botulinum toxin and before botulinum toxin re-injection. Although vocal quality improved after both RLN block and botulinum toxin injection, in general the botulinum toxin produced a more satisfactory voice. On laryngoscopy, behaviour of the vocal folds and supralaryngeal structures was seen to be less aberrant after botulinum toxin denervation than after RLN block; airflow and maximum phonation time measures were similarly superior after botulinum toxin injection. The results suggested that bilateral partial denervation by botulinum toxin was the most successful of the treatments assessed in improving phonatory physiology and in restoring vocal fold vibration closer to that seen in normal subjects.

Patients with mild vocal symptoms sometimes regard surgery or botulinum toxin injections as excessive intervention, particularly as these are symptomatic treatments that do not improve the underlying condition. They decide that, once a diagnosis has been made and explanations have been given, they would prefer to manage the situation by less invasive means. If vocal function is regarded by speakers as adequate for their lifestyle, there is no reason for them to be persuaded that they should undergo these treatments. Patients can be reassured that, if they change their minds, they will be considered for treatment subsequently. A course of voice therapy is helpful in ameliorating their symptoms and ensuring maintenance of optimal vocal function. The opportunity to discuss the practical and emotional effects of the condition within these treatment sessions provides valuable support.

It is recommended that botulinum toxin therapy for SD be implemented by a multidisciplinary team consisting of a laryngologist, speech–language pathologist, neurologist and a physician specialised in using EMG.

Voice evaluation and therapy

Voice therapy alone is generally regarded as being ineffective in treating SD but the speech–language pathologist does have a role in evaluating phonatory function, contributing to the diagnostic process and in helping the patient to manage the symptoms (Dedo and Shipp, 1980; Dedo and Izdebski, 1983b; Murry and Woodson, 1995). Evaluation using the usual range of tests (see Chapter 13) does not necessarily produce a true vocal profile because of the fluctuating severity of the symptoms and the adverse effect of stress on the intensity of the laryngospasm. A diagnostic battery of tests, which are capable of generating or eliminating adductor SD symptoms, as described by Izdebski (1992), is an essential contribution to the diagnostic process. The patient is asked to carry out the following speech tasks:

- sustained phonation at varied frequency and intensity levels
- all-voiced and voiced/voiceless speech
- modal, falsetto and whisper modes
- vegetative tasks.

Izdebski notes that the symptoms of adductor SD will occur predominantly in loud modal phonation and when speaking fundamental frequency is raised within 1 or 2 octaves above the original speaking fundamental frequency. In contrast, the laryngospasm is not apparent at very high pitch or in whisper, whatever the loudness level. Woodson et al. (1992) suggest the use of a functional status rating scale, which indicates the severity of the disorder:

- Class I patients: mildly concerned.
- Class II patients: significant problems, but could carry on their work and social activities.
- Class III patients: employment problems, career changes, restricted social activities.

Although these are broad ratings, they have been found to be useful in validating objective measures. Functional rating scales in this context are also described by Freeman, Cannito and Finitzo-Hiebert (1984) and Blitzer and Brin (1991).

Voice therapy cannot 'cure' SD (Schaeffer and Freeman, 1987), but it enables the patient to establish and maintain optimal voice and to reduce phonatory effort (Heuer, 1992). The patient can be helped to manage the symptoms, in particular by gaining insight into inappropriate compensatory strategies that might have evolved to overcome the laryngospasm. It is possible also to reduce hyperfunctional aspects of phonation by introducing improved speech–breathing and gentle onset techniques (see Chapter 14) After botulinum toxin injection, voice therapy helps the patient to manage the changed laryngeal behaviour and to ensure that optimal function is acquired. Emotional support and encouragement is also an important aspect of treatment.

Other treatment approaches

A technique of unilateral percutaneous electrical stimulation of the RLN by means of an implantable electrode and receiver to improve vocal quality in SD patients was reported by Friedman et al. (1987).

Case histories

RF

RF (38 years), a married man with two young children, was referred for speech therapy from the laryngologist with the diagnosis 'hoarse voice – vocal cords normal'. As he spoke there was frequent laryngospasm and speech involved great effort. The symptoms were those of spasmodic dysphonia. His manner was incongruously cheerful in the light of his obvious difficulty in phonating; laughter was normal.

The case history revealed that a 'catch' in his voice had become noticeable shortly after he was told that he was to be made redundant from his job as an accountant. Phonation had become increasingly effortful in the 5 weeks before seeing the laryngologist. He was now in the process of applying for another job. Although he found it difficult to believe that there was any connection between losing his job and his dysphonia, he was highly motivated to comply with therapy because of forthcoming interviews. Relaxation and breathing therapy, followed by work on voiceless/voiced sighs and the elimination of hard glottal attack to avoid inducing laryngospasm, proved to be the most effective method of remediation. Cheerfully and politely he rejected all attempts at discussion of the possible underlying aspects of his problem. As he became able to produce vowel strings with normal voice and his confidence increased in applying these principles to normal speech, carry-over was apparent. Although the voice was not completely normal he dealt with job interviews successfully, started his new job and eventually telephoned the therapist to report that his voice was fine, which it did indeed seem to be. There was no evidence of the psychogenic spasmodic dysphonia.

TM

TM (63-year-old female) was referred for speech therapy by the laryngologist with the diagnosis 'normal vocal cords but tremor on movement, typical of a functional voice disorder induced by stress'. The laryngospasm was of relatively modest severity, but concerned the patient because she wanted to know its cause and because she felt that it made her sound uncertain and older than her true age. She had retired from her administrative post at the normal retirement age (60 years) and had been divorced 30 years previously. She had excellent relationships with her adult children but lived alone. She was quietly assertive in seeking the resolution of her voice problems. While the case history was being taken, she recalled that she had noticed slight voice problems some years before she retired, particularly when attempting to initiate phonation and when trying to increase vocal loudness. These vocal features had not caused her concern at the time, but she realised in retrospect that they were the initial indications of her present problems. She reported that her maternal grandmother had had a head tremor and that her voice was 'wobbly'. It had been commented on by friends that TM's younger daughter was beginning to have the same 'catch' in her voice as her mother. A second opinion was sought from a laryngologist with a special interest in spasmodic dysphonia and a diagnosis of adductor laryngeal dystonia was made. TM felt that her symptoms did not warrant the botulinum toxin injections that were suggested and opted instead for a course of voice therapy in order to use her existing voice as effectively as possible.

LB

LB (35 years) worked as an office receptionist. She was referred with the diagnosis '?spastic dysphonia'. She presented with the typical vocal features of SD, predominantly severe laryngospasm at voice onset and during phonation, which had been present during the past 3 months. It was revealed that she had had a previous similar episode 6 months before, but that there had been a period of normal voice between the two episodes. As this was unlikely to be a laryngeal focal dystonia, therefore, a possible precipitating factor was sought. Gradually, it transpired that LB had a busy romantic life with at least two men, in addition to her husband. On each occasion when her voice had 'gone', her husband had almost discovered her extramarital activities. She accepted the correlation between her vocal problems and these stressful incidents, and normal voice was recovered during the initial consultation by the strategies used to restore voice in cases of conversion symptom aphonia. LB was relieved by the explanations for her voice problems and they did not recur.

GD

GD (42 years), a married man with an office job, was seen in the voice clinic after 18 months of voice therapy in another centre. He was extremely tense and rigid. Phonation was effortful and strained–strangled. He had been seen by two laryngologists before voice therapy and the diagnoses had been 'normal larynx' and 'functional dysphonia'. His voice problem had not responded to voice therapy. Oral examination revealed a fine tremor of the tongue and soft palate. On laryngoscopy, a similar laryngeal tremor was observed at rest. On phonation, marked hyperadduction of the true and false vocal folds occurred on initiation and throughout attempts to maintain a steady note. The patient was very distressed by his condition, which was affecting his work and social life. A diagnosis of spasmodic dysphonia was made and he responded well to botulinum toxin injections and further voice therapy.

Peripheral nervous system lesions

On account of the distribution of the superior and recurrent laryngeal nerves (see Chapter 2), a total unilateral paralysis of the larynx can result only if the lesion occurs at, or above, the level of the ganglion nodosum before the superior laryngeal nerve branches off from the vagus. This means that, in lesions involving the recurrent laryngeal nerves, the cricothyroid muscle will be spared. Nuclear lesions of the vagus, already described in connection with bulbar palsies, are caused by a variety of pathological conditions: multiple sclerosis, medullary tumours, focal thrombosis, encephalitis lethargica, tabes dorsalis and chronic bulbar palsy. Poliomyelitis (Bosma, 1953) is also a possible cause of a lesion because it confines itself to focal infection of motor nerve cells in the brain stem and spinal cord. Damage to the nucleus ambiguus may result in complete laryngeal paralysis because it involves both superior and recurrent laryngeal nerves.

VOCAL FOLD PARALYSIS AND PARESIS

Paralysis of the vocal folds can be unilateral or bilateral, depending on the neurological damage sustained and, as in all nerve paralyses, can be divided into three types (Table 10.16).

The most common PNS lesions are those of the recurrent laryngeal nerve (RLN) whereas a minority of PNS dysphonias are the result of superior laryngeal nerve lesions.

Table 10.16 Categories of nerve paralysis

Neuropraxia:
- The nerve is damaged so that nerve impulses are blocked temporarily
- Function is restored gradually
- No muscle atrophy

Axonotmesis:
- Axons of the nerve are sectioned

Neurotmesis:
- Nerve fibres are severed

In cases of axonotmesis and neurotmesis the affected muscle will atrophy if the nerve fibres do not regenerate. Complete recovery will not take place (Ford and Bless, 1991).

Superior laryngeal nerve lesion

Superior laryngeal nerve (SLN) lesions involve sensory loss in addition to paralysis of the cricothyroid muscle. Unilateral sensory loss gives rise to a vague sensation of a foreign body in the throat with associated throat clearing and paroxysmal coughing (Tucker and Lavertu, 1992). The rarer bilateral sensory loss can lead to aspiration and pneumonia. The paralysed vocal fold is flaccid and cannot be stretched and elongated. At rest and during inspiration, the fold may appear normal, but on phonation there is asymmetry of vibration. The paralysed fold is slightly lower than the healthy one and can even permit prolapse of the affected arytenoid forwards into the interior of the larynx (Tucker, 1987b). The fold is able to adduct, but there is an anterior shift of the fold and the epiglottis to the healthy side, presenting a characteristic askew appearance (Tucker, 1980) – the 'oblique glottis' (Luchsinger, 1965b). Hanson (1991) describes in detail the underlying factors that result in the typical appearance of the larynx after SLN paralysis, a form of laryngeal paralysis that is thought to be frequently unrecognised. The position of the paretic fold is either paramedian or intermediate, not median (Hirano, Shin and Nozoe, 1977). The voice may be weak and breathy and singing is seriously affected. Aphonia occurs in bilateral paralysis. (See Table 10.17 for a profile of voice disorder resulting from an SLN lesion.)

Recurrent laryngeal nerve lesions

Aetiology

Vocal fold paralysis arises most commonly because of damage to one or both of the RLNs supplying the larynx. The tortuous route of the left RLN (see Chapter 2) renders it particularly vulnerable to trauma. The causes of RLN paralyses are summarised in Table 10.18.

Pressure

This occurs from tumours in the neck or apex of the lungs (Jiu, Sobol and Grozea, 1985), enlarged bronchial glands, enlarged thyroid gland, aortic aneurysm, mitral stenosis and enlarged left auricle. Enlargement of the thyroid gland and penetration into the retro-oesophageal and tracheal areas can create pressure on the laryngeal nerve, and thus impair function of the muscles. This occurs rarely according to Sonninen (1960), who reported only one case of laryngeal palsy caused by compression preoperatively in a series of 131 patients. Patients may be referred with 'functional voice disorder' when suffering from real vocal weakness on account of such organic diseases.

Table 10.17 Dysphonia caused by superior laryngeal nerve lesions

Pathology	Weakness/paralysis of the cricothyroid muscle
Aetiology	Trauma
Signs and symptoms	Dysphonia Unilateral sensory loss: • sensation of foreign body • throat clearing • paroxysmal coughing Bilateral sensory loss: • aspiration • pneumonia
Laryngoscopic findings	Unilateral cricothyroid paresis: • both folds appear to adduct on phonation • paralysed fold is shorter and lower than healthy fold • skewed glottis to healthy side • at rest, paralysed fold in paramedian or intermediate position • asymmetrical mucosal waves Bilateral cricothyroid paresis: • overhanging epiglottis • vocal folds bowed
Expected vocal profile	Breathy, hoarse Reduced loudness Ability to alter pitch impaired
Acoustic analysis profile	Reduced harmonics-to-noise ratio Intensity reduced Jitter and shimmer increased Reduced pitch range
Airflow and volume measures	Increased transglottal airflow

Trauma

Trauma from external injuries such as gunshot wounds, or blows to the larynx in road traffic accidents, does occur but lesions can be incurred during surgery. The most common cause of vocal fold paralysis and pareses is trauma sustained during **thyroidectomy** (Holinger, Holinger and Holinger, 1976; Tucker, 1980). The thyroid gland is situated in the lower neck opposite cervical vertebrae C5–7 and the first thoracic vertebra. It consists of two lobes formed by an isthmus that crosses the second and third tracheal rings. The lobes are in close relation to the RLNs before they enter the larynx via the articulation of the cricoid and thyroid cartilages. These nerves are therefore at risk during thyroidectomy (De Souza, 1980), especially as the course

Table 10.18 Recurrent laryngeal nerve lesions: causes

Pressure	• tumours in neck/apex of lung • enlarged bronchial glands • enlarged thyroid gland • aortic aneurysm • enlarged left ventricle
Trauma	• injury • surgery
Endotracheal intubation	• causing RLN compression
Toxaemia	• causing peripheral neuritis
Systemic disease	• e.g. viral infections
Idiopathic disease	• 14% of all cases of laryngeal palsy

and branching of the nerves vary considerably between individuals and render their identification difficult during surgery. (Thyroid gland dysfunction, and its effects on the voice, are discussed in Chapter 11.)

Endotracheal intubation

This occurs on account of the tube being too large or being left in situ for a prolonged period (Hahn, Martin and Lillie, 1970; Ellis and Pallister, 1975; Ellis and Bennett, 1977). Peripheral nerve damage may also occur when the RLN is compressed between the inflated endotracheal tube cuff and the overlying thyroid cartilage (Cavo, 1985). Vocal fold paralysis can follow chest surgery, but there is evidence that it is more likely to result from endotracheal intubation (Hirano, Shin and Nozoe, 1977). Pre-term infants in intensive care, with endotracheal intubation and mechanical ventilation, can have vocal fold paralysis and tracheal stenosis as a result of this life-saving procedure (Papsidero and Pashley, 1980). (Cases of hereditary abductor vocal fold paralysis also occur in children. See below.)

Toxic conditions

Peripheral neuritis and a temporary paralysis may be caused by toxic conditions that prevent conveyance of neural impulses to the muscles. In these cases, a complete paralysis fixes the folds in the paramedian position. The condition is usually bilateral, and complete recovery is to be expected once the toxaemia subsides. Lead poisoning is a toxic condition causing laryngeal neuritis.

Systemic disease

Commonly cited examples of systemic disease causing neuritis and vocal fold paralysis are diphtheria and typhoid (Musgrove, 1952). Virus infections such as measles, pertussis (whooping cough) and influenza also cause neuritis. Acute localised inflammation in herpes zoster (shingles) can also reduce the efficiency of the RLN (Golden, Deeb and deFries, 1990).

Idiopathic

Congenital and/or unknown causes comprise 14% of all cases of laryngeal palsy (Tucker, 1980). It is possible that these cases are viral or caused by a central lesion (Ward, Hanson and Abemayer, 1985).

Childhood vocal paralysis

Vocal paralyses in children are the second most common laryngeal abnormality of the newborn (Swift and Rogers, 1987). Cavanagh (1955) reviewed the available literature on the subject and also reported on her personal examination of 107 children: 37 had laryngeal paralysis – most were unilateral but 10 were bilateral, some were congenital and others acquired. A wide degree of variation in improvement of the airway and recovery of vocal fold movement was noted. She observed that, in the cases of unilateral vocal fold paralysis, the healthy fold abducted three to five times to one abduction of the recovering fold. In several babies with congenital laryngeal stridor, one arytenoid was placed further forward than the other whereas the aryepiglottic fold on the affected side was usually rolled towards the midline and seemed shortened. Greene examined a 7-year-old boy with this condition, which was accompanied by a unilateral palatal palsy on the side opposite to that of the affected fold. He had an inspiratory stridor on effort and when speaking, but no hypernasality.

Van Thal (1962) reported an interesting case of familial laryngeal palsy with aphonia among four generations of the same family. This report appears to be unique in the literature on the subject of congenital laryngeal palsy. Gacek (1976) has also reported cases of hereditary abductor vocal fold paralysis.

Signs and symptoms

In addition to dysphonia, the patient with a unilateral vocal fold paralysis can achieve only a **weak cough** because of the inability to approximate the vocal folds firmly. Even when the vocal folds approximate in the midline, the flaccidity of the paralysed vocal fold fails to resist the increased pressure of the expiratory airstream required for clearing the airway. As a result, the relative incompetency of the laryngeal valve does not allow the necessary raised subglottal air pressure to be established. This is a distressing problem, particularly when laryngeal and tracheal secretions are increased during respiratory tract infections. In some cases, swallowing thin fluids, particularly if they are gaseous or drunk quickly, can cause paroxysmal coughing as liquid seeps through the poorly closed glottis.

Many patients report that they experience **dizziness** during conversation. This appears to be the result of using excessive effort in an attempt to maintain phonation and to increase vocal loudness. The rapid loss of air from the inefficient glottal closure results in frequent inhalations, usually achieved by shallow, upper chest breathing patterns. This over-breathing resembles hyperventilation and, as a result, the patient becomes dizzy. In some cases, the dizziness becomes an additional cause for concern if the sequence of events is not understood by the patient. Explanations and advice regarding less effortful phonation rapidly eliminate the problem in most cases. (See Table 10.19 for a profile of recurrent laryngeal nerve vocal fold paralysis.)

Laryngoscopic findings

Paralysis of the RLN affects the whole adductor and abductor phonatory mechanism. The paralysed fold assumes a paramedian position and is flaccid and bowed. The arytenoid cartilage tilts forward without the bracing action of the posterior cricoarytenoid. The interarytenoid muscle, although having a double innervation, is weak and only poorly able to assist in adduction. The immobile vocal fold is readily identified in the paramedian position on phonation whereas the healthy fold moves to the midline. There is incomplete vocal fold adduction and, although there might appear to be slight adduction on phonation, there is no abduction of the vocal fold. The vocal folds are not on the same plane in some cases. Stroboscopic examination shows that vibration is asymmetrical; the affected vocal fold behaves atypically because the body and cover act as one in large, irregular movements (Moore et al., 1987). Being an LMN lesion, muscles atrophy and are flaccid. As a result of the loss of muscle stiffness, the consistency of the mucosa and muscle is similar. Consequently, the normal mucosal wave of movement as a separate entity from the underlying muscle movement is lost. Absence of the mucosal wave on the affected vocal fold is evidence of a severely damaged fold and indicates poor prognosis (Hirano, Shin and Nozoe, 1977). Care should be taken to ensure that the affected vocal fold is not fixed, rather than paralysed. Sometimes fixation can be confirmed by stroboscopy because the vibratory characteristics of a paralysed vocal fold differ from those of a fixed fold, although palpation of the cricoarytenoid joint under general anaesthetic might be necessary to confirm the diagnosis (Tucker and Lavertu, 1992). In cases of several months standing, unilateral or bilateral hypertrophy of the false vocal folds can be observed in some patients who have developed supraglottal compensatory manoeuvres. Figure 10.1 shows a unilateral vocal fold paralysis.

The final position of the paralysed vocal fold over several months is determined by the site of the lesion. In the case of neck injuries and peripheral nerve damage, position and mobility of the affected vocal fold depend

Table 10.19 Recurrent laryngeal nerve dysphonia	
Pathology	Unilateral or bilateral vocal fold paresis/paralysis
Aetiology	Pressure, trauma, endotracheal intubation, toxicity, systemic disease, idiopathic disease
Signs and symptoms	Unilateral lesion: • weak cough • airway reduced • dizziness with prolonged talking Bilateral lesions: • stridor • airway significantly reduced and tracheostomy necessary
Laryngoscopic findings	Unilateral lesion: • one hypomobile or paralysed vocal fold in paramedian position • paralysed vocal fold mucosal waves chaotic and out of phase with healthy fold vibrations Bilateral lesions: • vocal folds in paramedian position, failing to abduct on inspiration
Expected vocal profile	Breathy Reduced loudness Diplophonia Low pitch or raised pitch Reduced pitch range Reduced maximum phonation time Reduced phrase length
Acoustic analysis profile	Reduced harmonics-to-noise ratio SFo: • primary feature – SFo lowered • secondary feature – SFo raised Intensity reduced Jitter and shimmer increased
Airflow and volume measures	Increased transglottal airflow

on whether the SLN (cricothyroid tensor) and/or the RLN is involved. The positions assumed by the vocal folds depend on the degree of damage suffered by the RLNs and SLNs and whether the damage is unilateral or bilateral. Aronson (1980) provides a clear account of the flaccid dysphonia problem in vagus nerve lesions. Luchsinger (1965b) analysed the vocal disorders in laryngeal paralysis (paralytic dysphonia) and dysfunction of individual muscles. Paralysed vocal folds can eventually assume the positions summarised in Table 10.20.

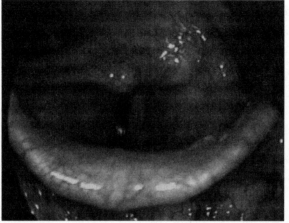

Photograph: Julian McGlashan

Figure 10.1 Right recurrent laryngeal nerve palsy following Cloward's procedure, a spinal operation to remove osteophytes or degenerative discs in the cervical spine during which the larynx and oesophagus are retracted and rotated to allow access to the vertebral bodies.

Paralysed vocal folds finally assume a particular position according to the site of the lesion. As a result of atrophic changes in the muscle fibres and perhaps partial recovery of some motor units, the position of the paralysed fold can move laterally for the following reasons:

- Even when weakened by unilateral paresis, the interarytenoid muscles, which are supplied by both the right and left RLNs, retain the possibility of adducting the fold towards the midline (from an intermediate to a paramedian position). In cases of unilateral paralyses, they do not atrophy like the other intrinsic laryngeal muscles and appear healthy and capable (Kirchner, 1966, 1983).
- Atrophy of muscle tissue and fibrosis of the thyroarytenoid muscles shortens the fold and may alter its position.
- Continued tensor action of the cricothyroid muscle, if there is no lesion of the SLN, may also assist in medial movement of the fold.
- The posterior cricoarytenoid is the sole abductor of the vocal fold and is in fact two muscles – the oblique and vertical fibres. Both may not be wholly impaired and the vertical muscle may retain some abductor action (Zemlin, Davis and Gaza, 1984).
- Besides the propensity in many cases for the paralysed vocal fold to move towards the centre, the healthy fold has a natural tendency, when unopposed, to pass over the midline. This is known as compensation.

Table 10.20 Positions of paralysed vocal folds

Median: adductor, phonatory and midline are synonymous with median	Vocal fold lies in the midline.
Glottic chink: occurs in bilateral abductor paralysis (see below)	The folds are adducted but flaccid, allowing minimal separation during respiration.
Paramedian	The fold lies slightly to the side of the midline. If both are paralysed they are separated posteriorly by a distance of 3.5 mm or 4.0 mm
Intermediate (cadaveric)	The fold lies in a position that is between paramedian and gentle abduction. The cord is flaccid and in the same position as in the cadaver
Gentle abduction	The fold is abducted further than in the cadaveric position, but not fully. This is the position of a healthy vocal fold during quiet respiration
Full abduction	The fold is abducted to its fullest extent. This is the position of a healthy vocal fold during forced inspiration when the maximal airway is necessary

The arytenoid of the healthy fold passes in front of the prolapsed (tilted) paralysed arytenoid. The voice can become almost normal (Williams, Farquharson and Anthony, 1975).

Note

A comprehensive review of old controversies about the phylogeny of neurological damage in relation to vocal fold position in paralysis and paresis can be found in Capps Semon Lecture (Capps, 1958), Arnold (1957) and Dedo (1976). In the past, interest concentrated on the positions assumed by the vocal folds in paralysis and endeavoured to relate these to neurological laws. Felix Semon propounded an evolutionary explanation about abductor and adductor action of the RLNs. Sir Victor Negus, the great authority on the larynges of all creatures great and small, meticulously examined the problem in his classic publication *The Comparative Anatomy and Physiology of the Larynx* (1949) and in his paper 'Observations on Semon's law derived from evidence of comparative anatomy and physiology' (1931). The end-result of his scholarly research was that the evidence supported Semon's law. Semon was a great laryngologist of his time who treated the Prime Minister, Gladstone, for hoarseness. Queen Victoria complained that the leader of her Government always addressed her like a public meeting, which probably accounted for his dysphonia (Hutzinga, 1966).

Expected vocal profile

The abnormal voice resulting from a paralysed vocal fold is the result of three major biomechanical features:

1. The inability of the vocal folds to approximate (glottal insufficiency or incompetency) which allows turbulent air to be generated in the glottis during phonation.

2. The loss of mass and stiffness of the paralysed fold as the thyroarytenoid atrophies, which alters the vibratory characteristics of the vocal fold. The vocalis muscle no longer provides a firm basement structure over which the mucosal wave is generated in the usual way and, as a result, there is loss of symmetry of vocal fold mucosal waves. The loss of innervation also results in dystrophic changes of the vocal fold cover which almost certainly affects vocal fold oscillation adversely.

3. The resistance of the affected vocal fold to the expiratory airstream is reduced (Crumley and Izdebski, 1986). This contributes to glottal insufficiency as the fold is literally blown out of the way during phonation, a feature that becomes more exaggerated as attempts are made to increase vocal loudness.

The vocal characteristics commonly associated with unilateral vocal fold paralysis are listed in Table 10.21.

The aetiology and duration of a unilateral paralysis will affect the voice, which also varies according to the position of the paralysed fold and the effectiveness of compensation achieved by the mobile fold (Ward, Hanson and Abemayer, 1985).

Acoustic analysis profile

The acoustic analysis profile is included in Table 10.19. There is a raised noise component of the vocal note, as a result of the turbulent glottic air, and higher mean flow rates than in normal speakers. A typical voice resulting from an RLN paralysis shows greater frequency and amplitude perturbation measures than in normal speakers (Colton and Casper, 1990).

Bilateral RLN paralysis

If the abductor (posterior cricoarytenoid) muscle is weak, the adductors will hold the vocal fold in the midline. In cases of bilateral abductor paralysis, when both vocal folds are fully adducted, the airway is seriously compromised and a tracheostomy is required. The voice is near to normal, but there is inspiratory stridor. Bilateral abductor paralysis is most frequently caused by total thyroidectomy (Holinger, Holinger and Holinger, 1976; Singer, Hamaker and Miller, 1985) or other trauma. It is an unusual complication after intubation and is immediately recognisable by the acute onset of respiratory distress and stridor after extubation (Brandwen,

Table 10.21 Expected vocal profile in unilateral vocal fold paralysis

Vocal feature	Laryngeal biomechanics
Breathy vocal note	Failure of the vocal folds to approximate competently allows turbulent air to 'leak' through the glottis during phonation
Reduced intensity (a particular problem when attempting to speak against background noise)	Glottal insufficiency results from inadequate vocal fold approximation and the inability of the paralysed fold to resist the expiratory airstream
Short maximum phonation time (resulting in reduced phrase length in connected speech)	Due to the incompetency of the laryngeal valve which allows rapid air escape on phonation
Lowered habitual pitch	Tension of the paralysed vocal fold cannot be increased and it vibrates at a lower frequency than a healthy vocal fold
Reduced pitch range	High notes in the range cannot be produced because the paralysed vocal fold cannot be tightened. Attempted phonation of lower notes is unsuccessful because, as the healthy fold also becomes more flaccid in order to vibrate at a lower frequency, glottal closure becomes even less efficient
Vocal fatigue	All aspects of the voice deteriorate as the speaking episode continues because increasing effort is required to improve glottic closure and to replenish the rapidly lost air pressure. The speaker may feel short of breath and dizzy
Diplophonia (double vocal note)	The effect of a double note, or two pitches, which can be heard simultaneously during phonation may be caused by the generation of more than one fundamental vocal note as the result of the asymmetrical vibrations of the vocal folds
Secondary feature: excessively high habitual pitch. This can occur in an attempt to increase vocal loudness	Greatly increased laryngeal and supraglottic tension

Abramson and Shikowitz, 1986). It is possible for some patients to manage without a tracheostomy, if a chink between the vocal folds occurs subsequently, but they are at risk of airway obstruction in the event of acute laryngitis. Younger, active individuals also find that vigorous exercise or even fast walking is impossible because of the restricted airway (see Case DN in Chapter 9).

Psychogenic 'abductor paralysis'

Occasionally, patients present with symptoms suggesting bilateral abductor vocal fold palsy, which are subsequently found to be psychogenic. This condition has been called Munchausen's stridor, factitious asthma and emotional wheezing (Myears et al., 1985), and can be so severe that a tracheostomy is performed. Paradoxical phonation, i.e. inspiratory phonation, can occur in these patients. Fibreoptic laryngoscopy before and after sedation is proposed by Myears et al. as a method of determining differential diagnosis. They report that, in their experience, a conversion reaction of this type responds well to psychotherapy, speech therapy and relaxation.

Clinical experience suggests that there is a related group of patients who are true asthmatics but who unintentionally compound their symptoms during an asthma attack by hyperadduction of the vocal folds. The resulting paradoxical phonation and noisy inspiratory stridor frighten the patient and those observing or treating the attack, with the effect of heightening the drama of the entire episode (see Case Mr P on page 224).

Laryngeal electromyography

Laryngeal electromyography (LEMG) is diagnostically valuable in the assessment of the residual, functional, electrical potential of laryngeal muscles (Hiroto, Hirano and Tomita, 1968). The insertion of needle electrodes into individual muscle fibre bundles is difficult and requires much experience. When accurate, the results pinpoint the site of nerve lesions, distinguishing myopathy from neuropathy (Parnes and Satya-Murti, 1985) and mechanical fixation from immobility arising from vocal fold paralysis (Hirano, 1981). The degree and extent of paralysis are identifiable and the information provided is useful as a basis for various surgical procedures. To a certain extent, prognostic information can be provided for evaluating future function (Hirose, 1985; Parnes and Satya-Murti, 1985). LEMG is also a means of distinguishing between organic and psychogenic disorders. The technique can therefore provide valuable guidelines for remedial speech therapy. The reader is referred to studies by Faaborg-Anderson and Nykobing (1965), Hirano, Shin and Nozoe (1977) and Hirose (1985).

Medicosurgical decisions

Recovery from paralytic damage to the intrinsic muscles of the larynx is unpredictable. Recovery from nerve damage frequently takes place and should be given time, from 6 months to a year (Tucker, 1980). Hirano,

Shin and Nozoe (1977), in examining the prognostic features of RLN paralysis, found that none of their group of 167 patients recovered after the 6-month period. Paralyses caused by pressure or contusion of the RLN have the best chance of recovery. Intratracheal intubation paralysis has a good prognosis. Neuritis will also resolve and, with disappearance of inflammation, neuroelectric impulses can travel along the nerve pathway again. Post-influenza laryngeal paralysis can be expected to resolve quickly unless the nucleus has been affected.

The more median the vocal fold position, the greater the action potential of the neuromotor unit and the better the chance of spontaneous recovery. If EMG reveals some electrical activity during volitional phonation soon after paralytic trauma, this is a favourable sign for recovery. Electrical activity has been registered years after the initial trauma but the vocal fold remains immobile on account of fibrosis and muscle atrophy. In such cases nerve regeneration must have occurred but too late to be functionally useful. Laryngostroboscopy is an important adjunct to EMG. The presence or absence of the mucosal wave over the surface of the paralysed vocal folds is a diagnostic indicator (Isshiki, 1980); when the mucosal wave is absent, the paralysis is severe and chance of recovery slight. Idiopathic paralysis is expected to recover spontaneously before 6 months.

Unilateral vocal fold paralysis: treatment options

The options for improving the voice in cases of unilateral vocal fold paralysis are summarised in Table 10.22.

Table 10.22 Medicosurgical treatment options in the management of unilateral vocal fold paralysis

Voice therapy:	• trial for 6 months + • proceed to other treatments if voice remains unsatisfactory
Phonosurgery: (laryngeal framework surgery)	• medialisation laryngoplasty to move the paralysed vocal fold towards the midline by inserting a silicon or cartilage wedge • arytenoid adduction
Injected implants:	• increase mass of paralysed vocal fold by injecting collagen, Teflon, Gelfoam or autologous fat
Ansa hypoglossi– *RLN anastomosis*	• reinnervation technique (not in general use)

Voice therapy

Voice therapy is frequently used as a trial treatment during the first 6 months while the patient is observed for possible recovery of the paretic vocal fold. Its primary goal is to improve vocal fold approximation either by capitalising on spontaneous recovery or by encouraging the healthy fold to make an excursion across the midline in order to approximate to the paralysed fold (see Chapter 15). Speech–breathing patterns are also developed to ensure appropriate subglottal air pressure. The secondary goal of therapy is to prevent the development of inappropriate compensatory vocal behaviours, which may reduce the functional effectiveness of the voice. This goal alone is an important justification for appropriate voice therapy in the early stages of recovery, even if it is thought that function will eventually return to the paralysed vocal fold spontaneously. When patients develop hyperfunctional phonation in an attempt to increase loudness, these behaviour patterns can be difficult to discard at a later stage. In addition, because it is tiring and distressing to conduct daily life with an RLN dysphonia, the support of voice therapy and knowledge of the most efficient methods of increasing vocal potential help the patient to deal with the situation.

Phonosurgery (laryngeal framework surgery)

Medialisation laryngoplasty or thyroplasty

Medialisation procedures are usually carried out when it has been established that the RLN is unlikely to recover, i.e. when the vocal fold shows no sign of normal movement after about 6 months. In some centres patients are operated on at an earlier stage. Terminal patients might also be given the option of medialisation, but many decide that they do not want to embark on surgery. The aim of this procedure, originally described by Isshiki, Morita and Okamura (1974), is to move the paralysed fold towards the midline. This is achieved by making a window in the ala of the thyroid cartilage on the affected side, so that a wedge of silicon or cartilage can be inserted between the thyroid cartilage and the perichondrium of the larynx. The operation can be carried out under local anaesthetic and the patient phonates while the surgeon finds the best position for the implant. (Practice varies, however, and the procedure is also performed under general anaesthetic.) Simultaneous vocal ligament tightening in addition to medialisation laryngoplasty is performed in some cases (Koufman, 1986).

Medialisation thyroplasty may be preferred over injected implants (see below) in cases of unilateral combined paralysis of the RLN and SLN, because the involved fold will be slack and the arytenoid tipped forwards and positioned at a lower level than the healthy fold. In these circumstances, an injected implant may be ineffective and it may be preferable to medialise the fold (Isshiki, Okamura and Ishikawa, 1975; Isshiki, Tanabe and Sawada, 1978). An important potential advantage of medialisation procedures over injected implants is that the layers of the lamina propria remain undisturbed. Consequently, the vocal fold mucosa has the potential for mucosal waves once the tension of the vocalis muscle has been increased by stretching the vocal fold over the inserted wedge.

Arytenoid adduction

In cases of damage to the vagus nerve, resulting in paralysis of the SLNs and RLNs, glottal incompetency of the posterior glottis is a common feature. Various procedures have been evolved to approximate the arytenoid cartilages in order to enhance glottal closure (Isshiki, Tanabe and Sawada, 1978; Zeitels, Hochman and Hillman, 1998). In certain cases where the vocal folds are on different planes, this approach has the advantage that the deficit can be corrected by appropriate manipulation of the arytenoid cartilages.

Injected implants

Teflon implant

Until comparatively recently, Teflon implant was the preferred method of improving glottic closure in cases of **unilateral vocal fold paralysis,** but this procedure has largely been abandoned in favour of alternative approaches. For many years, however, it was the most effective method of reducing glottal insufficiency in this group of patients and it continues to have a role in achieving a rapid method of improving the voice in terminally ill patients who have a paralysed vocal fold.

Teflon injection into the paralysed fold increases its bulk so that the healthy fold approximates more easily. The procedure takes a few minutes and can be done under local anaesthetic so that phonation is assessed immediately. Further injections can be given after an interval if further improvement of the voice is required. Oedema sets in almost at once after the injection, and the voice deteriorates and becomes hoarse until swelling and inflammation have subsided. This may take a few days or weeks and the larynx may be painful (Nassar, 1977). The patient requires referral to the speech–language pathologist for reassurance that the voice will recover, and should be advised to use the voice sparingly until the larynx is comfortable again (Mueller, 1973). After several years, a firm rubbery mass is still apparent at the site of the injection (Ward, Hanson and Abemayer, 1985).

Injection of Teflon is most successful when the fold lies in the paramedian or intermediate position. If the glottic aperture is greater it cannot be compensated for by the Teflon implant. If there is doubt about success of the procedure, a preliminary trial with injection of Gelfoam is advisable. This disperses after a few days (Tucker, 1980). The results of Teflon implant are generally good and the success of this treatment was reported in many reviews of patients treated by laryngologists. The principal benefits of Teflon injection are restoration of an efficient cough and increase in vocal intensity. Although it has been suggested that injection into the muscle body of the fold stiffens it while leaving the mucosa free, as in the normal fold (Moore et al., 1987), the voice is not restored to normal because the muscle mass and tension are not the same as those of the normal vocal fold (Crumley and Izdebski, 1986) As a result, the voice may be rough or hoarse with pitch breaks and other abnormalities. Bartelli, Ford and Bless (1986) analysed poor results in 17 adults after Teflon injection. They attributed failure to a number of causes: overfilling supra- and subglottic structures; migration of the Teflon from the vocal folds; granuloma and scar tissue; and stiffness of the injected vocal fold. Although they reported that the condition of the damaged fold was improved by removal of the Teflon and the injection of collagen, Teflon injection should be regarded as essentially irreversible because of the fibrous tissue that gradually fixes it in position (Crumley, 1990). It is the treatment of choice for elderly or terminally ill patients where immediate vocal improvement is needed and can be achieved most easily. It is generally well tolerated (Ward, Hanson and Abemayer, 1985).

Collagen-injected implant

Injectable collagen for **unilateral vocal fold paralysis** is regarded as possibly having certain advantages over Teflon although a cautious approach to its use is advocated (Ford and Bless, 1987; Spiegel, Sataloff and Gould, 1987). Whereas Teflon is an inert substance, collagen is biologically active (Ford, Gilchrist and Bartell, 1987). Adverse reactions such as swelling are reported in some cases, although it is generally well tolerated. Liquid collagen is more easily and accurately administered than Teflon, which is a thick paste. Collagen has the additional advantage of softening and reducing scar tissue in the treated area. The implant of collagen into the existing collagen layer of the lamina propria augments normal collagen and stimulates replacement. Ford, Bless and Campbell (1986) reported improvement in vibratory pattern and phonation in 80 patients receiving collagen implants.

Fat- and Gelfoam-injected implants

Fat and Gelfoam are gradually absorbed by the laryngeal tissue, so they can therefore be useful trial materials when deciding upon the treatment route.

The eventual choice of treatment depends on the following factors:

- The aetiology of the RLN lesion. In cases of terminal carcinoma of the lung, e.g. when the RLN is compressed, the objective of treatment is usually to restore functionally useful voice as rapidly as possible.
- Whether it has been possible to establish that the RLN has been severed or irretrievably damaged. If it is thought that there is some possibility of recovery, voice therapy ensures best voice care and most effective vocal behaviours while giving the patient positive support.
- The length of time since the RLN injury was incurred. Phonosurgery is probably the treatment of choice if there is no evidence of recovery 6 months or more post-onset.

Voice therapy is an important adjunct to medialisation procedures and to injected implants in order to help patients to adjust vocal behaviour and to avoid hyperfunction.

Bilateral abductor paralysis: treatment options

The severe respiratory difficulties resulting from bilateral paralysis of the vocal folds in the midline means that establishing and maintaining an adequate airway assume priority over phonatory needs. In most cases, the voice is functionally adequate, but procedures designed to improve the airway tend to compromise phonation. Ideally, management decisions attempt to balance these needs. The treatment options for bilateral abductor paralysis are summarised in Table 10.23.

Tracheotomy

Most patients with bilateral abductor vocal fold paralysis require a tracheostomy, even if breathing is adequate at rest because they are at risk of airway obstruction in the event of respiratory infection, and because the airway is inadequate on exertion. A speaking valve (see page 261), fitted to the tracheostomy tube, allows air to be directed through the larynx on expiration so that the patient can phonate.

Table 10.23 Bilateral abductor vocal fold paralysis: treatment options

---

Surgery

Tracheotomy:
- to ensure adequate airway while recovery is monitored and until decisions are made regarding further surgical options which allow closure of the stoma
- speaking valve (e.g. Rusch, Passy-Muir)

Unilateral arytenoidectomy:
- lateralisation of one vocal fold aims to preserve the airway and allow the membranous vocal folds to adduct for phonation. The tracheostomy is then closed

Transoral laser cordectomy and arytenoidectomy:
- aim: to lateralise one vocal fold to improve airway

Ansahypoglossi–RLN anastomosis:
- aim: reinnervation of posterior cricoarytenoid abductor muscle to improve airway and preserve voice

Voice therapy

- for support in managing communication after tracheostomy
- to facilitate optimum voice after surgical intervention

Surgical lateralisation, laryngofissure and arytenoidectomy

Surgical lateralisation procedures aim to enlarge the glottic airway. Laryngofissure and arytenoidectomy can improve the airway with minimal adverse effects on phonation. After laryngofissure, unilateral arytenoidectomy is performed without lateralisation of the vocal fold (Singer, Hamaker and Miller, 1985). This results in a posterior glottic chink which preserves the airway and competent adduction of the anterior glottis for phonation. Although aware of the possibility of using a carbon dioxide laser to perform arytenoidectomy, Singer, Hamaker and Miller (1985) advocate caution. There is danger of glottic scarring reported by some pioneers in this field.

Transoral laser cordectomy and arytenoidectomy

These procedures are used to lateralise one of the paralysed vocal folds in order to establish an improved airway (Eckel et al., 1994). Inevitably, phonation is compromised and the outcome is unpredictable. Respiratory parameters are improved but remain compromised. Voice therapy is necessary to ensure that the patient is phonating as efficiently as possible and that counterproductive, inappropriate, compensatory strategies do not evolve.

Ansa hypoglossi–RLN anastomosis

Tucker (1976, 1978, 1980) advocated nerve and muscle pedicle reinner-vation in cases of **bilateral abductor paralysis.** The procedure involves reinnervating the posterior cricoarytenoid abductor muscle by using a branch of the ansa hypoglossi to the omohyoid muscle. Tucker explains that, as the strap muscles are accessory inspiratory muscles, they contract on inspiration. The transplanted nerve grows to innervate the abductor muscle and opens the larynx on inspiration. This opens up the airway and remedies breathing difficulties on exertion and the danger of obstruction in respiratory infections. The provision of an adequate airway does not impair the voice. The operation is relatively easy and function returns to the pos-terior cricoarytenoid after between 6 and 12 weeks. Tucker (1980) reports an 88.6% success rate with subsequent removal of the tracheostomy and without compromising voice in 80% of cases (Tucker and Lavertu, 1992).

Crumley and Izdebski (1986) have reported the results of Tucker's technique for **unilateral vocal fold paresis,** using an ansa hypoglossi–RLN anastomosis. Their study confirmed that this is a simple procedure without serious side effects and that it is non-invasive in relation to the larynx. Subjective and objective assessment of phonation postoper-atively revealed that the resulting voice quality was superior to that obtained by Teflon implant, because it does not affect vocal fold structure. Crumley (1990) has confirmed his preference for this procedure in a subsequent discussion paper. This procedure is not in general use.

Summary

■   A voice disorder resulting from a lesion of the central nervous system is usually only one element of a range of neurological abnormalities.
■   The voice disorder may be the earliest indication of neuropathology (Ramig et al., 1988)
■   A voice disorder resulting from a lesion of the peripheral nervous system can exist in isolation.
■   The vocal profile is frequently highly variable in a neurologically dis-ordered voice and this fact must be taken into account during laryn-goscopic and acoustic evaluation, and during treatment.
■   Medication, fatigue and stress can affect a neurogenic voice problem significantly.
■   A multidisciplinary team approach consisting of neurologist, laryn-gologist and speech–language pathologist is particularly important for this patient group.

Further reading

Neurogenic voice disorders constitute a particularly complex subsection of voice disorders because of their pathophysiology. The following texts are recommended for more detailed reading:

Bhatnagar SC, Andy OJ (1995) *Neuroscience for the Study of Communicative Disorders*. Baltimore: Williams & Wilkins

Blitzer A, Brin M, Sasaki CT, Fahn S, Harris K, eds (1992) *Neurologic Disorders of the Larynx*. New York: Thième

Hanson DG (1991) Neuromuscular disorders of the larynx. *Otolaryngologic Clinics of North America* 24: 1035–1051

Special issue (1992) Spasmodic dysphonia. *Journal of Voice* 6(4).

CHAPTER

Diseases and conditions affecting the vocal tract

Numerous conditions apart from those discussed in the previous chapters can cause changes in the voice. In some instances the vocal change is the first indication of underlying pathology. This chapter describes some of these conditions which can be classified into three broad categories:

- Diseases and conditions that affect the larynx directly.
- Respiratory diseases and conditions that chiefly affect the voice because of inadequate subglottal air pressure, but that can also involve the larynx.
- Systemic diseases with laryngeal manifestations.

Laryngeal conditions and diseases (Table 11.1)

LARYNGEAL IRRITANTS

Laryngopharyngeal reflux

Reflux of stomach contents up the oesophagus with subsequent overspill into the larynx has been accepted as a major cause of laryngeal irritation since the publication of papers by Cherry and Margulies (1968) and Cherry and Delahunty (1968). These authors described three patients suffering from contact ulcers which failed to heal when treated by conventional voice rest and voice therapy. They hypothesised that pharyngo-oesophagitis caused by peptic acid reflux occurred when the patients were sleeping and that acid seeped into the posterior larynx, causing inflammation and ulceration. After treatment with antacids and patients being advised to sleep on raised pillows, the ulcers were cured after a period of 3–6 months. The hypothesis that contact ulcers are actually peptic ulcers of the larynx was further supported by

Table 11.1 Laryngeal disease, inflammatory conditions and diseases affecting the vocal tract

Laryngeal	Laryngeal irritants:	
		• gastric reflux
		• inhaled and ingested substances
	Laryngitis:	
		• acute infective
		• acute non-infective
		• chronic
		• chronic hyperplastic
		• hypertrophic posterior
		• fungal
	Neoplasms:	
		• malignant
		• benign: papillomas
		cysts
Respiratory		
		• asthma
		• bronchitis
		• emphysema
		• carcinoma
		• chronic obstructive airways/ pulmonary disease (COAD or COPD)
Systemic	Autoimmune diseases:	
		• laryngeal rheumatoid arthritis
		• systemic lupus erythematosus
		• relapsing polychondritis
		• sarcoidosis
		• Sjögren's syndrome
		• vasculitis, e.g. Wegener's granulomatosis
	Infection:	
		• TB
		• diphtheria
		• syphilis
	Endocrinological:	
		• hypothyroidism
		• hyperthyroidism
		• testosterone insufficiency
		• virilisation

COAD, chronic obstructive airway disease; COPD, chronic obstructive pulmonary disease.

the inflammation and ulceration which resulted from painting the vocal folds of dogs with gastric acid.

More recently, it has been estimated that almost two-thirds of patients attending ENT clinics with laryngeal and voice disorders may have gastro-oesophageal reflux disease (GERD) (Koufman, 1995). When acid from the stomach reaches the larynx (laryngopharyngeal reflux or LPR), the mucosa is subjected to irritation which can give rise to unpleasant sensory symptoms and to changes in the voice.

Signs and symptoms

Gastric reflux is now acknowledged to give rise to or to contribute to an extensive list of signs and symptoms (Table 11.2). It is commonly referred to as heartburn, a burning sensation that travels upwards from the area of the process of the sternum to the laryngeal area. In severe episodes, the sufferer is aware of regurgitation of stomach contents into the hypopharynx. In most cases, even when experiencing heartburn or indigestion at frequent intervals, the patient will not have considered that these episodes might be related to the voice disorder. More significantly, it is suggested that fewer than 50% of patients in whom reflux is a significant factor or primary contributory cause have overt symptoms of heartburn or regurgitation (Forrest and Weed, 1998). It is the role of the clinician, therefore, to consider and assess the possible contribution of gastric reflux to a voice problem through amassing details of diet and lifestyle, laryngoscopic examination and the appropriate investigations (see below).

Aetiology

The causal relationships between gastric reflux and voice disorders are only poorly understood and are probably wide ranging. It is possible that in some cases vocal abuse causes the initial laryngeal irritation, which is subsequently exacerbated by reflux. Alternatively, reflux causes irritation which is the basis of abusing the larynx as the speaker attempts to overcome the effects of the discomfort. The aetiology of reflux is related to incompetency of the lower oesophageal segment, which allows return of the stomach contents. Olson (1991), in a comprehensive review of the laryngeal manifestations of GERD, discusses its pathogenesis. It is known that fats, alcohol, chocolate and smoking all affect the lower oesophageal segment pressure. In addition, Olson refers to three mechanical causes of GERD resulting from alterations in stomach and lower oesophageal segment pressure:

- transient lower oesophageal segment relaxation
- increased intra-abdominal pressure
- spontaneous free reflux.

In many individuals, GERD is related to lifestyle. A diet consisting of a high intake of coffee and gaseous drinks (particularly diet beverages), meals taken late at night and rapid eating patterns will render many

Table 11.2 Disorders and symptoms that may be related to gastric reflux

- Posterior laryngitis
- Cricoarytenoid joint arthritis
- Subglottic stenosis
- Laryngeal carcinoma
- Non-productive, irritable coughing
- Hoarseness
- Hyperkeratosis of the posterior larynx (pachydermia laryngis)
- Laryngospasm
- Cervical oesophagitis and web formation (Plummer–Vinson syndrome)
- Excess salivation
- Aspiration pneumonia
- Zenker's diverticulum
- Dental caries
- Oral cavity ulceration
- Sore throat
- Intubation granuloma
- Globus sensation
- Choking sensation
- Throat clearing
- Weakness of the voice
- Neck and jaw pain
- Carcinoma of the larynx
- Subglottic stenosis
- Uni- or bilateral arytenoid fixation

Sources: Olson (1991); Koufman (1995).

individuals susceptible to reflux. This tendency is exacerbated when the eater is sitting in a crouched position – on a sofa, for example – rather than upright at a table. There is also evidence that vigorous physical exercise induces gastric reflux, which is most severe after running or when exercise is taken shortly after eating. The effects of acid reflux on the vocal folds can also be seen in association with bulimia when frequent self-induced vomiting causes laryngo-oesophagitis (Rothstein, 1998).

Laryngoscopic findings

The effect of acid irritation of the larynx in cases of GERD is classic and the literature is in agreement on the laryngoscopic findings (Koufman, 1995; Forrest and Weed, 1998; Ross, Noordzji and Woo, 1998; Rothstein, 1998) (Table 11.3).

Expected vocal profile

The vocal profiles of individuals with laryngopharyngeal reflux tend to resemble those with muscle tension dysphonia (see Chapter 7) and, as a result, the contribution of LPR to a voice disorder may be overlooked,

Table 11.3 Dysphonia associated with laryngopharyngeal reflux (LPR)

Pathology	Related to incompetency of the lower oesophageal segment allowing return of stomach contents
Aetiology	Either acid irritation of the laryngeal mucosa resulting in changed phonatory patterns or vocal abuse rendering laryngeal tissues susceptible to acid irritation.
Signs and symptoms	'Heartburn' and dysphonia Laryngeal irritation and soreness Throat clearing
Laryngoscopic findings	Reddened arytenoids Laryngeal oedema Vocal fold oedema Hypertrophy[a] of posterior glottis (pachydermia laryngis) Generalised/posterior erythema[a] Laryngeal telangiectasis[a] Leukoplakia[a] False vocal fold adduction on phonation
Expected vocal profile	Musculoskeletal tension Hard glottal attack Vocal creak Restricted resonance of the fundamental vocal note Hoarseness
Acoustic analysis	Reduced harmonics-to-noise ratio SFo possibly reduced Pitch range reduced
Airflow and volume measures	Reduced airflow if there is excessive vocal creak, but transglottal airflow may be excessive if there is glottal chink
Medicosurgical decisions	Management/medication for LPR (see Table 11.4) Voice therapy LPR should be considered in all cases of MTD that do not respond to voice therapy

Note: some or all of these laryngeal features can be present.
[a]**Hypertrophy**: an increase in volume of tissue produced entirely by enlargement of existing cells.
Erythema: redness caused by congestion of the capillaries occurring with infection or trauma.
Telangiectasia: dilatation of small blood vessels. **Leukoplakia**: white, thickened patches on the mucous membrane which have a tendency to become malignant. These conditions are not only associated with laryngopharyngeal reflux but can also occur when vocal fold trauma or infection has occurred.

particularly if the condition is occult and the patient is unaware of 'heartburn'. It has been suggested that patients with LPR consistently exhibit more specific vocal characteristics than patients with only generic voice disorders or hoarseness (Ross, Noordzji and Woo, 1998). These perceptual voice characteristics include hard glottal attack, glottal fry and restricted tone placement. Increased musculoskeletal tension is also a feature.

It should not be overlooked that varying degrees of LPR can contribute to vocal symptoms in a wide range of voice problems and is not necessarily itself the primary causative factor.

Management

The basis of the management of LPR in association with a voice disorder is the clinician's awareness that this might be an important factor in the aetiology of the presenting dysphonia. Definitive diagnosis depends on 24-hour ambulatory pH monitoring, during which oesophageal and pharyngeal acidity is monitored by a nasogastric tube attached to a small computer worn by the patient. In many instances, trial treatment with anti-reflux medication (e.g. omeprazole) and changes in lifestyle and diet are used to determine the presence of LPR. The treatment of GERD consists of lifestyle and dietary changes in combination with medical or surgical intervention as necessary (Table 11.4). Voice therapy is essential to overcome the damaging vocal behaviours that have developed and to reduce laryngeal discomfort.

Alcohol

Alcohol causes the larynx to become injected (i.e. congested with an abnormal accumulation of blood). These changes are seen particularly in the subglottic portion of the vocal folds, the anterior commissure, the ventricles and the

Table 11.4 Treatment of gastro-oesophageal reflux

Weight reduction	In obese individuals
Posture changes	Elevate bed-head by 6 inches (15 cm) Avoid slumping, kneeling, wearing constricting clothing

Diet changes	Do not eat for at least 2 hours before going to bed
	Do not overeat
	Avoid:
	    Cola and citrus/citrus drinks Fats
	    Chocolate Tea
	    Tomato products Mints
	    All coffee Chewing gum
	    Beer Sweets
	    Spirits Milk

Medication	Antacids 1 hour before eating Other medication: cimetidine, ranitidine, omeprazole
Surgery	In severe cases such as persistent oesophagitis or oesophageal stenosis

Sources: Olson (1991); Koufman (1995).

midportion of the true vocal folds. The posterior region of the larynx and the arytenoid cartilages also become reddened (Watanabe et al., 1994). As a result, vocal efficiency deteriorates but lack of inhibition during inebriation can lead to a significantly wider pitch and loudness range than usual. The anomaly arises that alcohol can seem to be soothing if the throat or larynx is sore. There are many traditional remedies for treating sore throats, or even supposedly preparing the larynx for a demanding vocal performance, that involve drinking or gargling with alcohol. Alcohol may be a main ingredient of 'over-the-counter' remedies. The use of these and various folk remedies is misguided and will aggravate or even cause laryngeal irritation.

Smoking

Tobacco smoking in the form of cigarettes, cigars and pipes dries and irritates the larynx, leading to changes in the laryngeal mucosa. The combined effects of smoking and alcohol can result in laryngeal carcinoma. Other substances, such as cannabis, also dry and irritate the larynx, and the behavioural changes associated with their use might predispose the user to further vocal misuse.

Chemicals

Laryngeal irritation caused by chemicals can occur in the workplace and home. Even low level exposure to formaldehyde, for example, is associated with changes in epithelial cells in the mouth and throat irritation (Chia et al., 1992; Kriebel, Sama and Cocanour, 1993; Suruda et al., 1993). Similar effects can occur when using ammonia or some oven cleaners in poorly ventilated rooms. Masks should be worn when using chemicals that can cause irritation.

LARYNGITIS

Speech and language therapists are so familiar with laryngitis caused by vocal misuse that there is a tendency to overlook the possibility of the pathologies that cause inflammatory diseases of the larynx (Vrabec and Davison, 1980). Laryngeal inflammation can be accompanied by oedema, which is a non-specific reaction to a variety of insults to the tissues resulting in swelling (Table 11.5).

Acute laryngitis

Infective

Acute infective laryngitis is usually viral and occurs in association with an upper respiratory tract infection. In most cases, it is self-limiting and resolves spontaneously, but in some cases secondary infections compound

Table 11.5 Laryngeal oedema: causes

Infection	
Vocal abuse	
Smoking	
Trauma	
Radiotherapy:	laryngeal perichondritis (inflammation of tissue covering the laryngeal cartilages)
Allergic angio-oedema:	can be provoked by food, inhalants and drugs (most common: aspirin, iodine and penicillin) (common: chicken, beef, bee stings, house dust, cosmetics)

Source: Teitel et al. (1992).

the primary problem. Laryngeal infections commonly cause acute mucosal inflammation which is sometimes accompanied by oedema. The degree to which the condition affects the voice is generally directly proportional to the severity of the condition, with voice problems ranging from aphonia to slight hoarseness. Depending on the severity and type of infection, the larynx can be extremely sore or there might be no discomfort even when the sufferer is severely dysphonic or aphonic. In some cases of infection the dysphonia may continue for up to a fortnight. Voice rest is important.

Non-infective

An acute inflammation of the laryngeal mucosa can also be caused by a range of laryngeal irritants from an episode of laryngeal abuse, such as shouting at a football game, to exposure to a polluted atmosphere. The voice will be hoarse and aphonia may occur. The condition usually improves after 2 or 3 days if the voice is rested and not subjected to further abuse.

Although acute laryngitis alone does not require voice therapy, it may be the precipitating factor for a clinical voice disorder that eventually requires treatment. In many instances, the inappropriate compensatory strategies that are employed in an attempt to overcome the vocal effects of the laryngitis are the basis for a voice disorder that continues when the initial laryngitis has resolved. Attempts to increase vocal loudness or the clarity of the vocal note can amount to vocal abuse that compounds the laryngitis. In some cases, the patient tries to 'protect' the voice by talking more quietly, but inadvertently lowers habitual pitch so that, although quiet, phonation becomes hyperfunctional. Consequently, these vocal behaviours tend to compound and prolong the acute laryngitis. It is also important to recognise that, in many instances, even when the laryngeal mucosa has fully recovered, the kinaesthetic model for normal phonation is compromised. Patients frequently comment that they cannot remember what it feels like to talk normally and as a result they might continue to use excessive phonatory effort or an abnormal speaking fundamental frequency. Recovery can also be delayed by the patient's conviction that a prolonged infection is the basis of the problem rather than changed vocal behaviour that can be modified. Acute laryngitis can also be the 'trigger' for conversion symptom aphonia and a range of psychogenic voice disorders.

Chronic non-specific laryngitis

Kleinsasser (1968) described the confusion of terms and conditions associated with the collective term 'chronic laryngitis' and remarked that laryngologists have differing concepts of the clinical picture presented by such terms as pachydermia, keratosis, leukoplakia, polyp, papilloma, etc. Ambiguity of terminology continues not only globally but also within each country. Vrabec and Davison (1980) advocated the term 'chronic non-specific laryngitis' to include a variety of long-standing inflammatory changes (laryngitis) in the laryngeal mucosa. Subdivisions can then be apportioned to chronic laryngitis, chronic hyperplastic laryngitis and hypertrophic posterior laryngitis.

Chronic laryngitis

Chronic laryngitis (Figure 11.1) results in generalised oedema and inflammation of the mucous membrane of the vocal folds. This condition is most commonly seen in men when the use of tobacco is associated with excessive alcohol consumption and vocal abuse. It may follow an acute infection, but more commonly it becomes established slowly and is a long-term condition

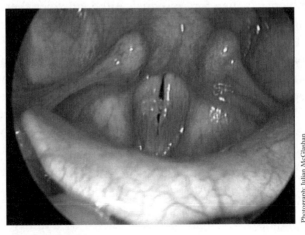

Figure 11.1 Chronic laryngitis.

resulting from physical and chemical irritants. It is associated with tobacco and alcohol in particular, but dust, fumes and continual coughing as a result of infection or allergic rhinitis can also contribute to the problem, with gastric reflux making a further contribution in some cases. The role of illegal substances is unclear but cannabis appears to cause marked drying of the vocal tract mucosa in addition to its irritant effect. Inhaled cocaine is also an irritant. Apart from their direct effect on the mucosal surface, mood-altering substances also cause behavioural changes. The resulting disinhibition allows the substance user to behave more expansively and possibly vocalise more vigorously. As a result, the irritant effect of the substance is compounded by vocal abuse. Atmospheric pollution, including dust and chemicals such as ammonia and oven cleaners, is probably also an important cause. In central heating, the dehydrated air dries out the mucous membrane and arrests the ciliary movement. This permits infective organisms to penetrate the mucosa and set up inflammation. Laryngitis is thus established. Allergic responses to certain drugs may be contributory. Faulty voice use also appears to be a factor; Morrison, Nichol and Rammage (1986) reported that they had usually observed the condition in adult males, particularly those at the beginning of a singing career without the benefit of good singing tuition. A summary of the causes of chronic laryngitis appears in Table 11.6.

The chief characteristics on laryngoscopy are viscid mucus, chronic inflammation and epithelial thickening. Remacle, Degols and Delos (1996) describe two stages in the development of chronic laryngitis. The first stage is of oedema or laryngitis, which can be reversed by conservative treatments. The second, irreversible stage consists of an extension of the oedema and fibrosis, with the ciliated mucous membrane being replaced by squamous epithelium. The histological changes may be precursors to malignant change and biopsy is therefore essential. Although voice therapy alone will not reverse the changes in the vocal fold mucosa, it is essential pre- and post-operatively for the cycle of abusive behaviour to be broken.

The patient may complain of a sore throat in the early stages of the condition, but with the onset of fibrosis discomfort is minimal. The voice is hoarse as a result of the changed vibratory and biomechanical characteristics of the vocal folds. Increased vocal fold mass causes significantly lowered pitch. In advanced cases volume is reduced, but at earlier stages the voice may be excessively loud as an element of vocal abuse. Phonation may be effortful and fatiguing as attempts are made to compensate for the laryngeal changes.

Chronic hyperplastic laryngitis

Chronic hyperplastic laryngitis is characterised by a diffuse inflammatory process that extends over a wide area of the laryngeal mucosa (Kleinsasser,

Table 11.6 Chronic laryngitis profile

Pathology	Diffuse, chronic inflammatory changes and oedema of the vocal fold mucosa
Aetiology	Prolonged irritation of the laryngeal mucosa by: • Vocal abuse • Smoking • Excessive alcohol • Repeated episodes of laryngitis • Atmospheric pollutants • Dry atmosphere • Extremes of climate • Chronic mouth breathing • Possibly infection
Signs and symptoms	Gradual onset of hoarseness, sometimes over many years Effortful phonation Laryngeal soreness initially which reduces as fibrotic changes become established

Laryngoscopic findings	• Bilateral and symmetrical vocal fold changes:
	  – Hyperaemia (pink or reddened according to severity of the condition)
	  – Hypertrophy (thickening, possibly in association with hypertrophy of other laryngeal areas)
	  – Oedema (vocal fold swelling)
	• Hyperadduction in early stages
	• Inadequate glottal closure in advanced stages of the condition because of rough free edges of the vocal folds
	• Reduced, asymmetrical mucosal waves because of stiffness of the mucosa
	• Prolonged closed phase in early stages leading to reduced or absent closed phase in advanced state
	• False vocal fold adduction may occur in effortful compensatory phonation
	• Leukoplakia (white patches) on vocal folds in some cases (see Figure 11.2)

Expected vocal profile	Hoarseness Marked roughness of the vocal note Reduced loudness Lowered vocal pitch Unstable vocal quality
Acoustic analysis	Reduced harmonics-to-noise ratio Reduced SFo Reduced intensity
Airflow and volume	Although glottal closure is incomplete, glottal resistance is frequently raised as the speaker attempts to overcome the increased inertia of the relatively stiff vocal folds by hyperfunctional phonation. Airflow measures vary according to the stage of the condition.
Medicosurgical decisions	Biopsy Antibiotics, if necessary Voice conservation and vocal hygiene advice If surgery necessary, pre- and postoperative voice therapy

1968). It is usually highly developed on the vocal folds and eventually leads to epithelial hyperplasia, characterised by white raised patches on the vocal folds called leukoplakia (Figure 11.2). This condition, unlike acute and chronic laryngitis, does not heal when infection or irritants are removed and it is potentially a pre-cancerous condition. Kleinsasser recommended stripping of the folds (decortication) and removal of the thickened epithelium because it arrests the disease and achieves voice improvement. It may also prevent malignancy developing. The new epithelium that forms after stripping of the vocal folds remains thin, smooth and non-inflamed for years afterwards in most patients, according to Vrabek and Davison (1980). On the other hand, Ballantyne and Groves (1982) reported that recurrence is usual. All possible laryngeal irritants must be eliminated, including vocal abuse (Shaw and Friedmann, 1964). Hyperfunctional phonation develops in an attempt to overcome the dysphonia that is secondary to inflammation. Most of these patients are or have been heavy smokers and they must be warned of the dangers of smoking and advised to stop. Air pollutants such as dust or fumes that may be inhaled regularly at work or in other situations should be avoided and masks worn.

Voice rest is recommended postoperatively, but if the patient must talk the use of gentle normal voice is less harmful than whispering. Only when the vocal folds have fully healed and re-epithelialised, usually after 3–4 weeks, is speech therapy prescribed if necessary. Considerable voice improvement can be achieved relatively quickly if the patient is cooperative

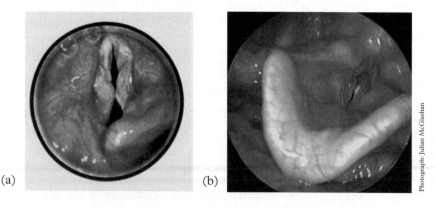

(a)　　　　　　　　　　　　　　(b)

Photograph: Julian McGlashan

Figure 11.2 (a) Chronic hyperplastic laryngitis (b) (Left vocal fold) Leukoplakia.

and complies with a programme of voice conservation and vocal hygiene. Restoration of normal voice is not generally a realistic goal.

Hypertrophic posterior laryngitis

This is another term for pachydermia and interarytenoid pachydermia which was discussed in connection with contact ulcers and intubation granuloma (see Chapter 7). The condition shown on indirect laryngoscopy is a mass of grey tissue in the posterior larynx, extending forwards over the arytenoids and usually symmetrical. No conclusive aetiology has been decided, but in the past smoking and alcohol were thought to be the chief factors. Delahunty and Ardran (1970) produced evidence of acid laryngeal and gastric reflux with oesophagitis occurring at night, resulting in reflux pachydermia. Attention to diet, elevation of the head at night and medication to reduce stomach acidity are recommended. Spicy and fried foods that cause 'heartburn' should be avoided especially. Delahunty (1972) reported good results after 6–8 weeks on this regimen. Goldberg, Noyek and Pritzker (1978) describe a case of laryngeal 'granuloma' on two-thirds of one vocal cord attributed to gastro-oesophageal reflux, which appeared to be identical with reflux pachydermia when the histological structure was examined.

Fungal infection

When voice disorders occur in an individual with compromised immunological status, fungal infection of the larynx should be considered. Fungal (mycotic) infections involving the larynx are relatively common in the immunocompromised host but rare in the immunocompetent individual (Forrest and Weed, 1998). If fungal infection is found in the larynx systemic disease is, therefore, a possibility. The predisposing factors are alterations in the mucosal barrier or in the immune status. The most commonly encountered predisposing factors are the previous administration of antibiotics or inhaled steroids. Patients who already have significant underlying disease, and who are receiving broad-spectrum antimicrobial therapy, are particularly vulnerable to candidiasis, an infection by fungi of the genus *Candida* (Figure 11.3) which occurs chiefly in warm moist areas.

Hoarseness and laryngitis caused by fungal infections may be indistinguishable initially from other causes of laryngitis. Candidiasis, which presents as diffuse erythema in conjunction with areas of white plaque adhering firmly to the laryngeal mucosa, can mimic other conditions such as gastric reflux changes, granulomatous disease and carcinoma. Isolated

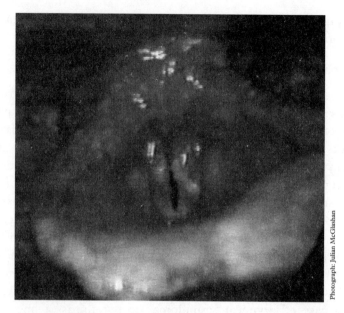

Photograph: Julian McGlashan

Figure 11.3 *Candida* involving the vocal folds.

laryngeal candidiasis gives rise to intense pain in the oropharynx and if allowed to progress will cause breathing difficulties or systemic fungal disease. If hoarseness and dysphagia occur in this patient group, laryngeal candidiasis should be considered as the cause (Tashjian and Peacock, 1984). Granulomas of the vocal fold may also occur secondary to fungal infection. Although extremely rare, fungal infections have been recorded in individuals dealing with plant matter such as sphagnum moss (Agger and Seager, 1985).

Biopsy and cultures of the affected area will indicate appropriate treatment. Forrest and Weed (1998) stress the importance of requesting a mucosal biopsy because of its much higher accuracy in revealing candida infection than the routinely used tests. Candidiasis is treated with anti-fungal agents such as nystatin, but these only suppress fungal growth and it is essential for the underlying problem to be addressed effectively. It is also important that good vocal hygiene is adhered to in order to ensure that the laryngeal mucosa is as healthy as possible, and therefore less susceptible to infection. Voice therapy is indicated to correct any patterns of vocal abuse that might have made the larynx particularly vulnerable to fungal infection when the spores were initially inhaled.

AIDS/HIV

Acquired immune deficiency syndrome (AIDS) is a spectrum of diseases associated with human immunodeficiency virus (HIV), a viral infection that causes a slowly progressive weakening in the cellular immune system. Patients with AIDS may present with manifestations in the head and neck as a result of the individual's compromised immune system (Gray and Rutka, 1988). These presentations tend to fall into three categories:

(1)   oral, pharyngeal, laryngeal and oesophageal candidiasis which is associated with painful swallowing and dysphagia
(2)   cutaneous, oral, pharyngeal and laryngeal lesions, such as Kaposi's sarcoma, a progressive malignant tumour
(3)   chronic cough and dyspnoea because the pulmonary system is the subject of repeated opportunistic infections.

NEOPLASMS

Laryngeal neoplasms are benign or malignant. This section is confined to benign growths. Malignant tumours are discussed in relation to laryngeal carcinoma and laryngectomy (see Chapter 17).

Benign

Papilloma

Papillomas are benign neoplasms consisting of a vascular connective tissue core, which may have several subdivisions, covered by stratified squamous epithelium. They are sessile or pedunculated and are attached to the mucous membrane of the respiratory tract. They occur mainly on the vocal folds but can invade the trachea. They are translucent and pinkish red and easily recognisable because multiple lesions form in clusters like warts. They have long been attributed, like warts, to viral infection (Bone, Feren and Nahum, 1976). The specific virus has not, however, been identified. Despite the assumption of viral infection, there is also a hormonal influence. Holinger, Schild and Mauriz (1968) drew attention to the fact that papilloma occurs more frequently in men than in women, although there is an equal distribution before puberty. Recession often occurs at puberty and during pregnancy, but the disease recurs later. Cook et al. (1973) reported papilloma incidence to be in the male:female ratio of 2:1. Recurrence may occur at the menopause.

Juvenile papillomas are the most common laryngeal tumours in children (Robbins and Howard, 1983) and occur most frequently between the ages of 4 and 6 years (Kleinsasser, 1968). Multiple laryngeal papillomatosis is more likely to occur in the child than in the adult. The condition usually involves the vocal folds and the ventricular bands, but may extend to the trachea, bronchi and epiglottis. Papillomas rarely make their first appearance later in childhood. In some children there is recession at 11 years of age (Senturia and Wilson, 1968), but regression may be delayed until puberty (Robbins and Howard, 1983). A distinction is made between juvenile and adult papilloma by some authorities, not so much by reason of their histological structure but

(a)

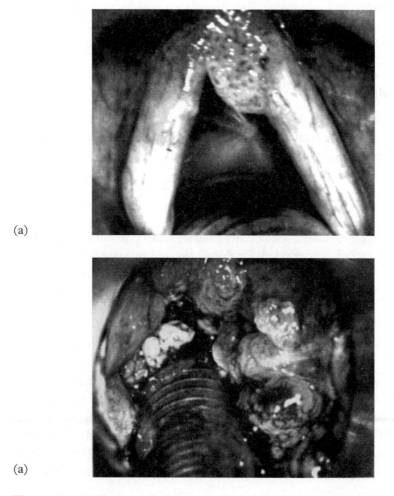

(a)

Figure 11.4 (a) Early papillomatosis involving the right vocal fold and anterior commissure (b) Advanced papillomatosis.

because of their clinical performance (Bone, 1986). Single papilloma occurs more frequently in adults and is rare in children.

The depressing feature of papillomatosis is that, despite the several forms of treatment practised, there is rarely a cure and recurrences occur at frequent intervals in childhood, and often after long intervals of remission in adulthood. It must be regarded as a potentially life-long condition (Brondbo, Alberti and Crowson, 1983). The efficacy of treatment can be judged only by immediate dispersal of papilloma, but long-term follow-up is required in assessment of real curative therapy. Some treatments seem to achieve longer intervals of remission than others. Varying degrees of hoarseness are present whenever the vocal folds are involved. In many cases, there is also a pattern of vocal abuse that arises as the individual attempts to increase the loudness and carrying power of the affected voice.

Treatment of papilloma

Numerous treatment procedures have been tried in an attempt to remove the papillomas efficiently while, if possible, reducing the recurrence rate. Methods include CO_2 laser surgery, ultrasonography, cryosurgery, hormones, steroids, antibiotics, chemotherapy, forceps removal, cauterization and vaccine (Robbins and Howard, 1983; Abramson, Steinberg and Winkler, 1987). Papilloma does not become malignant at any stage, although this was thought possible at one time. It was found, however, that irradiation of the larynx to disperse the growths of childhood led to later malignant degeneration (Rabbett, 1965; Vermeuling, 1966) or to damage of the laryngeal cartilages. Cauterisation is rejected on the grounds that it can cause scarring and stricture of the vocal folds (Abramson, Steinberg and Winkler, 1987).

- Surgery: in children the primary concern is to preserve the respiratory airway from obstruction (Holinger, 1959). Holinger, Schild and Mauriz (1968) advocated forceps removal and no tracheostomy, which presents problems with wearing the cannula and renders the child susceptible to respiratory infections and bronchitis. On the other hand, persistent recurrences cause anxiety about sudden onset of dyspnoea. Forceps removal also endangers the surfaces of the vocal folds and adjacent laryngeal structures.
- Laser surgery: laser surgery (Andrews and Moss, 1974) has been found to be more successful than excision, in that it provides longer periods of remission (Brondbo, Alberti and Crowson, 1983). There are some hazards attendant upon laser surgery because it requires considerable expertise to achieve the burn quickly and precisely

without damaging healthy tissue. However, there is no bleeding and immediate coagulation occurs, so that logopaedic intervention can start a day after surgery (Sorensen, 1982). Laser surgery is the preferred treatment for adults but, in childhood, excision may be preferred depending on the laryngologist's assessment.

Whatever surgical procedure is used, it is likely that it will be necessary to perform it on many occasions because of the frequent recurrence of the papillomatosis. In very rare cases of great severity, in which obstruction of the airway is a major problem, laryngectomy may be necessary. Robbins and Howard (1983) record that, of 63 patients aged over 24 years with papillomatosis, two were treated with laryngectomy because of severe disease.

- Drug therapy: the most encouraging development in treatment of papillomatosis of the larynx has been the administration of leukocyte interferon therapy. Haghund, Lundquist and Cantrell (1981) noted regression of plantar warts in a woman being treated with interferon for cervical cancer and carried out a study of seven patients with laryngeal papilloma. A further study was carried out by Bornholt (1983), which confirmed temporary regression of the growths. As Bone (1986) points out in his concise and valuable review of papillomatosis, the palliative effect of interferon appears to work only while the substance is being administered. This and the fact that interferon is exceedingly expensive means that the treatment cannot be generally applied as yet. Interferon was discovered by Alick Isaacs and Jean Lindenmann in Oxford in 1957. It is known to be effective against many viral diseases, including hepatitis B, and it arrests growth of malignant cells. It does not have the toxic side effects of chemotherapy.

- Voice therapy: hoarseness is the first sign of papilloma recurrence and may remain a problem after successful removal and arrest of neoplasm. The efficacy of remediation procedures depends on the existing surface structure of the vocal folds, and the correction of misuse arising out of the recurring periods of laryngeal obstruction and hoarseness. The efficacy of voice therapy for children who have papilloma of the larynx is not generally recognised. Boone (1977) stated categorically that such cases were not candidates for therapy for hyperfunction, a view that is omitted, however, in subsequent editions. Cooper (1971), on the other hand, is of the opinion that vocal rehabilitation can reduce or even eliminate papillomas. In a study of eight cases of biopsied papilloma, four of five who cooperated in treatment improved. Three who refused treatment made no improvement. Vocal abuse may well act as an irritant and help the spread of papilloma. Rabbett (1965) drew attention to the need to cure infections and to restore the larynx to health quickly, because this renders the mucosa less susceptible to invasion by viruses. Taking into account the resemblance that papillomas bear to warts, which are known to be contagious and prone to spread from one site to another, it seems plausible that hyperfunctional laryngitis and vocal abuse might promote the spread of papillomas in the larynx. Papillomas also resemble warts in their tendency to reduce or resolve spontaneously in some cases, possibly as the result of suggestion.

Case histories

Child W

A case confirming Cooper's view that speech therapy can reduce or even eliminate papillomas in children was encountered by Greene in Auckland. She was asked to examine a boy aged 9 years who had become hoarse and in whom papillomas had been diagnosed. He was under periodic review by the laryngologist and dreaded his visits and feared an operation. The speech therapist in charge wanted to know whether voice therapy was advisable because his voice production was very strained. She had told mother and child of the visiting therapist from England and they were impressed, especially the child who thought she must have royal connections. With an authoritative manner, the need for quiet speech and no shouting was emphasised. The importance of relaxation and adequate breath support during phonation was made clear. A happy and much less anxious boy and mother departed for home. Two weeks later, the speech therapist telephoned Greene in Dunedin to say that the laryngologist had seen the boy again and had been amazed to find that the clusters of papillomas were reduced in number and much smaller. He sent a message to the effect that the 'Queen's representative' must be congratulated on the 'magic' that she had worked. Suggestion and careful compliance with vocal hygiene advice appear to have influenced the improvement.

Mr F (67 years)

This patient had had laryngeal papillomatosis for many years and had undergone various procedures for removal of the papillomas. Eventually he had undergone successful laser surgery, which left only a small 'tag' of papillomatous tissue in the anterior commissure. The laryngologist referred Mr F for voice therapy in

(contd)

order to improve vocal efficiency and the patient's awareness of vocal hygiene and conservation.

Mr F was a cheerful and sociable person who talked incessantly in the clinic. His wife had died a year earlier; it had been a very happy marriage and he missed her company acutely. There were no children and he lived alone with his dog. His philosophy was that no one liked a miserable person and so he made great efforts to be cheerful and friendly. He had established a circle of acquaintances at his local pub, acted as a good neighbour to a number of people he regarded as less fortunate than himself, and went for long walks with his dog. His voice was inappropriately high-pitched and its production was obviously effortful, with visible tension of the external laryngeal muscles and a markedly raised larynx. Breathing was clavicular with noisy intake. Although listeners supposed that phonation must cause discomfort he was adamant that this was not so.

Mr F was not particularly concerned about his dysphonia but was prepared to cooperate with therapy because his surgeon, in whom he had great faith, had thought the referral was necessary. The therapeutic approach was based on helping the patient to have insight into his present method of voice production and why this might exacerbate laryngeal dysfunction, in addition to outlining ways of conserving the voice. The problem of the raised fundamental frequency was tackled early in treatment with a combination of relaxation and a firm, but gentle, cough to establish the natural pitch. The effects of grieving were gradually discussed when the occasion was appropriate. The responses of the vocal tract when the individual is under some stress but remaining stoical were also explained in relation to phonation.

Mr F responded positively to treatment, although he found it difficult to talk less when he had the opportunity to be with other people. Pitch gradually became more appropriate and phonation was less effortful. Initially, he attended for weekly treatments which were reduced over a period of 9 months as the voice improved. At this time, he was discharged when the laryngologist pronounced satisfaction with the larynx. There was no sign of inflammation and the voice was satisfactory although it remained breathy.

Laryngeal cysts

Cysts of the vocal folds are usually unilateral, although they can be multi-focal and bilateral (Figure 11.5). They arise from the superficial layer of the lamina propria, with some appearing to be congenital and others the result of vocal fold trauma. Almost all are retention cysts and develop secondary

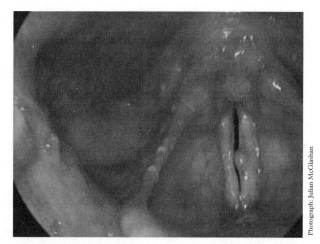

Photograph: Julian McGlashan

Figure 11.5 Epidermoid cyst.

Case notes

- A 10-year-old boy was diagnosed as having bilateral vocal fold nodules which were located in the classic position. After a course of voice therapy and careful compliance with advice regarding voice conservation and vocal hygiene, his voice improved. On re-examination with videostroboscopy, the right vocal fold nodule had resolved and the left nodule was reduced. Careful observation of the mucosal wave on the left fold revealed a submucosal cyst. The right 'nodule' had been the result of trauma to the contralateral vocal fold by the cyst.

- A woman of 45 years developed hoarseness and an anxiety state after the sudden enlargement of a cyst which obstructed breathing. Following its removal, she began to have difficulty with breathing on exertion after discharge from hospital, and then an inspiratory stridor developed in speech. She was given relaxation and diaphragmatic breathing exercises and was treated as a case of anxiety state and hyperventilation because there was no impairment of the vocal fold movements. Delay in being admitted into hospital for surgery and the subsequent delay in obtaining voice therapy had upset her.

- When a laryngeal cyst occurs in the posterior portion of the vocal fold, it may immobilise the vocal fold if it involves the arytenoid cartilage. As a result of the fixed cartilage being unable to rotate, a diagnosis of unilateral vocal fold paralysis may be made incorrectly. Laryngostroboscopy may be the only method of confirming the correct diagnosis as is described in the case in Chapter 15 (re changed diagnoses).

to degenerative processes in the ductal system of the mucous gland network. On videostroboscopy, the mucosal wave is reduced or absent over the site of the cyst. The voice is breathy if the cyst is sufficiently large to affect vocal fold adduction, but the quality of the vocal note is affected initially because the mucosal waves are out of phase, causing a rough vocal note or the inability to sing notes of a particular pitch. Treatment consists of aspirating the fluid from the cyst or surgical removal. The voice is usually dramatically improved postoperatively, but a short course of voice therapy is important in order to reduce hyperfunctional patterns that might have developed, and to re-establish efficient phonation.

Cysts also occur on the false vocal folds, most frequently in individuals over 50–60 years of age (Kleinsasser, 1968). They may hang from the inlet to the ventricle and obstruct the airway or may be situated deep within the false vocal fold; they are not painful. Although the removal of cysts on the false folds and ventricle should not disturb the voice, cases of dysphonia are sometimes referred for speech therapy postoperatively. Lymphatic cysts also occur on the free edges of the aryepiglottic folds and epiglottis, but are generally so small that they need not be removed.

Respiratory conditions

All speech–breathing requirements are met at a metabolic cost (Orlikoff, 1994), because they are in competition with the body's respiratory needs. Consequently, when lung function is compromised the voice is affected adversely because the process of ventilation takes priority. Respiratory disease can influence the speed and volume of inspiration and expiration, so that both the sound of the voice and the timing of phonation are affected. Adequate subglottic air pressure, appropriately controlled, is essential for a stable vocal note and for increasing and maintaining loudness. When it is compromised, therefore, loudness and stability of the voice become difficult to initiate and maintain. Reduced respiratory efficiency affects not only the sound of the voice but also the length of time for which voice can be sustained. Consequently, phrase length is reduced and the pauses between phrases might lengthen. In some cases, the speaker becomes increasingly breathless and fatigued as the attempt to maintain speech breathing competes with the process of gaseous exchange in the lungs (Table 11.7).

Respiratory conditions can be divided into those that are obstructive (such as asthma) and those that are restrictive (e.g. sarcoidosis) (see page 354). Conditions such as bronchitis, emphysema, carcinoma of the lung and chronic obstructive airway disease can all affect speech–breathing and the degree to which the voice is affected will reflect the severity of the disease.

Table 11.7 Effects of respiratory disease on phonation

- Breathlessness while speaking
- Reduced phrase length
- Reduced maximum phonation time
- Reduced inspiratory volume
- Reduced expiratory volume
- Reduced duration of breath cycle (i.e. inspiration/expiration)
- Increased speech rate
- Increased length of pauses between phrases
- Increased jitter and shimmer measures
- Reduced subglottic air pressure
- Reduced vocal loudness

Each of the vocal features listed in the table is the direct result of the need to replenish the breath supply because of the inefficiency of the diseased respiratory system. The reduced inspiratory volume means that the speaker cannot prolong the expiratory airflow required for speech. As a result phrase length is reduced and the speaker becomes breathless in an attempt quickly to replenish air repeatedly. There is a tendency to accelerate speech rate while trying to say as much as possible before the expiratory airflow fails but pauses between phrases lengthen as the speaker tries to meet the body's need for oxygen.

In general, it is not appropriate to treat the vocal deficiencies arising from severe respiratory disease alone by voice therapy, but in some instances voice disorders coexist with these conditions or the disease predisposes the patient to hyperfunctional phonation which requires treatment.

ASTHMA

When a patient with a clinical voice disorder also has asthma, the speech and language therapist encounters a number of related factors that will affect the progress of treatment. Asthma is a reversible obstructive airway disease that affects 5% of the adult population, but which can occur for the first time at any age. Its peak incidence is in young children in whom it is probably underdiagnosed (Johnson, 1990). There are three factors that contribute to airway obstruction in asthma:

- bronchial smooth muscle spasm
- bronchial wall oedema and inflammation
- increased mucus production.

As a result, airflow and vital capacity are reduced. The symptoms can be worse at certain times of the day and some individuals will have episodes of a severity that constitutes an asthma attack. The respiratory distress is accompanied in some cases by such forceful coughing that the vocal fold mucosa is traumatised. Common symptoms of asthma include:

- episodic shortness of breath
- audible wheezing
- coughing
- increased mucus production.

Voice changes associated with asthma can be directly related to the physical changes in the respiratory tract, but it should be remembered that most sufferers will be taking medication, which in itself can affect various aspects of the voice (see below). When chronic asthma becomes established, the airways become fibrotic and scarred and the condition does not respond to medication. Although asthma and asthma medication can be the primary causes of a voice problem, they can also be important contributory factors when someone with asthma develops a voice disorder for other reasons. Asthma itself reduces air volume and air pressure available for phonation whereas asthma medication may have a direct effect on the vocal folds. Table 11.8 shows the possible effects on the voice that can occur as the direct result of asthma.

Treatment of the condition is directed at dilating the airway with bronchodilators (agents that cause dilatation of the passages of the bronchial tree and relieve bronchospasm) and reducing inflammation by use of inhaled steroids. It is now recognised that the metered-dose administration by pressurised aerosol of inhaled corticosteroids causes local side effects and is associated with a high percentage of voice and throat symptoms after prolonged use (Watkin and Ewanowski, 1985). These are the result of changes in both vocal fold muscle and mucosa. The severity of these changes

Table 11.8 Asthma: potential effects on voice

Airway obstruction → (as a result of bronchial spasm oedema and inflammation, increased airway secretions)	Reduced vital capacity and airflow →	• Reduced subglottal airflow • Phonation on residual air • Reduced loudness potential	Hyperfunctional phonation
Oedema and inflammation →	Increased vocal fold mass →	Reduced SFo Reduced harmonics-to noise-ratio	
Increased airway secretions →	Mucus pooling in laryngeal area →	'Wet' voice/'frog in the throat'	

In a study by Lee et al. (1988), it was found that, although asthmatic speakers could meet the sound level requirements of loud counting and could generally produce speech segment durations similar to healthy subjects, they increased the pause time between speech segments, produced fewer syllables per breath and spent a larger percentage of time on non-speech breathing than the healthy subjects.

appears to depend partly on the pattern of deposition of the inhaled particles of the medication in the mouth and throat. Variations in the deposition
have been found to be the result of deviations in pharyngeal configuration
while inhaling. (This suggests that, as pharyngeal dimensions can be varied
to a degree, despite anatomical limitations, inhalation efficiency has the
potential to be improved.) Prolonged use of corticosteroids can cause
steroid myopathy, and consequently reduce the efficiency of vocal fold
approximation, as well as give rise to changes in the vocal fold mucosa. In a
study in which healthy subjects inhaled beclomethasone dipropionate, there
was an objective rise in speaking fundamental frequency within hours of the
substance being inhaled (Clarke et al., 1992). This suggests a reduction in
the mass of the vocal fold mucosa.

This study reflects the findings of Goldberg and Kovarsky (1983)
who described a reduction in vocal fold oedema in patients with rheumatoid disease when they used inhaled steroids. Frequent use of corticosteroids also renders the individual susceptible to oropharyngeal
candidiasis (see page 338). Use of a large-volume spacer does not appear
to reduce the laryngeal effects of inhaled steroids but a Turboinhaler can
be helpful. (A large volume spacer is an extension tube for a metered-dose
inhaler consisting of a plastic chamber, which allows small particles of
inhalant to stay in suspension and evaporation of the propellant so that
more particles of a respirable size are produced.) It is extremely important
that the mouth should be rinsed with water after use of the inhaler in order
to reduce the amount of excess inhalant lying in the vocal tract. Table
11.9 shows the potential effects of asthma medication on the voice. Voice
problems in individuals with asthma can be the result of a combination
of the effects of the asthma and the medication, as well as any other
coexisting vocal pathology.

Table 11.9 Asthma medication: potential effects on voice

Steroid myopathy →	Glottal insufficiency →	Breathiness Roughness
Vocal fold mucosa changes →	Reduction in mass (as a result of inhaled steroids) →	Increased SFo
Candidiasis →	Laryngitis	

Although inhaled steroids can reduce the mass of the vocal fold mucosa, the mucosa of the vocal tract
may be oedematous and therefore increased in mass in patients with asthma.
Asthma may coexist with functional airway obstruction (FAO) or be misdiagnosed in cases of FAO (see
Chapter 8).

Systemic conditions

AUTOIMMUNE DISEASES

Autoimmune diseases are those in which the body's aberrant immune response results in inflammation and destruction of the individual's own tissue. They develop when the regulatory systems, which normally prevent the body from reacting to its own antigens, break down. The conditions described in this section are those autoimmune diseases that frequently have head and neck manifestations. Many of these conditions are not common within the general population, but voice changes occur in a significant number of individuals with autoimmune diseases. Table 11.10 lists the laryngeal manifestations of various autoimmune diseases.

Laryngeal rheumatoid arthritis

Pathology

Rheumatoid arthritis can affect all organs and connective tissue throughout the body. The most common form affects articulating structures (joints),

Table 11.10 Laryngeal manifestations of various autoimmune diseases

Disease	Laryngeal manifestations
Rheumatoid arthritis	Cricoarytenoid arthritis Rheumatoid nodules of vocal folds Laryngeal myositis Vocal fold paralysis (ischaemic recurrent laryngeal nerve paralysis)
Systemic lupus erythematosus (SLE)	Epiglottitis Laryngitis Cricoarytenoid arthritis Sicca syndrome (also tracheitis)
Sjögren's syndrome	Laryngitis/tracheitis sicca (dryness)
Scleroderma	Voice changes of uncertain origin
Vasculitis	One type of vasculitis, Wegener's granulomatosis, is associated with ulcers, erosions and stenosis of larynx and trachea in 25% of patients presenting with the condition
Relapsing polychondritis	Collapse of laryngeal and tracheal cartilages
Sarcoidosis[a]	Oedema/thickening of epiglottis, aryepiglottic folds and arytenoids Granulomas, particularly in subglottis Vocal fold thickening anteriorly

[a]The pathogenesis of sarcoidosis is unclear but there appears to be a response by the body to an unknown stimulus. Therefore, it is possibly an autoimmune disease (Campbell, Montanaro and Bardana, 1983; Gallivan and Landis, 1993).

but it can also cause inflammatory changes in ligaments, tendons and fascia (Campbell, Montanaro and Bardana, 1983). When the cricoarytenoid joint is affected, aphonia or dysphonia occurs according to the degree of immobility imposed upon the vocal folds. Traditionally, it has been considered a comparatively rare condition, with various studies suggesting clinical signs of arthritis on laryngoscopy being found in 17–33% of patients with rheumatoid arthritis. Later studies, using low-voltage radiotherapy, reveal that 45% of patients with rheumatoid arthritis have erosions and destructive changes of the cricoarytenoid joints (Jurik, Pedersen and Norgard, 1985). Severity of symptoms varies; a 'flare-up' of symptoms can occur, especially with a respiratory infection, and subside spontaneously (Wolman, Dorke and Young, 1965). Mumps and gonorrhoea are also known to affect the cricoarytenoid joint and traumatic cricoarytenoid arthritis has been recorded.

Laryngoscopic findings

In the early stages of invasion of the larynx by the disease, there is acute local inflammation and extraordinary pain upon phonation. Great difficulty is experienced in moving the folds and there is pronounced hoarseness. Laryngeal stridor may also occur. During the acute stage, there is red swelling over the arytenoids, but the vocal folds may appear normal or only slightly oedematous. The throat feels tight and painful in swallowing, coughing and speaking, and there may be acute pain radiating up to the ear (Montgomery, 1963). Other effects of rheumatoid arthritis in the larynx include rheumatoid nodules within the vocal folds, laryngeal polymyositis and recurrent laryngeal nerve paralysis as a result of ischaemia.

In a small proportion of cases, however, total fusion of the cricoarytenoid joint (ankylosis) takes place, in which case there is no chance of recovery. The position of the vocal fold in unilateral ankylosis of the arytenoid joint resembles that of the abductor paralysis of the recurrent laryngeal nerve with the fold fixed in the paramedian position (see page 313). Occasionally, it is held in a position of extreme abduction by the fibrous bands which form through arthritic changes in the arytenoid joint.

Case note

Williams, Farquharson and Anthony (1975) described a patient with generalised rheumatoid arthritis who developed hoarseness but whose larynx was pronounced normal when examined by indirect and direct laryngoscopy. Stroboscopic nasendoscopy showed that the larynx was injected, although minimally. The folds moved abnormally in phonation with unequal and non-synchronous vibrations, confirming that this was not a psychogenic disorder.

Expected vocal profile

When vocal fold mobility is poor, the voice is hoarse and breathy because of glottal insufficiency. The harmonics-to-noise ratio is reduced and vocal intensity cannot be increased, because loss of air at the glottis prevents the necessary increase in subglottal air pressure.

Medicosurgical decisions

Medical

The principal treatment is medical, directed at alleviating the arthritic disease, which can be widespread throughout the individual's system before the larynx becomes involved. Steroid injection into the cricoarytenoid joint to relieve acute inflammation may be prescribed and may have good results (Habib, 1977). Local short-wave diathermy may also be helpful. Aspirin reduces pain and inflammation as well as gentle massage with a soothing embrocation (Aronson, 1980).

Surgical

When compensation by the opposite fold is impossible, surgical medialisation of the fixed vocal fold can be carried out. The most common form of laryngeal arthritis is, however, bilateral with both folds immobilised in the midline. If there is difficulty in breathing, a tracheotomy will be performed. If the condition is not alleviated by medication and both folds remain permanently fixed in the midline, a surgical or laser arytenoidectomy can be considered. An operation may not be feasible if the patient is elderly and fragile. A tracheostomy and use of a 'speaking valve' tracheostomy tube will be the preferred choice of the medical adviser in such cases.

Voice therapy

As the acute stage of the arthritis subsides and normal movement is again possible, voice therapy may be helpful in some cases. The importance of gentle onset of phonation and adequate breath support should be emphasised. Over-exertion should be avoided because this can aggravate any remaining inflammation, although discomfort monitors vocal behaviour. The value of voice therapy after surgery is debatable, because the fold not operated on remains immobile, but appropriate advice to ensure optimum voice can be helpful.

Case note

A female patient's voice was severely hoarse following a brief attack of arthritis of the larynx, which rendered adduction of the folds difficult; she quickly developed a normal voice through the practice of voice exercises. Movement of the folds was stimulated by attempting their rapid adduction and abduction in quick succession. The patient was instructed to 'drink' a gulp of cold air to obtain full abduction and then to shout a vowel to promote full adduction. Relaxation and diaphragmatic breathing exercises were necessary preliminaries.

Systemic lupus erythematosus

Systemic lupus erythematosus (SLE) is an autoimmune multi-system disease, the onset of which is associated particularly with young women between the ages of 15 and 25 years. The prevalence in all women is 1 in 700, but in the general population it is 1 in 2000 (Campbell, Montanaro and Bardana, 1983). Head and neck manifestations of the condition are seen in the face, oral mucosa, nasal septum and upper respiratory tract, in the form of eruptions, ulcers and perforations. Cranial neuropathies and gland enlargement also occur. The larynx is involved in approximately one-third of patients with the condition, resulting in varying degrees of hoarseness and dyspnoea (Teitel et al., 1992).There are indications that laryngeal symptoms can be the first sign that SLE is worsening. Teitel et al. (1992) concluded from a review of the literature that laryngeal involvement in SLE can be divided into nine overlapping categories:

1. **Mucosal inflammation**: the most common clinical findings are oral ulceration, erythema and oedema. As expected, smoking, excessive alcohol intake and gastric reflux will exacerbate these symptoms and might confuse the diagnosis.
2. **Infection.**
3. **Vasculitis.**
4. **Vocal fold immobility**: as a result of inflammatory changes in the cricoarytenoid joint, movement of the arytenoid cartilage can become restricted and mobility of the affected vocal fold is reduced. Clinical studies show that, in many cases, recovery of movement follows corticosteroid therapy.
5. **Cricoarytenoid arthritis**: the diagnostic test for cricoarytenoid arthritis is medial compression of the thyroid cartilage. The ankylosed

      cricoarytenoid joint remains immobile when the larynx is com-
pressed but, in other conditions, such as vocal fold paralysis, the
affected cord is temporarily medialised by the compression.

6.   **Subglottic stenosis**: granulomatous inflammation in the subglottis
causes stenosis of the airway.

7.   **Inflammatory laryngeal mass**.

8.   **Rheumatoid nodules**: nodular formation on the vocal folds is seen
in 5% of patients with SLE, usually in association with rheumatoid-
like changes in the joints.

9.   **Epiglottitis**: inflammatory changes in the epiglottis can cause
serious airway obstruction and are potentially life threatening.

Relapsing polychondritis

Relapsing polychondritis is a rare condition in which inflammatory changes
in the cartilages of the ear, nose and airway eventually lead to the collapse
of these structures (Bachynski and Vyas, 1976; Casselman et al., 1988;
Crockford and Kerr, 1988). These patients, therefore, frequently present
initially to the otolaryngologist. The destruction and subsequent collapse of
the upper respiratory tract cause hoarseness and airway obstruction. The
larynx is involved in more than 50% of cases, with laryngeal stenosis occurring even with steroids (Teitel et al., 1992). Painful swelling of the pinnae
of the ear is the most common presenting symptom, followed by middle- and
inner-ear involvement resulting in hearing loss and vertigo. Subsequently,
saddle deformity of the nose occurs as the septum collapses. Voice changes
are the result of the laryngeal cartilages being affected and the laryngeal
mucosa becoming red and swollen, sometimes in conjunction with hypertro-
phied false vocal folds. The larynx is frequently tender (Moloney, 1978). As
the condition progresses and the thyroid cartilage collapses and flattens, the
anteroposterior dimension of the larynx shortens. The vocal folds are consequently also shortened and adduction of the relatively flaccid folds is inefficient. As a result, speaking fundamental pitch is reduced and the voice is
breathy. The condition is potentially life threatening and intervention such as
biopsy or tracheotomy can exacerbate the airway changes.

Sarcoidosis

The pathogenesis of this multisystem granulomatous condition is unclear and
it is possible that the immunological features are secondary rather than primary
phenomena (Gallivan and Landis, 1993). It involves the larynx in about 5% of
cases, with the supraglottic laryngeal region being most commonly involved,
causing hypertrophy of the false vocal folds. The degree to which the larynx is
involved tends to be proportional to the extent of the systemic disease, with

granuloma formation, although rare in the larynx, causing hoarseness, dyspnoea and dysphagia. The typical laryngeal appearance of sarcoidosis is turban-
like, oedematous, pale pink, enlarged epiglottis, aryepiglottic folds and
arytenoid areas, with relatively normal vocal folds (Gallivan and Landis,
1993). This formation imparts a 'honking' voice quality which can be recognised as the presenting sign. Treatment consists of systemic corticosteroid
therapy but surgery may be required to ensure a patent airway.

Sjögren's syndrome

The classic definition of Sjögren's syndrome is the triad of xerophthalmia
(dry eyes), xerostomia (dry mouth) and an autoimmune disease, usually
rheumatoid arthritis. Laryngeal dryness can affect the vocal fold mucosal
wave with resulting hoarseness or lowered vocal pitch. Treatment is
primarily directed at the underlying autoimmune disease, but the use of
artificial saliva might be helpful symptomatic treatment.

SYSTEMIC INFECTION

Tuberculosis of the larynx (phthisis laryngea)

This is a secondary complication of advanced pulmonary infection.
Tuberculosis (TB) is highly infectious especially among children, but it is
relatively uncommon in affluent societies as a result of improved health
and living conditions and treatment with antibiotics. In recent years, however, there has been a resurgence of respiratory tuberculosis in elderly
people aged over 65 years and we have had two patients referred with a
diagnosis of laryngitis attributed initially to vocal misuse. Further tests led
to a correct diagnosis.

Travis, Hybels and Newman (1976) reported 13 cases of TB over a
period of 15 years. They warn that initial infiltration of the laryngeal
mucosa can be misleading and mistaken for chronic laryngitis. An early
report of the initial symptoms and progress of this laryngeal disease is of
interest because, in areas of the world deficient in medical services,
untreated phthisis laryngea is not a rarity. Smurthwaite (1919) noted that,
in the early stages of infiltration, an adductor paralysis (myopathic paresis) may appear before any positive signs of inflammation are visible, and
that asthenic voice may be incorrectly diagnosed as an 'hysterical' disorder with bowing of the vocal folds (see page 200). If infection progresses,
ulceration of the fold can develop, but anti-tuberculous chemotherapy
results in a rapid improvement in the laryngeal condition (Ballantyne and
Groves, 1982). Complete vocal rest is essential and this must be strictly
observed. Scarring and irregularity of the folds may occur during healing,

with resultant impairment of the voice dependent on the degree and site of the damage. Thickening of the mucous membrane cover of the vocal folds may remain along their length or in the arytenoid region. The voice is characteristically deep and husky with a rather hollow tone (Turner, 1952).

Case note

A female patient of 60 years was referred for speech therapy after treatment and cure of tuberculosis. She had developed considerable anxiety over her health and economic situation, besides tension in trying to obtain a louder voice. She responded well to relaxation, breathing exercises, hearing training and raising the vocal pitch.

Another patient had recovered from TB some years previously and had not been anxious about her impaired voice until domestic difficulties produced a functional aphonia. Vocal exercises and discussion of her difficulties brought her voice back. She said it improved in clarity and strength during treatment and was better than it had been since her tubercular illness.

In neither of these cases did the huskiness and 'veiling' of the voice disappear completely, because permanent changes and thickening of the vocal fold mucosa had taken place.

Syphilitic inflammation and ulceration of the larynx

Syphilis of the larynx may occur as a congenital infection or as an acquired condition, secondary to primary infection. The disease may produce acute inflammation of the larynx with similar involvement of the pharynx and, in advanced stages of the disease, ulceration occurs. The symptom of hoarseness is a prominent feature of syphilitic laryngitis; the voice is strong with a distinctive rough quality and generally causes no discomfort (Turner, 1952). In the early stages, the intractable laryngitis and pharyngitis can easily be mistaken for a simple infection. In very advanced stages, the formation of syphilomas may resemble cancerous tumours. Ballantyne and Groves (1982) noted that syphilis can mimic all other laryngeal diseases and for this reason may cause diagnostic problems. Accurate diagnosis depends on a positive Wasserman reaction being obtained from a test of the patient's serum, but in a small proportion of cases in the tertiary stages of syphilis a positive reaction is not obtained. Scarring of the vocal folds after ulceration is generally severe and may cause stenosis of the larynx and breathing difficulty (dyspnoea). Treatment must obviously be directed to cure of the disease, and only after this has been achieved and the laryngeal symptoms alleviated can any attempt at improvement of the voice be undertaken. The patient can then be helped to develop vocal potential. Prognosis is unfavourable unless cicatricial tissue is minimal or can be removed surgically, so that the vocal folds present even edges in adduction.

ENDOCRINOLOGICAL CONDITIONS

The endocrine glands secrete hormones that regulate bodily growth, development of sexual and reproductive functions, and the emotional stability of the individual. The chief endocrine glands controlling normal development and relating to normal voice are the thyroid, ovaries and testes. The mutual interdependence of the various endocrine glands is complex and only the voice disorders that are predominantly related to particular hormonal systems are described in this section.

Endocrine dysphonia in males

Development of male characteristics is dependent on the release of male hormones during puberty. The growth of facial and pubic hair and of the larynx may be delayed by several years in 'late developers'. The youth then retains a boy's voice while growing in normal bodily dimensions. In many cases, normal development of masculine maturity without recourse to hormone treatment takes place (Luchsinger and Arnold, 1965). Significant gonadal failure results in the absence of the secondary sexual characteristics with the pre-pubertal voice being maintained. Trauma and disease are both causes of reduced testosterone secretion. Damage to the testes before puberty can cause atrophy and prevent development of male sexual features altogether, but accidents involving the testes are rare. Tuberculosis is also a comparatively rare cause, although tumours of the testes are less rare, representing the second most common form of malignancy in young males.

Evaluation and treatment by an endocrinologist are essential when secondary sexual characteristics fail to develop.

It is doubtful whether voice therapy directed at lowering the pitch of the voice can produce a marked change in cases where insufficient androgens are being secreted. Isshiki (1980) suggests a thyroplasty under local anaesthetic, suitable for a female-to-male sex change. This may be suitable for physically determined puberphonia. The anteroposterior distance of the thyroid ala is reduced by excision of a vertical rectangular slice of cartilage. Excision on one side may be sufficient. The vocal fold is shortened by this procedure and relaxation and bunching of muscle take place as the thyroid angle is moved backwards.

Historical note

Chaucer's Pardoner in the Canterbury Tales is a classic example of this condition, although we have no information regarding aetiology except that he had strong connections with Rome:

> A voys he hadde as small as hath a goot
> No berd hadde he, ne never sholde have
> As smothe it was as it were late y-shave.

The connection between the testes and male sexuality has been recognised throughout the ages. Castration of male children was practised in the Orient in order to provide impotent domestic staff for harems. In the seventeenth and eighteenth centuries, the practice of castration was an accepted social and cultural procedure in order to satisfy the demand for the admired 'castrati' singers. The Vatican choir, not allowing female singers, engaged castrati singers as late as the nineteenth century until Pope Leo XIII (1878–1903) banned them (Luchsinger and Arnold, 1965). Moses (1960) draws attention to the fact that early castration resulted in abnormal growth of the long bones as a characteristic: the individual grows tall and thin. This is clearly displayed in the paintings of Farinelli (1705–1782), a famous castrato singer who was renowned throughout Europe for his marvellous voice and brilliant technique. He settled in Spain for 25 years, gaining great political power at court through his employment by the Queen to sing every night to Philip V to cure him of melancholy madness. Farinelli utilised his ascendancy to establish Italian opera in Madrid.

Female endocrine dysphonia

The female endocrine system controls the reproductive system, initiating puberty and the menstrual cycle, and maintaining pregnancies. The reproductive glands finally reduce and cease activity at the menopause.

Menstruation

At the onset of menstruation, vocal changes can occur as a result of congestion and reduced tonicity of the vocal folds. Oedematous changes result in a slightly lowered speaking fundamental frequency and reduced pitch range, in conjunction with a breathy vocal note. The vocal folds are more vulnerable to the effects of vocal misuse at this time and effortful singing, acting, shouting and cheering can exacerbate vocal problems. A deterioration in the voice and huskiness may recur every month with the vocal folds exhibiting hyperaemia, oedema and, in some cases, haemorrhage

(Van Gelder, 1974). It is advisable, therefore, for women to avoid taking aspirin premenstrually unless there are medical reasons for its prescription. There is some objective evidence of similarities between histological changes in the mucosa of the larynx and the cervix during the menstrual cycle (Abitbol et al., 1989). Oestrogen stimulation causes a thickening of the superficial epithelium of the vocal folds whereas progesterone stimulation develops the intermediate layer of the lamina propria. Abitbol et al. (1989) point out that the degree of water retention, oedema of the interstitial tissue and venous dilatation is the result of the ratio of oestrogen to progesterone. These vocal changes do not occur in all women and, even when they do, they are not a significant problem. For the actor or singer, however, the vocal limitation and unpredictability can cause performance difficulties. For this reason, some professional singers have a clause in their contracts excluding performance during the premenstrual period.

Pregnancy

During pregnancy the voice can also be affected by the influence of hormones on the larynx. Tarneaud (1961) claimed that these symptoms during menstruation and pregnancy cease after childbirth. Flach, Schwickardi and Simon (1969) reported assessment of 136 professional singers among whom 80 were engaged to sing large operatic parts. Their voices all deteriorated in the premenstrual and menstrual period. Two-thirds of the singers experienced vocal deterioration when they became pregnant, and in a quarter of these cases the voice change persisted after delivery. In addition to the hormonal changes that accompany pregnancy, the increasing size of the fetus as pregnancy progresses obstructs the descent of the diaphragm on inspiration. As a result, capacity and control of speech breathing are reduced. It also becomes impossible to brace the abdominal wall in order to provide additional support to the expiratory airstream. The combined effects of the hormonal and mechanical changes during pregnancy usually severely restricts the capacity of the professional singer.

Sexual excitement

Sexual excitement can evoke vocal change and the 'sexy voice' may be related to the fact that the recurrent laryngeal nerves contain both sympathetic and parasympathetic fibres (Rethi, 1963).

Menopause

At the menopause, cyclical menstruation ceases as a result of the reduction in the secretion of female hormones by the ovaries. Postmenopausally, androgens (male hormones) are secreted by the ovaries and the adrenal cortex. The lack of oestrogens and relative excess of androgens result in the vocal folds becoming oedematous, so that the voice may become noticeably deeper and hoarse. Changes in the voice are often accompanied by vaso-motor rhinitis. It is a time of life when the middle-aged woman may feel unwell, irritable and excessively tired with a tendency to nervousness and depression. The most troublesome symptom is the 'hot flush' and, at night, sweating that disturbs sleep. Women may also put on weight at this time and need to manage their diet carefully if they are to remain slim. This can be another cause of anxiety and also fatigue. Increasingly, perimenopausal and menopausal women are prescribed hormone replacement therapy (HRT) in order to counteract the range of symptoms resulting from the reduction in oestrogen secretion. Theoretically, HRT should preserve the premenopausal voice, but objective research has not yet been carried out to clarify this issue. It has to be remembered that, at the same time as the menopausal changes occur, other age-related factors that affect the voice adversely, such as the loss of elastic and collagen fibres in the lamina pro-pria, laryngeal muscle changes and reduction in vital capacity, are also taking place. It is presumed that the oestrogens in HRT help to retain the premenopausal voice, but the effects of progesterone are less predictable. There is anecdotal evidence that some progestogens might even affect the voice adversely because they have relatively high androgenic properties.

Menopausal voice changes are aggravated by excessive smoking which produces a chronic laryngitis, cough and considerable drop in vocal pitch. If the woman has to use her voice a great deal at work, the laryngeal condition may be aggravated by vocal strain. No improvement will be achieved without drastically reducing the number of cigarettes smoked each day. Women complaining of voice problems at this time need sympa-thy and support, and it may be necessary to explain to partners and adolescent children the difficulties that are being experienced.

Androphonia (virilisation of the female voice)

Hormonal treatments are used in the management of various conditions in women such as endometriosis, hormonal imbalance, fibrocystic disease, men-strual dysfunction, gynaecological carcinoma and menopausal symptoms. Synthetic derivatives of testosterone, such as androgenic progestogens (see above), are incorporated into hormonal treatments and, when they are included in prescribed drugs, various unwanted side effects can occur, includ-ing irreversible voice changes (Pattie et al., 1998). These effects have been known for several decades. In 1964, Damsté reported on six female patients with testosterone-induced dysphonia, resulting from drugs containing testosterone that had been administered by doctors who were unaware of the possible effects on the voice. These women's voices became 'unsteady', with pitch instability, before finally settling at a male pitch. Similar results were observed by Shepperd (1966) in five women whose menopausal symptoms had been treated with methyltestosterone and oestradiol for periods ranging from 6 months to 2 years. All the women developed hirsutism and deep voices. On withdrawal of the drugs, excess hair diminished but their voices remained at a low pitch. Shepperd noted that the women's voices were not hoarse, but strong and deep. There is little noise in the fundamental note in a virilised female voice, unlike that of women who smoke heavily and the low-pitched, rough vocal note caused by Reinke's oedema.

The female patient whose medication incorporates male hormones may develop male characteristics with growth of the clitoris, and hair on the face, legs and arms, as well as development of a male voice (Table 11.11). The changes in the larynx are irreversible and treatment with oestrogens (female hormones) does not lead to any improvement. Some patients, especially the younger ones, can be helped by voice therapy during which it is possible to learn to obtain a new balance between glottic tension and respiratory pressure and to use the upper vocal range.

Anabolic steroids have become notorious because of their use by sportsmen and sportswomen in order to increase muscle bulk and strength. Women who use anabolic steroids, which contain androgenic components, become increasingly masculine in appearance. Muscular hypertrophy and the development of a deep voice are common features (Van Gelder, 1974). Similar changes occur in women who are prescribed these substances in some cases of back pain and polymyalgia. The voice changes, which consist of lowering of pitch and subsequent narrowing of register, are generally regarded as irreversible (Van Gelder, 1974; Tanabe et al., 1985). However, voice quality may be considerably improved by voice therapy and by eliminating features of abuse which may have evolved.

Table 11.11 Possible androgen-related changes in women

Voice changes:
- Speaking fundamental frequency lowered
- Hoarseness
- Vocal weakness
- Pitch fluctuation before settling into male pitch

Physical changes:
- Excessive hair growth (hirsutism) on face, legs, arms, etc.
- Growth of clitoris
- Connective tissue changes

The development of male characteristics is naturally very distressing to the female patient. The phonosurgery recommended by Isshiki (1980) in connection with the myxoedematous voice may provide a solution.

Thyroid gland dysfunction

The effects of surgical trauma involving the recurrent laryngeal nerve during thyroidectomy are discussed in Chapter 10. The systemic effects of thyroid dysfunction can also involve the larynx and phonation (Ritter, 1967).

The thyroid gland, which is controlled by the anterior pituitary gland, is concerned with the maintenance of the metabolism of the body by discharging thyroxine into the blood. The regulation of all life functions, as Arnold (1962) pointed out, is dependent on the hypothalamic–pituitary–thyroid–adrenal system. Disturbance of thyroid function upsets the chemical and emotional balance of the body. As 'the thyroid hormone is primarily a stimulator of cell metabolism and as such it promotes intellectual activity and performance and increases sensitivity and alertness' (Wittkower and Mandelbrote, 1955), the physical and emotional symptoms overlap. Under-secretion causes myxoedema and excessive secretion causes thyrotoxicosis or hyperthyroidism.

Hypothyroidism

Cretinism

The congenital form of thyroid deficiency, when the normal secretion of thyroxine is diminished in children, causes physical handicap and learning difficulties known as cretinism. If recognised and treated with thyroxine early in childhood, the condition can be arrested. The cry of the baby with this condition is recognisably abnormal at birth, with a pitch conspicuously lower than normal and with constricted pitch range (Michelsson and Sirvio, 1976).

Myxoedema

Myxoedema is the disorder of metabolism that results from underactivity of the thyroid gland.

Juvenile myxoedema may arise from failure of thyroid function in childhood but this is not as serious as cretinism because normal development will have taken place in the fetus and in early childhood. The vocal folds appear oedematous and the voice is hoarse. The gradual onset of the disease may at first go unrecognised but early diagnosis and treatment are essential. A lifelong regime of thyroxine therapy has satisfactory results.

Case history

A girl aged 6 years 6 months was referred for voice therapy with a diagnosis of oedematous vocal folds and hoarseness. She was not noisy at home or school and did not get on well with other children, and at times was quarrelsome and aggressive. Her laryngeal condition did not appear to be caused by vocal strain. She was short, thick-set and overweight, slow in her movements and suffered from nasal catarrh. Her cheeks were noticeably rough. She was having reading difficulties and her IQ was estimated to be in the region of 80. She presented, in fact, the typical symptoms of hypothyroidism and was referred for investigation.

Myxoedema can also occur in normal individuals later in life. The skin becomes rough and dry and the hair thin; the individual may gain weight and become slow in movements and thought. An early sign is a slowly progressive deepening of the voice and a slight huskiness which is less conspicuous in men than in women. The vocal fold movements remain intact, but the folds increase in bulk as a result of deposits of mucopolysaccharides in the submucosa. Ritter (1967) advocated stripping the vocal folds along their edges, with the aim of reducing bulk or inducing scarring that increases tension – procedures that might jeopardise the quality of the vocal note. Isshiki (1980) also suggested various surgical procedures to improve voice, but the administration of thyroxine, and voice therapy, is the preferred course of treatment in most cases if the diagnosis is made early.

Heinemann (1969) investigated 42 cases of myxoedema and noted that, if the voice has been allowed to deteriorate substantially, administering thyroxine does not result in improved voice quality. Elderly people, particularly if living alone, may not realise or care that their health is slowly deteriorating. If there are no acute symptoms to alert them, any changes may be attributed to natural ageing.

Underactivity of the thyroid gland can cause unpleasant symptoms before there are overt signs of myxoedema. As the onset of thyroid underactivity may coincide with menopausal changes in women, the physical signs of weight gain, fatigue and sleepiness may not be recognised unless thyroid function tests are carried out.

Hyperthyroidism

When the secretion of thyroxine is excessive the individual has thyrotoxicosis. Enlargement of the gland may be minimal or visible and palpable. Nodular enlargement may prove to be malignant (De Souza, 1980;

Allen, 1984). The popular term for enlarged thyroid gland is 'goitre' and it is caused by deficiency of iodine in drinking water in many parts of the world. The addition of iodine salt in the diet prevents the occurrence of simple goitre.

If enlargement of the thyroid gland is associated with protrusion of the eyes (caused by fatty deposits behind the eyes), it is called exophthalmic goitre or Graves' disease. Women are more often affected than men in the ratio 8:1, and the age of onset is between 16 and 40 years. There is a familial history and the symptoms can be greatly aggravated by shock and stress (Thomson, 1976). Graves' disease is characterised by well-recognised symptoms: tachycardia (abnormally rapid pulse); a warm moist skin, heat intolerance, increased sweating, tremor, insomnia and diarrhoea. Appetite is increased but there is loss of weight as a result of increased body metabolism. There is also a pronounced nervousness and excitability associated with the physical condition (Wittkower and Mandelbrote, 1955), so that women may become tearful as well as having to deal with the menstrual changes that occur in both hyper- and hypothyroidism. The anxiety symptoms are comparable to those described under discussion about anxiety state (page 189). Increased metabolic rate disturbs the function of the whole organism and is a true example of systemic disease (Falk and Birken, 1985).

In the early stages of hyperthyroidism, it is difficult to distinguish between symptoms associated with thyrotoxicosis and disorders resulting from hormonal disturbance accompanying the menopause. It is possible that the anxiety and apparent hypochondria with complaints of discomfort or a lump in the throat and vocal weakness will be incorrectly diagnosed as psychogenic. Compression from the gland and systemic disturbance may be the cause, however, and the speech–language pathologist must be aware of this possibility in assessment of 'functional' cases of dysphonia referred for treatment. Sonninen (1960) listed the following symptoms of tracheal compression:

- constant desire to clear the throat
- sensations of pressure and pain
- paraesthesia
- difficulty in swallowing
- lowered speaking fundamental frequency
- lack of volume
- difficulty singing high notes.

The clinical picture of thyrotoxicosis so often closely resembles an anxiety state that diagnosis is extremely difficult. Here we see the psychosomatic 'servo-system' of the body at its most complex. Thyro-toxicosis can be precipitated by shock, and it should be remembered that conversion symptom aphonia and dysphonia frequently develop after shock or periods of ill-health, overwork and mental strain. Voice disorders within this patient group tend to be hyperfunctional and can be helped by voice therapy as an adjunct to medical or surgical treatment of the condition.

Anti-thyroxine medication may control excessive thyroxine in the blood but, if unsuccessful, thyroidectomy is performed. The entire gland is not removed, but a portion is left which it is anticipated will provide normal secretion of thyroxine. If this is underestimated, the patient will develop myx-oedema and will require life-long thyroxine treatment. The development of myxoedema can be detected a few days after surgery from the characteristic dysphonia: hoarseness and lowered pitch. Preoperatively, patients should undergo laryngoscopy and should be warned of the possibility of voice prob-lems after surgery (see Recurrent laryngeal nerve lesions, Chapter 10).

Pseudo-hyperthyroidism

It is not easy to distinguish between genuine hyperthyroidism resulting from over-secretion of thyroxine, and pseudo-hyperthyroidism that is largely psychogenic but with psychosomatic symptoms. Enlargement of the gland may be minimal and blood tests are not positive for thyrotoxico-sis but vocal changes may be present (Sonninen, 1960).

Summary

- Changes in vocal fold mucosa can be the result of inhaled and ingested substances, and can be caused by systemic disease or conditions.
- Voice disorders caused by these underlying factors may be mistaken for muscle tension dysphonia.
- When muscle tension dysphonia does not respond to voice therapy, some of the conditions described in this chapter might be considered and investigated.
- The vocal fold changes that result from certain systemic conditions and medications will become permanent if the condition is not man-aged appropriately at an early stage.
- Voice therapy facilitates best voice care and reduces the potential for damaging vocal behaviours.

Part III
Voice Therapy

Voice therapy: the process

'Begin at the beginning,' the King said gravely, 'and go on till you come to the end; then stop.'

Alice in Wonderland, Lewis Carroll

Clinical voice disorders can be treated by voice therapy or by a combination of medicine, surgery and voice therapy, according to the aetiology of the dysphonia. Voice therapy alone is the preferred route for treating the majority of voice disorders and is carried out in some countries by specialist speech–language pathologists (or therapists) and in others, chiefly mainland Europe, by phoniatricians. Surgical procedures to improve phonation are referred to as phonosurgery. In many cases, following the diagnostic evaluation, the preferred treatment route is obvious, but in others a coordinated decision-making pathway should be taken by the laryngologist and speech and language pathologist in order to ensure the best outcome. In the broadest terms, voice therapy is concerned with changing vocal behaviour whereas phonosurgery aims to normalise deviant laryngeal structures. Even when an excellent surgical result is achieved, voice therapy is an essential part of the rehabilitation process if the patient is to achieve optimum voice with the restored or repaired laryngeal structure.

The route by which an individual with a voice disorder reaches appropriate care is outlined in Figure 12.1. As with all disorders, the problem may be at an early or late stage when the patient first visits the general practitioner, but referral for laryngological examination is essential if the voice has been abnormal for more than 3 weeks in the absence of an upper respiratory tract infection. There is always a reason for a voice disorder and the aetiology can be determined only by competent examination (see Chapter 13). Table 12.1 gives the aims of voice therapy and phonosurgery.

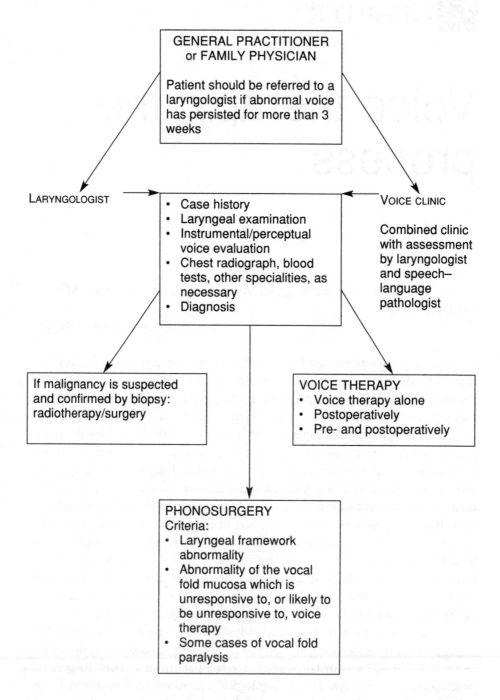

Figure 12.1 Treatment pathway for a patient with a clinical voice disorder. Preoperative voice therapy is used for two purposes: (1) to reduce hyperfunctional phonation in order to ensure that the vocal fold mucosa is in an optimal state before surgery; and (2) as a trial treatment to assess whether voice therapy can resolve a condition that might otherwise require surgical intervention.

Table 12.1 Aims of voice therapy and phonosurgery in the treatment of voice disorders

Voice therapy	Phonosurgery
• Restore 'normal voice'	Improve laryngeal structure and potential function by:
• Improve vocal profile	• removing diseased/abnormal laryngeal tissue
• Improve/restore laryngeal function	
• Eliminate/reduce some benign mass lesions	• normalising laryngeal framework abnormalities
• Protect the patient from regressing or causing further vocal problems	• re-positioning paralysed vocal fold
• Eliminate vocal tract discomfort associated with phonation	
• Enable patient to reach vocal potential and assist in communication adjustments in irreversible conditions	

This chapter outlines the process of voice therapy; an overall pattern of the elements involved from the speech–language pathologist's first contact with the patient until discharge (treatment techniques are discussed in Chapters 14 and 15). Unfortunately, this process is not necessarily as simple as the King's advice to Alice. Decisions have to be made, ranging from whether or not the patient's condition is likely to respond to treatment to whether the end of the treatment programme has been reached. Is the patient's larynx the object of treatment, or the voice? Or the person? The clinician's awareness of the decision-making processes involved and the variables that might have to be considered at any stage increase the likelihood of a successful treatment outcome. Although there are certain underlying tenets for treating the various types of voice disorders, it is essential that each course of treatment and its delivery is carefully designed to encompass the multifactorial nature of the vocal problem presented by each patient. Table 12.2 lists some important principles of voice therapy that are fundamental to the successful outcome of treatment.

The referral

The route by which the patient reaches the speech–language pathologist varies from country to country. In the UK, the dysphonic patient is initially referred by the general practitioner to the laryngologist who is responsible for the medical diagnosis and any medical or surgical treatment. As it is

Table 12.2 Principles of voice therapy

Sufficient information to plan and institute a valid treatment programme	A successful treatment outcome depends on comprehensive information re:
	• laryngeal pathology (structure and function) • instrumental and perceptual evaluation of the voice • the patient
Decision-making approach	Each programme of treatment must be specifically designed for the patient
Patient should understand the therapeutic process	An important aspect of successful treatment. Explanations at each stage of treatment enable the patient to take an active part in progress and then generalise new vocal behaviours
Patient shares responsibility for progress	The clinician cannot resolve the voice disorder without the patient's compliance and motivation. Patients who mentally 'hand over' the voice problem to the clinician should be helped to realise the importance of their active role
Holistic treatment	Even normal voices reflect many aspects of the speaker's life, health and emotional status. These elements are all relevant to a voice disorder and must be considered in assessment and treatment
Multidisciplinary approach	Treatment is most effectively delivered when the laryngologist and speech–language pathologist, and other related professionals, work closely together
Hierarchical treatment plan	Techniques should be introduced in a logical sequence with each new element of therapy based on foundation skills
Instrumental/perceptual monitoring	This provides feedback re: effectiveness of therapy and can indicate when a course of treatment should be revised
Maximum improvement in minimum time	Treatment should be delivered as efficiently as possible so that the voice is restored with minimal delay. Treatment must not be rushed, however, and the underlying factors must be fully addressed

imperative that malignancy should be excluded, it is generally accepted that dysphonia that lasts for more than 2–3 weeks after onset, in the absence of an upper respiratory tract infection, should be fully investigated. It still happens, however, that some patients return to their GPs repeatedly complaining of voice and vocal tract symptoms, but are not referred for a laryngological examination. In most of these cases, although the voice disorder steadily worsens and causes practical problems and some distress, the consequences to health are not significant. As hoarseness can indicate serious underlying disease, however, it should be fully investigated (see Chapter 13) and the speech–language pathologist must regard a laryngological examination and report as mandatory before accepting a patient for treatment.

Many speech–language pathologists who treat patients with voice disorders do not work in a voice clinic team and may be geographically remote from the laryngologist's clinic. Detailed findings of laryngeal structure and function are essential when these clinicians have little or no opportunity of viewing their patients' vocal tracts. There is the possibility of placing both children and adults at risk by accepting even the mildest case of hoarseness without a laryngological examination and diagnosis. Symptoms that appear to result from vocal abuse can be the first signs of

Case notes

Case 1

A hospital secretary asked the speech therapist to see her husband who had persistent hoarseness after flu. He did not like hospitals and thought that it might be possible to visit the speech therapy department on his way home from work in order to receive some helpful advice and so avoid an appointment in the ENT department. This request was refused on the grounds that a laryngological examination and report were essential initially. The couple resented this response and regarded it as uncooperative professionalism. Eventually the husband agreed to see the laryngologist and laryngeal carcinoma was diagnosed. After a course of radiotherapy, there was still no recurrence of the disease several years later. If diagnosis had been delayed, laryngectomy would probably have been necessary.

Case 2

A general surgeon referred one of his patients to the speech–language pathologist because of her weak voice. She had undergone a mastectomy for carcinoma of the breast 5 months earlier. The surgeon considered that her voice had changed because of the stress of her illness. The speech–language pathologist responded to the referral by recommending that the patient should be referred to the voice clinic. Examination revealed that one vocal fold was hypomobile and further investigation revealed a metastatic growth involving the recurrent laryngeal nerve. As a result, appropriate treatment for dealing with the secondary growth was instituted immediately and non-productive voice therapy, while the disease progressed, was avoided.

neurological or systemic disease, particularly carcinoma. Any pressure by patients or doctors to begin treatment without the laryngologist's report must be resisted because of the possibility of serious disease being overlooked. Apart from excluding disease, a valid remediation programme cannot be evolved without clear information about laryngeal function and the type and site of any mucosal changes.

> **Case note**
>
> It should be remembered that, even when an individual works in a vocally demanding job, this is not necessarily the cause of the voice problem. It can never be presumed that the context of voice use or a particular sequence of events indicates conclusively that the vocal symptoms are the result of vocal abuse. Laryngoscopic examination is essential. Teachers fall into this group and, although vocal abuse is frequently the cause of their problems, other underlying factors must not be overlooked.

The clinicians

The laryngologist and speech–language pathologist are the core members of the team with whom the voice-disordered patient comes into contact. The team may also include a singing teacher, physiotherapist or osteopath, voice scientist, psychiatrist and social worker, with referrals being made to a neurologist and others, as required. The laryngologist is responsible for the medical diagnosis and overall medical and surgical management of patients. The speech–language pathologist evaluates phonatory behaviour and the underlying factors that might be involved in precipitating and maintaining the voice disorder, before evolving a treatment plan and carrying out a treatment programme. Diagnosis and assessment of a voice disorder requires collaboration between all the professional specialists who can contribute information about the patient's problems. Since the advent of multidisciplinary voice clinics 15–20 years ago, the roles of laryngologists and speech–language pathologists have become increasingly cooperative and supportive in many centres. The shared expertise and discussion about the best management route in each case are to the patient's benefit.

When a laryngologist and speech pathologist work closely together in a voice clinic, the patient and team begin to build a constructive relationship which gives the patient confidence. The mutual respect of the clinicians for each other and the coordinated expertise from the integrated disciplines help to reassure the patient and to ensure that informed explanations regarding the various aspects of the voice problem and its treatment are available. Even when the clinicians do not work together in a voice clinic setting, the way in which the laryngologist explains the need for a referral for voice therapy to the patient can have a significant effect on the patient's attitude to treatment or whether he or she attends at all. If the need for speech therapy is explained and its importance is indicated, the patient is more likely to embark on remediation appropriately motivated and with confidence. Many people are unaware of the speech–language pathologist's role in treating voice disorders, and some are horrified or amused that they are being referred for treatment by someone, as they mistakenly believe, who treats only children who lisp or stammer. Voice therapy is also considered to be too time-consuming by some patients, particularly if the voice

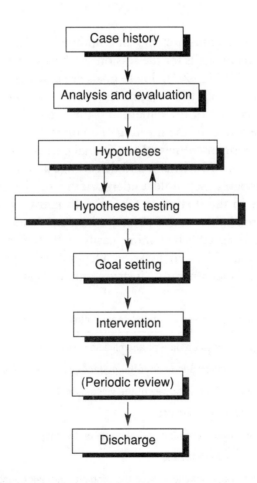

Figure 12.2 Voice therapy: The process. These key stages of the therapeutic process are hierarchical and interdependent. For example, carefully delivered treatment is worthless if the hypotheses on which it is based are invalid. Similarly, goal setting is fundamental to deciding when treatment should be concluded.

apparently returns to normal after surgery. In the long run, avoidance of therapy does not necessarily save time, but can lead to recurrence of the problem and more prolonged investigation and treatment.

The process of therapy comprises certain key elements that can present the clinician with dilemmas as well as resolutions at each stage of the decision-making process. These key elements of treatment evolve logically and are summarised in Figure 12.2. Although the time taken for each element and for the overall process will vary from patient to patient, no stage can be omitted if treatment is to be successful.

Initial consultation

GOALS

When the patient attends for the first interview, the speech–language pathologist has certain goals for the session as a basis for initiating the treatment programme (Table 12.3). These goals are essentially the same whatever the aetiology of the voice disorder. The compilation of a comprehensive account of the patient and the voice disorder is a priority, but it is only one aspect of the meeting. To concentrate entirely on asking questions and making instrumental and formal perceptual evaluation of the voice at this stage may overwhelm and discourage a patient, who is already anxious and probably has little understanding of the speech–language pathologist's role in the treatment schedule. In many cases, however, the patient is reassured by the use of objective instrumentation and the clinical relationship can be established more easily with the instrumental tasks acting as an element of the initial session. Depending on patients' views and prejudices about voice therapy, instrumentation can demonstrate that

Table 12.3 Voice pathologist's aims at initial consultation

To facilitate good rapport between patient and clinician

To obtain comprehensive information about the patient and the voice disorder

To explain normal voice and the aetiology of the voice disorder

To give the patient realistic reassurance

To outline the proposed treatment plan, its rationale and timing

To give the patient self-help strategies

To give the patient the opportunity to explain the problem and ask questions

In practice, these aims are achieved as an integrated process during the interview and are not approached sequentially. The voice pathologist keeps them in mind while maintaining a relaxed and empathetic manner.

treatment will be based on suitable data. Consequently, an organised but pragmatic approach is probably the best route and clinical judgement should determine the balance of the session. It is important to ensure that the passage of information should not be from patient to clinician only, however well intentioned the careful compilation of data. By the end of the session, the patient should have a greater understanding of the voice disorder and be reassured by explanations and the proposed treatment plan.

By the end of the initial consultation, the patient should understand the role of the speech–language pathologist and the goals of therapy should have been agreed. In practical and therapeutic terms, it can be helpful to arrange a fixed number of sessions initially, rather than embark on an open-ended treatment programme. This allows patient and clinician to aim for certain improvements in a set time period with a review of progress at the end of the period, as well as ensuring that clinic time is not overbooked. It should be made clear to the patient that this is not a method of rationing treatment because the course of treatment will be extended or shortened according to the rate of progress. Agreeing to a provisional number of treatments initially can indicate positively to the patient that treatment has a beginning, a middle and an end, and that it will not be unnecessarily prolonged. It has to be remembered that most patients with voice disorders are otherwise socially active and trying to pursue their employment. Consequently, it is helpful for them to have some indication of the time they will need to commit to treatment.

ELICITING INFORMATION

Eliciting information from the patient requires considerable clinical skill and the effectiveness of this process can fundamentally affect the outcome of treatment. Many of the necessary skills are used intuitively on a daily basis in social situations, but can be overwhelmed by the pressure to amass as many data as possible in the clinical situation. A direct question-and-answer approach can inhibit the patient and possibly reduce the information given. As a result, relevant facts may be omitted and the opportunity to observe the voice in general conversation is reduced. There should be a clear awareness of the information that needs to be collated, but initially, in many cases, the most productive approach for the clinician and the most comfortable for the patient is to ask for an account of the problem from the time of the first symptoms. In this way, a chronological account emerges in conjunction with a pattern of the voice disorder that can be related to events. The patient's beliefs and perceptions regarding the causes and effects of the voice problem are revealed in association with paralinguistic features and body language, which clarify the content of the account. This approach also ensures that patients feel that they have been listened to and had the opportunity to express their concerns. The speech–language pathologist can ask closed questions to obtain specific facts, but open-ended questions will help to overcome any diffidence on the patient's part, together with prompting by encouraging remarks and questions that explore new areas of information. When an individual has difficulty relating the relevant events, because of strong emotions or a reluctance to talk, expansion can be encouraged by not intervening with a further question, but affirming the account so far by nodding or saying 'mm', and waiting for a short period. This pause should produce a further response within a few seconds but must not be so long as to be uncomfortable.

The amount and quality of the information given by the patient are affected by the overall pace at which the interview is conducted. Sufficient time must be allowed for the patient to give an account of the voice disorder and to answer questions fully; when the account becomes repetitive or rambling, however, the interviewer should move the conversation to its next stage. The patient will speak more freely if the speech–language pathologist appears relaxed and interested, whatever the time constraints in a busy clinic. Allowing sufficient time for collating information at this early stage of treatment reduces the possibility of overlooking important contributory factors to the voice problem. Information will often be given more freely if it is made clear to the patient that personal information will remain confidential. Although most patients presume that this will be the case, many will respond by relating relevant information when this assurance is given voluntarily by the clinician.

As in all conversations, the characteristics and behaviour of the speech–language pathologist will influence the interaction and affect the relationship with the patient throughout evaluation and treatment. It should be remembered that the patient is also conducting a process of evaluation, even if intuitively, which will contribute to decisions concerning the clinician's competence, understanding and ability to establish a supportive and productive relationship. If the patient reaches negative conclusions at this early stage, the effectiveness of the treatment will be undermined, even if intervention is theoretically sound and skilfully delivered.

DOES THE PATIENT UNDERSTAND?

The patient's understanding, or misconceptions, regarding a voice disorder can affect the success of treatment. Consequently, useful clinic time can be spent in listening, explaining and asking questions to ascertain what the patient thinks. If the situation is not clarified early in treatment, the patient's unfounded theories can influence vocal tract behaviour and obstruct progress.

The diagnosis

During the initial consultation, the patient's understanding of the laryngo-scopic findings and the results of any tests should be clarified. It is a common experience among professionals to encounter patients who emphatically deny that they have been given explanations about their con-dition and the treatment that has been planned for them so far. There are a number of reasons for this. In some cases, the patient has not actually received explanations, sometimes because assumptions are made that another member of the team has covered this aspect. More frequently, when an explanation has been given it is not meaningful to the patient. This may be because the language used is inappropriate. Professional people sometimes fail to realise that the jargon that they use with each other is incomprehensible to those who have no knowledge of anatomy and physi-ology. Patients can soon become lost in a linguistic limbo.

Language may also be inappropriate because of the speaker's socio-linguistic and cultural assumptions. In general, the patient's anxiety and apprehension may have prevented explanations being understood, and there may be fears that asking for the information to be repeated runs the risk of looking foolish.

Voice therapy

It should be established whether or not the patient understands why a referral to the speech–language pathologist has been made. As a result of misconceptions, reactions may include willing compliance purely because the laryngologist has made the referral or surprise because 'I can speak all right, it's just my voice'. The dysphonic patient who has no mucosal changes in the larynx, and who has been told by the laryngologist that the larynx is normal, may be concerned that voice therapy is a type of psychi-atry. For the therapist to gain the patient's confidence, any such misun-derstandings must be discussed. It should be made clear that the purpose of the initial interview is assessment of the voice problem in the light of the laryngological findings and that this is the basis for planning suitable treatment.

Normal voice production

Although not wanting to be patronisingly simple in explanations of how the patient's laryngeal function differs from normal, the extent of the patient's knowledge should be established. The individual who visualises the larynx as a harp-like structure with several vibrating 'cords' in a vertical position is not well equipped to have insight into the condition.

CASE HISTORY

The case history should provide a comprehensive picture of the individual in addition to the factual information relevant to the voice disorder. The detailed information required is described as part of the process of analysis and evaluation in the next chapter. As the process of acquiring the information can be as informative and revealing as the information obtained, this section considers factors that contribute to a valuable case history. During this interview, the speech–language pathologist's own voice quality and communication skills affect the type and amount of information acquired. A friendly and sympathetic, but professional, manner helps the patient to describe the voice disorder and associated problems confidently.

Environment

Ideally this interview should take place in a quiet room without interruption from other colleagues or the telephone, and where the patient knows that there is no likelihood of being overheard. The patient's previous contacts, unless attending a private office, will have been in the limited privacy of an ENT clinic or a general ward. In the privacy of the first interview, patients will frequently divulge significant information, previously unrevealed, and admit to not understanding aspects of their condition that are fundamental to treatment. Care should be taken to help the patient to feel as relaxed and confident as possible. This is partly out of respect for the patient's immediate needs, but it is also the most effective clinical strategy. A comfortable situation tends to elicit more information and to allow vocal potential to be revealed.

Recording data

Thought also has to be given to the method of recording data. Writing down every fact as it is given will certainly reduce the flow of information because both spontaneity and eye contact are lost. An audio-tape recording is intimidating and must not be made without the patient's agreement. The most productive approach is usually a combination of careful listening and writing down factual details, such as dates, during the interview. Immediately writing up the case details after the interview is appropriate in most instances. Other opportunities to acquire case history information occur and are sometimes more productive because of the relative informality of the conversation. Details concerning domestic relationships and apparently unrelated facts are often gleaned during informal conversation as the session ends or while equipment is being prepared. The skilful clinician does not consider them unimportant because they are not part of the formal case history taking, but notes their relevance or the way in which they affect the information already collated.

ANALYSIS AND EVALUATION

Evaluation and analysis of the various factors that have contributed to and maintained the voice disorder, together with the collation of information regarding its current status, are the basis of remediation. (Perceptual and instrumental evaluation is described in Chapter 13.) The quality of this essential, foundation information is fundamental to the success of therapy, but even more important is the clinician's ability to identify the most significant factors and synthesise them into valid hypotheses. The collection of information and data requires clinical skills that elicit representative information about the patient's disorder and the potential of the vocal tract. Useful material is less likely to be obtained if the patient is intimidated by procedures or the clinician's manner. When clinicians become so involved with the technicalities of an instrumental task or a certain line of questioning that the patient feels a mere appendage to the process, not only is there an increased probability of less useful information being acquired, but the clinical relationship is eroded, which may reduce the effectiveness of treatment. Explanations, encouragement and reassurance generally elicit a more realistic profile of the patient and the voice disorder while fostering a productive clinical relationship. Although it is essential that sufficient information is obtained to provide a sound basis for the treatment programme, the process of evaluation should not unduly delay the onset of treatment. Most of the essential facts and data can usually be obtained in the initial consultation and, by the end of this session, the patient should be given explanations and advice that are the first stages in treatment. Patients are discouraged by prolonged assessment protocols over a number of visits to the clinic if they feel that they have not received any 'treatment' (see Goals of initial consultation above).

Note

Instrumental and time constraints in many settings mean that clinicians have to choose the instrumentation and instrumental measures that they consider will be most valuable to their clinical population, while excluding those that might be interesting but not essential. Generally, clinics attached to academic institutions, where research is a high priority, tend to have more equipment together with essential technical support than those in general hospitals. Lack of extensive measurement equipment does not necessarily mean that effective treatment cannot be delivered, but in some cases patients should be referred to another centre if it becomes clear that more sophisticated investigations or measurements are essential.

HYPOTHESES

Intervention can only usefully begin when hypotheses have been formulated about the factors contributing to the voice disorder. The primary cause of the dysphonia might be obvious, but the clinician must take a broad view that acknowledges the multifactorial background of many dysphonias. Equipped with laryngoscopic information, perceptual and instrumental profiles, and a comprehensive case history, the speech–language therapist considers the interrelationships between the various elements. Hypotheses are based on the compatibilities and anomalies between the various facts that have been amassed. When facts appear to be incompatible, it is either because the information is wrong or because a variable behavioural pattern is contributing to the symptom. Information may need to be revisited, so that it is amplified and clarified to obtain the full picture. As hypotheses are formed, they can be tested by treatment trials and subsequently reconsidered if a particular route confounds the hypothesis and is unsuccessful. The following examples demonstrate how elements of a hypothesis may evolve.

Case histories

FY

A teacher (FY), who had been qualified for 3 years, developed voice problems that appeared to correlate directly with the amount of voice use and vocal loading. She reported that her voice deteriorated towards the end of the day and at the end of the term, but that her voice was almost non-existent before going to school each morning. She had experienced episodes of total loss of voice following upper respiratory tract infections on five occasions during the year before seeking help for her symptoms. Laryngoscopic examination and her acoustic profile were within normal limits on initial examination. She was quietly spoken and not a classic vocal abuser in general conversation, and she was concerned that her recurrent voice problem would affect her chances of promotion. The way in which she presented was compatible with a diagnosis of vocal misuse resulting from teaching a large class of 5 and 6 year olds. An apparently minor anomaly in her behaviour was an excessive amount of smiling throughout the session, which obscured nuances of facial expression and which the speech–language pathologist felt acted as a barrier to 'reading' the patient accurately. People may smile a great deal when they are nervous or apprehensive, but in this instance the amount of smiling was exceptional, particularly as the patient was expressing concern about her symptoms. The speech–language pathologist began to query whether the hypothesis of vocal misuse that had been developing was the whole story. Further questions were asked about the episodes of total voice loss after upper respiratory infections. It appeared that the first aphonic episode had occurred suddenly in the absence of infection and had lasted for 2 weeks. Subsequent episodes happened near the beginning of each term or shortly after returning to school following the half-term holiday. The symptoms of the apparent infections were usually a slightly sore throat before the voice disappeared suddenly. It usually returned equally suddenly about 2 weeks later. The hypothesis was changing. The pattern of aphonic episodes suggested a psychogenic aphonia rather than straightforward vocal misuse. Initially, as the speech–language pathologist introduced general discussion about the effects of stress on the voice and the stresses associated with teaching in particular, FY described how much she loved her job. Gentle questioning revealed, however, that there were many pressures related to additional duties, working relationships and demands on her to perform. FY set high standards for herself and wanted to do well. The hypothesis was revised: although there were possibly elements of vocal misuse as a basis for the voice problem, they must be minimal because there was no evidence of changes on the vocal fold mucosa despite a prolonged history of vocal symptoms. The aphonic episodes tended to occur in anticipation of being in the teaching situation, at the beginning of a term or the second half of the term, and any dysphonia was worse at the beginning of the day. It was decided that she had a stress-related voice problem which was exacerbated and highlighted by the demands made on her vocally in her work. Establishing the correct hypothesis significantly affected the treatment programme. Emphasis was placed on developing FY's insight into the factors affecting her voice and helping her to develop coping strategies, with some time being spent on developing vocal skills and stamina. If treated as a problem of vocal misuse, intervention would have disregarded primary aetiological factors.

BD

BD (54-year-old male) was referred for speech therapy from a routine ENT clinic by a junior doctor with the diagnosis 'NAD larynx' (no abnormality detected). The dominant perceptual and instrumental features of his voice were roughness, extremely deep pitch and reduced loudness. His work as an electrician was not vocally demanding and he had stopped smoking 18 months earlier. Throughout a range of tasks, his vocal features remained consistent and the vocal note did not improve on vegetative behaviour. In most cases of dysphonia, when the diagnosis is 'NAD larynx', the voice is variable and it is possible to elicit a normal, or more normal, vocal note by various strategies. The speech–language pathologist concluded that BD's voice and vocal behaviour reflected a structural abnormality of the vocal folds. Consequently, after the initial consultation, BD was referred to the voice clinic for further

(contd)

laryngoscopic examination. Well-established carcinoma was found on the anterior left vocal fold. Voice therapy was inappropriate and he was referred for radiotherapy.

This case demonstrates the importance of the speech–language pathologist maintaining an analytical view of all data and information received from patients and other members of the team. Incongruities should be questioned whenever they occur because they may be highly significant. In the case of BD, the speech–language pathologist's data and experience suggested that the patient's voice could not emanate from a normal larynx. It appears that an inexperienced doctor had not seen the carcinoma because the anterior part of the vocal fold was obscured by the epiglottis. If a course of speech therapy had been embarked upon and persisted with, the consequences for the patient could have been disastrous. It is important, therefore, in all cases that the speech–language pathologist remains alert to the significance of the various features that emerge during assessment and treatment, and does not slip into a purely reactive or accepting mind set.

CL

CL (42-year-old male) had become increasingly hoarse over a period of 9 months, and was referred for speech therapy with reddened and oedematous true and false vocal folds. He was the head of department in a large insurance company and had an imposing and authoritative manner, which included speaking loudly as if he were giving a presentation to an audience, even in one-to-one conversation. As expected, speaking fundamental frequency was lowered because of the increased mass of the vocal folds, and there was a significant noise component to the fundamental vocal note. Deciding on a reasonable hypothesis involved considering whether his very deep voice was a primary or secondary feature, i.e. was the lowered pitch the direct result of vocal abuse arising from his overloud phonation, so causing the vocal folds to increase in mass? Alternatively, before his voice problems, had he spoken on an unduly low pitch and so increased phonatory effort and caused changes in the vocal folds? From his general behaviour the speech–language pathologist postulated that the latter sequence of events was probable. He attempted to convey authority in the way in which he talked about his work and on a range of subjects that were introduced. It was suggested to him that attempts to convey authority are sometimes reflected in lowered vocal pitch, in some cases deliberately and in others without awareness, and that this might be the basis of his voice problems. He expressed amazement that this point had been raised and gradually disclosed his feelings of inadequacy socially and at work. He had risen to a high position in his company, although he had left school aged 16 years. He did not have a degree and was overwhelmed by the bright graduates on his staff, although there was no suggestion that anyone doubted his competency. Using an authoritative manner had become his protection. The hypothesis that provided the basis of treatment was that his dysphonia had a sociolinguistic basis which had eventually resulted in changes in the vocal fold mucosa. Addressing this underlying fact through discussion and explanation, in conjunction with a treatment programme directed at establishing a new kinaesthetic model and improved vocal skills, resolved the problem.

KS

KS (72-year-old male) complained that he had noticed that his voice continued to be breathy and weak after a flu-like illness. He waited for some months before seeking medical advice because he hoped the problem would resolve. On nasendoscopic examination of the larynx, the left vocal fold was immobile. Various examinations, including chest radiographs, excluded disease and it was concluded that the cause of his vocal fold paralysis was idiopathic, probably viral. During the first session with the speech–language pathologist, he was shown how to carry out laryngeal valving exercises (see page 496) and he performed these without excessive effort. On his second visit, 1 week later, he began by saying that he was making good progress and he thought that his voice was improving. His enthusiasm for complying with treatment and his positive attitude regarding his progress were professionally gratifying. It was only when he was asked if he had had any problems or difficulties that he mentioned that his throat felt rather sore after practising his exercises, but he did not mind as long as his voice was improving. Clinical experience suggested that laryngeal soreness was an uncommon symptom in cases of vocal fold paralysis because the flaccid, immobile vocal fold militates against hyperfunctional vocal fold adduction. The paralysed fold does not allow sufficiently forceful vocal fold impact to cause soreness. A possible source of discomfort might be effortful false vocal fold adduction which can occur in compensation for glottal insufficiency. The speech–language pathologist arranged for the patient to be examined using videostroboscopy (see page 432). The absence of mucosal waves over the posterior part of the left vocal fold and the deflection of wave around the area confirmed a diagnosis of a vocal fold cyst involving the arytenoid cartilage. Consequently, the vocal fold was fixed, not paralysed. The cyst was aspirated and after one session of voice therapy his voice returned to normal.

The case of KS is another instance of an anomaly leading to reconsideration of the problem and various lessons can be learned from this case:

* The way in which the vocal folds should be functioning, according to the given diagnosis, must be borne in mind during evaluation of the

voice and during treatment. An explanation should be sought for unexplained symptoms.

• Patients' enthusiasm, thanks and pleasure at their progress do not necessarily mean that all is well. Careful questioning can reveal negative factors that might be significant.

• Stroboscopic examination provides information about laryngeal structure and function, which is not apparent on mirror or routine nasendoscopy (see page 427).

• Time spent on carefully formulating a valid hypothesis can save time and resources spent on inappropriate treatment routes. If treatment had continued on the presumption of a vocal fold paralysis, a considerable number of treatment sessions might have been spent incorrectly on therapy directed at improving vocal fold adduction. In the light of the laryngeal discomfort that occurred after 1 week, it is possible that vocal fold trauma would have been incurred.

GOAL SETTING

The simply stated aim of voice therapy would appear to be to cure the voice disorder and to return the patient's voice to normal. The reality is more complex. Is the aim of normality defined by what is normal for the patient or according to normative data? If the patient's 'normal' voice was the abusive phonation that resulted in vocal nodules, they will regenerate if those vocal patterns are not eliminated. If a larynx has been irreparably damaged in a road traffic accident or there is laryngeal neuropathology, normal voice by any definition might not be a realistic goal. Consequently, goals have to be set with regard to a number of parameters. The goals decided on enable the speech–language pathologist to make decisions regarding the patient's discharge from treatment; if they have not been carefully established, the point at which treatment has been completed is unclear. The categories into which treatment goals can be classified are discussed below and summarised in Table 12.4.

Laryngoscopic findings

The goals under this heading fall into two broad categories: structural and functional. In cases where there is inflammation of the vocal folds as the result of hyperfunctional phonation, a treatment goal should be the resolution of these inflammatory changes. Similarly, certain benign mass lesions of the vocal folds can be reduced or eliminated by changing vocal behaviour. Soft vocal nodules, for example, fall into this category, but decisions

Table 12.4 Treatment goals

Bases of goal setting	Goals
Laryngoscopic findings	To reduce vocal fold mass or inflammation
	To improve laryngeal function
Acoustic profile:	
• instrumental	To establish vocal parameter norms
• perceptual	To establish a voice that is within normal limits and fulfils the speaker's demands
Vocal tract discomfort and phonatory effort	To reduce or eliminate soreness, aching, tightness and other sensory symptoms
	To achieve effortless phonation throughout pitch and loudness range
Emotional status	To reduce distress as an element of voice therapy or to refer for counselling
Non-phonatory vocal tract behaviours	To eliminate vigorous throat clearing and other potentially damaging vocal tract manoeuvres
Occupational demands	To develop the patient's vocal skills so that the voice meets employment needs whenever possible

Goals can be set in each of the categories listed. Within each category there are likely to be subgoals as explained in the text.

may have to be made as to whether the goal of treatment is to eliminate the nodules entirely or to establish a voice within normal limits and which the patient regards as satisfactory.

In all cases, improved laryngeal function is an essential goal, whether or not there have been structural abnormalities. The subgoals are likely to be elimination of aberrant or damaging vocal fold (and in some cases false vocal fold) behaviour, followed by the development of improved phonatory biomechanics.

Acoustic profile (perceptual and instrumental).

Key goals are set in relation to the sound of the voice. For most patients, the abnormal sound of the voice causes them to seek treatment, and their goal is to produce a voice that sounds normal. The clinician's goals are set on the basis of the instrumental and perceptual findings (see Chapter 13). Whenever possible, the goal of treatment is to achieve an acoustic profile that falls within established vocal parameter norms, when using instrumental measures. Perceptually, in cases of reversible voice disorder, the ideal treatment goal is a voice that sounds normal to the patient, and the patient's family and friends, as well as to the speech–language pathologist. If it is a realistic goal, the voice should also fulfil the patient's particular needs by the end of the treatment pro-gramme. The goal for a teacher, for example, should be a voice that not only meets the normative data and sounds normal in general conversation, but that can achieve considerable loudness and has the stamina to perform at this level as required.

Vocal tract discomfort and phonatory effort

Voice disorders are frequently associated with sensory symptoms (see page 124) and for many people the effort or discomfort is a significant problem. (There are also those whose voices are measurably within normal limits, but whose vocal tract discomfort causes considerable distress.) Decisions have to be made as to whether these symptoms will resolve spontaneously as treatment aimed at improving the voice progresses, or whether symp-tom-specific strategies can bring the patient relief more quickly. There is evidence that various manual strategies reduce tension in the intrinsic and extrinsic laryngeal musculature (Aronson, 1990; Mathieson, 1993a; Roy and Leeper, 1993; Lieberman, 1998) (see page 498). Consequently, it might be decided that this should be an early treatment goal in appropriate cases. When discomfort can be dealt with quickly, patients become less anxious and are able to comply with and benefit from treatment more effec-tively. Effort on phonation is also frequently experienced by patients and can be observed as they speak. It may be both a primary and a secondary feature of the dysphonia (see page 121), and it is important to deal with this problem as soon as possible if satisfactory progress is to be made. The ulti-mate goal is to achieve effortless phonation throughout the patient's pitch and loudness range.

Emotional status

Patients who have voice disorders are often distressed because of the way in which the quality of their lives is affected by the problem. It can be antic-ipated, therefore, that as the dysphonia responds to treatment their con-cerns resolve and the improvement of their emotional status is a subsidiary goal, attached to vocal improvement. When the voice problem is primarily psychogenic or reflects a patient's emotional status, however, it is essential to address the underlying factors. It must be decided whether counselling and advice from the speech–language pathologist is appropriate or, as in cases of persistent emotional symptoms or significant psychiatric illness, the patient should be referred to a counsellor, psychologist or psychiatrist. The speech–language pathologist's goal in this area might be to enable the patient to improve emotional status rather than attempt to provide solutions. In the clinical situation, identifying the point at which further referral should take place can be difficult to determine, particularly if clinicians find that they have inadvertently taken on the task of trying to resolve a wide range of a patient's difficulties. It is arguable that, when the dysphonia has been successfully treated, continuing emotional issues should be dealt with by other professionals.

Non-phonatory vocal tract behaviours

Another goal, which should be achieved as soon as possible after the onset of treatment, is the eradication of potentially damaging vocal tract behaviours that are not related to voice production. The most common is probably vigorous throat clearing, particularly in cases of vocal misuse or abuse and also when gastric reflux is contributing to the problem. Constant throat clearing irritates the mucosa of the vocal folds and, as a result, further mucus is secreted so that still more throat clearing is required. Unless this vicious circle is broken, the behaviour and its damaging effects will persist. Any hyperfunctional behaviours, particularly those involving the vocal folds, such as grunting on bearing weights or coughing with unnecessary force, should also be discouraged early in treatment.

The professional voice user

The goals for this group are similar to those for all patients, but the clinician should be aware that many people who fall into this category are 'vocal athletes'. Their vocal requirements in all vocal parameters may far exceed those of most people and treatment goals should reflect the superior skills required. Many professional voice users must be able to achieve extremes of pitch and loudness ranges while maintaining vocal note quality and stability. High levels of vocal flexibility and stamina can be essential.

In practice, each goal category will include a number of subgoals which are intended to resolve the vocal pathology and suit the patient's needs. Successful remediation of the voice problem depends on the selection of sufficient, appropriate goals as a focus for treatment. As treatment progresses, it may become clear that some goals have been wrongly identified or that additional goals should be included. As a result, they should be revised as necessary.

Treatment plan

The treatment plan is derived from the various goals that have been decided on. For maximum treatment effectiveness, consideration should be given not only to the therapeutic strategies that will be used, but also to the sequence in which they will be introduced. By following a logical, but flexible, hierarchy, the patient is able to make steady, comprehensible progress. This allows for appropriate back-tracking to an earlier stage, and consolidation before moving to the next stage, when necessary. The overall structure of the treatment plan can follow this pattern:

- explanations/education/reassurance
- voice conservation/vocal hygiene advice where appropriate
- vocal re-education programme.

The overall hierarchy of the treatment plan includes a hierarchy of tasks to implement voice change (Figure 12.3). In most cases, therapy will be directed initially at improving the quality of the vocal note. There is little point in attempting to increase vocal loudness if the quality of the vocal note is abnormal, for example, even if the patient perceives lack of volume as the main problem. When vocal note quality has been improved, strategies can be introduced to stabilise the vocal note before vocal flexibility, loudness and vocal stamina are addressed.

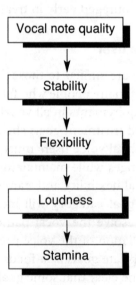

Figure 12.3 Treatment hierarchy: the overall treatment pattern usually follows this hierarchy, whatever treatment techniques are used. Each stage of vocal improvement is dependent on the previous stage.

INTERVENTION

Successful voice therapy depends on the relationship between the speech–language pathologist and the patient. As Andrews and Schmidt (1995) point out:

> Effective voice therapy requires knowledge and skill on the part of the clinician and motivation and trust on the part of the client. Both the clinician and client are partners in the therapeutic process, and it is the quality of the collaboration, rather than the skill of the clinician alone, that predisposes a successful outcome.

It is incumbent on the clinician, however, to provide the situation that allows and encourages this interaction to develop effectively. The clinician is working in a familiar subject area and environment that can intimidate and cause anxiety to the person who is experiencing the voice disorder. The situation is influenced by the personality characteristics of both the clinician and the patient, but good clinicians tend to develop a flexibility in their behaviours that allows them to adapt their behaviour from one patient to another (Andrews and Schmidt, 1995). It is essential that the patient is helped to feel that the clinician is giving full attention to the problem and is making every attempt to understand its significance to the sufferer.

Treatment techniques during voice therapy fall broadly into two categories: direct and indirect. Indirect strategies include explanations, advice and counselling. These enable patients to increase their understanding of the problem and the process of therapy. In this way they can develop some control over their voices and the recovery process. Direct strategies employed by speech–language pathologists include techniques that are used to change vocal behaviour. Therapeutic techniques are described in detail in the following chapters.

To answer patients' questions about how long treatment will take and the number of sessions required, the speech–language pathologist generally has to rely on personal experience and that of colleagues because of a paucity of definitive data in the literature. Although information about treatment efficacy is gradually increasing (Pannbacker, 1998; Ramig and Verdolini, 1998) (see page 469), information about treatment duration is generally inconsistent and unsatisfactory. Many studies do not record treatment duration and even when this time is noted it may be in hours, weeks, months or number of sessions, so that it is not possible to compare studies reliably. Prospective studies of treatment efficacy are usually for a set period, so they are not relevant to clinical practice in terms of how long treatment might take until the patient can be discharged. A few studies, however, do record treatment time (Stemple et al., 1994; Gordon et al., 1997; Lockart, Paton and Pearson, 1997). To be relevant to clinical practice, reports of treatment should include all aspects of timing: the number of treatment sessions, the length of each session, and the period of time over which they are administered. Some conditions, for example, may require intensive treatment on a daily basis for 2 weeks whereas others should be treated weekly or fortnightly over 2 or 3 months. At the moment, there is some informal agreement on treatment times, but variations between treatment centres suggest that clinician's preferences, rather than objective data, dictate frequency and length of treatment. Financial constraints in public health services and in private medicine funded by medical insurance will continue to necessitate value for money with regard to all treatments. As a result, there is pressure for speech–language pathologists to ensure that patients receive the most effective treatment in the shortest period of time. This is also to the benefit of the patient.

In cases of muscle tension dysphonia (MTD) and vocal misuse or abuse (the largest group of voice disorders), patients frequently respond to therapy relatively quickly, in about two to six treatment sessions. Although treatment may be undertaken on a weekly basis, it may be extended over 2–3 months (Lockart, Paton and Pearson, 1997). Unpleasant sensory symptoms can improve within a few days of the first session, and this may be accompanied by a reduction in vocal symptoms during the same period, with lasting effect (Mathieson, 1993a). Certain categories of voice disorder, such as conversion symptom aphonia and mutational falsetto (puberphonia), can respond to intervention so rapidly that normal voice can be elicited during the initial session. These early improvements are developed and consolidated as the treatment programme progresses (Boone and McFarlane, 1988; Aronson, 1990). The longest periods of treatment are usually involved in cases of neurogenic voice disorders and where vocal tract trauma has been sustained (see Chapters 9 and 10). In all instances, it is the speech–language pathologist's responsibility to ensure that, while carrying out a focused, efficient programme of treatment, the patient is enabled to feel as relaxed and as much at ease as possible.

Lack of progress during a course of therapy is significant and its reasons must be explored. Two major patterns can occur: some patients do not show any appreciable improvement from the onset of therapy whereas others improve in the early stages of treatment and then their progress plateaus. A small group makes good progress initially and subsequently regresses. The reasons for lack of progress are summarised in Table 12.5.

When a patient's voice disorder fails to respond to therapy from the outset, it is possible that there is insufficient information about the

Table 12.5 Voice therapy: reasons for lack of progress

- Insufficient information re: laryngopathology or other significant details
- A condition that will not respond to voice therapy alone
- Lack of patient commitment to therapy
- Dysphonia serving patient's needs
- Poorly conceived, directed and executed therapy

laryngopathology. Unless there are other circumstances that obviously account for the lack of progress, further laryngoscopic examination is essential. Videostroboscopy should be arranged if less informative laryngoscopic examination has been used initially (see page 432). Speech–language pathologists must also make realistic judgements as to whether or not a particular voice disorder is likely to respond to voice therapy. Certain conditions, such as cysts, pedunculated polyps and established Reinke's oedema, cannot be reversed by voice therapy alone, although it is essential postoperatively and can be beneficial preoperatively in some cases. Surgery is the primary treatment approach in these cases. Other conditions can merit a trial course of therapy. In this way, it can be assessed whether the vocal fold changes can be reversed by therapy, even if it is thought that surgery might be required. Progress will also be limited if the patient is deriving certain benefits from the voice disorder, such as being unable to continue with an unpleasant job or gaining considerable attention and sympathy not usually received. Finally, it must be remembered that voice therapy that is inappropriate or inadequate in any element might be the cause of lack of progress. Consequently, when a patient fails to make progress, the speech–language therapist should review each element of the voice therapy process to ensure that the most effective treatment is being given.

A skilful clinician not only will deliver treatment efficiently, but can also help the patient to enjoy the process. Initially, and understandably, many patients are concerned, anxious or distressed by their symptoms. As these concerns recede in the early stages of treatment, the restoration of vocal function and the acquisition of new vocal skills can be satisfying and pleasurable. It is not uncommon for patients to comment, on being discharged, that they have enjoyed the treatment sessions.

PERIODIC REASSESSMENT

Throughout the treatment programme, reassessment is necessary to monitor the path and rate of progress. Informally, this is carried out in conversation with the patient at each session. Questions concerning vocal function since the previous appointment are an important part of monitoring progress. Formally, instrumental methods are used in order to make comparisons with baseline measurements taken at the onset of treatment. It is also helpful to review laryngeal status periodically during treatment in order to monitor changes in vocal fold and supraglottic phonatory behaviour and the response of vocal fold pathology to therapy.

Discharge

The aim of voice therapy is ultimately to discharge the patient with the voice problem resolved, improved and compensated for, or to the care of another professional (see below). Whichever outcome is reached, the process of discharge from treatment should not come as a surprise to the patient, but be carefully prepared for by the speech–language pathologist. Throughout treatment, the patient should receive feedback about progress and have some awareness that treatment is progressing through a hierarchy. As each stage is completed it should be apparent that therapeutic tasks increasingly resemble the vocal requirements of everyday usage.

If the treatment goals have been correctly identified, the clinician and patient should agree that the treatment programme is complete when the goals have been reached. The patient can then be discharged. In many cases the decision to discharge is unequivocal but there are common dilemmas that have to be considered if unnecessarily protracted treatment or disappointed patients are to be avoided. These are summarised in Table 12.6 and discussed below.

Table 12.6 Discharge from voice therapy: common dilemmas

- The normal/disordered voice continuum
- Patient/clinician evaluation mismatch
- Patient wants 'better' voice than before onset of voice disorder
- Laryngeal potential limits recovery
- Voice within normal limits but phonation feels abnormal to patient
- Larynx and voice are normal but the voice lacks stamina
- Patient or voice pathologist reluctant to terminate treatment
- Poor patient compliance
- The professional voice user

The normal–disordered voice continuum

As a result of the infinite variations of normal voices (see Chapter 4), it can be difficult to judge reliably when normal voice has been reached for a particular individual. The achievement of instrumental norms for each parameter is not conclusive because it does not reflect the voice in conversation. Similarly, controlled speech samples might be regarded as normal on perceptual evaluation but do not cover the range of vocal behaviours used in spontaneous speech in a range of contexts. If voice samples can be rated as within normal limits perceptually and instrumentally, this indicates that a vocal tract is capable of producing normal voice, but it does not confirm that normal voice is actually being used in all spontaneous speech. Clinical decisions have to be made regarding the appropriate point of discharge, according to the aetiology of the voice disorder and the patient's needs.

Patient/clinician evaluation mismatch

The patient and speech–language pathologist may vary in their views about the extent of progress and readiness for discharge. When the clinician thinks that the point of discharging the patient has been reached, but the patient disagrees, the reasons for the differences probably lie in relatively covert factors. For example, the patient may be aware that there is some discomfort after prolonged talking or that the voice does not reflect paralinguistic features with the same subtlety as before the onset of the problem. Alternatively, when the patient feels ready to be discharged from therapy, although the clinician thinks that further treatment is necessary, it can be the result of the patient's overconfidence, a lack of understanding of the need to conserve the voice or limited appreciation of the inadequacies of vocal function. (Of course, the patient might just have found the treatment programme tedious and wishes to complete it as quickly as possible!) The reasons for the different perceptions of the situation should be identified and discussed, so that the patient is not discharged prematurely and does not subsequently regress.

The patient wants a 'better' voice than before the onset of the voice disorder

In some respects, this might be a valid expectation. If inadequate vocal skills or a pattern of vocal abuse have led to the voice disorder, treatment will have been directed at improving vocal behaviour. The dilemma regarding discharge can arise when the patient seeks to improve aesthetic aspects of the voice to a superior level, beyond the point when vocal function is considered within normal limits in all respects. The speech–language pathologist can help to resolve the situation by encouraging the patient to enrol for singing lessons or coaching by a voice teacher.

Laryngeal potential limits recovery

When laryngeal abnormality, and other conditions, limit the amount of possible vocal improvement, difficult judgements might have to be made regarding the conclusion of treatment. These will depend on the type and extent of structural or functional impairment and the patient's needs and wishes. Consideration must also be given to whether or not the full potential appears to have been reached. This situation can frequently be met by not formally discharging patients while they still hope for further improvement. Regular treatment sessions can be suspended when progress plateaus; review appointments then continue to monitor the patient and provide support. In this way, the patient does not feel abandoned and it reduces the possibility of regression. At the same time, clinical resources are being used efficiently by limiting the amount of non-productive treatment time. If there appears to be a change in laryngeal potential, or in the voice, a short course of trial treatment can be arranged to explore whether or not further improvement is possible. If there are signs that treatment is producing further improvement, further treatment can be arranged. Over a long period of regular review appointments, new surgical procedures sometimes emerge from which the patient will benefit. In many cases, such as road traffic accident survivors, following the support of review appointments with the laryngologist and speech–language pathologist over a considerable period, patients adjust to their changed voices when no further treatment can be offered. They become rehabilitated at work and socially so that they no longer feel the need for medical and therapeutic support which can finally be withdrawn.

The voice sounds normal but the patient complains that phonation does not feel normal

This situation can arise either when all aspects of voice production are satisfactory but the patient has not adjusted to the new behaviour pattern, or when some organic pathology persists but phonatory behaviour has been adapted in order to achieve a voice that falls within normal limits. The first category is observed in some patients who achieve voice after a conversion symptom aphonia and they need time to adjust to the changed kinaesthetic feedback of producing normal voice, as well as dealing with the underlying psychological reasons for their problem (see page 512). Also falling into this first category are some patients who achieve normal voice after a hyperfunctional voice disorder. Not only may it feel strange to produce voice without effort, but there may be a tendency to speak more quietly than before therapy. In these cases, treatment is not complete until accept-ably loud, effortless voice can be produced which allows the speaker to communicate as vigorously as desired. In the second category, some patients with soft vocal nodules, for example, can produce relatively normal voice by increased hyperadduction of their vocal folds, which over-rides the effect of the nodules. If this pattern of phonation persists the vocal fold mucosa sustains further damage.

It is advisable, therefore, to ask a patient if the throat feels comfort-able or back to normal as normal voice is achieved, and to take seriously complaints of unusual or uncomfortable throat sensations, even when the voice is well within normal limits. Laryngoscopic examination will help to clarify the basis of the problem. The patient should not be discharged until the sensory symptoms are resolved.

The larynx and voice are within normal limits but vocal stamina is limited

The degree of vocal stamina required varies from one patient to another according to personality, lifestyle and occupation. Patients should be helped to achieve the vocal skills necessary to sustain a normal vocal note to meet their requirements throughout extensive pitch and loudness ranges, if physiologically possible. In some cases, further regular treatment sessions are required whereas, in others, if the patient is able to develop the tech-niques practised in treatment, regular review appointments until discharge can provide support. There is a danger of patients developing effortful voice production in a misguided attempt to sustain voice if they are discharged before sufficient vocal stamina to meet their needs has been established.

The patient is reluctant to conclude treatment

As in many clinical relationships, complex factors which are well recog-nised in the psychology literature can contribute to interdependence between the patient and speech–language pathologist. The patient, fre-quently anxious and distressed, initially seeks a solution to the voice prob-lem and, as treatment progresses, may form an attachment to the clinician. The support, concern and sensitivity arising from professional commit-ment are sometimes perceived by vulnerable or emotionally isolated patients as having a deeper personal basis. It is for these reasons that, while taking account of patients' feelings and emotions, the speech–language therapist should retain a certain professional distance so that the risk of caring behaviour being misinterpreted is minimised. Even when these factors are taken into account, some patients are reluctant to be discharged despite normal vocal function having been achieved, and they may present a number of reasons why they are not yet ready to conclude treatment. These arguments should be addressed positively and care should be taken to ensure that there are no significant problems before the patient is discharged. Referral to a psychologist or counsellor may be necessary.

Patients who lack confidence in their newly established voices sometimes want to delay discharge. In these circumstances, if the speech–language pathologist concludes that the voice is satisfactory, a gradual withdrawal of treatment can be helpful. If the time between each appointment is increased, the patient feels supported while re-establishing voice use on a daily basis. Referral to a singing or voice teacher, in order to further develop the voice that has returned to normal, should be arranged when patients feel that they need further help.

Poor patient compliance

If a patient does not comply with voice therapy, treatment is unlikely to be successful. Professionally, this is unsatisfactory and frustrating because of the time that is wasted when other patients might benefit from treatment. Although the number of patients who do not comply with treatment is probably small, it is important to discover the reasons for non-compliance before deciding to discharge those who fail to cooperate. Some of these reasons are summarised in Table 12.7.

- When patients are unconvinced of the need for voice therapy, it is usually because they do not understand what it is, why it is necessary and what it can achieve. Explanations by the laryngologist and speech–language therapist at the time of referral and the initial session can change misconceptions and enable the patient to begin treatment with conviction.

Table 12.7 Voice therapy: reasons for poor compliance

- Patient unconvinced of need for voice therapy
- Lack of concern about the disordered voice
- Lack of insight into own vocal and general behaviour
- Emotional factors
- Patient thinks voice pathologist is unable to help

- Lack of concern about an abnormal voice is based on various factors: it does not present a problem functionally; the patient does not realise that it might deteriorate further or, on having been told that there is no disease, the patient is no longer concerned. The clinician's course of action will vary according to the aetiology of the voice disorder. Most importantly, in conditions where the lack of voice therapy is likely to result in damage or further damage to the vocal fold mucosa, the possible consequences should be explained to the patient. In cases such as presbyphonia (see page 563), where a degree of age-related muscle atrophy and changes in the vocal fold mucosa cause voice changes, patients sometimes decide not to embark on therapy when they have been reassured that there is no disease causing their voice changes. It seems unnecessary to compel such patients to attend for treatment. Explanations and reassurances that treatment will be available if the patient would like to proceed with therapy at a later date are sufficient.
- When patients have poor insight into their own vocal and general behaviour, their lack of compliance with treatment may be unintentional. Consequently, if they are unaware that their loud, effortful phonation is only one aspect of a generally aggressive manner, or that a 'pressed', low-pitched voice reflects pomposity, they will find it difficult to change vocally. Compliance can be achieved by helping patients to understand the context in which their vocal behaviour occurs.
- Significant emotional factors can prevent a patient from complying with treatment. The help of a psychologist or counsellor should be sought if distress, anxiety or depression, which is more fundamental than a reaction to the voice problem, prevents the patient from complying.
- It should not be forgotten that non-compliance might be the fault of the speech–language pathologist and not patient based. If the patient doubts the clinician's competency, if treatment sessions are poorly focused and appear to have an uncertain theoretical base, or if patients are given the impression that they are not being listened to, they are unlikely to respect the clinician sufficiently to comply with therapy. Patients comply with professional advice most readily when they respect and like the clinician.

The professional voice user

The professional voice user can present particular issues with regard to being discharged. The demands on vocal performance exceed those of most speakers in terms of vocal loading and skills required. As a result, treatment of disordered voices in this group is directed at higher levels of performance, so that professional requirements can be consistently met without causing vocal fold trauma. Singers and actors have particular vocal demands (see Chapter 16). The final stages of treatment ideally take place concurrently with singing or voice lessons so that, on discharge from therapy, the patient's instruction continues seamlessly. Some singers and actors find it helpful to have review appointments in the voice clinic from time to time. In this way, they can discuss any difficulties or concerns that they are experiencing with their voices, as a preventive procedure.

After successful treatment, patients can usually be placed in one of the categories listed in Table 12.8 when they are finally discharged from a course of voice therapy.

Table 12.8 Discharge categories after voice therapy

Voice problem resolved
Some aspects of the voice problem remain but:
• the patient regards the voice as functionally satisfactory
• the laryngologist is satisfied that the larynx is healthy
• the speech–language pathologist is satisfied that the new phonatory behaviours are secure and not potentially damaging
Maximum improvement or compensation in an irreversible condition

It is perhaps even more important that a suitable course of action is taken when it becomes evident that voice therapy is unsuccessful. The speech–language pathologist must consider that intervention might not produce a satisfactory outcome when one or more of the following factors occurs:

- The vocal profile shows no improvement, even when the expected timescale for improvement in a particular condition has passed.
- Progress plateaus at a level below satisfactory vocal function.
- Vocal behaviours remain unchanged.
- Voice therapy appears to be associated with further deterioration.
- No therapeutic or management route produces positive results.

In some cases, allowing further time will produce a favourable solution, but it is a matter of clinical judgement to recognise when intervention should be concluded if progress plateaus or regresses. It is important that the patient's needs are taken into account and that treatment does not merely cease. There are three courses of action that can be taken if voice therapy is finally judged to be unsuccessful.

- Laryngeal status should be reviewed using videostrobolaryngoscopy. This is the most revealing laryngeal examination and will reveal abnormalities of vocal fold structure and function, which cannot be observed on any other laryngeal examination (see page 432).
- The voice therapy treatment programme should be comprehensively reviewed and revised, if necessary.
- Referral to another professional (e.g. neurologist, psychiatrist) may be necessary either for further diagnostic information or to deal with other causative factors.

After review of the situation, it may be possible to recommence voice therapy and progress to a successful outcome. Ultimately, it is important that all routes are explored before a patient is discharged if the voice continues to be abnormal.

Outcome measures

An outcome is the amount of change in the physical, mental and social states, which comprise health, as the result of treatment or non-treatment (World Health Organization, 1971). Measuring outcomes is an essential element of ascertaining the effectiveness of treatment. For many years, outcome measures in many clinical disciplines have concentrated on the physical aspects of a given condition, which can be measured objectively. This has also applied to the treatment of voice disorders. The acquisition of objective information through the procedures described in Chapter 13 (e.g. laryngoscopy, acoustic analysis, electroglottography) provides an essential baseline against which outcomes can be measured. This physical model of outcome measurement has, however, tended to overlook the patient's mental and social state (Benninger et al., 1998). In recent years, there has been increasing recognition of the importance of measuring changes in a patient's quality of life as the result of treatment. Outcome measures, such as the Voice Handicap Index (VHI) (see page 465) address this issue (Jacobson et al., 1997) and should be incorporated into the battery of outcome measures used by the voice clinician.

Summary

■ Voice therapy alone is the preferred treatment for most voice disorders.

■ Voice therapy is an essential adjunct to phonosurgery pre- and postoperatively.

■ A team approach, with a laryngologist and specialist speech–language pathologist working closely together, provides the most comprehensive analysis, evaluation and treatment of the voice-disordered patient.

■ Laryngoscopic examination is mandatory before accepting patients with voice disorders for treatment.

■ The process of voice therapy consists of a hierarchy of key stages that are interdependent.

■ Voice therapy is an interactive process to which the speech–language pathologist and the patient both contribute.

13 CHAPTER

Analysis and evaluation: instrumental and perceptual

In clinical practice, the purpose of analysis and evaluation is to collect information about the patient and his or her voice disorder in order to compile a comprehensive description of the problem and the relevant issues. Subsequently, the diagnosis and management plan are based on this essential information. Certain aspects enable the laryngologist and speech–language pathologist to quantify the deviation of vocal function from the norm and so to establish a baseline that will act as a point of reference as treatment progresses. The most effective assessments are those where the results of each investigation are finally synthesised to produce a diagnosis and a cohesive hypothesis for the patient's voice disorder. Amassing large amounts of data is not an effective basis in itself for resolving voice disorders. It is the informed and careful interpretation of salient facts and observations that enables the clinician to come to valid conclusions which contribute to an improvement.

Procedures vary from one centre to another, but protocols ensure that a suitable procedure is followed. Throughout the entire process, it must be remembered that the evaluation is being carried out for the benefit of the patient, not of the examining clinician. To disregard the patient's feelings and concerns throughout the process of information gathering and data collection is not only insensitive, but can subsequently adversely affect treatment if confidence and goodwill are lost. Conversely, if the patient comes to trust the examining clinicians, information might be collected that would otherwise have been withheld. The patient is entitled to explanations about the purpose of each aspect of the investigations and should be informed of the findings in appropriate terms. Some procedures, such as laryngoscopic examination, can cause considerable anxiety and this can be exacerbated by the way in which clinicians relate to patients. As a result, the true picture of the problem is distorted and the information does not necessarily reflect the actual situation. A maximally productive process of compiling comprehensive information also depends on a proactive and analytical attitude to the emerging information by the clinician. Anomalies between apparent facts and points of information that are incongruous should be explored, expanded and verified to ensure that the information reflects reality.

The process of assessment begins from the first contact, whether hearing patients on the telephone, seeing them in the waiting room or watching how they relate to others. These are the opportunities for evaluating vocal function, and other factors, outside the constraints of clinical tasks. Patients' reactions and responses to assessment procedures can be informative in themselves and are discussed in the following sections. Bless (1991a, 1991b) lists the five basic steps of voice evaluation as:

- interviewing
- observing
- describing the voice
- comparing observations to standards and normal values
- integrating the information to determine treatment.

There are four broad categories of assessment for voice disorders described and discussed in this chapter (Table 13.1).

THE CASE HISTORY

Information relating to each patient is compiled on a form, which varies from one centre to another. A scheme followed routinely ensures that important information about each patient is not omitted and it also acts as a standard guide to all members of a department. (Comprehensive case history information can also be a valuable resource for retrospective research and for audit studies designed to improve patient care.) Some of the reasons for the information requested on the case history form (Figure 13.1) are discussed below.

Table 13.1 Analysis and evaluation procedures

- Case history
- Laryngoscopic examination
- Evaluation of voice: perceptual and instrumental
- Patient self-rating

VOICE DISORDER: CASE HISTORY FORM

Name...   Date of Birth....................................

Address......................................   Hospital number..............................

....   General practitioner.........................

....   Laryngologist.................................

Tel.(home)....................................   Voice pathologist
Tel.(work)....................................   ....

Other professional staff
....
....
....

Occupation....................................

DIAGNOSIS ....

Laryngoscopic examination(s)

Date(s)   Type:
   (• mirror laryngoscopy
   • nasendoscopy / nasendoscopy +
    stroboscopy
   • rigid endoscopy / rigid endoscopy +
    stroboscopy
   • direct laryngoscopy
    under general anaesthetic)

....
....
....
....

Audio recordings ....
....
....

Video recordings ....
....
....

VOICE HISTORY

1. Chronology of voice disorder (e.g. date of onset, remissions / recurrences, etc.)
....
....
....
....

(continued)

2. Patient's reaction to voice disorder/ opinion re: cause

....

....

....

....

3. Voice variability

....

....

....

....

4. Vocal tract discomfort

Burning, soreness, tickling, irritation (i.e. inflammatory symptoms)

....

Aching, tightness (i.e. musculoskeletal symptoms)

....

5. Patient's report of listener reactions to voice disorder

....

....

....

....

6. Previous voice problems

....

....

....

....

7. Previous voice therapy

....

....

....

....

MEDICAL HISTORY

1. Operations...

   Illnesses..

   Neuropathology...

   Other conditions..

   ....

   ....

2. Specific respiratory tract problems (e.g. asthma, allergies, etc.)

   ....

   ....

   ....

   ....

(continued)

3. Gastric/laryngopharyngeal reflux..
   Medication...

4. Psychiatric / psychological treatment and / or counselling
   ....

5. Hormonal status (e.g. peri-/postmenopausal; hypo-/hyperthyroidism)
   ....
   ....

6. Back/neck problems..
   ....

7. Hearing...

8. Current medication...
   ....
   ....

VOCAL TRACT HYGIENE

1. Does patient smoke?   Yes / No

   Cigarettes / cigars / pipe / other..

   How many / much?..

   Past smoker? Yes / No   How many?..............   How long ago?............

2. Alcohol intake and type..

3. Coffee / tea / canned drinks intake ....

4. Water intake..

OCCUPATIONAL DEMANDS ON VOICE

1. Professional voice user?..

2. Amount of voice use..

3. Type of voice use (eg telephone, vocal projection required, high levels of
   background noise, etc.)
   ....
   ....
   ....

4. Levels of stress / tension..
   ....

(continued)

DOMESTIC SITUATION

1. **Number of people in household** (note number of children; individuals with hearing loss, etc.)
    ....
    ....

2   **Housing conditions**
    ....

LEISURE ACTIVITIES

1. **Vocal hobbies** (e.g. singing, acting)..
    ....

2. **Significant vocal demands** (eg clubs, pubs, some restaurants, shouting / grunting during sport)

EMOTIONAL STATUS

....
....
....

SUMMARY OF DIAGNOSTIC LISTENING AND OBSERVATION

....
....
....
....

ATTACHED REPORTS

1. Videostroboscopy

2. Formal perceptual evaluation (e.g. GRBAS, VPA, Buffalo III)

3. (a) Palpatory findings
    (b) Patient self-rating scale of vocal tract discomfort.

4. Instrumental evaluation:
    (i)   electroglottography
    (ii)   acoustic analysis
    (iii) aerodynamic measurements
    (iv)   vocal tract imaging
    (v)   electrophysiology

5. Patient self-rating protocol (e.g. Voice Handicap Index)

(continued)

CONCLUSIONS

....

....

....

....

....

MANAGEMENT PLAN

Goals...   Strategies...

....

....

....

....

DISCHARGE: SUMMARY OF MANAGEMENT

- Number of treatment sessions   ....
- Length of each treatment session   ....
- Length of treatment period   ....
- Type of discharge:
    - voice within normal limits   ....
    - voice functionally satisfactory   ....
    - maximum improvement in
      irreversible condition   ....

Figure 13.1 Case history form.

Laryngoscopic examination

The way in which the larynx has been examined is significant because of the very different quality and clarity of the images of laryngeal structure and function that are obtained by the various procedures (see below). Ideally, speech–language pathologists view the larynx with laryngologists or carry out laryngoscopic examination themselves. If the speech–language pathologist has not been present during the laryngoscopic examination and is dependent on a written report, it is particularly important that the method of laryngeal examination is known. It might influence whether further or more sophisticated laryngoscopy is requested to clarify the biomechanical basis of the dysphonia. Further complications can also arise because of the lack of consistency in the terminology used to describe laryngeal pathology, even by laryngologists in the same country or the same hospital. A small, unilateral, benign mass lesion might be called a nodule by one laryngologist but a sessile polyp by another who regards nodules as always being bilateral lesions. The speech–language pathologist who does not view and discuss the findings with the laryngologist must clarify these details because they can affect the treatment approach and possible timescale of treatment.

Voice history

Chronological account of voice disorder

The chronology of the voice disorder reveals the progressive stages of the problem and the timespan over which the voice has deteriorated. It is frequently possible to relate the onset to a precipitating factor or an event that the patient considers as the cause. It is relevant whether the voice deteriorated steadily, or disappeared suddenly. If the problem is episodic, the frequency and length of each dysphonic episode should be noted, together with periods of normal or greatly improved vocal function.

The patient's reaction to the problem

The patient's view of the voice disorder reveals its significance in relation to working, social and family life, and may not concur with the clinician's perceptual or objective evaluation of the problem. The actor whose voice becomes mildly hoarse by the end of a performance may view his voice disorder as severe, whereas a market trader who is severely dysphonic by the end of the day's trading considers that there is a problem only when he loses his voice completely. The obvious anxiety of the professional voice user and all those whose ability to communicate effectively depends on an efficient voice, making maximum use of paralinguistic features, should not be dismissed as neurotic. The concerns may be well founded for that person. The patient's perception of the ways in which the voice has changed can help to clarify the problem and contribute to treatment goals.

Voice variability

The pattern of vocal deterioration can give diagnostic information. For example, if a voice deteriorates as it is used throughout the day, but tends to recover when rested, it is reasonable to suppose that it is being misused or that excessive demands are being made which it is unable to meet. A voice that is worse in the morning may have been misused during the previous evening and affected by gastric reflux during the night. Alternatively, in some cases where there is significant psychological aetiology, there is a pattern of vocal deterioration at the start of the day or before a stressful event. When this information is considered in conjunction with the laryngoscopic findings, the aetiology of the dysphonia emerges. Previous voice problems and their relationship with the current symptoms must be explored and previous voice therapy reports should be requested.

Vocal tract discomfort

Patients with voice disorders frequently experience vocal tract discomfort (Mathieson, 1993a) (see page 124). For some, these sensory symptoms are more distressing and cause more concern than the vocal changes. Discomfort cannot be quantified objectively but it is important to form an impression of the patient's perception of the experience to avoid disregarding an aspect of the problem that the patient considers to be important. Linear self-ratings of severity of discomfort at the initial assessment, and subsequently as progress is reviewed, give useful insights into a particular patient's experience of the problem, although they cannot be regarded as reliable indicators of the severity of the discomfort across a population (see Figure 13.3 on page 421). Qualitative information should be collected because it can help to direct treatment strategies according to the type of discomfort (Mathieson, 1993a). It can be standardised by supplying perceptual terms related to vocal tract discomfort that fall into two broad categories: inflammation and musculoskeletal tension (see Figure 13.3 on page 421). The severity of the musculoskeletal tension can be investigated by palpation of the extrinsic laryngeal musculature and laryngeal cartilages (see below).

Patient's report of listener reactions to the voice disorder

This information provides useful insights into everyday vocal function and into the patient's relationships with family, colleagues and friends.

Occupational vocal demands

Professional voice users, such as teachers, lecturers, preachers, singers, actors and aerobics instructors, and those who work in noisy surroundings, are at risk of vocal misuse and abuse. Environmental conditions in the place of work may include irritants that aggravate the mild chronic laryngeal inflammation. A smoky, dusty or over-dry atmosphere with non-humidified central heating can be harmful. The sensitive mucous membrane of the larynx becomes dry and irritants provoke coughing which, in turn, further aggravates the condition. The importance of voice to the patient's job, and whether or not employment is in jeopardy because of the dysphonia, must be established. 'Rationalisation' and 'down-sizing' of the workforce as a result of increasing technology and financial pressures means that unemployment hangs over the heads of many people. The individual who anticipates being made redundant, or who is in a career backwater because of a take-over, can experience the same level of anxiety as someone who is unemployed. These stresses will affect treatment progress.

Domestic situation

Information is required about the patient's home life, encompassing the physical environment and other members of the family or those with whom the home is shared. Shouting at a dog can have a traumatising effect on the larynx, but is frequently less forceful than shouting at a difficult child when frustration and anger are powerful components. The laryngeal effect of shouting at a deaf relative is aggravated by irritation and guilt, with which it is frequently associated. In any relationship that is unsatisfactory, the effect of severe dysphonia on communication can increase the existing problems. More detailed information about domestic relationships is usually acquired during later sessions.

Leisure activities

The patient's social life may be vocally demanding, with activities such as choral singing and amateur dramatics, or considerable time being spent in the smoky and noisy atmosphere of a pub or club, or shouting at football matches. During the past decade, karaoke singing appears to be a factor in some cases of vocal abuse and training with weights can encourage grunting with forceful vocal fold adduction. In some households talking is against the constant background noise of television or radio. In addition, a more complete profile of the individual is compiled by discovering interests and hobbies.

Emotional status

Observation of patients may provide substantial information about their psychological state during the initial consultation, but direct questioning at a subsequent interview, if appropriate or necessary, often yields more representative information.

Diagnostic listening and observation

From the moment of first meeting and throughout the patient's account, considerable information can be collected by the speech–language pathologist by observing non-verbal communication and listening to vocal features. Levels of motivation and potential cooperation become apparent and influence the therapeutic approach. Posture reflects tension both generally in the body and specifically in the neck and face. It will also provide information about the individual's personality and feelings of self-worth. Eye contact, facial expression and hand movements give clues to the emotional state. The speech–language pathologist should be alert to the patient who gives out ambiguous messages; an assurance that all is well at home may be accompanied by a facial expression that 'says' the opposite and by eye avoidance. Minimal facial expression can signal a negative response to the clinician or it may indicate depression or intense emotion. The mask-like face of the Parkinson's disease patient, which is neurologically based, conceals emotions that must not be overlooked. Every attempt should be made to put the patient at ease. Apparently negative emotions and a 'difficult' manner are not necessarily a true reflection of the patient's usual behaviour, but arise from anxiety and concern. A negative response by the clinician compounds the problem; acceptance and encouragement are generally more constructive.

The way in which patients describe voice problems can range from the dramatically histrionic, although the symptoms are minimal, to the unnaturally stoic despite considerable handicap. These factors should be observed and noted because they may be relevant to diagnosis and must be taken into consideration during treatment.

Evaluation of voice and vocal function

Methods of assessment can be classified broadly into subjective (or perceptual) and objective (or instrumental). The two processes are complementary and each is composed of a number of elements that constitute a comprehensive profile of the problem when results are amassed. In practice, perceptual and objective analyses overlap in some areas because the interpretation of some instrumentally acquired information is essentially subjective. Although the most advanced laryngovideostroboscopic equipment (see below) provides an excellent image of laryngeal structure and function, for example, the interpretation of its fine detail ultimately depends on the skill and experience of the clinician.

The reasons for analysis and evaluation of the voice and vocal function are summarised in Table 13.2.

Table 13.2 Reasons for analysis and evaluation of voice

- Description
- Diagnosis
- Comparisons with normative data
- Formulate management plan
- Determine treatment strategies
- Monitor treatment progress
- Provide outcome measures
- Clinical research

PERCEPTUAL EVALUATION OF VOICE

The assessment of dysphonia which relies on auditory perception ('the ear') of the therapist is, in the final analysis, the most telling evaluation possible. When objective acoustic measures alone are used to analyse vocal quality, they appear to 'represent only a fraction of the set of all measures used by the human listener' (Eskenazi, Childers and Hicks, 1990). How a voice sounds and how far the voice meets the speaker's needs is the ultimate dictum in the rehabilitation programme. Perceptual evaluation is an integrated process of listening to and describing a particular voice. The clinician needs intensive training in the vocal dimensions that identify pathology most effectively. Rating voice quality perceptually is universally acknowledged as a difficult task and one that requires considerable experience (Bassich and Ludlow, 1986). Although it is generally recognised that no electronic instrument can replace 'the ear', instruments provide accurate measurement of specific parameters in voice production such as volume, pitch and airflow. The conclusion of the evaluation and the subsequent treatment route depends on the amalgamation of perceptual and instrumental information with other physical, psychological and lifestyle findings. Subjective and instrumental assessment results form the baseline on which progress is evaluated.

A major issue in the perceptual evaluation of voice is the problem of description. There are no reliable verbal terms defining vocal characteristics, although there is a continuous struggle to produce a definitive descriptive terminology. Adjectives may have different meanings for different people. Fairbanks (1960) thought the great variety of perceptible vocal symptoms could be classified under three headings: harshness, breathiness and hoarseness, and given ratings on a scale of 0–5. Few experts can agree with this: hoarseness is breathy and harshness may mean metallic (Aronson, 1980). Case (1991) listed over 40 vocal misuse and abuse characteristics and what amounts in reality to 40 bones of contention.

A universally acceptable and understood nomenclature would be of great value in writing reports, assessing treatment and progress, and comparing research results of other workers in the field. Nevertheless, researchers endeavour to overcome the difficulties of compiling an accurate verbal profile that is universally acceptable. Wynter and Martin (1981) spent 5 years in an attempt at training speech pathology students to remember and identify characteristics of dysphonia by listening to sample recordings. A team of experienced speech therapists had classified and agreed on the description of 100 recordings. The categories were: creaky, husky, hoarse, harsh, disordered pitch, disordered resonance and 'others'. The 'others' included voices that 'defied any attempt to be categorised under present terminology'. This admission, of course, caused complications from the outset but the final concession of defeat took 5 years to materialise. The results of the research were disappointing because the auditory perception of the trained students failed to match closely the perception of the researchers.

Subsequently, research conducted by Hammarberg (1986) was directed at correlating perceptual vocal characteristics of vocal dysfunction with acoustic characteristics. Initial studies showed that speech pathologists who were experienced in the diagnosis and therapy of voice disorders could agree on 12 voice quality parameters:

•	aphonic/intermittent aphonic	•	breathy
•	hyperfunctional/tense	•	hypofunctional/lax
•	vocal fry/creaky	•	rough
•	grating	•	diplophonic
•	voice breaks	•	instability
•	register	•	pitch.

Acoustic correlates were found for nine of these voice qualities. Hammarberg (1986) pointed out that perceptual voice evaluation by clinically well-trained listeners can be reliable if based on standardised rating procedures, and that training for voice therapists can be more effective if perceptual–acoustic relationships are identified. In the same year, these issues were addressed by Wendler and Anders (1986). Hammarberg and Gauffin (1995), and Wolfe and Martin (1997) have subsequently developed this work.

As a result of the problems associated with descriptive terminology, a scheme of phonetic symbols for transcribing vocal quality has been developed (Ball, 1996; Ball, Esling and Dickson, 2000) in an attempt to overcome the problems of impressionistic labelling (Figure 13.2). The VoQS (Voice Quality Symbols) system is divided into three main parts: airstream types, phonation types and supralaryngeal settings. The symbols can represent both normal and disordered voice.

Perceptual evaluation can be conducted informally in general conversation and formally, using a protocol based on standard terms and categories. Both processes are important components in describing the disordered voice and one is not used to the exclusion of the other.

Informal perceptual evaluation

The speech–language pathologist specialising in the treatment of voice disorders gradually develops skills of perceptual evaluation, which are employed automatically when listening to any voice, particularly patients'

VoQS: Voice Quality Symbols

AIRSTREAM TYPES

Œ	oesophageal speech	И	electrolarynx speech
ɪO	tracheo-oesophageal speech	↓	pulmonic ingressive speech

PHONATION TYPES

V	modal voice	F	falsetto
W	whisper	C	creak
V̤	whispery voice (murmur)	V̰	creaky voice
C̬	whispery creak	V!	harsh voice
V!!	ventricular phonation	V̰!!	diplophonia
V̪	anterior or pressed phonation	W̠	posterior whisper

SUPRALARYNGEAL SETTINGS

L̝	raised larynx	L̞	lowered larynx
Vœ	labialised voice (open round)	Vʷ	labialised voice (close round)
V̈	spread-lip voice	Vᵛ	labio-dentalised voice
V̺	linguo-apicalised voice	V̻	linguo-laminalised voice
V˞	retroflex voice	V̪	dentalized voice
V̳	alveolarized voice	V̲ʲ	palatoalveolarised voice
Vʲ	palatalized voice	Vˠ	velarized voice
Vʁ	uvularized voice	Vˤ	pharyngealized voice
V̰ˤ	laryngo-pharyngealised voice	Vᴴ	faucalised voice
Ṽ	nasalised voice	V̷	denasalised voice
J̞	open jaw voice	J̝	close jaw voice
J̪	right offset jaw voice	J̠	left offset jaw voice
J̟	protruded jaw voice	⊖	protruded tongue voice

Use of labelled braces and numerals to mark stretches of speech
and degrees and combinations of voice quality

[ˈðɪs ɪz ˈnɔˑməl ˈvɔɪs {3V! ˈðɪs ɪz ˈveɹi ˈhɑˑʃ ˈvɔɪs 3V!} ˈðɪs ɪz ˈnɔˑməl ˈvɔɪs
wʌns ˈmɔˑ {L̝1V! ˈðɪs ɪz ˈles ˈhɑˑʃ ˈvɔɪs wɪð ˈloʊəd ˈlæɪŋks 1V!L̝}]

Figure 13.2 The VoQS System. (by permission of Professor Martin J. Ball)

voices. Consequently, informal perceptual evaluation takes place from the moment of meeting the patient and throughout assessment and treatment. Observations of spontaneous speech can be organised into the following categories.

Speech–breathing patterns

Habitual breathing patterns at rest and during connected speech are observed. If the patient appears to be breathless on entering the room or at rest, phonation will almost certainly be compromised as metabolic needs will have priority over breathing for speech. A 'noisy' chest, either wheezing or 'bubbly', may accompany shortness of breath and breathing may be effortful and rapid. Air intake can also be noisy at the laryngeal level. In its most extreme form, when there is laryngeal obstruction, this is known as inspiratory stridor and can be present at rest and on exertion as well as before speaking. In the absence of laryngeal obstruction, noisy air intake in the form of a slight gasp can indicate tense laryngeal musculature, with the vocal folds not fully abducted on inspiration. Some speakers appear to run out of air and to use residual air towards the end of phrases and sentences. This may be caused by shallow, upper chest breathing and, as a result, insufficient volume of air to maintain adequate subglottic air pressure. In some individuals, with normal air capacity, there is a tendency to continue to speak although they have run out of air. It seems that their need to continue until the end of the sentence, to inhibit interjection from others or the urgency of their communication overrides their need to replenish air intake. Speech rate is usually very rapid and anxiety may be high. As with all symptoms, the underlying aetiology, whether organic or behavioural, must be clarified to ensure that appropriate treatment is instituted.

Phonation

Informal perceptual evaluation of the patient's voice in connected speech during general conversation can be organised into categories that comprise a vocal profile, in the same way in which the more formal subjective and instrumental profiles are compiled (see below). The voice in conversation is the best example of the patient's voice in daily life and, in most cases, most accurately represents the communication deficit. Table 13.3 indicates aspects of the voice and vocal behaviour that should be considered.

Articulation

Articulatory patterns and observation of oromotor movements can provide important diagnostic clues regarding organic and behavioural elements of voice disorders. Neurogenic voice disorders arising from central nervous system lesions are frequently accompanied by dysarthria, which indicates muscle tone and levels of effort required to initiate movement. In other categories of voice disorder, excessive muscular tension is apparent through over-articulation or marked mouth closure during speech. The latter may

Table 13.3 Informal perceptual evaluation of phonation

Vocal behaviours and parameters	Possible features observed
Fundamental vocal note quality	Rough Breathy 'Wet' Consistent quality Varies according to pitch/loudness/phonation/or vegetative behaviour/emotion
Habitual pitch	Too high/low Unstable
Pitch range	Monopitch Limited in upper range Flexible intonation Extremes of pitch range
Loudness	Too quiet/loud Loudness decay, i.e. Voice becomes quieter at end of utterance, or as conversation progresses
Resonance	Hyper-/hyponasal
Onset	Hard glottal attack may coexist with breathy output
Vocal habits	Vigorous throat-clearing and coughing
Extrinsic laryngeal muscles	Observation of the neck during conversation can reveal tense strap muscles Excessive/restricted laryngeal vertical excursions
Vocal stamina/fatigue	Voice deteriorates/improves with use during interview

Aberrations	Normal voice may be heard on vegetative tasks,
	  e.g. laughing, but not during phonation
	Voice does not reflect laryngoscopic findings, or is
	  much better/worse than expected

Posture	Excessive chin raising or lowering affecting
	  laryngeal position and movement
	Jutting head forward affecting laryngeal movement
	  and dimensions of supralaryngeal spaces
	Stooped, rounded shoulders affecting chest
	  expansion

The aspects of phonation can be observed informally in general conversation with the patient.

give a hypernasal quality to the voice. The speaker may also clench the teeth when at rest. Marked tongue bunching in these individuals can lead to supraglottic tension and a raised larynx. The individual with aspirations to higher social status may assume an accent that is accompanied by considerable tension. In any case, different accents require different articulatory movements, such as more or less lip-rounding, which can affect vocal quality.

Formal perceptual evaluation

Formal perceptual evaluation enables the speech–language pathologist to quantify the problem as well as describe the voice in an organised profile (Carding et al., 2000). By confining the description to a set number of terms, the formal assessment attempts to minimise the confusion that can arise from a plethora of synonyms and ambiguous descriptors. The rationale for carrying out formal perceptual evaluation of voice in a clinical setting is outlined in Table 13.4. The fact that perceptual evaluations do not produce hard data and no single protocol is universal mean that certain problems are intrinsic to the process. First, there a great many different schemes globally. In the USA alone, it appears that there are 57 different schemes (Kreiman et al., 1993). Each scheme uses different terminology and even when similar terminology is used it may not have the same definition. The three schemes described below illustrate some of these issues. They are the most commonly used scales in the UK and are also used internationally.

Table 13.4 Formal perceptual evaluation of voice: rationale

Description of the disordered voice	Identification of disordered features Severity rating
Comparison of findings with other elements of evaluation (e.g. acoustic analysis, laryngoscopic findings)	e.g. a 'breathy' voice will be associated with a reduced HNR and glottal insufficiency Comparisons allow clinicians to confirm or refute the emerging clinical picture
Indicates intervention strategies	e.g. a 'breathy' voice indicates poor vocal fold approximation and strategies must aim to improve closure
Provides baseline vocal profile	As treatment progresses, it can be monitored against the findings of the formal perceptual evaluation
Clinical outcome measure	The effectiveness of treatment approaches can be evaluated in a clinical population
Facilitates communication about the problem with colleagues and the patient	By reducing the number of terms and having definitions of the terms used, discussions are more meaningful and confusions are less likely to arise

HNR, harmonics-to-noise ratio.

The 'GRBAS' scale

This simple scale was developed by the Committee of Phonatory Function Tests of the Japan Society of Logopedics and Phoniatrics (Hirano, 1981). The 'GRBAS' scale for evaluating hoarseness on five scales – grade (i.e. degree of voice abnormality), rough, breathy, asthenic (weak) and strained – is accompanied by a standard tape of voice samples. Each parameter is rated on a 4-point scale ranging from 0 (normal) to 3 (extreme). Although problems inevitably arise as to the exact meaning of this terminology, as in all perceptual schemes, this has been shown to be a reliable measure and is recommended for clinical and research purposes by the European Research Group on the Larynx (Dejonckere et al., 1993, 1996).

The Vocal Profile Analysis Protocol

The search for a verbal blueprint was pursued by Laver (1980) who endeavoured to establish a phonetic description of voice quality. He charted the positions of labial, mandibular, lingual, velopharyngeal and laryngeal structures to which he gave tension ratings. Phonation types are classified as harshness, whispery, breathiness, creaky, falsetto and modal. Originally, Laver thought that writing a book and producing a cassette of illustrative phonation types would produce clinicians who could complete the Vocal Profile Analysis (VPA) without further training. It became evident, however, that seminars and specific training in labelling of Laver's phonation types were essential. The VPA presents a formidable list of items and demonstrates the immense variety of vocal qualities and phonetic gestures possible. This list alone provides a useful indicator of vocal features to be considered during assessment of the dysphonic patient. The charting of phonetic positions is based on listening and visual observation of articulatory sets unsupported by lateral radiographs. The emphasis on articulatory gestures is valuable in alerting the speech–language pathologist to these important aspects of phonation and sites of excessive tension described above (see Appendix B). A 2-day training course has to be attended before the VPA can be used.

Buffalo III Voice Profile

The Buffalo III Voice Profile developed by Wilson (1987) is probably the most commonly used scheme in the USA (Kreiman et al., 1993). It rates the following parameters – laryngeal tone, loudness, pitch, nasal resonance, oral resonance, breath supply, muscles, voice abuse, rate, speech anxiety, speech intelligibility and overall voice efficiency – on a 5-point scale, with appropriate descriptive terms listed for marking with each category. Speech samples should include connected speech, oral reading, individual

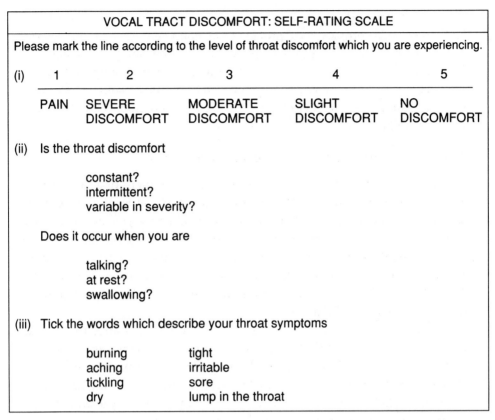

Figure 13.3 Vocal tract discomfort: self-rating scale. Burning, tickling, dry, irritable and sore tend to indicate inflammatory changes. Aching and tight usually relate to musculoskeletal tension. 'Lump in the throat': if this is ticked it might mean pharyngeal tension but some patients use this description when they feel laryngeal secretions accumulating, i.e. 'frog in the throat' (see globus symptoms [page 218]): there are many possible causes of this sensation and these should be investigated and excluded.

phonemes and counting. This scheme rates more general behaviour related to phonation than the VPA and GRBAS.

The speech–language pathologist's decision regarding the most suitable scheme to use will depend on various factors:

- The clinical setting: for routine evaluation of patients with voice problems, it is helpful if all clinicians within a department use the same protocol as a minimum standard. This facilitates communication, develops perceptual skills in relation to a particular scheme and enables them to evaluate each other's patients when necessary in order to maintain continuity. The GRBAS can fulfil this role as a basic, relatively reliable scheme.

- Information that will direct treatment: in addition to a foundation scheme, a complex vocal profile can be compiled using a more detailed scheme. The VPA and the Buffalo have the advantage of giving clear indications of vocal behaviour that might be contributing to or maintaining the dysphonia, and therefore can be useful in planning treatment.
- Reliability: in clinical practice, and for research, inter- and intrajudge reliability is an important factor.

Palpation of the extrinsic laryngeal musculature

Palpatory examination of the neck during the assessment of a patient with a voice disorder provides information about the status of the extrinsic laryngeal musculature and the positions of the major laryngeal cartilages at rest. Its purpose when carried out by the speech–language pathologist is not to determine the presence of disease (e.g. neoplasms), which is the responsibility of the laryngologist. Palpation can be carried out in various ways (Roy, Ford and Bless, 1998; Lieberman, 1998). A relatively straightforward method is described below.

Before the examination, it is helpful for the examiner to have an impression of the patient's perception of any sensory symptoms associated with the vocal tract. The patient who is experiencing marked discomfort should be palpated very gently initially, because pressure on the tense muscles can highlight extreme tenderness. A self-rating form is shown in Figure 13.3; this can be incorporated into the case history form.

Standing behind the patient, the examiner uses the finger-tips of the first three fingers of each hand to examine the sternocleidomastoid muscles, initially starting at the mastoid processes. Very gentle, slowly rotating pressure is gradually applied down the length of these muscles. When the muscles are relaxed, the finger-tips meet little resistance and the muscles are soft and malleable. Tense muscles feel firm and can resemble cables stretching from the mastoid process to the sternum. Palpation is approached gently because extremely tense muscles can be exquisitely tender and even moderate pressure can cause the patient extreme pain. Asymmetries should be noted. The examiner should be prepared that some patients will cough when even gentle pressure is applied to the inferior two-thirds of the sternocleidomastoid muscles. Palpation of the supralaryngeal area will be soft and yielding in a relaxed subject, but can be hard and resistant if the supralaryngeal muscles are tense, and this is frequently associated with a raised larynx elevated by the tense muscles. When the chin is lowered, the larynx may be forced down in the vocal tract and in some speakers this is a habitual posture. In this position, the hyoid bone may be concertinaed on to the thyroid cartilage, so eliminating the usual space between these structures. (Patients presenting with a forcefully lowered larynx tend to speak on a particularly low pitch and have considerable difficulty in using the middle and upper parts of their pitch range because they are inhibiting the usual vertical excursions of the larynx.)

Gentle, lateral digital pressure on each lamina of the thyroid cartilage alternately can give further information about whether or not the larynx is being held rigidly by tense surrounding muscles. In a relaxed individual, the larynx moves from side to side easily in response to gentle finger-tip pressure. In extreme tension, there is obvious resistance or complete immobility. Increased pressure should not be used to move the larynx laterally. Some patients may flinch or 'jump' if muscles are tense and tender but others are particularly stoic. It is advisable, therefore, to ask the patient to say if and where there is tenderness. Relaxed neck musculature is not tender on palpation, so tenderness is a useful indication of increased tension. A particularly tender area may be noted in the area of the hyoid bone.

The muscle tension may be the primary cause of the voice disorder and arise from a number of factors discussed elsewhere (see page 152), or have arisen as a secondary feature as the patient has attempted to overcome vocal dysfunction. In many cases, it will be the result of a combination of primary and secondary factors. In addition to the palpatory information, the clinician can gain further insights into patients by their responses to the examination. Those in considerable discomfort are understandably tense initially, but many find the palpation soothing as it progresses gently. Clinical experience suggests that, when patients remain rigid and resistant throughout, there may be other underlying emotional issues.

Note 1

Care should be taken when carrying out this examination because of the major blood vessels in the region, particularly the carotid bifurcation. The voice pathologist should ensure that any pressure is confined to the muscles and cartilages being examined. This examination should be avoided in individuals with cardiovascular problems and those who are very frail. It should be stopped if the patient feels dizzy or 'light-headed'. Patients should be asked to agree to the palpatory examination which should be explained briefly beforehand. Patients tend to be more relaxed if the examiner talks to them during palpation, explaining which structures are being felt and how they are responding.

Note 2

In addition to the intended information collected during palpation, the clinician frequently finds that the patient discloses information not previously volunteered. This appears to be a combination of touching the patient, which is presumably reassuring, and standing behind them so that any stresses arising from face-to-face contact are overcome. For this reason, delaying palpation until evaluation is well advanced, and a relationship has been established, is frequently the most productive approach. These advantages also apply during laryngeal manual therapy (see page 498).

Note 3

Palpatory examination of the laryngeal area has been discussed in considerable detail by Roy, Ford and Bless (1998) and Lieberman (1998).

OBJECTIVE/INSTRUMENTAL EVALUATION OF VOICE

An extensive range of technology is available to analyse the voice and the physiology of phonation. It has become an essential part of assessment and monitoring, and is also used for biofeedback during voice therapy. Instrumentation now contributes significantly to making diagnoses and to documenting treatment outcomes (Sataloff et al., 1990; Bless, 1991a, 1991b; Karnell and Finnegan, 1994). As with all technology, the usefulness of the information it produces depends on the equipment functioning properly, the knowledge and skill of the operator, the information that is put into the equipment ('garbage in, garbage out') and, perhaps most importantly, the ability of the person interpreting the information to make informed, valid judgements. Instrumentation does not, therefore, provide all the answers just because it gives quantified, objective data. In the clinical situation, it is helpful to remember that it is providing information about vocal activity at a particular moment, i.e. what the patient did on that occasion is not necessarily what the patient generally does or is capable of doing vocally. This is an important issue when collating baseline data and care should be taken to ensure that the vocal behaviours and voice samples that are analysed are representative of the current status of the voice disorder. It is also important to compare results with normative data and to control the variables surrounding the performance of a particular task if instrumental measures are to be meaningful. Raes and Clement (1996) consider that the following factors should be taken into account when considering test results:

- age
- sex
- type, pitch and loudness of phonation task
- number of trials
- modelling of the task
- amount of task instruction, encouragement and coaching provided.

The last three factors in this list also have implications for establishing protocols, particularly in a given department. Stemple, Stanley and Lee (1995) view the variation of protocols from one research team to another as having a significant negative effect on the value of many studies of normative values. These differences are probably compounded by the use of a range of instruments of varying efficiency from one study to another.

Stemple and his co-authors recommend that 'local norms' should be established using volunteers with normal voices, the same equipment, the same methods of eliciting the required vocal behaviour, and the same recording techniques as those used with speakers with vocal pathologies.

In summary, valid assessment requires, among other things, valid and reliable selection and application of tests and instrumentation, and valid interpretation of results in order to establish a diagnosis and to appraise the problem. These, in turn, demand good understanding of the instrumentation and of the underlying physiological and physical principles.

Technology in this field is constantly developing and, although it is capable of providing an increasing amount of valuable information, it is only one aspect of the complete process of information gathering and evaluation. Some of the most commonly used methods of instrumentation are described below and summarised in Table 13.5. Although an increasing number of voice clinics and ENT departments are acquiring more sophisticated equipment for viewing the larynx, the majority are unlikely to use the extensive range of instruments that would constitute a voice laboratory because it is expensive to purchase and maintain. However, it is necessary to be aware of their potential if opportunities do arise for them to be used in the clinic, both during treatment and research, and in order to evaluate reports emanating from research laboratories and well-equipped voice clinics. An increasing emphasis on outcome measures and the efficacy of treatment by the medical and paramedical professions, health authorities and medical insurers means that objective data are increasingly important. They can provide objective information regarding the initial problem, progress can be plotted and the outcome can be measured. A degree of caution should be observed, however, with apparently objective processes that require subjective interpretation. This applies particularly to videostrobolaryngoscopy (see below), where the knowledge and experience of the examiner determine the observations and diagnosis that are made in each case. This does not detract from the importance of an examination but highlights the fact that the visual image obtained can be interpreted differently by different practitioners, particularly in cases of difficult diagnoses such as unusual manifestations. If the examiner does not know of the existence of a certain condition, he or she cannot make that diagnosis. The primary aims of instrumental assessments are listed in Table 13.6.

Lack of extensive instrumentation does not necessarily prevent voice pathologists from carrying out successful treatment, using professional knowledge and experience, but ideally this expertise is supported by the appropriate instrumentation. There are few comparative studies about the

Table 13.5 Instrumental evaluation of voice and vocal function

Method/Instrumentation	Information
Laryngoscopy (laryngeal examination)	
Mirror	
Fibreoptic flexible nasendoscopy	Laryngeal structure and function
Rigid endoscopy	
Videostroboscopy (with flexible or rigid endoscopy)	Vocal fold vibratory characteristics
Direct laryngoscopy under general anaesthetic	Laryngeal structure/biopsy if necessary
Electroglottography (laryngography, EGG)	Vocal fold contact
Vocal tract imaging	
Videofluoroscopy	Lateral and anteroposterior images of
Xeroradiography	vocal tract
MRI	
Ultra-high-speed photography	
Videokymography	
Acoustic analysis	
Audio recording	Frequency
Sound spectrography	Intensity
Acoustic analysis software	Harmonics-to-noise ratio (HNR)
	Voice range profile
Aerodynamic measurements	
Spirometer	Airflow rate and volume
Pneumotachograph	Chest wall movements
Pneumography	Subglottal air pressure
Magnetometry	Glottal resistance
	Phonation quotient
	Phonation threshold pressure
	Maximum phonation time
Electrophysiology	
Electromyography (EMG)	Muscle activity
Neurography (ENG)	

Table 13.6 Aims of instrumental assessments

- To provide objective information regarding the voice, the anatomy/physiology of the larynx and vocal tract, and respiratory function for phonation

- To provide baseline measurements of the voice and vocal function

- To monitor treatment progress

- To provide outcome measures

effectiveness of biofeedback and traditional strategies, but those available are far from producing conclusive evidence regarding instrumental biofeedback (Andrews, Warner and Stewart, 1986). The aim of therapy is to achieve the maximum improvement in the shortest period of time. If instruments are available for assessment and treatment, they must be used if they accelerate the rate of improvement. Instruments are tools that supplement a clinician's pragmatic treatment and that can provide objective evidence of change.

Instrumental examinations

LARYNGOSCOPIC EXAMINATION

Detailed information about laryngeal structure and function, and the supraglottic vocal tract, is essential for the diagnosis of voice disorders and as a basis for making decisions about appropriate intervention. Laryngoscopy is, therefore, a mandatory examination before treating any patients with a voice disorder. Laryngeal pathology can never be presumed, whatever the apparent indicators. Primarily, disease must be identified or excluded, but observation of vocal tract behaviour during phonation is also an important basis for voice therapy. Although the medical diagnosis is the responsibility of the laryngologist, the voice pathologist should regard viewing the larynx as fundamental to the evaluation, treatment planning and monitoring, and outcome measurement of voice disorders, whether or not he or she also conducts the procedure. The primary role of the laryngologist is to identify disease whereas the speech–language pathologist is concerned with evaluating phonatory behaviour. The various methods of laryngoscopic examination are described below.

Mirror laryngoscopy (Figure 13.4)

Mirror examination of the larynx is the oldest form of indirect laryngoscopy. It is the standard clinical procedure in use by laryngologists for examination of the interior larynx. It is a mandatory routine examination which, as with all laryngoscopic procedures, provides instant information regarding gross changes of the laryngeal mucosa and gross vocal fold movement. The laryngoscope consists of a small laryngeal mirror on a handle. The mirror is placed against the elevated soft palate as the patient says 'ee' at a relatively high pitch, while the laryngologist holds the patient's tongue, wrapped in gauze. Light from an external source is reflected from the laryngologist's head mirror on to the laryngeal mirror and subsequently into the pharynx and larynx. The reflection of the vocal folds in the laryngeal mirror enables them to be viewed at rest and in phonation, so that their

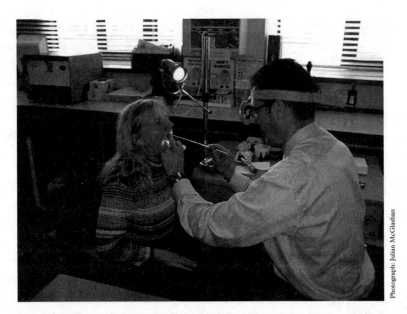

Figure 13.4 Mirror laryngoscopy.

appearance and movement can be carefully examined. In the mirror image, the right and left vocal folds are reversed and the anterior commissure appears in a posterior position. This image is the one that the laryngologist will record in the medical notes. The vocal folds cannot be viewed during continuous speech because the mirror is in the mouth. Figure 13.5 is the diagrammatic representation of the interior of the larynx used by laryngologists to illustrate laryngoscopic findings in the medical notes following mirror examination.

Direct laryngoscopy under general anaesthetic

Direct laryngoscopy under general anaesthetic is used when obvious laryngeal pathology needs to be examined more closely, and a biopsy taken (Figure 13.6). It also makes subglottal examination possible. With the development of videostroboscopy, which enables clinicians to examine laryngeal function in more detail than with the mirror, this procedure is carried out less frequently than in the past. A direct laryngoscope is inserted into the airway and the larynx is viewed with a microscope of long focal length outside the body. In this procedure, the larynx is only seen at rest, with the vocal folds moving towards the midline and away in a rhythmic movement generated by the respiratory cycle. A thorough examination of the vocal tract is possible but the actual function of the larynx in phonation, which can be so significant diagnostically, is not seen because the patient is unconscious.

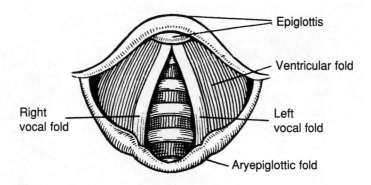

Figure 13.5 Mirror image of the interior of the larynx.

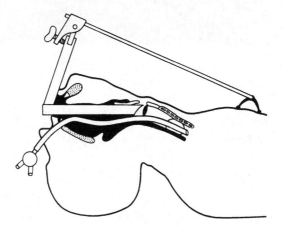

Figure 13.6 Direct laryngoscopy.

Fibreoptic laryngoscopy (Figure 13.7)

Fibreoptic laryngoscopy is a form of direct laryngoscopy because the optic is positioned just above the vocal folds. The fibreoptic laryngoscope consists of a thin flexible bundle of glass fibres containing a light source and a magnifying lens. The images are viewed through an eye piece. There is often also an additional eye piece which enables a colleague to view the larynx during the examination. The fibrescope can be attached to a camera for recording and for viewing on a TV monitor. Before the cable is inserted through the nose and passed down to an appropriate position in the pharynx, a local anaesthetic spray is administered. (The insertion of the flexible endoscope may be obstructed if the patient has a deflected septum.) An uninterrupted view is obtained of the vocal folds. At a higher level in the

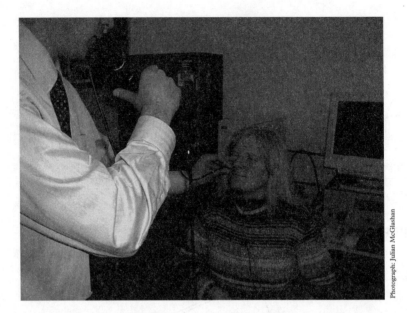

Photograph: Julian McGlashan

Figure 13.7 Fibreoptic nasendoscopy. In addition to its roles in viewing laryngeal and palatopharyngeal structure and function, the flexible fibreoptic endoscope is used in the assessment of swallowing safety in some cases of dysphagia (Langmore, Schatz and Olsen, 1988). The examination of the pharyngeal stage of swallowing, known as FEESS (fibreoptic endoscopic examination of swallowing safety) is used to detect aspiration and determine the safety of oral feeding in patients who cannot be examined with videofluoroscopy (see below).

vocal tract, the competency of the velopharyngeal sphincter can be observed when the optic is positioned just above the soft palate. The hand control on the equipment enables the examiner to move the flexible end of the tube so that vocal tract structures may be thoroughly examined. This procedure allows the patient to phonate and speak almost unimpeded. Patients frequently do not like the idea of having the flexible laryngoscope inserted into the nose but it is generally well tolerated, although the topical anaesthetic tastes unpleasant. However, this examination is frequently a successful alternative for use with patients who are unable to cooperate with rigid endoscopy. The fibreoptic laryngoscope can be used alone or in conjunction with videostroboscopy.

Rigid endoscopy (Figure 13.8)

Rigid endoscopy is a form of indirect laryngoscopy in which the endo-scope, with a 70° or 90° lens, conveys the image of the larynx to a televi-sion monitor and video recorder via a camera. It has certain advantages over the fibreoptic laryngoscope but it also has important limitations

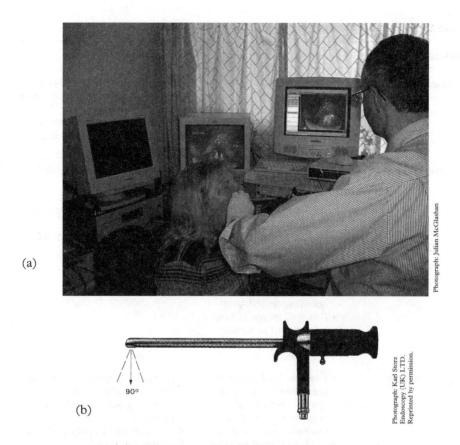

(a)

(b)

90°

Photograph: Julian McGlashan

Photograph: Karl Storz Endoscopy (UK) LTD. Reprinted by permission.

Figure 13.8 Rigid endoscopy. As Remacle (1996) points out, it is now possible to examine children below the traditional 'cut-off' point of 8 years. This is partly because of the available equipment but the examiner's methods and skills are of paramount importance. A study by Lotz et al. (1993) indicated that nasendoscopy can be carried out with relative ease in children as young as 2 years. They concluded that failures to complete examinations might relate more to the examiner's methods and skills than to the child's tolerance of the instrumentation. Some children may tolerate either the rigid or the flexible endoscope more easily than the other. A sympathetic and skilful clinician can view larynges in young children if suitable explanations are given without rushing. When an endoscope is used, children are intrigued by viewing a number of objects, their clothes, hands, hair, tongue, etc. on the monitor before the actual examination.

(Table 13.7). In clinical practice, it should not be a case of choosing either the rigid or flexible laryngoscope. Their roles are complementary and the most suitable equipment for a particular patient should be chosen.

Videolaryngoscopy

Flexible and rigid laryngoscopes can be used in conjunction with video recording in order to obtain a permanent record of the laryngeal

Table 13.7 Advantages and disadvantages of various laryngoscopic examinations

Method	Advantages	Disadvantages
Laryngoscopic mirror	• Inexpensive • Easy to use • Vocal folds can be viewed at rest and on phonation	Vocal folds can be viewed only on steady-state vowel, not continuous speech Small image, no magnification Fleeting view of larynx, no video recording potential
Flexible nasendoscopy	• Patient can speak and sing during examination • Tolerated well by most patients • Illuminated image • Can be linked to video-recorder for permanent record • Supraglottal tract activity can be observed during speaking and singing • Enlarged image can be viewed on TV monitor • Can be linked to stroboscope	Small, unmagnified image when used alone Patients may not like *idea* of nasendoscopy, but most tolerate it well Powerful light source needed for videoing
Rigid endoscopy	• Provides best image of vocal folds and supra-glottis – clearer, sharper, brighter picture than flexible nasendoscope • Linked to video-recorder • Enlarged image can be viewed on TV monitor • Easily used with stroboscope because of high-definition images • Minor/early mucosal changes easily detected	Presence of endoscope in mouth limits laryngeal examination to vowels; connected speech is impossible Poorly tolerated by patients with sensitive gag reflex Tends to distort vocal behaviour and change vocal tract configuration on phonation

Laryngoscopic mirror examination provides gross information about laryngeal structure and function. Flexible and rigid endoscopy are essential for more detailed information and their uses are complementary rather than mutually exclusive. Both can be used in conjunction with video-recorders and stroboscopy.

examination which can be viewed repeatedly. The main purposes of videolaryngoscopy are listed in Table 13.8.

Videostrobolaryngoscopy

Only gross disorders of vocal fold movement are discernible by mirror and fibreoptic laryngoscopy alone because the vocal folds vibrate too rapidly for the eye to resolve the individual vibratory cycles. The stroboscope helps to

Table 13.8 Purposes of videolaryngoscopy

- To assist in identifying the physiological basis of voice disorders: diagnosis and review
- To evaluate laryngeal behaviour during phonation:
    - as a basis for treatment planning
    - to monitor treatment and effectiveness
    - to provide biofeedback

- To document laryngeal and supraglottic status
- To clarify explanations to patients
- To support teaching and clinical discussion:
    - repeated viewing for valid clinical opinion and increasing clinical expertise

---

resolve this problem by providing a light source with intermittent flashes of light, which can be synchronised with the vibratory cycles and are instantly responsive to the subject's vocal pitch changes via a neck microphone. Flashes emitted at a slower rate than the phonation frequency produce the effect of simulated slow motion. The flash frequency can be adjusted so that the vocal folds appear to stand still and the timing of the flash can be manoeuvred to fix the image at different stages in the vibratory cycle (Baken, 1987). The image is not real time because it is composed of 'snapshots' of a sequence of vocal fold vibratory cycles, each 'snapshot' having been taken at a different stage in each cycle. Interpretation of the videostroboscopic image depends on an understanding of the histological structure of the vocal fold, the cover-body theory, the concept of closed and open phases of the vibratory cycle (Bless, 1991a, 1991b; Hirano and Bless, 1993), and the characteristics of normal larynges under stroboscopic examination (Pemberton et al., 1993).

A rigid endoscope or flexible nasendoscope is used to deliver stroboscopic illumination and to give magnification of the image so that even minute lesions and the effect that they have on the mucosal wave can be seen clearly. The flexible or rigid endoscope is attached to a camera which conveys the image to a TV monitor and a video-recorder. To gain maximum benefit from the equipment, a frame-by-frame viewing mode is essential. As a result of this greatly magnified, recorded image, the larynx and supraglottis can be examined repeatedly in considerable detail by the multidisciplinary team. Videostroboscopy reveals information that is not available by other clinical methods of laryngeal examination and is the definitive tool in differential diagnoses of laryngeal pathology. In certain cases, the information obtained with stroboscopy can establish a diagnosis that might otherwise only have been presumed or overlooked entirely (Kitzing, 1985; Sataloff et al., 1988). Studies by Woo et al. (1991) and Remacle (1996) suggest that 10–13% of diagnoses are changed when stroboscopy is used. Standard terminology used in stroboscopic examination is given in Table 13.9.

Table 13.9 Videostroboscopic examination: terminology

Vocal fold edge	Normal vocal fold edge is straight and smooth
Glottic closure	When assessed at point of maximum closure, normal vocal folds are fully approximated
Phase closure	Open and closed phases are roughly equal in each normal vibratory cycle
Presence/extent of mucosal wave	Normal wave travels from inferior surface of the vocal folds, vertically over the medial surface and spreads laterally across superior surface
Amplitude of vibration	The extent of lateral displacement of the vocal fold Amplitude normally varies from cycle to cycle
Phase symmetry	Both vocal folds reaching the midline and point of maximum glottic opening at the same time
Periodicity/regularity	The fundamental period is the time-span of one complete vibratory cycle Periodicity refers to a sequence of cycles: periodicity may be regular, irregular or inconsistent
Supraglottic activity	Activity of the vocal tract, including the false vocal folds, during phonation
Vertical level of vocal fold approximation	Vocal folds are normally on the same plane

Bless, Hirano and Feder (1987); Hirano and Bless (1993); Karnell (1994); Remacle (1996).

The increasing availability of videostrobolaryngoscopy has enabled clinicians to make more soundly based diagnoses, and medical and surgical treatment decisions, because of the increased information available regarding the behaviour of the vocal fold mucosa during phonation and the capability of repeatedly viewing the examination frame by frame. The important advantages of using stroboscopy are listed in Table 13.11, together with some disadvantages and Table 13.10 lists the observations of the disordered larynx.

LARYNGEAL EXAMINATION: CLINICAL ISSUES

Detailed laryngoscopic examination in the voice clinic, particularly in unusual or difficult cases, is fascinating and absorbing for the clinicians involved. It must always be remembered that the patient's perspective can be very different and that levels of anxiety before, during and immediately after the examination might be high. Patients are frequently fearful of both the procedure and the potential findings. Many find the idea of instruments being inserted into the mouth extremely invasive, with similarities to visits

Table 13.10 Videostroboscopic observations of the disordered larynx

Vocal fold edge	Deviations from a smooth, straight vocal fold edge may denote mass lesions or other structural abnormalities of the affected vocal fold
Glottic closure	Closure may be complete, incomplete or inconsistent The pattern of closure is noted: – longitudinal gap[a] – anterior gap – posterior gap – complete glottal closure – bowed vocal folds – irregular closure – hour-glass gap
Phase closure	A prolonged closed phase indicates hyperadduction, e.g. muscle tension dysphonia, spasmodic dysphonia A prolonged open phase indicates hypoadduction, e.g. unilateral vocal fold paralysis
Presence/extent of mucosal wave	The mucosal waves of both vocal folds are assessed according to the degree by which they are decreased from the expected norm. Non-vibrating segments indicate a lesion
Amplitude of vibration	Differences in the amplitude of vocal fold vibration may indicate differences in the vocal fold tissue Amplitude increases during increased intensity and subglottal air pressure and decreases with increased Fo, vocal fold stiffness and when the mucosal wave encounters obstacles, e.g. lesions
Phase symmetry	Phase asymmetry can indicate tissue differences between the vocal folds
Periodicity/regularity	The pattern of periodicity (regular, irregular, inconsistent) is noted. Irregular and inconsistent periodicity may be the result of a range of laryngeal pathology but can also occur in a structurally normal larynx
Supraglottic activity	Medial constriction of the false vocal folds is associated with hyperfunctional phonation. False vocal fold activity may also be seen in cases of glottal insufficiency when attempts to increase vocal loudness result in hyperfunction
Vertical level of vocal fold approximation	In cases of dislocation of an arytenoid cartilage and in some cases of trauma to the larynx or unilateral vocal fold paralysis, the vocal folds might not be on the same plane and approximation is compromised

Bless, Hirano and Feder (1987); Hirano and Bless (1993); Karnell (1994); Remacle (1996).
Patients are asked to carry out a number of vocal tasks while these observations are being made because vocal fold vibratory characteristics change according to intensity and frequency.
[a]The term 'chink' (as in ' posterior glottic chink') is also commonly used.

Table 13.11 Stroboscopy: advantages and disadvantages

Advantages	Disadvantages

Differential diagnosis, e.g.
  • identifying sulcus
  • differentiating vocal fold paralysis from cord fixation by cyst
  • identifying extent of mucosal oedema
	Cannot be used with aphonic or severely dysphonic patients; the poor vocal signal results in a poor image (consequently it is more useful in cases of mild-to-moderate dysphonia)

Reduces need for repeated biopsy	The image depends on a succession of vibrations and does not provide information about a single vibratory cycle
Changes diagnosis in 10–13% of patients previously examined by laryngologists not using stroboscopy	Irregular vibrations cannot be studied
Contributes to identification of early carcinoma	
Can help to avoid unnecessary surgery	
Documents progress	
Clarifies treatment route, either medical or surgical	
Useful or critical in 65% of cases (Woo et al., 1991)	
Particularly important in patients with difficult diagnoses	

to the dentist, and those with a sensitive gag reflex anticipate the unpleasant sensation. On the first occasion, it is also understandable that patients should be concerned about an unknown procedure. Clinicians should respect these apprehensions not only out of consideration for the individual in their care, but also because the examination of an unnecessarily anxious patient does not give the best results.

It is helpful to observe signs of the patient's tension as the case history is taken and to be alert to clues that indicate high levels of concern, even if the patient appears to be relaxed superficially. Reduced facial expression with fairly rapid eye movements or, alternatively, excessive laughing and joking can indicate anxiety. The equipment of endoscopes, stroboscope, TV monitors and video recorders, which is so familiar and comprehensible to the voice clinic team, can appear daunting and overwhelming to the examinee. Consequently, the process should be clearly and briefly explained before it begins. In particular, it is helpful to explain that the rigid endoscope will be placed only in the mouth. (Many patients view the length of the endoscope with concern and think that it will have to go into the throat to reach the larynx.) Some clinicians use a topical anaesthetic spray in order to reduce sensitivity. The unusual sensations that this causes, and their duration, should be explained. Many patients feel as if they have a lump in their throats and that they cannot swallow. They should be reassured that they can swallow and that the effects of the anaesthetic spray will disappear in approximately 10–15 minutes. A quiet, relaxed approach helps to put patients at their ease and enables them to cooperate fully throughout the examination. In some cases, where the patient has a very sensitive gag reflex or is excessively anxious, the larynx cannot be viewed successfully with a rigid endoscope, and attempts to view the larynx can cause obvious distress and should not be pursued. In these cases it is usually possible to use flexible nasendoscopy successfully.

As with all medical examinations, patients are listening for clues of the examiner's findings and conclusions. The discussion between members of the voice clinic team during observation of the vocal tract can be misconstrued, so care must be taken not to cause the patient unnecessary concern. After the examination, the findings are discussed by the team. Subsequently, they are discussed with the patient as the video-recording is viewed and the proposed management plan, and its rationale, is outlined. For many patients, the issue of primary importance is whether or not there are signs of cancer in the larynx and they seek reassurance regarding this, even if they feel unable to ask the question directly. Similarly, although terms such as 'nodules' and 'polyps' clearly indicate non-malignant vocal fold changes to the laryngologist and speech–language pathologist, patients need the reassurance of knowing the aetiology of these lesions and that they are benign. Many patients have been distressed by the term 'growths on the vocal cords' in explanations of benign mass lesions because of association of 'growth' with carcinomas. It should be made clear, therefore, when vocal fold mucosa changes are the result of mechanical damage.

Although the overall aim of the clinicians and patient is to restore 'normal' voice, the differing perspectives must be taken into account in the way in which the laryngeal examination is conducted. Although the voice clinic team wants to achieve a clear image of laryngeal structure and function, patients generally want to know what has been found, whether it is 'serious', and whether or not it can be resolved, with or without surgery. As far as the patient is concerned, the examination process is not completed until these questions have been resolved. It does not end when the laryngeal findings have been amassed.

Note 1

Laryngoscopy is an invasive procedure and clinical standards and infection control procedures laid down by professional bodies and employers must be adhered to in each case. In particular, as increasing numbers of speech–language pathologists carry out flexible and rigid endoscopic laryngeal examinations themselves, they must ensure that resuscitation personnel and equipment are available and that they protect patients, colleagues and themselves from cross-infection with approved sterilisation and cleaning procedures. These issues are discussed and described clearly by Karnell (1994) and Orlikoff and Baken (1993b). The speech–language pathologist should also be aware of the medicolegal implications of carrying out these procedures.

Note 2

The Interactive Video Textbook, 'Phonosurgery for Benign Vocal Fold Lesions', illustrates the collaborative work of Dr. Marc Bouchayer and Dr. Guy Cornut during laryngoscopic examinations and surgical procedures. (Appendix C)

ELECTROGLOTTOGRAPHY (LARYNGOGRAPHY, ELECTROLARYNGOGRAPHY)

This non-invasive technique provides information about vocal fold contact (Fourcin and Abberton, 1971; Abberton, Howard and Fourcin, 1989; Titze, 1990). Two small electrodes are placed on the neck, one on the skin overlying each lamina of the thyroid cartilage. As a weak electrical current is passed from one electrode to the other across the larynx at the level of the vocal folds, the instrument responds to changes in electrical impedance caused by their increasing and decreasing contact. The waveform produced is dependent on the degree of vocal fold contact (Figure 13.9): when the vocal folds are in contact, conductance is greater than when there is air in between them. The Laryngograph output is known as the Lx waveform. In a typical Lx waveform for a normal voice, the closing phase of the vocal

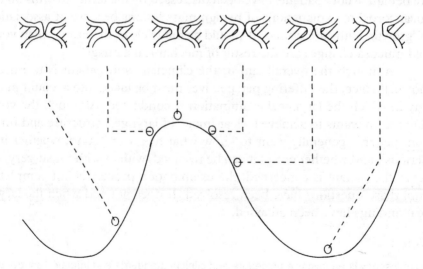

Figure 13.9 EGG waveform and its relationship to vocal fold contact in one vibratory cycle. (After MacCurtain and Fourcin, 1982.)

folds is indicated by a steep rise in the trace which culminates in the apex of the wave, indicating the point of maximum contact, after which the opening phase is represented by the right-sided slope of the waveform. The closing phase, the point of maximum contact and the opening phase together constitute the closed phase of the vocal fold vibratory cycle. The subsequent trough is termed the 'open phase'. As the vocal folds meet more rapidly than they part in each cycle in normal voices, and the closing phase is more rapid than the opening phase, the left-sided slope is steeper than that following the peak. The closed quotient (CQ) is a ratio that indicates the proportion of time the glottis is closed in one vibratory cycle (CQ = closed time divided by total cycle time).

The amplitude of the Lx waveform relates to the degree of vocal fold contact. In pathological voices its reduced amplitude can be a significant indication of poor vocal fold contact. Care has to be taken in interpreting this parameter, however, because variations can occur for other reasons that do not reflect abnormal function. In women and children, who have small larynges, and during low-intensity phonation, where glottal closure might be incomplete, the relative amplitude is reduced. Amplitude may also be low because the electrodes are poorly positioned or there is a significant subcutaneous fat layer. This parameter of the waveform should also be regarded with some caution because there is a gain control on the instrument which can affect the amplitude of the wave. The advantages and possible problems involved in using this instrumentation are summarised in Tables 13.12 and 13.13.

Vocal fundamental frequency can be derived from the individual vocal fold contacts on a steady note and speaking fundamental frequency measures can be made during connected speech in spontaneous conversation and in reading. The Lx waveform also provides extensive information regarding the laryngeal aspects of voice quality. As a result, Lx waveform information has been used in combination with stroboscopy so that each

Table 13.12 Electroglottography (electrolaryngography): advantages

---

- Non-invasive instrument, quickly and easily used in clinical setting
- Assessment and biofeedback
- Signal not affected by surrounding acoustic conditions
- Can be used in conversation, reading and with steady vowels
- Monitors change
- Fundamental frequency analysis
- Voice quality information
- Can be used simultaneously with stroboscopy

Table 13.13 Electroglottography (electrolaryngography): potential difficulties

Practical problems	
Placement of electrodes	Excessive adipose or muscular tissue can obscure the best site
	The electrodes might move or the laryngeal vertical excursions cause the larynx to move away from the electrodes in connected speech
	Skin oils can reduce electrode-to-skin contact
Greater difficulty in obtaining satisfactory EGG signals from women and children	Possibly caused by smaller vocal fold mass and wider thyroid cartilage angle in women and children
	May be the result of more adipose tissue in women
Waveform interpretation problems	
Vocal fold contact	The exact site of contact, either along length or depth of vocal fold, cannot be determined by EGG
	The waveform cannot indicate unilateral vocal fold behaviour, only the effect of bilateral vocal fold contact
Open phase of larynx less useful than closed phase	Because it depends on the absence of electrical data
Amplitude of larynx waveform not reliable	This parameter can be varied by the gain control and therefore is not a reliable representation
Non-vocal fold contact	The signal can be misleading if mucus spans the glottis or the false vocal folds approximate and act as a pathway for the current

Larynx waveform cannot be obtained in cases of very breathy voice or aphonia because there is no vocal fold contact.
Baken (1987); Abberton, Howard and Fourcin (1989); Childers et al. (1990); Colton and Conture (1990); Howard (1998); Fourcin (2000).

element of the stroboscopic image can be correlated with its corresponding point in the Lx waveform. This helps to overcome the problem of variable periodicity, which occurs in pathological voices and complicates analysis of the stroboscopic image (Karnell, 1989; Fourcin, 2000). (Figure 13.10)

Although the equipment is easily used, care must be taken in the placement of the electrodes if a useful Lx waveform is to be acquired. Each electrode should be sited on the middle of each thyroid cartilage lamina. In some subjects it is more difficult to locate the exact position and this can be complicated further in children and small women where the thyroid cartilage is small. By asking the patient to produce a steady vowel, it is usually possible carefully to reposition the electrodes until a suitable signal is obtained. The electrodes can then be stabilised either by holding them in position or by fixing them with a Velcro neck band. Some patients find having a band round their necks, even when not unduly tight, very difficult to tolerate and, in these cases, the electrodes can be held in position (Colton and Conture, 1990).

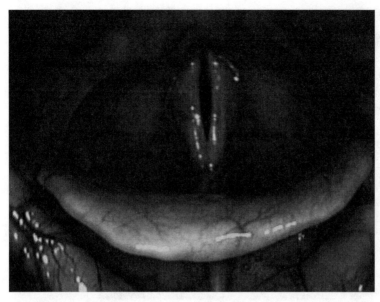

A high preci-
sion view of
the vibrating
folds taken
with a 5µs
flash, shows
essentially
perfect sym-
metry both of
the folds
themselves
and of their
supporting
structures

Figure 13.10(1) Normal vocal fold vibration 26yr woman. 264 Hz open phase *see the seventh image below*

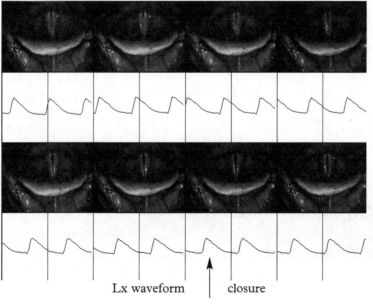

Each digital
image stored
automatically
by LxStrobe
with 5µs light
flashes for
each flash
uniformly
spaced for
successive
steps within
Tx. The flash
instant is
shown at the
centre of
each Lx
waveform.

Lx waveform   closure

Figure 13.10(2) Normal vibratory sequence within a single vocal fold period, Tx. Normal 26yr woman as above. *The progression shown by the markers on the Lx waveforms is from immediately before complete closure through opening to the open phase*

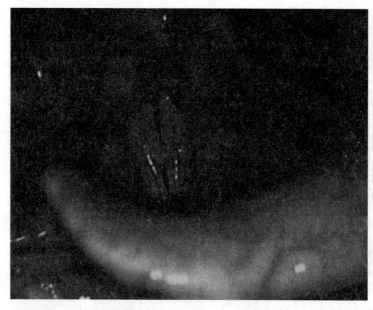

Asymmetry both of the vocal folds and of their supporting structures is shown. This often does not lead to irregular bimodal vibration in sustained sounds but image based interpretation alone can be inadequate

Figure 13.10(3) Abormal vocal folds 31yr woman 179 Hz Polypoid right vocal fold, left fold oedema *see the fifth image below*

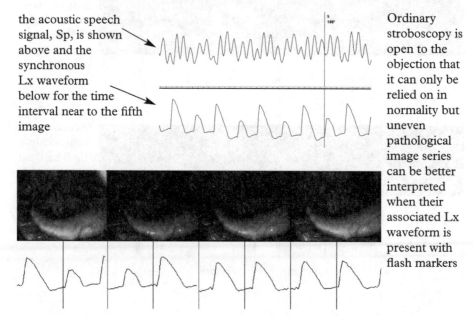

the acoustic speech signal, Sp, is shown above and the synchronous Lx waveform below for the time interval near to the fifth image

Ordinary stroboscopy is open to the objection that it can only be relied on in normality but uneven pathological image series can be better interpreted when their associated Lx waveform is present with flash markers

Figure 13.10(4) Polypoid right vocal fold, left oedema 31yr woman 121 Hz and 244 Hz bimodal vibratory sequence *links between sustained voice and speech become evident when images are linked to Lx*

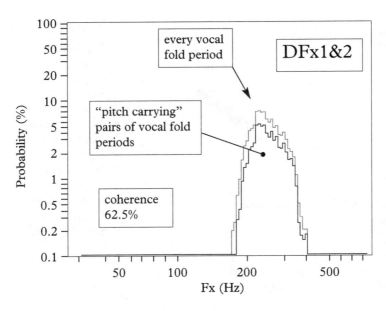

Figure 13.10(5) First and second order vocal fold frequency distributions, DFx1 and DFx2, for a 2m read text by the normal speaker of figure 13.10(1)

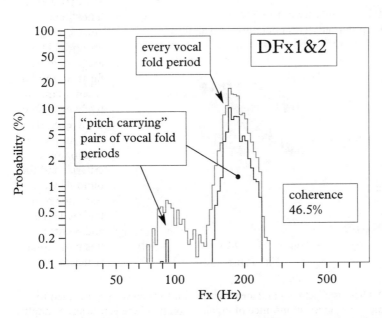

Figure 13.10(6) First and second order distributions are very different when irregular phonation is analysed. 'Coherence' here refers to the ratio between the number of larynx periods included in DFx2 relative to those in the whole speech sample – DFx1

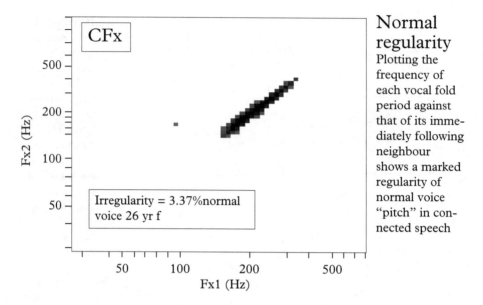

Normal regularity
Plotting the frequency of each vocal fold period against that of its immediately following neighbour shows a marked regularity of normal voice "pitch" in connected speech

Figure 13.10(7) Vocal fold period crossplot, CFx – although range is not as clearly shown as in DFx1 and 2, regularity is easily seen and measured

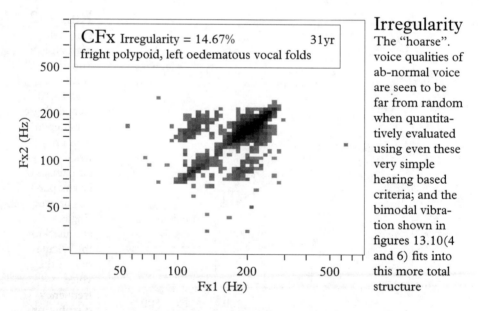

Irregularity
The "hoarse". voice qualities of ab-normal voice are seen to be far from random when quantitatively evaluated using even these very simple hearing based criteria; and the bimodal vibration shown in figures 13.10(4 and 6) fits into this more total structure

Figure 13.10(8) There is a richness and structure in voice which we are designed to hear and this simple plot gives an instance of organisation that here is measured simply but which can lead to greater clinical insights

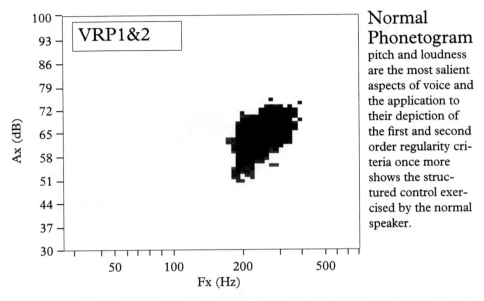

Normal Phonetogram pitch and loudness are the most salient aspects of voice and the application to their depiction of the first and second order regularity criteria once more shows the structured control exercised by the normal speaker.

Figure 13.10(9) 'Loudness plotted against pitch' for connected speech gives a natural communication version of the classic sung phonetogram

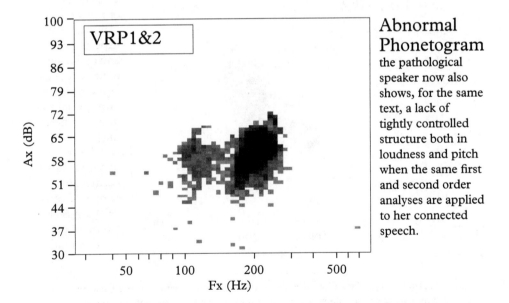

Abnormal Phonetogram the pathological speaker now also shows, for the same text, a lack of tightly controlled structure both in loudness and pitch when the same first and second order analyses are applied to her connected speech.

Figure 13.10(10) Bimodal clusters are expected for this speaker but the structure of amplitude as a function of instantaneous larynx frequency Fx reveals a lack of period to period consistency in speech pressure which is also perceptually of outcome consequence

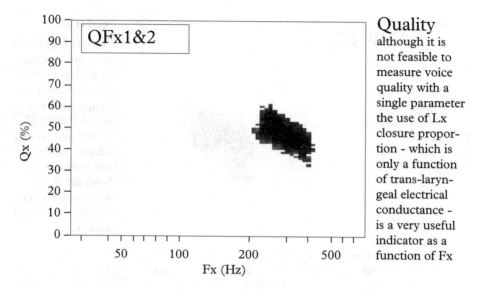

Quality although it is not feasible to measure voice quality with a single parameter the use of Lx closure proportion - which is only a function of trans-laryngeal electrical conductance - is a very useful indicator as a function of Fx

Figure 13.10(11) The superposition of the first and second order analyses reveals the degree of structured control normally present in closed phase control

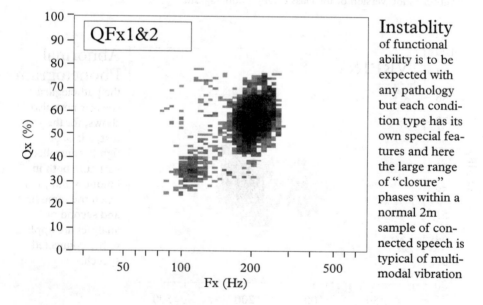

Instablity of functional ability is to be expected with any pathology but each condition type has its own special features and here the large range of "closure" phases within a normal 2m sample of connected speech is typical of multi-modal vibration

Figure 13.10(12) The data plotted is derived once more from the same basic recording but the dimensions chosen illustrate the depth of understanding that is potentially possible when listening is linked to quantitative analysis since a range of pressed to breathy phonation types are shown by this simple linking of Qx to Fx

Figure 13.10 Laryngograph data and analysis (analysis contributed by Professor Adrian Fourcin and images by Mr Julian McGlashan).

Synchronised videostroboscopy and electroglottography (EGG) can be used for cross-validation of the data acquired by each procedure (Karnell, 1989; Fourcin, 2000). The Lx waveform appears on the TV monitor at the same time as the laryngoscopic image.

VOCAL TRACT IMAGING

Radiography (videofluoroscopy)

Radiography allows the visualisation of internal body structures by projection of X-rays through, for example, the pharynx on to a fluoroscopic screen. The image can be observed directly, or photographed and recorded on video-tape and synchronised with phonation. An image intensifier can be used to strengthen the image and the examination can be viewed on a TV monitor. Videofluoroscopy is not suitable for the observation of the vocal folds because it is possible only to obtain lateral or anteroposterior views of the vocal tract. It is invaluable for the observation of pharyngeal, soft palate and tongue postures and movements. Its capability of imaging swallowing movements and the passage of solids and liquids of different consistencies through the oral cavity, pharynx and related structures has resulted in videofluoroscopy becoming the gold standard in the assessment of dysphagia (Logemann, 1983a; Dikeman and Kazandjian, 1995). It can also form an element of the various assessments of certain voice disorders, particularly those involving neurogenic deficits that affect the vocal tract, which may be associated with potential swallowing problems. Lateral radiographs with barium outline, used in the past (Calnan, 1955) to obtain sagittal stills of the soft palate in emission of vowel sounds, have been replaced by flexible nasendoscopy and videofluoroscopy. Video recordings of the examination can be used in treatment but direct fluoroscopy cannot be used routinely in therapy (McWilliams, Morris and Shelton, 1984). Exposure to radiation must be carefully controlled at all times.

Xeroradiography

This radiological process, originally developed for mammography, has been used for imaging the vocal tract. An electrostatic (still) image is produced on a xerographic plate, which registers X-rays on an electrically charged plate instead of the conventional radiographic screen (see Chapter 2). Lateral life-sized views are photographed, showing clearly the edge enhancement of soft tissues in three-dimensional depth as well as the contours of soft tissues, bones and cartilages seen on ordinary radiographs. Pharyngeal, lingual, soft palate and laryngeal 'gestures' are shown and are useful in observing undesirable muscular tensions and constriction. After therapy, restoration of relaxed positions can be shown to the patient and compared with previous tense gestures (Julian, MacCurtain and Noscoe, 1981; Berry et al., 1982). The technique is expensive and, because it subjects the patient to higher dosage of X-rays than conventional procedures, it has strictly limited use. Gordon (1986) drew attention to the fact that there were other procedures that were cheaper and safer to administer, and readily available. The combination of xeroradiography and electrolaryngography (XEL) to provide objective analysis of vocal tract function was used by Berry et al. (1982) and others, but because of the significant limitations there have been no further developments.

Magnetic resonance imaging (MRI)

Magnetic resonance imaging (MRI) is a non-invasive nuclear procedure for imaging tissues of high fat and water content that cannot be seen with other radiological techniques. It is not used routinely in the assessment of voice disorders but to investigate some cases of laryngeal disease.

Ultra-high-speed photography

Digital high-speed systems can be used for imaging but are time-consuming and expensive. Consequently, they are not a realistic possibility for most voice science laboratories (Švec and Schutte, 1996) and are not suitable for a clinical setting.

Videokymography

Videokymography is a relatively new digital technique, developed by Švec and Schutte (1996) for high-speed visualisation of the vibratory patterns of the vocal folds. It is not yet in general clinical use. The system uses a modified video camera that is able to function in two modes: high speed (nearly 8000 images/s) and standard (50 images/s). In high-speed mode, the camera selects one active horizontal line (i.e. transverse to the glottis) from the whole laryngeal image. Successive line images can then be seen on a TV monitor in real time and fill each video frame from top to bottom. Švec and Schutte (1996) report that this system allows observation of left/right asymmetry of vocal fold vibration, propagation of mucosal waves, and the movements of the upper and lower margins of the vocal folds. Videokymography appears to overcome certain problems associated with stroboscopy (see above).

Acoustic analysis

Acoustic analysis is the process of objective identification and description of the voice. Evaluation of the various parameters of the vocal signal can be carried out by individual instruments designed for the particular purpose or, increasingly, by software packages that can analyse each parameter and subsequently integrate the data acquired regarding these individual aspects. An acoustic analysis profile emerges, which can indicate the extent to which each parameter deviates from normative values and which acts as a baseline as treatment progresses. This section reviews the vocal features that can be examined and some of the instrumentation available. Acoustic analysis profiles have been referred to in earlier chapters and the parameters are outlined in Chapter 4.

Professionals working in the field of voice are increasingly aware of the need for identifying and establishing standards in acoustic analysis. At the moment, the way in which acoustic analysis is carried out varies between countries, centres and individuals. Global standards might be the ideal but, as a minimum, standards should be set in all centres assessing and treating voice disorders. Titze (1994a) cites four reasons for establishing standards in acoustic analysis of the voice:

1. Education: the process of writing standards encourages the professionals involved to define terms and consider details. Future ideals frequently emerge as these matters are considered.
2. Simplification: the most useful processes can be identified and improved while others are discarded.
3. Conservation: Titze describes standards as saving time, effort and money in clinical practice.
4. Certification: standards develop into the criteria by which the task is carried out. The professional and the patient are then more likely to have a clear structure in which they can feel confident.

Titze acknowledges the possible constraints of standards and stresses that they must be reviewed and revised regularly, and that they are reached by a process of consensus. Standards can be applied to all aspects of the acoustic analysis from the definition of the tasks to be undertaken, to the equipment used, the procedures adopted and the technical criteria for the equipment used. Hirano and Bless (1993) note five principles of test selection that can also be applied to perceptual acoustic evaluation:

1. Tests should include conditions that replicate typical habitual speaking and performance activities.
2. A standard test protocol and recording procedure.
3. The conditions should be constant.
4. The tests should elicit new information.
5. Restrictions on vocal behaviour should be minimal.

AUDIO RECORDING

Audio recording, with the patient's permission, is essential as a baseline record of the voice in spontaneous speech, as material for acoustic analysis and for biofeedback during treatment. It can be used for perceptual and instrumental voice analysis. Analogue recording is becoming redundant because digital audio tape (DAT) has become less expensive. DAT recording has higher fidelity and the quality does not deteriorate over time. It also has the advantage that the data collected can be fed into a computer for analysis. Minidisc systems have similar advantages and because they are so small they are ideal for recording patients on hospital wards and/or away from the voice laboratory or clinic. Ideally, a good quality microphone is head mounted to ensure that mouth-to-microphone distance is constant on repeated recordings. A set of speakers should also be the best quality that can be funded, for subjective evaluation and for patient feedback during treatment. Good audio recordings become an important element of patient documentation and a standard protocol of voice tasks used routinely during the initial assessment can be repeated at intervals during treatment to record and monitor progress. Table 13.14 lists tasks that can be incorporated into a protocol for audio recording.

SOUND SPECTROGRAPHY

The spectrograph analyses the periodic waveform produced by the vocal signal into a series of sine waves, each with a different frequency and amplitude. The resulting spectrogram converts the acoustic waveform into its component parts so that it is possible to visualise the interrelationship of the amplitude, frequency and time of each component. The most common displays show **frequency** on the vertical axis of the graph and **time** on the horizontal axis. **Intensity** is shown by the degree of blackening of the trace. The standard spectrogram (Figure 13.11) provides a graphic representation of the harmonics-to-noise ratio and Bless (1991a) cites a number of studies that show positive correlations between perceptual judgements of voice qualities and spectral analyses. Although spectrography is an important research tool, it can also provide significant clinical information with the measures and displays being used to document changes in vocal quality.

VOICE RANGE PROFILE (PHONETOGRAM)

The Voice Range Profile (VRP; previously known as a phonetogram) is a display of **vocal intensity range** versus **fundamental frequency**, i.e. it displays the intensity limits of phonation as a function of frequency (Figure 13.12). The phonetogram is compiled from individual vocal notes

Table 13.14 Audio recording protocol

spontaneous speech in conversation	within the clinical setting this gives the truest example of patient's vocal function, particularly paralinguistic features, rate, prosody and airflow
	note overall vocal impression and each parameter of vocal profile
	note non-phonatory vocal behaviours, e.g. throat clearing and quality of voice on vegetative behaviours, e.g. laughing, crying
	note vocal fatigue by end of recording and loudness decay at end of sentence
solo connected speech	e.g. a description of a standard picture note features as above
reading aloud	e.g. standard passage such as 'The Rainbow Passage' (Fairbanks, 1960)
	SFo is usually higher during reading (Baken, 1987)
maximum phonation time (MPT)[a]	sustained vowel /a:/ at a comfortable pitch on one exhalation timed in seconds (best of three attempts)
	provides information re: glottal efficiency (in combination with s/z ratio results)
	delayed voice onset may be noted
s/z ratio[b] **(Eckel & Boone, 1981)**	voiceless and voiced equivalents each sustained for as long as possible on one exhalation. Vocal fold pathology and abnormal laryngeal function will cause /z/, the voiced phoneme, to be much shorter
vocal glides (falling, rising, repeated fall–rise)	not sung glissandos
	note pitch breaks and where they occur, limitations in pitch range, quality throughout range
rapid repetition of short voiceless vowel	provides information re laryngeal diadochokinetic rate (see Baken, 1987)

Recording can be used for many instrumental acoustic analyses and for formal and informal perceptual voice analysis.

[a]MPT is discussed below. The reader is referred to a detailed account by Raes and Clement (1996) of MPT as an aerodynamic measure.

[b]Normal speakers produce similar duration times when asked to sustain /s/ and /z/ for as long as possible, with /z/ usually being slightly longer. Vocal fold pathology function will cause /z/, the voiced phoneme, to be much shorter than in normal subjects, although /s/ is unaffected. The s/z ratio is obtained by dividing the maximum /z/ time into the maximum /s/ time. Eckel and Boone (1981) found that more than 95% of their patients with laryngeal pathologies demonstrated s/z ratios in excess of 1.4.

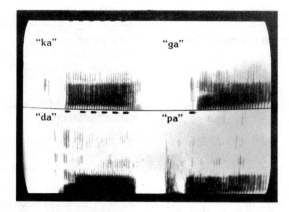

(a)

Note consonant differences.

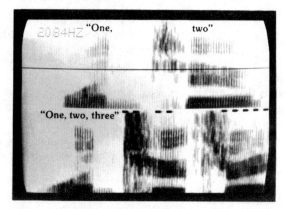

(b)

Cursor positioned at 3rd format and digital display of cursor position.

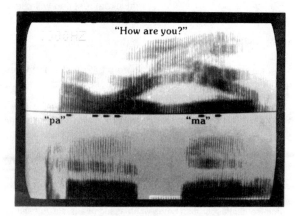

(c)

Note difficulty in word segmentation in running speech.

Figure 13.11 Spectrogram.

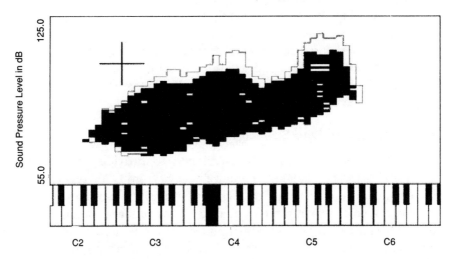

Figure 13.12 Voice Range Profile (phonetogram). Voice Range Profiling is a technique used to measure a client's voice capabilities by mapping the patient's complete range of amplitudes and fundamental frequencies. By measuring the complete range, VRP provides a uniquely revealing picture of the patient's vocal capabilities. © Kay Elemetrics Corp. Reprinted by permission.

produced at different pitches, each 1 semitone apart and produced at maximum and minimum intensity levels. As the frequencies are plotted against the intensity levels, a profile of the range of the voice emerges in graphic form, showing all the combinations of frequency and intensity at which a speaker can phonate (Orlikoff and Baken, 1993a). It is to be expected that pathological voices cover a much smaller field than normal voices, whereas professional singers have the largest range profiles. The Union of European Phoniatricians recommends a protocol for the VRP in an attempt to standardise this measurement, with patients being instructed to produce voice at its physiological boundaries without injury. The phonetogram can provide effective evidence of change in vocal function as a response to treatment.

Note

Schuttte and Seidner (1983) reported on the recommendations of the Union of European Phoniatricians regarding standardisation of phonetography.

INSTRUMENTS

Some of the commercial instruments available for acoustic analysis are listed below, but it is not realistic to provide an exhaustive list of available equipment because of constant changes and developments. Clinicians need reliable, robust and easily used instruments from manufacturers who provide good support in the form of knowledgeable, easily contacted technicians. The following pieces of equipment are in current use and have developed from earlier models. They are examples of the types of instruments on the market. Current developments are tending to produce integrated packages for clinical use, such as EGG with stroboscopy or multi-faceted hardware and software combinations which can provide complex analyses of multiple aspects of voice.

Kay CSL Computerized Speech Lab

This PC-based system has been developed to provide comprehensive speech analysis which can acquire data direct or from DAT recordings. Its facilities include spectrography, pitch and intensity analysis, voice range profile and a voice programme to quantify 22 vocal parameters. Although these data can be graphically and numerically compared with a built-in database, it is important to note that this system uses only a single norm for all analyses, ignoring the fact that norms vary by age, sex and other factors. The CSL (Figure 13.13) can show the EGG waveform. It is also intended to provide biofeedback in treatment.

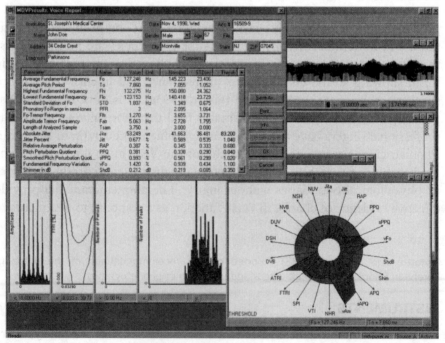

Figure 13.13 Kay CSL: Multi-Dimensional Voice Program (MDVP) MDVP provides a radial graph display that plots patient results on a database, numerical results and graphic contours of all voice parameters. © Kay Elemetrics Corp. Reprinted by permission.

VisiSpeech

This display system was developed by the RNID (Royal National Institute for Deaf People). It displays frequency, intensity and phonation time and can be used for assessment and to provide feedback during treatment. The analysis programme generates speaking fundamental frequency, pitch range and voiced/voiceless ratio. A split-screen capability allows the speech–language pathologist to model vocal behaviours that the patient can attempt to match. As the trace is sensitive to changes in vocal quality, particularly roughness of the vocal note, this equipment is useful for monitoring and reducing some types of noise. Breathy voices do not, however, produce a trace.

Kay Visi-Pitch

This equipment extracts fundamental frequency and amplitude of the input signal and can be used for assessment and biofeedback procedures. The latest models of this electronic instrument are computer assisted and automatically perform statistical calculations such as average pitch, average intensity, pitch perturbation and pitch range. A printout of the statistical data or the speech contours can form part of the patient's documentation. Clear visual displays of voice quality, intonation, timing and stress patterns are displayed in real time. It also has the potential to display the Laryngograph waveform.

Tunemaster III

This instrument registers fundamental pitch and is strongly recommended by Boone and McFarlane (1988) for pitch assessment and remediation programmes.

Glottal Frequency Analyser

This compact equipment provides information about fundamental frequency and has the facility for providing a hard copy. It is manufactured by Entomed AB.

Sound Level Recorder (Bruel and Kjaer Instruments)

A strip-chart record is produced by this complex instrument which is able to record rapid changes in intensity.

Sound Level Meter (Bruel and Kjaer Instruments)

Intensity level is shown on a meter but there is no permanent output record. Baken (1987) suggests that it is best for measuring the intensity of steady-state sounds such as prolonged vowels. (The VU [volume unit] meter on a tape recorder is useful for providing visual feedback of loudness when measurement is not required.)

AERODYNAMIC MEASUREMENTS

Respiratory function and speech–breathing patterns are of such direct relevance to normal voice production and dysphonia that aerodynamic studies have been the basis of a considerable number of research projects. Respiratory volumes, control of expiration and temporal aspects are an essential feature of assessment (Kelman et al., 1975). Gordon, Morton and Simpson (1978) reported that, in a corpus of 73 cases of 'mechanical dysphonia' (vocal misuse), 47.9% showed disturbed breathing patterns at rest and 79.5% were unable to maintain steady flow rate in phonation. Respiratory abnormalities can be a primary cause of voice disorders but disordered speech–breathing patterns can also result from laryngeal valving abnormalities. Objective evaluation provides clarification and quantifiable data about the efficiency of respiratory function, including air volume, and also airflow and subglottic air pressure measures during phonation. The value of aerodynamic measures is in monitoring changes as a result of treatment, rather than in providing a particular diagnosis.

Air volume measurement (Spirometry)

Air volume refers to the amount of air in the lungs. The volume of air used in speaking refers to the amount by which the total lung volume is reduced (Baken, 1987). Patients with diseases of the respiratory system, or neurological disorders affecting breathing movements, will have lower lung volumes than normal because of their reduced inspiratory ability. It is also extremely difficult to regulate the pressure of a small volume of air. Such difficulties can contribute to or exacerbate voice disorders.

The first spirometer was built in 1846 by John Hutchison who wanted to measure the amount of air that an individual could exhale after full inspiration. These simple instruments are still used in hospital respiratory function tests (Boone, 1977). Vital capacity, tidal capacity and complemental air are measurable.

Wet spirometer

This simple instrument works on the gasometer principle and is also known as a pulmometer. An inverted glass cylinder is situated inside a calibrated cylinder containing water. As the patient blows air through a rubber tube into the inverted cylinder, its displacement is measured against the calibrations, indicating the volume of air that has been expired. As Baken (1987) points out, although wet spirometers provide an excellent method of measuring ventilatory volumes, their usefulness is limited for measuring the small, rapid changes that occur during speech because of their sluggish response.

Dry spirometer

Mechanical and electronic dry spirometers that are hand held also provide air volume measures. They tend to be less reliable than wet spirometers because they are sensitive to the force with which breath is exhaled (Steer and Hanley, 1959; Boone, 1977). Simple spirometers measure expiratory volumes and can provide a useful measure of some aspects of respiratory function, but in the light of present electronic technology they are somewhat primitive and limited in the information they provide. However, they are inexpensive and reliable, and easily available from hospital respiratory departments.

Electrospirometer

Electrospirometers provide an accurate measure of lung capacity and function, e.g. vital capacity, reserve volume. A mask is worn by the subject during this procedure (which children may not tolerate) and airflow measurement in speech is not easy. Airflow studies during vowel production in measurement of maximum phonation time have tended to be the focus of assessment (Isshiki, 1965; Isshiki, Okamura and Morimoto, 1967; Yanagihara and Koike, 1967).

Airflow rate

Airflow rate refers to the rate at which air passes through the glottis during phonation and represents the change of volume. It is measured in units of cm^3/s or ml/s.

When mean airflow rate during a sample of voice is calculated from a spirometric record, the volume of air used is divided by the period of time for which voicing lasted on that exhalation (Baken, 1987), i.e. if 1 litre of volume change takes place in 10 seconds of voicing, the mean flow is 100 ml/s.

Pneumotachograph

A pneumotachograph is one type of airflow transducer. It generates a pressure which must then be converted to an electrical signal (Gould and Korovin, 1994). It is used for calculating airflow rate. The airflow volume over a given time can also be established. When these measurements are being made in relation to phonation, a mask is worn in order to leave the mouth as free as possible, although even this can constrict mandibular movement and affect the sound. It is important to ensure that air cannot leak from the mask. A specially designed facemask allows separate mea-surement of airflow from nose and mouth. Some investigators prefer to use a modified body plethysmograph, in which the subject is completely sealed within a box, to overcome the constraints of a facemask (Proctor, 1980; Baken, 1987).

A Mercury Electronic pneumotachograph system incorporating a spirometer was used by Gordon (1977) to measure breath flow rates and volumes. The flow-head attached to a rubber facemask was fitted with a microphone; sound was recorded on a Ferrograph audio-tape recorder and a Laryngograph was also used to monitor Lx waveform in production of vowels. This instrument has been updated and is now computer assisted. Mercury (Scotland) Ltd produce an extensive range of lung function analysers that use screen pneumotachographs. Certain models are com-puter based and are designed to extract relevant values from the maximal expiratory flow/volume curve. The displays are in numerical form.

Chest wall movements

In addition to air volume and airflow measures, it is helpful in some cases to measure the expansion and contraction of the chest wall. It is particularly important to evaluate the coordination of the chest and abdominal walls. The true relevance of such movements in phonation, however, requires linkage with lung volume and pressure measurements used in phonation (Baken 1977).

Two types of instrumentation are used in registration of respiratory movement of the rib cage and abdominal wall at rest and during speech. These are magnetometry and inductance plethysmography. Both methods are non-invasive.

Magnetometry

Magnetometer coils, which are encased in polyethylene, are glued to the chest wall. The basic principle is that of sensing, with one coil, the strength of a magnetic field that has been produced by the other, as a means of esti-mating body diameter (Baken, 1987). Hixon, Goldman and Mead (1973) measured anteroposterior diameters of the rib cage and abdomen in upright and supine postures during conversation, reading and singing. Among many pertinent observations, they noted that the abdominal wall occupies an especially important role in running conversation. The abdominal wall mechanically times the rise of the diaphragm to express air for speech.

Inductance plethysmography

This equipment, the 'Respitrace', was developed – and is primarily used – for monitoring neonatal vegetative respiratory movements of the chest and abdominal walls. Normal changes in the position of the baby do not disturb the equipment.

Maximum phonation time

This is the time in seconds for which a vowel can be maintained at a comfortable pitch and loudness after taking a deep breath. Maximum phonation time (MPT) is greater in males than in females; in males it falls within limits of 25–35 seconds and in females within 15–25 seconds. It is markedly reduced in many cases of laryngeal pathology (Hirano, 1981). Although it does not have diagnostic value, it is clinically useful for determining the degree of the voice disorder and monitoring progress over time. Raes and Clement (1996) deduced from their study of aerodynamic measurements of voice production that MPT is a more sensitive measure than phonation quotient (see below).

Subglottal air pressure

Subglottal air pressure during phonation is a potentially difficult measurement to make because instruments cannot be introduced into the trachea while the subject is speaking. This problem can be overcome by the speaker repeating the CV syllable /pi/ with an oral catheter, which is attached to a pressure transducer, placed in the mouth (Smitheran and Hixon, 1981). As the lips close for the bilateral consonant, the glottis opens, allowing the pressure in the mouth to rise to the value of the pressure below the vocal folds (Hirano and Bless, 1993). Air pressure recorded during production of the plosive consonant is therefore regarded as equal to the pressure within the trachea, if certain precautions are taken. Baken (1987) cautions that the length, diameter and angle of the tube can influence the pressure measurement.

A simple, non-invasive, home-made device has been suggested by Hixon, Hawley and Wilson (1982) in order to assess whether an individual has sufficient 'respiratory driving pressure' for speech. This method is easy and inexpensive to use in the clinic and provides some useful information about the speaker's speech–breathing potential. Its limitation is that it cannot be used during voice production.

Phonation threshold pressure

Phonation threshold pressure (PTP) is the minimum subglottal pressure required to initiate vocal fold oscillation (Titze, 1991, 1992). It is dependent on fundamental frequency and vocal intensity. Potentially, it is a useful measure in assessing pathological voices, but it is generally impractical because most methods used to obtain it are invasive (Fisher and Swank, 1997). Jiang et al. (1999) have reported on their development of a non-invasive system for estimating PTP at different levels of vocal intensity. The subjects in this study sustained a constant tone and the airflow was directed into a section of pipe with an airtight mask over the mouth and nose. The PTP for each subject was predicted from a difference between an estimate of the subglottal pressure and the vocal tract pressure at the point that phonation ceased after interruption of the airflow. This study showed that patients with vocal fold polyps had significantly higher estimations of PTP than for the control subjects. In many cases of vocal pathology, the relative inertia of the vocal folds is increased because of increased vocal fold mass. Consequently, higher air pressure levels are needed to initiate vocal fold vibration in these cases.

Glottal resistance

Glottal resistance reflects the force and duration of vocal fold closure. It is calculated by dividing subglottal air pressure by the mean airflow. It varies according to the vocal task, increasing with increased vocal intensity and pitch in normal voices (Bless, 1991a). In pathological voices, glottal resistance is affected by the structural and functional abnormalities, so that measurements can be particularly high in some cases of hyperfunctional dysphonia, for example, but lower than normal for unilateral vocal fold paralysis. Hirano and Bless (1993) regard measures of glottal resistance as more informative than those of airflow or pressure alone.

Phonation quotient

The phonation quotient approximately indicates air consumption during phonation per unit of time. This measure is obtained by dividing vital capacity by the MTP. Raes and Clement (1996) cite a number of studies that confirm that the phonation quotient tends to increase in pathological voices, with the highest mean phonation quotient values occurring in cases of unilateral vocal fold paralysis. The phonation quotient is, therefore, an indicator of glottal efficiency which can help to measure the severity of the dysphonia and which can be used for monitoring progress after surgery and voice therapy.

Note

Integrated systems for aerodynamic measurements are available commercially, e.g. the Kay airflow measurement system, the Aerophone, analyses and displays graphical and numerical data of peak flow, vital capacity, duration, phonation quotient, mean airflow rate, loudest tone level, mean tone level, softest tone level, sound pressure level, subglottal air pressure, intraoral pressure, glottal efficiency and glottal resistance.

ELECTROPHYSIOLOGY

Electromyography

Electromyography (EMG) is based on the fact that, when a muscle fibre contracts, there is electrical activity.

The magnitude of the electrical wave is called a muscle action potential (MAP). MAPs are detected and recorded during EMG by two methods (Baken, 1987). During *surface* EMG, electrodes are placed on the skin and the amplitude of the electrical impulses is displayed on an oscilloscope. Surface myography supplies only limited information about muscular activity, but can be used to record levels of generalised excessive laryngeal muscle tension (Andrews, 1995). It is a non-invasive method of assessment and biofeedback. *Intrinsic laryngeal muscle* EMG is carried out by inserting a needle or wire electrode into the muscle being investigated; it measures the potential of individual muscles. This potentially uncomfortable invasive technique is carried out by physicians and physiologists. It is used in cases of vocal fold paralysis and during the injection of botulinum toxin in the treatment of spasmodic dysphonia. Diagnosis, proposed surgical intervention and prognosis can be clarified by the use of EMG (Hirose, 1977; Hirano, 1981) but identification of abnormal laryngeal EMG activity is complicated by considerable variability in the muscle firing patterns within and between normal subjects (Ludlow et al., 1993; Karnell and Finnegan, 1994).

Neurography

Neurography (ENG) measures the velocities of sensory and motor nerve impulses. As such, it provides further detail regarding EMG measurements. The site and severity of nerve damage (e.g. the recurrent laryngeal nerve) and diagnosis of laryngeal neuromuscular conditions can be clarified by ENG. Kotby et al. (1992) have discussed the use of EMG and ENG in neurolaryngology.

NASAL ANEMOMETRY

Objective measures of nasalisation can be obtained by measuring the acoustic energy from the nasal and oral cavities to obtain a sound intensity ratio. This ratio was referred to as 'nasalance' by Fletcher (1970, 1972) and is the acoustic correlate of perceived nasality. Earlier instruments included the TONAR (The Oral Nasal Acoustic Ratio) in which microphones placed in the oral and nasal cavities processed frequencies from 50 to 20 kHz (Fletcher, 1970). This instrument was designed for assessment and to provide biofeedback, but was expensive, bulky and technically demanding for clinical use (McWilliams, Morris and Shelton, 1984). The Kay Nasometer used currently to assess nasality employs an input device consisting of two directional microphones and a nasal/oral separator. The nasal:oral ratio is calculated and displayed on the computer screen instantly. The software calculates mean nasality, standard deviation and range. It can be used to measure and document nasality before and after voice therapy and surgery, as well as to provide feedback.

Measures of nasal airflow can be obtained by instruments such as the Exeter Nasal Anemometry System (Ellis et al., 1978). This instrument measures nasal airflow during speech and provides an index of palatal efficiency by means of a digital display. A dual trace chart shows sound pressure on the upper trace and associated airflow on the lower trace (Ellis, 1979). In addition to acquiring baseline measures, the anemometer can be used to measure improvements in palatal efficiency after using a palatal training device produced by the same team (Curle, 1979). The less expensive Exeter Biofeedback Nasal Anemometer (EBNA) is designed specifically for feedback during treatment. The SeeScape (Winslow) also detects nasal emission of air, rather than nasality, during speech. Feedback is provided by the nasal tip of a catheter being placed in one of the patient's nostrils, so that any nasal emission of air causes a float to rise in the rigid calibrated plastic tube.

For more detailed information and discussion on the instruments that can be used, the reader is recommended the definitive text on the clinical measurement of speech and voice by Baken and Orlikoff (2000).

Patient self-rating

For many years, there has been an emphasis on the importance of instrumental evaluation of voice disorders for baseline data and on-going assessment. This continues to be an essential aspect of the assessment of patients with dysphonia. Experienced clinicians working in this field have, however, stressed the importance of more extensive evaluation of the patient. This is partly because many instrumental assessments do not reflect the patient's everyday speech patterns and are often based on the analysis of a steady vowel alone. In addition, the strictly clinical approach of judging the success of treatment by the methods described in this chapter does not take into account the patient's feelings of well-being and quality of life. It is now being acknowledged in the literature that the patient's subjective opinion about the disorder and the changes that result from treatment should be taken into account, along with improvement in biological and physiological status (Benninger et al., 1998). Voice disorders represent a significant degree of handicap and an improvement in quality of life with treatment is an important element to monitor. The Voice Handicap Index (VHI; Jacobson et al., 1997; Figure 13.14 on pages 465–6) has been developed as a psychometrically validated tool for measuring the psychosocial handicapping effects of voice disorders. Thirty statements about the effect of the voice disorder on the individual are divided into three subsections: functional, physical and emotional. The patient completes the form by marking the frequency with which each statement applies and points are allotted for each category: never (0 point), almost never (1 point), sometimes (2 points), almost always (3 points) or always (4 points). Each subsection is totalled and then a total for the entire scale is calculated. The VHI can help the clinician to understand the impact of the voice disorder on the patient's quality of life, contribute to treatment planning and provide outcome measures. It can also be of use in evaluating the effectiveness of specific treatments.

Report writing

After the assessment procedures described in this chapter, conclusions are drawn and decisions are made regarding future management. A written report should be sent to referring clinicians and to other professionals involved in the patient's care, where appropriate. It summarises the assessment findings, the conclusions that have been drawn from the collated information and data, the course of intervention that has been decided upon and the rationale for this course of action. This report is an essential part of the case documentation and serves as a point of reference as treatment proceeds, particularly if recovery does not progress as expected.

Summary

- Comprehensive evaluation of the patient, the physiological basis of the voice disorder, and its presentation are fundamental to the treatment of voice disorders.
- Laryngoscopic examination is a mandatory procedure before treatment.
- Correct conclusions regarding the problem can be reached only when the information and data from these assessments have been integrated.

■   Assessment procedures can be used as a basis for treatment and for measuring treatment outcomes.

■   The patient's view of the voice problem, how it affects quality of life and its response to treatment must be taken into account during assessments.

	Never	Almost Never	Sometimes	Almost Always	Always
F1. My voice makes it difficult for people to hear me.					
P2. I run out of air when I talk.					
F3. People have difficulty under-standing me in a noisy room.					
P4. The sound of my voice varies throughout the day.					
F5. My family has difficulty hearing me when I call them throughout the house.					
F6. I use the phone less often than I would like.					
E7. I'm tense when talking with others because of my voice.					
F8. I tend to avoid groups of people because of my voice.					
E9. People seem irritated with my voice.					
P10. People ask, 'What's wrong with your voice?'					
F11. I speak with friends, neighbors, or relatives less often because of my voice.					
F12. people ask me to repeat myself when speaking face-to-face.					
P13. My voice sounds creaky and dry.					
P14. I feel as though I have to strain to produce voice					
E15. I find other people don't understand my voice problem.					
F16. My voice difficulties restrict my personal and social life.					

(contd)

	Never	Almost Never	Sometimes	Almost Always	Always
P17. The clarity of my voice is unpredictable.					
P18. I try to change my voice to sound different.					
F19. I feel left out of conversations because of my voice.					
P20. I use a great deal of effort to speak.					
P21. My voice is worse in the evening.					
F22. My voice problem causes me to lose income.					
E23. My voice problem upsets me.					
E24. I am less out-going because of my voice my voice problem.					
E25. My voice makes me feel handicapped.					
P26. My voice 'gives out' on me in the middle of speaking.					
E27. I feel annoyed when people ask me to repeat.					
E28. I feel embarrassed when people ask me to repeat.					
E29. My voice makes me feel incompetent.					
E30. I'm ashamed of my voice problem.					

P Scale
F Scale
E Scale
Total Scale

Please circle the number that matches how you feel your voice is today.

Normal		Mild		Moderate		Severe	
1	2	3	4	5	6	7	

Instructions: These are statements that many people have used to describe their voices and the effects of their voices on their lives. Check the response that indicates how frequently you have the same experience. (Never = 0 points; Almost Never = 1 point; Sometimes = 2 points; Almost Always = 3 points; Always = 4 points)

Figure 13.14 Voice Handicap Index (VHI) self-rating form. © American Speech-Language-Hearing Association. Reprinted by permission.

14 CHAPTER

Management and treatment: principles and techniques

The majority of voice disorders are treated by voice therapy. Voice therapy includes various strategies aimed at changing vocal behaviours in order to minimise or resolve the voice disorder. The underlying aetiological factors are addressed whenever possible, but symptomatic treatment is also employed. A combination of both approaches is the clinical reality in many instances. Within the disciplines of otorhinolaryngology and speech–language pathology, there is general acceptance that voice therapy is effective in treating many voice disorders (Mackenzie et al., 1998; Pannbacker, 1998; Ramig and Verdolini, 1998; Carding, Horsley and Docherty, 1999; Hicks, 1999). It is only comparatively recently, however, that studies have been conducted to investigate the efficacy of various treatment techniques. In the past, acknowledged texts and articles have tended to be based on the 'how I do it' principle (Ramig and Verdolini, 1998), with clinicians describing various treatment approaches that they find helpful in their own clinical practice. Treatment outcomes of particular types of intervention have not generally been investigated. Voice pathologists generally choose techniques on an eclectic basis, according to a rationale arising from the aetiology of the voice disorder, observed or reported laryngeal findings, aberrant features of the vocal profile and aerodynamic deficiencies. Personal or departmental preferences also influence the choice of techniques. Most clinicians probably select treatment techniques on the basis of experience rather than research evidence.

The reason for the lack of evidence-based clinical practice in voice pathology is unclear. It is possible that, if the outcome of a process seems obvious, there is little motivation to prove cause and effect. For example, if it is observed that every time people jump off a cliff they hit the beach below, the effect of jumping off cliffs seems obvious. (The process only becomes interesting when someone jumps off the cliff and then flies.) Similarly, experienced clinicians know that a large proportion of their patients with voice disorders improve during the time that they are in treatment, even when the problem has been long-standing and previously showed no sign of spontaneous improvement. The process of therapy, therefore, appears to produce a satisfactory outcome, but as yet there is little evidence as to which techniques and elements of treatment bring about this improvement. Is it the advice that is given? Are some techniques intrinsically more effective than others? To what extent does the speech–language pathologist's demeanour and interpersonal skills affect the outcome? Are techniques that are used effectively by one clinician ineffective when used by someone else? Why?

The current emphasis on evidence-based practice is founded on a number of factors. Most importantly, the patient is entitled to receive treatment that will produce the best outcome as quickly as possible. This is also the best use of resources. Whether funded by the state, medical insurance or patient self-payment, value for money in clinical practice is best achieved by delivering care by methods that are known to be effective. This reduces expensive waste of time using ineffective procedures which either do not produce the required results or take much longer to resolve the condition. In an increasingly litigious society, professionals also need the protection of knowing which techniques have proven worth and which might be regarded as ineffective or even damaging.

Evidence-based practice is founded on research into treatment **efficacy**, **efficiency** and **effectiveness** (Kearns and Simmons, 1990; Rosenberg and Donald, 1995; Benninger et al., 1998):

- Treatment **efficacy** is the ability of a particular treatment strategy to achieve a predicted result directly.
- Treatment **efficiency** refers to the relative performance of treatment approaches, i.e. whether one strategy works more effectively than another.
- Treatment **effectiveness** is a broader concept. It relates to the effects of the treatment and their worth when generalised to everyday life. It includes the patient's subjective opinion about the overall improvement as a result of the treatment. The generalisation of treatment effects to the patient's domestic and social life as well as to employment is of paramount importance in evaluating the value of treatment in any communication disorder, including voice pathology.

Ideally, speech–language pathologists should conduct voice therapy on the basis of procedures that are known, through research evidence, to be effective. This involves systematically finding, appraising and using current research results and conclusions as the basis for clinical decisions (Rosenberg and Donald, 1995), and implementing useful findings in clinical practice (Table 14.1). As Pannbacker (1998) states in her review of outcome studies of voice treatment techniques: 'Clinical practice should be guided by data about outcome; it should be based on what is proven, not on what is popular.' Where evidence exists that validates certain

Table 14.1 Studies demonstrating the value of voice therapy

Disorder	Study	Treatments
Muscle tension dysphonia (MTD)	Bridger and Epstein (1983) Koufman and Blalock (1988) Carding and Horsley (1992) Carding, Horsley and Docherty (1999)	Combination of treatments/ traditional voice therapy
	Roy and Leeper (1993)	Manual therapy
	Fex et al. (1994)	Accent method
Vocal fold nodules	Stemple et al. (1980)	EMG feedback
	Andrews, Warner and Stewart (1986)	EMG feedback and relaxation
	Lancer et al. (1988)	Combination of treatments/
	Blood (1994) Verdolini-Marston et al. (1995)	traditional voice therapy
	Verdolini-Marston, Sandage and Titze (1994)	Hydration
Surgery for benign and malignant vocal fold lesions	Koufman and Blalock (1989)	Incidence of prolonged post-operative dysphonia significantly lower in group receiving preoperative voice therapy
Psychogenic voice disorders	Andersson and Schalen (1998)	Vocal exercises and communication skills training

Sources: Ramig and Verdolini (1998); Pannbacker (1998).

Most of these studies used a combination of treatment approaches and this reflects general clinical practice. The minimum duration of treatment was one session of 1–3 hours (Roy and Leeper, 1993: manual therapy.) The maximum treatment time in the papers cited was 10 weeks.

It is interesting to note that, even when subjects do not have a voice disorder, studies indicate that normal vocal function can be improved by methods used to treat clinical voice disorders (Kotby, Shiromoto and Hirano, 1993: Accent method; Chan, 1994: vocal hygiene; Stemple et al., 1994: vocal function exercises).

It has also been found that, when healthy singers without voice problems carry out vocal function exercises in addition to their regular singing practice regimen, there are significant improvements in phonation volume, maximum phonation times and flow rate. These improvements suggest an increase in glottal efficiency (Sabol, Lee and Stemple, 1995).

techniques, it can provide a sound basis for clinical practice. At the moment, however, evidence has not been amassed for many of the techniques currently used. This does not mean that they are to be avoided but that they should be employed with critical awareness by the voice pathologist.

It has to be remembered that the validation of treatment efficacy is a complex process, which can be affected by a multiplicity of variables related to the patient, the clinician and the treatment process. Pannbacker (1998) notes that the effectiveness of treatment can be affected by:

- speaker variables, e.g. age, sex
- the techniques employed
- the length of treatment sessions
- the duration of treatment
- the aetiology of the condition
- the duration of the symptoms
- the severity of the problem.

In addition, little research has been carried out on the effect of the clinician on the effectiveness of treatment (Andrews and Schmidt, 1995). It is reasonable to presume from clinical experience that this can be a profoundly positive or negative influence on the process and outcome of therapy.

This chapter discusses some of the treatment strategies that are used by speech–language pathologists specialising in voice disorders. Efficacy studies have been conducted on some of these approaches whereas others are popular but their effectiveness is unproven. Many can be applied to a range of disorders but, where specific approaches are required, these are included under the relevant headings. Table 14.2 lists some of the treatments that can be used in voice therapy. It demonstrates clearly the wide range of treatment options and the problem of choosing the most suitable technique that confronts the clinician. In clinical practice, successful treatment outcome depends on accurate and comprehensive information about laryngeal structure and function, the speech–language pathologist's skill at evaluating patients and their voice disorders, the selection of appropriate treatment techniques and the way in which treatment is developed and executed. It also depends on the patient's compliance and motivation.

Treatment approaches tend to fall into categories but elements of the various categories overlap. In many cases, an element from one category will be a precursor to an element of another category. For example, reduction of vocal abuse will usually precede the introduction of improved vocal techniques in cases of hyperfunctional dysphonia. Facilitation techniques,

Table 14.2 Treatment approaches in voice therapy

Voice therapy Treatment categories	
Education and explanation	Normal anatomy/physiology Patient's laryngeal status Aetiological factors Realistic reassurance
Vocal tract care	Adequate hydration (systemic and atmospheric) Reduction/elimination of laryngeal irritants
Voice conservation/vocal hygiene	Reduction of vocal abuse Reduced vocal loudness Phonation without effort Reduced speech rate Reduction of hard glottal attack 'Confidential voice' Voice rest
Improved vocal techniques	Vocal function exercises (physiological voice therapy) Speech–breathing techniques
Pedagogic strategies	Modification of vocal behaviours Biofeedback Imagery Negative practice Treatment schemes, e.g. Accent method; LSVT
Facilitating techniques	Yawn/sigh Pushing exercises Laryngeal valving exercises Froeschels' chewing method Manual techniques Vegetative techniques Inspiratory phonation
Indirect treatments	Relaxation Psychological counselling Specialised techniques, e.g. Alexander, Feldenkrais techniques

such as laughing or throat clearing, can restore voice in conversion symptom aphonia but psychological counselling may be necessary subsequently.

Education and explanation

It is essential for patients to understand the normal anatomy and physiology of the vocal tract, their laryngeal status and the causative factors. The clinician's skill is to give explanations at an appropriate level so that the situation is clarified and the management plan can be recognised by the patient as a logical strategy for overcoming the voice disorder. Explanations should take account of patients' emotional status, whatever their educational or intellectual levels. High levels of anxiety impair the absorption of complex information which can increase anxiety and concern. It is helpful to use three-dimensional models of the larynx and vocal tract as well as clear anatomical drawings which are commercially available. A video of normal laryngeal structure and function, and of the patient's larynx, can be helpful, but care must be taken to establish that the patient is happy to view this material. Some individuals particularly dislike the idea of viewing their internal workings and these feelings should be respected by the clinician. As these explanations are given, soundly based reassurance can be combined with the information. This can help to reduce anxiety and establish an attitude in the patient that recovery is possible. It is indefensible to give unrealistic reassurance, but in most cases it is possible to give a degree of reassurance regarding the outcome which helps the patient to cooperate with treatment. This is particularly so in cases such as muscle tension dysphonia where there is no laryngeal pathology. It should be explained to the patient that, as there is no organic reason for the voice disorder, there is no reason theoretically why vocal function should not be improved, i.e. there is nothing wrong with the equipment but it is being used incorrectly.

Vocal tract care

Cases of vocal misuse and abuse recover more quickly if the patient takes the best care of the larynx and vocal tract by keeping adequately hydrated and by reducing exposure to substances that can irritate and damage the larynx and vocal tract. Pannbacker (1998) cites a number of studies that indicate that increasing systemic hydration has a beneficial effect, and the patient should be encouraged to drink at least 2 litres of water each day. Atmospheric hydration by steam inhalation can also reduce laryngeal irritability. It is unnecessary and inadvisable to add menthol and other substances, which can be counterproductive by increasing laryngeal irritability. The adverse effects of smoking cigarettes and other substances, as well as the inflammatory and dehydrating results of drinking excessive alcohol, should also be addressed. Tea and coffee intake should be reduced because of their dehydrating effect and simple advice to eliminate gastric reflux should be given (see page 325). Factory workers in dusty or fume-laden atmospheres should be encouraged to wear masks whenever possible. The advice regarding good vocal tract and voice care is summarised in Figure 14.1 in the form of a leaflet that can be given to patients. It seems that this written information is more effective if

---

VOICE CARE

When a voice problem is the result of vocal misuse or abuse, it is important to change the vocal behaviour and to reduce or eliminate anything that causes damage to the vocal tract.

The majority of voice care advice falls into two categories: voice conservation and vocal tract hygiene.

VOICE CONSERVATION

The changes in the abused vocal folds – inflammation, thickening, nodules, etc. – must be allowed to settle and reduce. Consequently, it is essential that you should **use your voice without effort** even if this means that it is quiet and breathy.

The following points should be remembered:

- talk gently
- avoid talking against background noise
- no shouting
- no singing
- no whispering
- no calling from room to room
- keep telephone calls to a minimum
- reduce hard glottal attack.

If your throat starts to hurt or your voice deteriorates, stop talking and rest your voice for 30 minutes to an hour. Ideally, try not to talk more than necessary but do not put yourself on complete voice rest over a long period, as this might lead to more voice problems.

It is very common for mucus to accumulate in the larynx when the vocal folds are inflamed. As a result you might feel the need to clear your throat frequently. When this collection of mucus occurs, try to clear it first by a firm swallow or, if this fails, by gentle throat clearing so that the vocal folds are not damaged further by vigorous coughing.

Most importantly, observe the way you use your voice – this is almost certainly the main cause of the voice problem – and use less vocal force.

VOCAL TRACT HYGIENE

Vocal hygiene includes reducing the intake of laryngeal irritants and also taking positive measures to maintain a healthy larynx and vocal tract.

It is best to avoid:

- smoking cigarettes, cigars, pipes
- spirits: whisky and other spirits might feel soothing but they only anaesthetise the throat while causing further irritation
- smoky, dusty or dry atmospheres
- coffee
- very hot, very cold or very spicy food and drink
- gargling
- indigestion and heartburn.

It is helpful to:

- drink plenty of water (your urine should be clear)
- have steam inhalations
- keep the atmosphere moist: open the window; have plants in the room.

Figure 14.1 Voice care leaflet for patients with hyperfunctional dysphonia resulting in changes to the vocal fold mucosa, ranging from laryngeal irritation to benign mass lesions as the result of vocal abuse. The reverse side of the leaflet can include a diagram of the vocal folds; when relevant and appropriate, the patient's laryngeal abnormality can be drawn onto the image by the clinician. It is also useful to have a 'personal information' box on the reverse so that key points of advice can be noted.

each item, and the reason for its inclusion, are discussed. On the reverse side of the leaflet, there is a panel where personal notes can be made for the patient, e.g. 'Remember to breathe – don't try to continue talking when you have run out of air!' and a simple diagram of the vocal folds, where the site of lesions can be marked, for example.

Voice conservation/vocal hygiene

Voice conservation, or vocal hygiene, is important when the vocal fold mucosa has been traumatised with resulting inflammation, oedema, nodules, polyps and other lesions; these are the result of mechanical damage arising from forceful vocal fold adduction. It can also be important to conserve the voice after trauma to the vocal folds by external sources, such as intubation for general anaesthetic, and after phonosurgery. In both cases, it might be necessary to allow for re-epithelialisation of the damaged area of the vocal fold by gentle voice use. The aim of voice conservation is to allow the traumatised mucosa to recover by using the voice gently and with minimal effort, so reducing vocal abuse.

The speech–language pathologist may have to demonstrate the use of effortless, gentle voice. Patients frequently think that reduced effort means speaking more quietly and, although these two features are linked, it is important to ensure that further abusive vocal behaviours do not occur as the patient attempts to comply. A common problem arises because of the correlation between loudness and pitch. In an attempt to speak more gently, and therefore more quietly, patients sometimes reduce their speaking pitch. If they are not carefully monitored, they can then cause further vocal fold damage or vocal tract discomfort as they attempt to speak on an unduly low pitch. Although encouraging the patient to speak less loudly is a reasonable strategy with the forceful, ebullient speaker, it should be remembered that hyperadducted vocal folds can also occur in the quiet tense speaker. The exhortation to speak more gently and with minimal effort applies generally to patients in the vocal misuse and abuse category. The patient needs clinical time to practise and stabilise this skill with guidance, before it can be generalised and can be helped by imagery (see below). In their attempts to comply with the advice that they have been given, patients may attempt to 'save' their voices by whispering and this must be discouraged because it can be effortful with relatively high-pressure air passing through, and irritating, the glottis.

When very rapid speech rate is part of the general picture of forceful, 'driven' communication, encouraging the speaker to reduce excessive speed can be helpful in producing more relaxed phonation. Many speakers find that this is extremely difficult to maintain in spontaneous speech, however, and they should be shown that it is possible to speak rapidly with minimal effort using light articulatory contacts and 'flowing' phonation.

REDUCTION OF HARD GLOTTAL ATTACK

When hard glottal attack is prevalent, patients are usually unaware of this feature of their vocal behaviour. Even when identified, it is such an integral part of phonation that they may have great difficulty in eliminating it voluntarily. The following hierarchy of techniques can be used to achieve easy onset:

- The patient inspires and then breathes out on a gentle voiceless vowel. When this is being achieved with a relatively relaxed vocal tract, voiced vowels preceded by /h/ are attempted. The vowel /a:/ is usually the easiest to produce without tension.
- The patient inspires and then produces strings of vowels with continuous voice. Although it might still be difficult to use easy onset on the initial vowel, the following vowels should be free of hard glottal attack as the vocal folds are vibrating continuously. The vocal tract and mandible should be as relaxed as possible. When the sensation of easy, unforced onset becomes established, each vowel is produced in isolation without hard attack.
- If these methods do not work, the problem can be overcome if the patient is encouraged to phonate in unison with the speech–language pathologist. It appears that the auditory and kinaesthetic patterns have become so entrenched in these patients that they have difficulty in changing their vocal behaviour. The simultaneous feedback of the clinician's phonation appears to disturb the usual feedback patterns and allows a change in vocal patterns. Following this, the vowel can be produced unaccompanied.
- When it has been achieved at the onset of isolated vowels, easy onset can be produced on words beginning with vowels, in words and in phrases. The sensation of effortless phonation can be strange after years of using hard glottal attack, and patients frequently comment that it feels as if they are singing (when they are speaking).

'CONFIDENTIAL VOICE'

This technique encourages use of the voice at the quietest intensity that can be used, as if exchanging a confidence with a friend (Pannbacker, 1998). In this way, a new kinaesthetic image for phonation can be established and patients are frequently surprised that they can still be heard in conversation. This is a technique that can be used in the clinic as a means of reducing excessive loudness in general conversation. Many over-loud, forceful speakers appear to think that they will not be heard unless they speak excessively loudly. Care must be taken, however, to ensure that hyperfunctional patterns are not transferred to confidential voice, and the way in which the technique is modelled by the speech–language pathologist is crucial.

VOICE REST

The rationale for total voice rest is that it allows traumatic damage of the vocal fold mucosa to resolve. It is most commonly used after microsurgery so that re-epithelialisation can occur as rapidly as possible; it is also recommended when there are severe inflammatory or haemorrhagic changes in the vocal fold mucosa. Koufman and Blalock (1991) consider that voice rest is mandatory only in cases of vocal fold haemorrhage. Its validity as a technique is queried for a number of reasons. Total voice rest, at best, is effective only while it is being observed, because the patient will revert to abusive vocal behaviours immediately voice is used, unless modified by therapy. In addition, it is almost impossible for most patients to maintain complete voice rest for long. The period of recommended voice rest varies from one surgeon to another and is based on opinion rather than evidence. In the UK, recommended voice rest tends to range from 48 hours to 5 days. Prolonged total voice rest is difficult to justify. There is little doubt, however, that patients rapidly cause further damage if they do not conserve their voices and eliminate abusive vocal behaviours immediately after surgery involving the vocal fold mucosa. From their study of voice rest in microlaryngeal surgical cases, Koufman and Blalock (1989) concluded that absolute voice rest provided no greater protection against postoperative dysphonia than a programme of voice conservation incorporating limited speaking for 7–10 days, use of soft glottal attack, reduced loudness and avoidance of abusive behaviours such as throat clearing. They acknowledged the importance of preoperative voice therapy as an effective preventive measure and stressed that patient compliance and motivation are the key to successful outcome.

Improved vocal techniques

Voice therapy is aimed at changing vocal behaviour in order to maximise vocal effectiveness, given the existing disorder, and to reduce the handicapping effect of the voice problem (Ramig and Verdolini, 1998). It includes eliminating counterproductive or damaging vocal behaviours and helping patients to establish vocal skills commensurate with their professional and social requirements, whenever possible. In the process of therapy, the patient's kinaesthetic model of phonation is modified while changes are being made to the acoustic profile. It is essential to choose a technique based on a viable rationale. This depends on understanding the aetiology of the voice disorder and on having accurate information about the laryngeal biomechanics in each case. The reasons for the use of various techniques should be explained carefully to patients with clear instructions as to how they should be carried out. These activities become comfortably familiar to the voice pathologist but, to the average patient, already contending with the problems of a voice disorder, vocal function exercises and other techniques frequently seem bizarre and even embarrassing. Consequently, the way in which they are introduced can significantly affect their effectiveness.

VOCAL FUNCTION EXERCISES/PHYSIOLOGICAL VOICE THERAPY

Improved vocal skills can be acquired through what have been termed 'vocal function exercises' or 'physiological voice therapy' (Stemple et al., 1994), which can have a pronounced effect on phonation. Stemple et al. (1994) verified the efficacy of such exercises in healthy, young women without laryngeal pathology in whom the exercise programme enhanced normal vocal function, particularly the extremes of pitch level. In patients with voice disorders, particular exercises are chosen according to observed laryngeal function abnormalities, such as hyperadduction, glottal insufficiency or whether the larynx is held at an unusually high or lowered position in the vocal tract. It is frequently helpful to use simple techniques based on sung or chanted vowels initially, to overcome the habituated speaking behaviour. (Patients who say that they cannot sing should be encouraged to comply and are often pleased by what they can achieve. Occasionally, patients are reduced to helpless laughter, sometimes by embarrassment but also because they are suddenly amused by the situation. Using speech-based exercises usually overcomes this reaction.) To be maximally effective, clinical experience indicates that, while these tasks must be well focused and carried out efficiently, they should also be enjoyable and even fun if possible. There is little point in the treatment if it compounds the intensity and anxiety that have caused or maintained the voice problem. A hierarchy of tasks should be designed which enables patients to be successful initially so that confidence develops and they are able to relax.

Exercises to counteract hyperfunctional phonation are directed at helping the patient to achieve competent vocal fold adduction without excessive effort. As the patient may have strong sensations of phonation in the laryngeal area, shifting the focus of sensation to the lips, front of face and oral cavity can help to reduce hyperfunction. At the same time, this encourages easy resonance of the fundamental vocal note and a perceived increase in vocal loudness, which the patient has previously attempted to achieve by excessive laryngeal effort. Vocal function exercises are directed at the following targets (see Table 14.3).

Table 14.3 Target behaviours for improved vocal function exercises

---

- Vocal note quality modification
- Soft/easy onset of vocal note
- Pitch modification
- Development of resonance
- Reduction of articulatory tension
- Vocal fold adduction in hyperfunctional glottic chink
- Reduction of supraglottic activity: inspiratory phonation

Vocal note quality modification

Imitation of various vocal qualities increases the patient's awareness of possible variations and also helps to change vocal behaviour. The speech–language pathologist demonstrates a voice with a 'sharp edge', a 'rounded edge' and weak, breathy voice (see 'Imagery' below). As the patient attempts to produce what amounts to different degrees of adduction, awareness of varying levels of effort and its relationship to changes in the sound of the voice develop. A new kinaesthetic model emerges and the patient begins to appreciate the excessive phonatory effort that has been used habitually.

Soft/easy vocal onset

The patient works through vowels and diphthongs on a sigh, introducing voice after /h/ to ensure a soft attack:

- single vowels are sung on a steady note with an evenly sustained breath
- unbroken chains of different vowels are sung on one note
- interruption of phonation is introduced between each vowel in the chain, ensuring that hard glottal attack does not recur.

Throughout these exercises there is emphasis on easy onset, reduced volume, a clear vocal note and open, relaxed articulation. If avoidance of hard attack is still found difficult, more time must be spent on 'sighing' vowels and 'gliding' into phonation with an uninterrupted breath. Vowels may be preceded by /h/ or a voiceless fricative lasting 3 or 4 seconds. Some vowels cause more difficulty than others, depending on individual patients, the voice cracking on these long after all others have become strong and clear. It is sometimes found helpful to preface a difficult vowel with a vowel that is easy for the patient, and then to isolate the 'difficult' one.

Pitch modification

When inappropriate speaking pitch, either too high or too low, is an aspect of a disordered voice, pitch glides enable the patient to explore the potential of the pitch range and experience the ease of producing notes at a more suitable frequency. The vocal note is immediately clearer and appears to be louder when this is reached. The resonance change is far more obvious in strained than in normal voices (Laguaite and Waldrop, 1963), and the appropriate speaking pitch can be established during subsequent exercises. Most patients appear to find a rising glide easier to start with. (Starting high in the vocal range encourages hyperadduction as a result of the increased tension required for higher notes.) A single vowel is used for the glide; the vowel /a:/ can be used to encourage an open mouth and relaxed mandible. Falling glides are initially achieved most easily if they are produced as continuations of a rising glide. A tendency to produce vocal creak as the glide falls to the lower part of the range indicates hyperadduction and the patient can be helped by being encouraged to 'let your voice happen rather than trying to make it happen'. Finally, continuous rising–falling glides give a sensation of effortlessness and the extent of the range can gradually be expanded.

Patients usually recognise the vocal improvement but in the early stages find it difficult to initiate the appropriate frequency. The speech–language pathologist can help the patient to return to the identified pitch by monitoring when it has been lost. This facilitates auditory perception and motor skills. It appears that, when habitual pitch has been unduly high, patients are pleased or not concerned when it has been lowered. In contrast, men with excessively low pitch, as in cases of contact ulcers, can be reluctant to raise their pitch because of fears that a higher pitch will affect the image of their masculinity. They may acknowledge that their voices must be raised out of the vocal fry register (Nahum, 1967), but care has to be taken through discussion and feedback techniques to ensure that the higher pitch is accepted.

Developing resonance

Vocal resonance can be developed with exercises based on humming. The sensation and auditory feedback of achieving increased loudness with minimal effort reduces hyperfunctional behaviour:

- Humming is sustained on a single note at a comfortable pitch, with the aim of feeling vibration on the lips and front of the face.

- The hands are placed lightly over the face and nose while humming so that vibrations may be felt by the fingers. The vibrations become much stronger when the optimum pitch is reached. The patient can feel the therapist's face for comparison (Zaliouk, 1960, 1963).
- A finger-tip can be placed on lax lips and the vibrations felt as a gentle hum is produced. Relaxed lips will tingle during humming. Children can use a comb covered with tissue paper held to the lips to feel this effect when humming.
- Ear cupping: humming with the palms of the hands cupped over the ears amplifies the resonance of the voice and is also a useful device for determining the best vocal range. Vibrations can be felt in the ears, jaws, and by the hands, as well as heard.
- Chest resonance: tactile clues can be used when treating men whose habitual pitch is too high and women who have immature voices. Chest vibration can be felt by placing the hand lightly on the throat, with the thumb and first finger touching the larynx and the lower edge of the hand resting on the clavicles. Tactile sensations should be felt when high and low notes are contrasted.
- When a note is produced that is not hyperfunctional and that has improved resonance, humming on /m/ is followed by vowels, e.g. /ma/, /moʉ/, /meɪ/, /mi/. Each syllable is then produced throughout the scale in *arpeggios* with various intervals. A relaxed tongue and awareness of a relaxed, open pharynx are encouraged.

Reducing articulatory tension

Specific work on articulation may be necessary for patients whose articulatory patterns adversely affect phonation, as in the individual with little mouth-opening and a tense jaw. Relaxed but accurate articulation is the aim of therapy. Consonants are practised in various combinations and rhythms, in order to develop both coordination of fine muscle movements and kinaesthetic and auditory awareness. Eventually tongue twisters and alliterative sentences can be used for developing effortless articulatory expertise without hyperfunctional phonation.

Vocal fold adduction in hyperfunctional glottic chink

Insufficient approximation of the vocal folds, in contrast to hyperadduction, occurs in some cases of muscle tension dysphonia supposedly caused by internal tensor weakness. Treatment is generally directed at reducing excessive effort, as described above. In cases that do not respond, direct strategies for improving adduction might be necessary, but these must be used with care and discarded as soon as possible to avoid exacerbating the situation or traumatising the vocal folds. The patient should practise these exercises only with the speech–language pathologist and not as home practice:

- Coughing in order to obtain complete approximation of the folds and to obtain a hard attack can be used to develop kinaesthetic and tactile awareness of appropriate laryngeal tonicity.
- The previous exercise is followed by clear articulation of vowels which are initiated with a glottal stop. Each vowel is sustained clearly for several seconds. The vowels are then repeated without the glottal stop onset.
- Strings of vowels are intoned on one breath, each preceded by hard attack. These are then repeated without hard attack while there are still clear auditory and kinaesthetic images of strong voice.
- Consonant–vowel syllables are practised using exaggerated plosives.
- Singing exercises are useful, build confidence and help to overcome inhibitions.
- Reading and speaking against ambient noise should be practised as described in the voice exercises (see 'Prosody').

In all these methods for obtaining closer approximation of the vocal folds and correcting air wastage during phonation, care must be taken to avoid any increase of generalised tension in the patient and interference with breathing technique. The hard attack should be discarded as soon as possible, especially with patients who have a history of vocal abuse.

Inspiratory phonation

The above strategies help to reduce supraglottic activity accompanying true vocal fold approximation, but a more specific strategy may be required to overcome false vocal fold adduction. Inspiratory phonation or reversed phonation (Lehmann, 1965; Williams, Farquharson and Anthony, 1975) causes the laryngeal ventricles to open and the false folds to be drawn away from the midline. After prolonged inspiratory phonation, voice is produced on expiration in a continuous process. Boone (1977) also recommended this exercise for treating conversion symptom aphonia and puberphonia.

SPEECH–BREATHING TECHNIQUES

Considerable discussion has been generated among those who treat dysphonic patients about work on breathing technique. Many believe (Wilson, 1987; Aronson, 1980; Stemple, 1984; Fawcus, 1986b) that the teaching of breathing techniques is usually unnecessary in cases of hyperkinetic dysphonia, where relaxed, natural breathing patterns are all that is required as a basis for vocal recovery. It is argued that the introduction of 'breathing exercises' into the treatment programme will create awareness and a resulting increase in tension which will be counterproductive. All these writers agree, however, that there are cases where this approach is insufficient and that, if breathing patterns are markedly disturbed by tension and anxiety, a more direct approach is required. There is general agreement that, for those patients whose voice disorders are the result of neurological involvement, the teaching of improved breathing techniques is valuable. The beneficial effects on phonation of training in breathing techniques is noted by a number of writers (Proctor, 1980; Gould, 1981; Bunch, 1982; Wilder, 1983; Hixon, 1987) and should not be disregarded in voice therapy.

The therapist must adapt explanations and suggestions for changes in breathing technique to each patient's needs. The patient will gradually develop an awareness of respiratory function as appropriate patterns are practised. In addition, many patients discover that to practise improved breathing techniques in a relaxed environment has a calming effect, which provides an ideal basis for voice therapy as well as a surprising and revealing contrast to their normal respiratory patterns for speech. Patients with habitual patterns of breathing that adversely affect phonation have forgotten the sensation of normal breathing and need help in restoring these breathing patterns.

Objectives of breathing techniques

The chief object of teaching breathing technique is to enable the patient to control the volume and expiratory flow of air, thus providing the means of controlling phonation effortlessly and easily. Increase in vital capacity is not the aim, but control of expiration in relation to vocal fold resistance. This requires complex muscular coordination, which can be developed through an amalgam of kinaesthetic and tactile sensations.

Preparation for breathing techniques

Posture must be checked because a relaxed upright carriage of the torso, head and neck is essential. Cotes (1979) gives a clear account of changes in lung volume induced by postural changes. Round shoulders, and a sagging posture that folds the chest at an angle upon the abdomen in a crease at waist level, will not allow good expansion of the lungs or control of expiration. Posture is also allied to personality and confidence (Lieberman, 1998). Bunch (1982), in discussing the 'dynamics of the singing voice', defines posture as alignment. The position of the head establishes the carriage of the long axis of the spine. The balance of muscular forces conserves energy and enhances resonance.

Explanation and demonstration

The speech–language pathologist first describes to the patient how difficult it is for the pear-shaped lungs to expand within the upper thoracic region which is encased in a bony cage, whereas it is easier to expand the lower region where the lungs are larger and the ribs free in front and separated by a large area of elastic muscle. A demonstration is given of the correct breathing action, showing how the abdomen wall moves forward and the ribs lift in order to fill the lungs. The abdominal wall flattens and the ribs fall to empty them. The thoracic and abdominal movements can be imitated with the hands, finger-tips touching, and palms adducting and abducting on expiration and inspiration.

Exercises are best demonstrated while the patient is standing so that the speech–language pathologist can gently manipulate the necessary movement of ribs and abdominal wall. The clinician can demonstrate the desired movement as the patient practises before a mirror. One hand on the clavicle and the other on the abdominal wall just above waist level reinforces the tactile, kinaesthetic and visual sensations. The patient now takes a small easy breath with one hand on the abdominal wall just above waist level and the other on the rib cage, so that the forward and lateral expansion of the thorax can be felt. The instructions 'swell up' with air and then 'squeeze it out' may be given. The verbal cues are important. The simple instruction to breathe 'in' and breathe 'out' may produce the reverse of the desired action, with the patient pulling in the abdomen on the instruction to breathe 'in' and pushing it out on breathing 'out'. This pattern is known as 'reverse breathing'. There is a widespread and firmly held but mistaken belief that, for inspiration, the abdominal wall should be well pulled in and the chest thrown out.

Problem-solving

It is sometimes difficult in cases of habitual dysphonia to obtain the correct response. In such cases the following procedures are helpful:

- The patient is instructed to breathe out, then sigh noisily on the remaining air. At the same time the therapist should apply manual pressure to the abdominal wall in the area of the diaphragm which is at the base of the sternum. This pressure is relaxed as inspiration begins, then applied again during the sigh. Manipulation of the abdominal wall in this way assists in the establishment of the easy rhythmic swing on inspiration and expiration, which is difficult for some to achieve voluntarily.
- The patient imitates a panting dog by pushing out the abdominal wall and then pulling it in. The breath is not held by a closed glottis

and the breathing is not thought about consciously until the sharp oral intake and output of air is heard. Then, attention can be drawn to the breathing and voluntary control gradually achieved, and the movement slowed down to a normal respiratory rhythm.

• The patient breathes out and then pretends to blow out a candle with the remaining air; this is produced by the rapid ascent of the diaphragm in the need to provide further airflow.

• The patient is asked to 'empty the lungs completely' by breathing out for as long as possible. Inspiration should then be delayed until the patient feels the need to inspire. When inspiration does eventually occur, expansion of the abdominal wall and rib cage takes place.

Home practice

Once the patient is able to perform the required breathing patterns, they should be practised several times each day, preferably in front of a mirror so that any movement in the upper thorax can be monitored and corrected. A week's home practice may be sufficient time for the individual to learn to produce central breathing. Frequently, there is no improvement by the second treatment, but the temptation to progress rapidly to the next stage should be resisted if steady progress is to be made with each step having been securely mastered.

Hyperventilation

Deep breathing when first practised by shallow breathers frequently induces dizziness and the patient should be warned of the possibility and reassured. A short rest should be taken after dizziness before continuing with practice which should be carried out only for short periods initially. Any tight clothing should be loosened to allow full expansion at the waist.

Common faults

It is important that the speech–language pathologist should be aware of the most common faults that may occur during acquisition of improved breathing patterns and correct them as soon as they occur:

• Tension generally occurs at each attempt to perform any new exercise demanding concentration and voluntary effort.

• Nearly all patients lapse into old breathing patterns when initially asked to phonate during exercises.

• Poor posture may prevent adequate thoracic movement.

• Inspiration may be noisy as a result of laryngeal tension and approximation of the vocal folds.

- The patient may mistakenly think that a large volume of air is required and this will result in excessive effort being used during the breathing exercises. The emphasis should be on effortless control of both correct respiratory movements and expiration for phonation.

Oral breathing and phonation

Oral inspiration of air should be used during these exercises because this is the normal method of inspiration for speech and allows air to be inspired rapidly and imperceptibly between phrases. The coordination of expiration with phonation can now be introduced in treatment by production of a clear sustained vowel of appropriate pitch as soon as a correct breathing pattern is established.

Breathing and voice control – preliminary strategy

- With the hand flat on the abdominal wall just above waist level, the patient breathes in slowly. On the out-going breath, count quietly up to four at the rate of one per second. No breath should escape between each count. This is practised, gradually increasing the count.
- Rib reserve: as counting above 10 develops, the patient often quite unconsciously holds the ribs in an elevated position and lowers them only near the end of the breath. This can be taught as a voluntary pattern to the professional voice user: the singer, actor or public speaker. A deep breath should be taken; the ribs are elevated while counting aloud up to 15 and then gradually relaxed. For ordinary purposes a count of 20, one per second, should be the target, but for singers and actors a count of 30 is appropriate.
- The patient breathes in and then counts aloud in groups of three while holding the breath for a mental count of three between each group.
- After inspiration, breath is emitted on a loud sustained voiceless fricative: /ʃ/, /s/, /f/. The fricative should be maintained at a steady volume and not fluctuate or fade towards the end. The gradual contraction of the abdominal wall is felt with the hand as the breath is expired.
- Voiceless fricatives are practised on a crescendo and diminuendo of volume: sssssSSSSSSSSsssss.
- Voiceless fricatives are emitted in rhythmic patterns.
- Maximum phonation time: once a reasonable degree of respiratory control has been achieved, the aim is to produce a prolonged vowel on a steady note and in the middle of the range of the patient's voice. The quality of the vocal note is as important as the length of time for

which it can be maintained. As the voice improves, the phonation can be extended and timed until a comfortable maximum phonation time is achieved. Increasing phonation time is a good indication of progress and a matter of encouragement to the patient. This can be followed by practising inflected vowels and intonation exercises.

Speech–breathing rhythm

- The patient breathes in and out slowly several times and then imitates the speech–language pathologist's demonstration of quick intake and slow expiration. The abdominal wall should jump forward on inspiration and subside very gradually on expiration.
- The patient takes a quick breath in and then breathes out, slowly counting six. The natural tendency to count too fast should be corrected. Repeat six times, until the new rhythmic swing is performed easily. A suggestion of the movement required may be given by the clinician by a quick hand movement to one side and a slow, drawn-out movement to the other.
- Gradually, the patient increases the count on expiration until able to count to 20 using quick inspiration.
- The patient practises sustaining a trilled /r/ at constant pitch and volume – this is a real test of breath control, necessitating a constant breath pressure to maintain vibration of the tip of the tongue and relaxation of the oral musculature.

Pedagogic strategies

Throughout the process of modifying vocal behaviour, certain teaching strategies can be employed to elicit, establish and stabilise the new phonatory patterns. These strategies facilitate the change and underpin the introduction of the various methods of improving vocal technique. Each clinician's use of these methods will vary, but they are fundamental to therapeutic intervention.

MODIFYING VOCAL BEHAVIOUR: METHOD

The voice pathologist guides the patient through a standard route consisting of five elements as each vocal task is attempted: explanation, modelling, imitation, generation and generalisation.

Explanation

In most instances, an explanation is given to the patient about the type of task that is about to be attempted, with its rationale. This enables patients to comply as well as possible and to feel that they have some control over the process.

Modelling

The voice pathologist cannot rely on instructions alone when introducing the patient to treatment techniques. It is necessary to model or demonstrate the vocal task and so provide a target for the patient. The way in which this is done can significantly affect the patient's performance and the outcome will be influenced by the vocal skills of the clinician. A good model guides and encourages the patient while the voice pathologist's inability to provide a good model reduces the credibility of the clinician. Patients cannot be expected to modify and control vocal behaviour if the clinician has not developed these skills satisfactorily.

Imitation

The patient attempts to imitate the task and receives feedback from the clinician and various types of biofeedback (see below), which confirms when the model has been matched. It is important that encouragement and constructive advice should be given so that confidence is maintained and performance improves.

Generation

When a task can be imitated reliably, modelling is withdrawn and the patient attempts to generate the behaviour in the clinical setting.

Generalisation

Finally, the new vocal behaviour, which has previously been used only in the controlled clinical situation, is generalised to other contexts.

A programme of home practice can be used once the patient has reached the stage where the desired vocal behaviour can be generated spontaneously and reliably. Self-practice at an earlier stage can lead to the habituation of potentially damaging patterns of phonation and should be avoided. Patients appear to take home practice more seriously if it is recommended that they should practise for a given period each day. Twice or three times daily, depending on work schedules, for 10 minutes on each occasion is a minimum amount of practice that is possible for most people. This does not exclude odd occasions of spontaneous practice which many patients enjoy once they have some control over their voices and are aware of improvement.

BIOFEEDBACK

This term originated from biological engineering to describe the process whereby physiological activity of which subjects are unaware is fed back to them by presentation of visual, auditory or tactile signals. The rationale is that, by monitoring the signals, the unconscious function can be brought under voluntary control. Biofeedback systems are used in psychiatry to treat anxiety that is unresponsive to drug therapy, with patients watching alpha rhythm from the electroencephalogram. Surface electromyography (EMG) without needles is also used by physiotherapists to induce relaxation.

Audio recording

Audio recording is the most commonly used biofeedback in voice therapy and enables the patient to analyse and monitor the disordered voice and its progress. Hearing training is an intrinsic part of treatment, which gives patients the opportunity to listen to their voices objectively and critically, in a way that is impossible when actively participating in voice production.

Many patients have difficulty in distinguishing between 'good' and 'bad' voice, changes in pitch, resonance, volume and breathiness. It is often thought that tone deafness, or at least poor musicality, is common to these individuals but research fails to prove this. The speech–language pathologist's 'ear' is trained so acutely that it can be difficult to appreciate how little most people listen to their own voices and how little awareness there is of their speech mannerisms. Tapes consisting of different samples of dysphonic and normal speech can be compiled easily in a voice clinic and given to patients to evaluate as exercises in developing listening skills. This may usefully precede introduction of evaluation of the patient's own recordings. Children enjoy this exercise, especially if recordings include funny voices and those of popular television characters (but note that consent from the copyright holder must be obtained).

After therapy, audio recording can provide reassurance that the voice does not sound peculiar, even if it sounds strange to the patient who has not yet adjusted to the change. Recordings of vocal tasks made by the speech–language therapist provide a target behaviour which can be practised away from the clinic.

Video recording

Video recording of laryngeal behaviour during various vocal tasks can provide feedback instantaneously or, more usually, after the laryngeal examination. Many patients appear to find it extremely helpful to see exactly what is happening, so that they have a laryngeal image when carrying out various vocal function tasks, although they do not have proprioceptive control over laryngeal movements. At the moment, there is little evidence to support the use of videoendoscopy as biofeedback on a routine clinical basis, but practice indicates that it can be a valuable tool (Bastian and Nagorsky, 1987; Karnell, 1994). Care has to be taken, however, as those who are very anxious can have their anxiety increased as yet another facet of the problem is presented to them. In these cases, the video may raise more questions than it answers as they become unduly concerned and attach sinister significance to details that are not a cause for concern.

Professional voice users and some other patients also find it helpful to see video-recordings of themselves speaking or singing. Counterproductive postures, ineffectual breathing patterns, and signs of neck and body tension can be identified. When these have been addressed, the changes are monitored by re-recording.

Note

In some countries, the patient's written consent must be obtained before recordings are made. This usually takes the form of a document that explains the purposes for which any recordings might be used, to be signed by the patient. Failure to obtain written consent may result in legal action against the clinician.

Visual display

Video display is a feature of much of the instrumentation described in Chapter 13. Software packages can provide real-time screens for frequency and loudness as well as giving some indication of vocal quality. This objective feedback is valuable not only for the information it provides, but because some patients are much more at ease performing vocal tasks with computerised equipment that is so familiar. It also enables many people to be less self-conscious as the clinical focus of attention moves from themselves to the display screen. Increasingly, patients appreciate objective information about their behaviour which provides a target and registers their improvement. It also has to be admitted that the use of instrumentation increases the credibility of voice therapy for many patients, and for this reason is useful when patients are sceptical about their referral to a voice pathologist and where a 'low-tech' approach might confirm their views. The screen display of vocal features reinforces auditory and sensory feedback and these systems can be a useful adjunct to therapy. The patient can work alone at times and monitor performance without constant intervention by the voice pathologist. The behaviour elicited by biofeedback is unlikely to be generalised without further reinforcement.

It is essential, therefore, that the clinician continues to adhere to the basic principles of treatment when such equipment is used and is aware of possible pitfalls. Tasks should be modelled clearly and the chances of significant failure should be minimised. The visual display that demonstrates success so clearly also provides irrefutable evidence of failure which can discourage the patient and, as confidence is lost, the lack of success on subsequent attempts is obvious. Imagery can also be used effectively. For example, when working with equipment that displays the frequency of the fundamental note and the patient is required to produce a vocal glide or frequency pattern, a patient's intense approach can limit performance. When encouraged to 'draw with the voice', pitch range and vocal quality usually improve considerably as the patient begins to relax and 'play' with the voice.

Amplification

Amplification can be used in certain cases to provide feedback during therapy. When the voice is excessively quiet, as in parkinsonism, amplification provides an auditory model of intensity which can continue to be targeted by the patient as the amplification is gradually reduced and withdrawn. In cases of unduly loud voice, the speaker tends to reduce volume if there is simultaneous amplification and experiences a changed kinaesthetic model of phonation during quieter speech. The aim is for reduced vocal intensity to carry over without this feedback.

TAM (tactile acoustic monitor)

TAM is a biofeedback device which provides tactile stimulation from a small instrument strapped to the wrist (Summers and Martin, 1980). Incoming sounds are amplified and these signals operate a vibrator which is sensitive to a frequency range of 100 Hz to 10 kHz. In conjunction with the temporal pattern of sounds in the environment, it renders sound sources recognisable to the profoundly deaf, the blind and cochlear implant patients, for whom the instrument was designed by the medical physics group at the University of Exeter in collaboration with the RNID. It has a volume control that can be adjusted to the requirements of the wearer against ambient noise. There is also a light that flickers on and off in unison with sound stimuli. A battery charger is provided. Although primarily an invaluable generator of warning signals for the deaf, it may also be used in voice therapy to monitor voice amplitude and prosodic accent patterns in dysphonic patients.

Voice Loudness Indicator (Jedcom)

This portable, battery-operated biofeedback device displays relative levels of vocal intensity on a display of eight lights. It has an integral microphone and a sensitivity control for adjustment.

Vocal Intensity Controller

A portable instrument used by Holbrook, Rolnick and Bailey (1974), in which a throat microphone activates a tone generator which sends signals to earphones, registering excessive vocal intensity. It can be worn continuously. Eleven of 32 patients in this experiment experienced complete resolution of vocal abuse.

Facilitator™ Model 3500

This equipment, devised by Professor Emeritus Daniel R. Boone and manufactured by Kay Elemetrics, is an auditory feedback device which offers amplification, looping, delayed auditory feedback, masking and metronomic pacing.

Electromyography

Electromyography (EMG) feedback is also potentially useful because it can monitor muscle tone in cases of dysphonia (Boone, 1977). Although there is some evidence that it can be beneficial in encouraging relaxation (Allen, Bernstein and Chait, 1991), it is not in general use. Prosek et al. (1978) studied EMG biofeedback treatment in six cases of hyperfunctional voice disorders with laryngitis, oedema, hoarseness and aphonia. The subjects received 14 training sessions of 30 minutes each. Electrodes placed on the thyroid cartilage were linked to a noise generator, which was activated when EMG activity exceeded the value selected from a control group of normal speakers. After 14 sessions, three patients had improved and three were unchanged. This would be an unsatisfactory result after 14 treatments of traditional therapy. A study undertaken by Andrews, Warner and Stewart (1986) concluded that EMG feedback was useful in detecting global increases in laryngeal tension and in demonstrating this to the patient. Unfortunately, it did not detect adductor tension in hard glottal attack and some subjects were so irritated when tension increases were registered, that their tension increased further. The importance of a competent and caring clinician and the acknowledgement of the patient as an individual were stressed in this study.

Biofeedback augments other treatment techniques in voice therapy. Guidance and encouragement are important whichever method or combination of methods is used in treating voice disorders.

IMAGERY

Imagery can be used to help patients, and students, to understand normal vocal tract function and to complement descriptions of vocal behaviours that are to be targeted in therapy. Images appear to be most useful when they reflect the reality of laryngeal and vocal tract biomechanics. Some examples are given below, but clinicians evolve the imagery that they find most useful.

Subglottic air pressure

It is understandable that many individuals with voice disorders attempt to improve the situation, and to increase loudness, by increasing expiratory effort. They perceive that high airflow through the larynx will produce more effective and louder voice. The clinician needs to explain that it is subglottic air pressure that is required for efficient phonation, not increased transglottic airflow.

The image

The relationship of vocal loudness to the expiratory airflow is like a ping-pong ball on a fountain. A steady pressure is required to keep the ball in one position. The height of the ball depends on the pressure of the water. Increases in pressure cause the ball to rise, loss of pressure causes it to reduce height. Variable pressure results in the position of the ball being unstable.

Effect of dehydration on vocal fold vibration

Reasons for advice that is given are helpful; this applies to requests for patients to increase systemic hydration.

The image

The mucosal surface of the vocal folds can be compared with canned plums, which retain their moisture, and dried fruits, with stiff unyielding skins. If a jet of air were blown over the surface of a moist fruit, the skin would respond instantly with waves of movement across its surface. The greater stiffness of the skin of the dried fruit skin would need much higher air pressure to set it in motion.

Reducing transglottic airflow

This image can help to reduce breathiness and roughness in the early stages of vocal function tasks when single vowels are being attempted. It encourages a controlled expiratory airflow and helps to maintain stable subglottal air pressure.

The image

The adducted vocal folds comprise a valve which controls the amount of air that can be released. As a vocal note is produced, imagine that only a thin thread of air is leaving the valve and that most of the air remains below it.

Reducing laryngeal effort

Effortful phonation is inevitably associated with the sensation that the voice has to be forced from the throat. As the voice deteriorates, the speaker increases the laryngeal effort in a counterproductive attempt to maintain voice.

The image

Imagine that the voice is produced in the mouth, almost on the lips. Aim for the sensation that the throat is open and that there is very little activity in the throat.

Case notes

- A patient who had been using her voice forcefully for many years was encouraged to use this image. Initially, she had considerable difficulty but suddenly managed to achieve this sensation. 'Oh, I see! When you talk it should feel as if there is nothing between your chest and your head.'

- An extremely energetic, tense and voluble patient used excessive muscular effort for all tasks, including phonation. She also maintained high levels of muscular tension even when she was apparently at rest. It was pointed out to her that her face muscles were contracted, and that she was obviously maintaining vocal fold adduction when carrying out various tasks, because the release of air could be heard from time to time. It was explained that this indicated considerable laryngeal tension. This was a revelation to her and she accurately summed up the situation – 'I hadn't realised; I've been frowning with my vocal folds.'

NEGATIVE PRACTICE

Negative practice is a treatment method that was pioneered by Mostafa Fahmy, a psychologist (1950), and Van Riper (1947) in the treatment of stammering and articulation disorders. Wilson (1987) stressed its importance in the remediation of children's voice disorders. When used in the treatment of dysphonia, negative practice is based on the hypothesis that, if a patient is made aware of a particular fault in vocal behaviour and it is then brought under conscious control, it may be used as a contrast to reinforce desirable vocal behaviour. It cannot be used as a therapeutic strategy until good voice is readily produced under voluntary control. It is a useful method of dealing with hard glottal attack. When the patient is able to produce a vowel with soft onset, the production of the same sound with hard attack highlights the kinaesthetic and auditory differences. Obviously, care must be taken not to use this practice if there is any danger of exacerbating symptoms of vocal abuse by reinforcement of bad voice production.

TREATMENT SCHEMES

Accent method

The Accent method is a dynamic, holistic approach to voice therapy which was developed by Svend Smith in Denmark in the 1930s. It has been widely used in Scandinavia for many years and there appears to be an increasing interest in this method globally. It involves the respiratory and phonatory muscles, with particular attention to the abdominal muscles, and total body movement in rhythmic sequences. The aim is to increase flexibility and elasticity of the vocal folds and ultimately to produce optimal voice function. The voice training is followed by speech training directed at accentuating prosody. There are three fundamental elements to the Accent method: dynamism, rhythmic intonation (accent) and expiratory breath control (Kotby, 1995). Breathing exercises are taught initially, and subsequently combined with voice exercises. As breath is expressed, a stream of sounds is uttered in varied rhythms and pitch changes, e.g. 'ha-ha-haha-ha', etc. Rhythmic beating of a drum and rhythmic body movements accompany voice exercises. Finally, texts are used to establish various vocal patterns. Psychologically, this method can release inhibitions and self-consciousness, and is suitable for use with children as well as adults. The patient relaxes when the therapy is undertaken in unison with the therapist. It is essential that the therapist and patient should enjoy the Accent Method and not feel foolish if it is to be effective. Smith and Thyme (1976), Damsté and Lerman (1975), Thyme (1980) and Kotby (1995) have described this method and its application.

Lee Silverman Voice Treatment programme

Lee Silverman Voice Treatment (LSVT) programme is one of the most commonly used voice treatment methods in America (Pannbacker, 1998). It is designed to increase phonatory effort, reduce vocal fold bowing and improve loudness. This intensive programme of four treatment sessions per week for 1 month is used in cases of neurological glottal insufficiency such as parkinsonism. Treatment strategies include increasing loudness, maximum phonatory effort and voice awareness through a hierarchy of increasingly complex vocal drills. Smith et al. (1995), in a study of patients with parkinsonism, found that LSVT (incorporating respiratory and phonatory tasks) proved to be more effective than respiratory treatment alone. Pannbacker (1998) reports further studies using LSVT that have also produced favourable results (see Chapter 15).

The Boone Voice Programmes for Adults and Children

These programmes are available in kits containing manuals for screening and evaluating voice disorders and for remediation. The programme for children includes step-by-step procedures for the reduction of vocal abuse based on approaches such as yawn/sigh, changing loudness, mouth opening and eliminating hard glottal attack. The adult programme is based on a similar approach and provides self-practice materials.

Estill Method of Compulsory Voice Figures

This teaching programme for developing vocal skills is based on gaining control over 11 parts of the phonatory anatomy by mastering 11 'figures' or manoeuvres. Control is directed at the false vocal folds, vocal fold mass, soft palate control, the width and length of the vocal tract, the tongue, the aryepiglottic folds and the degree of laryngeal tilting with reduced emphasis on breathing. The aim is to move each structure into two or three possible positions, such as raised or lowered or relaxed or active, so that the potential for changing vocal quality is increased. Clinicians intending to use this method attend a 5-day intensive course.

Facilitating techniques

A facilitating technique enables the patient to experience a change in vocal function which appears to produce optimum voice (Boone and McFarlane, 1988). The subsequent aim is for the patient to generate the vocal change when the facilitating technique has been withdrawn.

YAWN/SIGH

The yawn/sigh technique is a popular strategy which is used as one of a number of approaches in the treatment of hyperfunctional dysphonia. It is based on the fact that, during the prolonged inspiration at the onset of a yawn, the pharyngeal constrictors relax and there is maximum widening of the supraglottal airway. Gentle phonation is encouraged on the subsequent expiration and the patient should feel easy, relaxed phonation (Boone and McFarlane, 1988). When patients are able to cooperate with this procedure, it can be extremely effective in eliciting normal, or greatly improved, voice. As with any good facilitating technique, the vocal change can be a dramatic revelation to the patient who may be surprised that it is possible to produce such a sound. Repetition of this adapted vegetative behaviour then allows the patient to experience the sensation of normal voice until it can be translated into a gentle vowel – 'hah' – and into words.

It is essential to introduce this strategy with care if it is to work at the first attempt. Some patients are easily embarrassed by being asked to perform an expansive behaviour which generally occurs only when they are relaxed and at ease, or even in relative privacy. As a result, a tense 'ah' is produced. The clinician must demonstrate the yawn and it can be helpful if speech–language pathologist and patient yawn together. This frequently triggers genuine yawning (in both!) and easy phonation can be achieved.

PUSHING EXERCISES

Pushing exercises have been used for many years in voice therapy to encourage glottal closure through effort. Patients are asked to push down on the chair on which they are sitting or to push against a wall while simultaneously saying a vowel with a hard glottal attack. As they do so, closure of the glottis is facilitated (Wilson, 1987; Boone and McFarlane, 1988; Colton and Casper, 1990). Pushing exercises have been particularly associated with the treatment of unilateral vocal fold paralyses, the aim of treatment being to encourage maximum movement in the healthy fold and, in cases of neuropraxia of the affected fold (see page 305), to accelerate recovery. This relatively forceful strategy should not be used in cases of existing vocal fold trauma or where glottal closure is adequate. Although a study by Yamaguchi et al. (1993) confirmed that this strategy could be effective 'in select cases of glottal incompetence', the clinician should be aware of its potential hazards. It is inherent within this approach that there is a risk of hyperfunctional phonation. If patients are not carefully monitored, false vocal fold activity and considerable supraglottal activity will become associated with vocalisation. We have considerably reduced the use of 'pushing' in our clinical practice in recent years because of these potential problems and because this approach does not necessarily produce the best results. We agree with Yamaguchi et al. (1993) that alternative techniques can be more effective or, at least, equally successful (see 'Laryngeal valving' below).

LARYNGEAL VALVING

Laryngeal valving is a more subtle approach at achieving vocal fold closure than pushing or effort closure and is directed at the vocal folds specifically, rather than achieving a complete sphincteric action of the larynx. The stages are as follows:

• With the mouth open and relaxed, and without using voice, the patient attempts to obstruct a gentle expiratory airstream by adduction of the vocal folds, however fleetingly. A quiet plosion can be heard as the air is released when closure has been achieved. This stage helps the patient to identify the site of the vocal fold closure as well as to achieve glottal competency.

• When a competent closure has been achieved, the patient attempts to build up air pressure below the vocal folds and maintain the vocal fold closure. This is done silently.

• Subsequently, voicing is attempted *on release of the closure only* on the vowel /ɜ/. This is done with quiet voice.

• Vowels are produced with firm but gentle glottal closure on quiet voice and this is extended to words and phrases.

This technique appears to be helpful because the task is controlled in terms of airflow and pressure, as well as glottal closure. Patients seem less tempted to use excessive effort than in pushing exercises because the focus initially is on accurate, voiceless, vocal fold adduction rather than voice.

FROESCHELS' CHEWING METHOD

The teaching of Froeschels (1948) has never been used extensively in the UK and attempts at introducing chewing therapy have been discouraged by the marked resistance and even ridicule from patients. This was also the experience of Van Riper and Irwin (1958) who nevertheless found the method successful in lowering vocal pitch in some cases of boys with pitch breaks and in some cases of vocal nodules, when other methods had failed. They commented on the possible psychological value of the method, in addition to its manifest achievement in obtaining relaxation of the vocal and speech mechanism. The technique allows for a reversion to an infantile form of behaviour and some of Van Riper and Irwin's cases improved with the practice of vocalised thumb sucking!

The enthusiasm for the method among Froeschels' followers is impressive. The fact that it has been widely practised in America and Europe with good results would seem to indicate its value. Practically any technique in teaching, however, will achieve good results in a certain proportion of cases, but all cure also depends on the faith that the therapist has in the methods used and the faith that can be inspired in the patient. Froeschels was not only a great therapist but a great teacher, judging by the faith with which he inspired his disciples and such medical experts as Weiss (1964) and Brodnitz (1959). Froeschels' method was described in *Twentieth Century Voice Correction* (Froeschels, 1948) and *Practice of Voice and Speech Therapy* (Froeschels and Jellinek, 1941). He advocated the method chiefly as a cure for stammering. His method is based on the untested hypothesis that the movements for chewing and talking are almost identical and that chewing is the origin of human speech. He noted that, as primitive peoples chew, the movements of the articulators are accompanied by vocalisation and that babies, during the babbling stage, also move their lips and tongues as if chewing while simultaneously vocalising. Froeschels recommended that, after this explanation of the theory has been given, the patient should attempt to use voice while chewing. Nonsense syllables are produced with varied intonation used so that the voiced chewing resembles human speech. The therapist and patient have 'chewing conversations' so that 'the patient becomes aware of the fact that there is no fundamental difference between this kind of language and his natural tongue, as far as the use of muscles is concerned'. The patient is instructed to use voiced chewing for a few moments each day as a reminder. Froeschels did recognise, however, that, in some cases where there is an important psychogenic contribution to the voice disorder, more fundamental, psychological help is necessary.

MANUAL TECHNIQUES FOR REDUCING LARYNGEAL TENSION

The rationale for manual therapy is that excessive tension of the intrinsic and extrinsic laryngeal muscles affects phonation adversely and can cause considerable discomfort (see pages 124–5). Relaxing these muscles manually allows the larynx to return to a better position and posture. As a result, optimum voice can be produced and discomfort is reduced or eliminated. The stages of reducing laryngeal muscle tension by this method have been described by Aronson (1980, 1990), Roy and Leeper (1993) and Mathieson (1993a). The way in which these manual techniques are carried out varies, with the clinician either standing behind the patient or sitting in front. There is an emphasis on lowering the larynx, because the larynx is held high in the vocal tract in many hyperfunctional voice disorders. There are a significant number of patients, however, with extremely tense laryngeal musculature whose larynges are forced down as they speak on a very low speaking fundamental frequency. The larynx can be exceptionally resistant to lateral digital pressure when the larynx is held in such a depressed position. In these cases, the extrinsic laryngeal muscle tension can be reduced by massage of the sternocleidomastoid muscles (Mathieson, 1993a), in addition to the technique described by Aronson. Clinical experience shows that patients value this approach for a number of reasons. As it is highly effective in most cases, patients welcome the rapid relief from discomfort. Many patients also comment on how they enjoy the process and that massage of the tense muscles is a very pleasant sensation. It seems that an additional benefit, particularly from the clinician's point of view, is that many patients value the manual intervention because it is an

Table 14.4 Manual therapy for the laryngeal area: Aronson protocol

- The thumb and middle finger encircle the hyoid bone until the major horns can be felt. Light, rotating digital pressure is applied over the tips of the hyoid bone. The patient is carefully monitored for signs of discomfort.

- The procedure is repeated in the thyrohyoid space; the rotating digital pressure starts at the thyroid notch and moves posteriorly.

- The procedure is then repeated medially to the sternocleidomastoid muscles at the posterior borders of the thyroid cartilage.

- The larynx is gently worked downwards by applying pressure to the superior border of the thyroid cartilage. The thyrohyoid space enlarges as the larynx is lowered. The larynx should occasionally be moved laterally during this process.

- During these procedures, the patient is asked to produce steady vowels so that the reduction in tension in the laryngeal musculature is manifested in clearer vocal quality and lowered pitch. These vocal changes are then practised by the patient.

After Aronson (1990).
Aronson points out that as these procedures are fatiguing for the patient, rest periods should be provided. The patient's laryngeal area may feel sore and tender afterwards but this discomfort disappears over 1 or 2 days.

active 'hands-on' process. Finally, a subsidiary advantage of standing behind the patient while massaging the laryngeal musculature is that many patients begin to talk freely about issues as they relax and when they do not have to deal with face-to-face contact.

An alternative method of laryngeal manual therapy to Aronson's technique (Table 14.4) can also be used as described below:

- The process is described to the patient and the patient's permission is sought before starting manual therapy.
- The voice pathologist stands behind the patient who is seated in an upright chair with a low back.
- The fingers of both hands are placed on the mastoid process behind each ear and the attachment of the sternocleidomastoid muscle is located. The finger-tips are rotated in a massaging movement over the upper part of this muscle, and this movement is continued as they slowly descend along its length. Initially, only very gentle pressure must be used on this tense, tender musculature. Care must be taken when massaging the lower third of the sternocleidomastoids because coughing may be caused in the tense patient. The length of time spent on massaging the sternocleidomastoids varies from one patient to another, according to the degree of tension. As tension reduces, the muscles are noticeably softer and greater pressure can be applied without causing the patient any discomfort.

- The supralaryngeal area can then be gently kneaded with the finger tips. At first this may be hard and unyielding. The patient should be asked to relax the mandible and allow the tongue to lie in the floor of the mouth. (The habitual tongue posture in many patients with muscle tension dysphonia [MTD] is for it to be pressed upwards onto the hard palate.)
- The finger-tips then move in a circular motion over the hyoid bone. This area may be exquisitely tender and should be approached gently.
- When the sternocleidomastoid muscles and the supralaryngeal area have relaxed, the larynx can be moved with lateral digital pressure.
- Finally, the patient is asked to swallow and then to vocalise.

In cases of muscle tension dysphonia (MTD), the voice frequently improves dramatically after approximately 10 or 15 minutes' use of this technique, and it is realistic to aim for normal voice or a significant improvement within the first treatment session using this method (Aronson, 1990; Mathieson, 1993a; Roy and Leeper, 1993). Patients tend to notice a reduction in discomfort initially and make very similar descriptive comments. They remark that their throats feel more open or wider, that they can swallow more easily and that the sensation of a lump in the throat has gone. They comment that the neck is softer. During massage of the sternocleidomastoid muscles, the reduction in muscle tension can be felt by the practitioner as the muscles change from being firm and resistant to being softer and more malleable. Kneading of the supralaryngeal area produces similar changes with a transition in tension from a firm or hard oral cavity floor to one that allows the thumbs to intrude beyond the boundaries of the mandible. These changes are observable even in obese patients where the tense musculature can be felt beneath the soft covering tissue.

Many patients who have had a history of vocal tract discomfort over weeks or months respond immediately to this treatment, which appears to have the benefit of causing a significant change in the kinaesthetic image of phonation. This sensory change then acts as a positive basis for vocal function exercises. Aronson (1990) points out that this approach can be successful where less aggressive methods fail and he regards it as a primary therapy, not an alternative one. This does not disregard the importance of underlying emotional factors, which can be explored once the vocal tract is more comfortable and the vocal symptoms have been improved. In some cases, the immediate improvement remains and the patient's sensory symptoms do not return throughout the programme of vocal function exercises. Other patients report improvement for some hours or days afterwards, but that symptoms subsequently return. Following sessions generally resolve the problem. Lack of response to this approach may indicate, when organic factors have been excluded, that there is a significant psychological reason for the voice problem. Manual therapy for the laryngeal area is a powerful clinical approach which can rapidly improve vocal function and reduce or eliminate vocal tract discomfort (Mathieson, 1993a). The experience of clinicians who use this technique is that it produces beneficial results more rapidly and more permanently in many cases than the use of relaxation techniques (see below).

Note 1

As in examination of the extrinsic laryngeal musculature (see page 422), care must be taken not to apply pressure in the area of major blood vessels in the neck. It is advisable to avoid using this approach in patients with a history of cardiovascular disease and frail elderly people. Patients with neck problems might also be at risk. In all patients with whom this technique is used, digital pressure should be applied only to identified cartilages and muscles. The procedure should be stopped if patients report or exhibit any signs of 'light-headedness' or dizziness.

Note 2

A comprehensive account of an osteopath's method of manual therapy in the treatment of voice disorders has been given by Lieberman (1998), but extends beyond the competencies of speech–language pathologists.

VEGETATIVE TECHNIQUES

These techniques are those that elicit and capitalise on vegetative behaviours in order to produce normal voice. The rationale behind this approach is that such behaviours are frequently unaffected by the laryngeal tensions associated with phonation in communication. When a normal vocal note is apparent on a laugh or cough in spontaneous conversation, this can be used to convince patients that they are capable of normal voice and as a basis for the production of vowels and words before being generalised. The use of vegetative behaviours in treating conversion symptom aphonia and puberphonia are discussed below (see pages 514 and 520).

INSPIRATORY PHONATION

Inspiratory phonation can be used to bring the vocal folds to the midline, and this gives the patient sensory and acoustic feedback of a type of phonation that is free of any effortful compensatory features of normal phonation. Patients with vocal fold paralysis may find this a helpful approach, particularly if they have been using excessive expiratory effort in an attempt to produce voice. It can be used as a precursor to laryngeal valving. The vocal folds are drawn to the midline during prolonged, voiced inspiration. Just before expiration, the vocal folds are firmly adducted and the stages of the laryngeal valving routine are started (see above).

Indirect treatments for voice disorders

All the treatments that have been described above are focused directly on improving vocal function, but because the voice reflects many aspects of individuals and their behaviour the treatment of voice disorders frequently necessitates additional approaches. The significant underlying fact is that voice disorders can be the result, and the cause, of musculoskeletal tension that impairs recovery. Some patients require help in addition to direct voice treatment, some of which can be given by the speech–language pathologist but some of which involve other professionals. Some of these approaches can be one element of therapy in combination with other strategies, whereas others are used as ongoing treatment when vocal function has reached maximum improvement. It is usually speech–language pathologists, of all the voice professionals, who have most contact with each patient with a clinical voice disorder. Consequently, they are often in the best position to identify when additional care should be considered although this issue should be discussed with the laryngologist who has the ultimate medical responsibility for the patient.

RELAXATION TECHNIQUES

Relaxation used to be regarded as a cornerstone of treatment for many speech and voice disorders, but it is now used far less than formerly. The reduction in its use possibly began during the 1960s and 1970s when laryngologists began to prescribe tranquillisers for anxious patients and there appeared to be less need for working intensively on physical relaxation. Diazepam (Valium) and chlordiazepoxide (Librium), two of the commonly described drugs, were subsequently found to be addictive; when they were withdrawn, their effect generally ceased and tension and anxiety remained. As a result, they were no longer prescribed for tense and anxious patients with voice disorders. Relaxation as a technique, however, did not return to its former popularity, partly because its beneficial effect does not generalise to everyday life particularly well. More recently, manual therapy to reduce laryngeal tension has been shown to produce results in many cases without the need for full relaxation (see above). This should not detract from the fact that relaxation can be a useful adjunct to voice therapy in some cases, particularly in the treatment of hyperfunctional dysphonia (Boone and McFarlane, 1988), although there are no significant changes in vocal function when it is used alone (Blood, 1994).

Relaxation techniques are relatively time-consuming and are probably not necessary for most patients with whom other techniques can be used to achieve relaxation of the laryngeal musculature equally, if not more, effectively. Consequently, it is realistic to give particularly careful consideration to patient selection for this approach. Clinical experience suggests that there are certain indicators for using general relaxation approaches:

- Extreme tension reflected in body posture, which pervades all movements and does not lessen on familiarity with the clinician and the clinical setting.
- Lack of insight into marked tension which is obvious to observers. Patients in this group are not necessarily unhappy about high tension levels which might even be a reflection of a driving, energetic personality which is viewed positively by the patient and others. These individuals frequently use excessive effort for all activities, including phonation – 'a sledgehammer to crack a nut' approach to life. For this group, the opportunity to experience a degree of relaxation can highlight the possibility of continuing to achieve their goals without excessive effort.
- The very tense, talkative patient. A small minority of patients, particularly from the category of hyperfunctional voice disorders, talk so excessively and rapidly that this behaviour significantly interferes with and inhibits voice therapy. Frequently, these patients do not listen to the clinician because of their constant talking. Consequently, advice and instruction are not absorbed. In some cases, this behaviour is a reflection of tension and anxiety whereas in others there appears to be little awareness that their garrulousness is interfering with the remediation that they have sought. Relaxation can be used to introduce the experience of stillness and quietness before proceeding with voice therapy.

There is well-documented evidence that reaction to stress is far less when a patient is relaxed and at ease than when tense and upset. For example, in a controlled experiment (Linford Rees, 1982), the reaction of patients suffering from allergic asthma and hay fever to artificially introduced pollen was found to be measurably greater when tense than when relaxed. Relaxation does not remove anxiety and conflict, but alleviates the bodily somatic accompaniment. Relaxation can be deliberately cultivated; it eases panic and allows the intellect to take stock of situations and analyse problems more rationally. Suggestions are then received from the clinician more readily. This is the psychological value of relaxation, but there are also mechanical and physiological effects.

Physiology of muscular tension

Bodily movement requires the rhythmic coordination of three groups of muscles: the agonists, the antagonists and the synergists. The agonists (the prime movers) initiate the voluntary movement. The antagonists are responsible for the opposing movement and have to relax in order to allow the agonists freedom to act. The synergists are bracing muscles which hold the limb in position. A classic example is the clenching of the fist. The agonists are the flexors of the fingers, the antagonists extend the fingers and the wrist extensors act as the synergists. Alternatively, when limb extension is the goal, the extensors are the prime movers and the flexors provide the braking force. For example, when reaching for an object, the agonists are the elbow extensors and the antagonists are the flexors.

Excessively tense muscles oppose each other rather than coordinate. This gives rise to fatigue and energy is wasted. The individual is not necessarily aware of the resulting tension which affects all activities. It often produces harmful postures and strained muscles (Barlow, 1959; Linford Rees, 1982), but aching shoulders, neck and back may also be the result of arthritis and other conditions that require medical investigations. Conversely, poor posture, particularly for long periods (e.g. working at a computer) can lead to neck and back discomfort.

Relaxation strategies

The therapist should explain the reasons for using relaxation strategies so that the patient is able to cooperate. It is essential that the patient is comfortable and that any embarrassment is minimised. The fundamental principle of relaxation strategies is the development of kinaesthetic and proprioceptive awareness by contrasting muscular tension with muscular relaxation. Relaxation can be carried out with the patient in a supine or sitting position, sometimes progressing from the former to the latter. In practice, manual therapy and relaxation in a sitting position have virtually supplanted supine relaxation but some clinicians might consider that this approach is appropriate in certain cases.

Supine relaxation

The patient lies in a supine position with the head supported by a low pillow. The therapist encourages a feeling of heaviness and slowing down. Relaxation is encouraged by:

- suggestion through the description of a peaceful scene and/or soothing music (audio tapes for relaxation are available commercially and patients can use these at home).

- physical manipulation of the limbs, i.e. lifting and gently dropping the limb, until the patient no longer controls the limb but allows it to drop.
- contrasting tense and relaxed muscle states with the patient deliberately tensing all muscles and then releasing.

When the patient is relaxed, closed eyelids are still (and do not flicker) and breathing rate is slowed. As the period of relaxation ends, the patient is encouraged to remember the sensation and to retain it as conversation with the clinician is resumed.

Relaxation when sitting

Some people feel particularly vulnerable if asked to lie down in order to relax and will achieve a relaxed state much more easily if they are sitting in a comfortable chair:

- The patient's eyes are closed and the clinician, using a suitably gentle voice and slow rate of speech, asks the patient to breathe slowly and deeply as if becoming drowsy before sleep. The head should be dropped forward onto the chest with an increasing sensation of heaviness.
- The therapist describes each part of the body – feet, legs, trunk, arms, shoulders, face – as becoming increasingly heavy and immobile. The patient should be observed carefully for signs that full relaxation has not been achieved, e.g. rapid breathing rate, flickering eyelids, tense facial expression, movements of the hands and feet, and these areas should be talked through again.
- When maximum relaxation has been reached, the patient is asked to remain in the same position with eyes closed and the therapist explains that he or she is going to move the patient's head and neck gently.
- The therapist places one cupped hand under the patient's chin and the other supports the back of the head. Tension will frequently be felt in the neck. If fully relaxed, the head is very heavy to lift and move. The patient remains passive while the therapist gently lifts the head and moves it from left to right. As the neck relaxes, the head may be gently tilted backwards and forwards while fully supported. The therapist must not remove this support without warning the patient. If the patient has arthritis of the cervical spine, this procedure must be discussed with the patient's doctor before its use.

- The patient remains in a quiet relaxed state for a short period after head and neck relaxation is complete.

It is important that the therapist explains that, after periods of relaxation, the expectation is not for the patient to retain this state in everyday life. The aims are for the patient to develop the skill of releasing excessively tense muscles and to establish a kinaesthetic model of relaxed musculature, which acts as a baseline by which the patient can monitor excessive tension.

PSYCHOLOGICAL COUNSELLING

Awareness of patients' emotional status, from an aetiological perspective and with regard to their distress, is fundamental to understanding voice disorders and to their treatment (see page 186). The term 'counselling' is used differently in various contexts. It may refer to the general advice given by the speech–language pathologist about the voice disorder and ways that it can be managed, or to dealing with aspects of the distress linked to the problem. Speech–language pathologists undertake both roles on a daily basis. A proportion of patients with voice disorders, however, exhibit anxiety, distress or other emotional symptoms which need psychological counselling from a trained counsellor, psychotherapist or psychiatrist. Some patients recognise the need for such help and are relieved when a referral is suggested. The idea has to be introduced with care, however, because it can cause distress or anger if patients reject or deny that further professional help is necessary. Insensitive handling of the situation by the speech–language pathologist or laryngologist can drive the patient away, not only from the suggested psychological help but also from voice therapy. Consequently, the suggested referral should emerge as a logical step from the discussions occurring in treatment between the voice pathologist and the patient. Although speech–language pathologists can give constructive emotional support in many cases, they should be aware of their limitations in this area when more complex psychodynamics underpin the voice disorder and associated symptoms.

SPECIALISED TECHNIQUES

Formalised techniques for improving body alignment, and encouraging relaxed posture and movement, can be helpful for some patients because of their effect on phonation. These include the Alexander technique (Alexander, 1942; Macdonald, 1994) and the Feldenkrais method which are taught by accredited teachers.

Development and carry-over

Throughout treatment the ultimate aim is to restore voice for daily life. This must be considered not only in the structure of the treatment programme, but also in the way in which the various strategies are presented to patients. It should be explained that the early breathing exercises are a means to an end, for example, not the way in which the patient is expected to breathe when chatting with friends. Whichever strategies are used in treatment, they are incorporated into a hierarchy (see Chapter 12) directed at moving from the pathological voice to improved or normal voice in the clinic, and finally to spontaneous speech in the patient's usual settings. Therapy tends to be delivered in a continuum consisting of the following stages:

- explanation and reassurance
- vocal tract care and muscle tension reduction
- breathing and vocal skills
- vocal note quality and appropriate pitch
- articulation and resonance
- vocal flexibility, prosody and interpretation.

Naturally the above is an artificial demarcation of function and early in treatment all these aspects begin to be fused. A vocal note involves a balance between relaxation, tension and confidence, besides breath control. Flexibility involves control of expiration and glottal tension, besides self-expression. Treatment depends on the needs of the patient after careful assessment of difficulties and faults in voice production. A sufferer from slight vocal strain will need different treatment from one with vocal nodules or contact ulcers. One patient may need little instruction in breathing technique and concentration upon laryngeal tensions, another may be found to have recovered from laryngeal tension when breathing technique has improved. Treatment must be flexible and imaginative and suited to the patient's needs because these change during the course of treatment.

Every treatment should allow time for a discussion of how the patient is coping. This gives opportunities for making suggestions about lifestyle and for counselling as problems in the family or at work are exposed. Some individuals will show excellent adjustment and are simple casualties of their personalities and of driving themselves too hard, trying to get the utmost out of work, sports and social activities. Others will need encouragement, the building of confidence to participate in activities and to live life more fully. A sympathetic and understanding yet impartial confidante found in the therapist may bring about recovery far more successfully than a series of voice training exercises.

Throughout therapy, the procedures involved should never be regarded as drills that will bring about improvement purely because they are practised regularly. They have validity only if the patient fully understands the rationale behind them and realises their importance in establishing tactile, kinaesthetic and proprioceptive awareness of appropriate methods of healthy voice production.

A strong clear voice is achieved first in exercises and only later will this standard of voice production be maintained during connected speech. At first the old speech patterns prevail because of habit, and the practice in mechanical speech has to be carried over into spontaneous conversation. An important aim in the latter stages of treatment must be the provision of interest and variety so that the patient's interest is held and enthusiasm sustained. Some patients do not need this stage and rapidly integrate their new vocal behaviour into connected speech without help. The following approaches can help those who find the transition more difficult.

SPEECH BREATHING

Once patients have mastered the basic speech–breathing skills, these exercises and their variations develop the rhythms and speed required in connected speech:

- With quick inspiration before each line the patient chants a jingle, concentrating on good tone and articulation.
- Breath intake is adjusted to phrase length. The patient chants and then speaks: 'One is all I need; one, two is all I need; one, two, three is all I need', etc. The count is increased until full capacity is reached, but reserve or residual air must not be used. Discomfort and tension are immediately felt. The patient must learn to recognise the danger signals and to replenish the breath supply immediately the necessity arises.
- The patient composes phrases of increasing length:
     'It was a cold day'
     'It was a cold and windy day'
     'It was a cold, windy and wet day'.

These exercises should introduce the particular vowels and consonants in which the individual needs practice. Accurate articulation should be encouraged while the vowels must be slightly prolonged in order to develop their full resonance.

PROSODY

The development of vocal flexibility and the prevention of a monotonous and limited pitch range should be an integral part of all vocal exercises:

* Phrases can be marked with an intonation pattern. The same phrase can be spoken with as many different meanings as possible. Saying a sentence with a different word being stressed each time produces similar results and is helpful when the speaker has difficulty in voluntarily making the pitch changes to change intonation. This has the effect of also changing intonation, e.g.

  'I'm going for a **walk**.'
  '**I'm** going for a walk.'
  'I'm **going** for a walk.'

  The patient learns to be expressive and animated without relying on increased loudness and effort.
* The lines of a poem, or of prose suitably phrased, are repeated after the therapist with careful attention to tone, intonation, rhythm and rate. The patient's faults should be imitated by the therapist and the patient asked to correct them. When this exercise has been worked through, the patient reads the passage alone attempting to rectify previous faults. Playback of tape-recordings reinforces learning.
* Practice in reading aloud is a much more difficult exercise and should not be introduced until the new vocal patterns are secure. The patient should be stopped immediately if poor phonation patterns recur. Inability to self-correct necessitates further practice of earlier exercises with recording and playback. Some individuals find that it is easier to read poetry and blank verse than prose.
* Exercises for the correction of a considerable drop in pitch at the ends of phrases are often necessary. Although this is a characteristic of English intonation, it may be excessive, the voice dropping into vocal fry register as volume and breath pressure fall. The patient can practise the following:

  – speak the last word of a phrase with exaggerated rising intonation
  – speak a phrase on a monotone and then repeat with normal intonation pattern
  – speak a phrase with 'and' tagged onto the end as if the utterance were going to continue.

- Spontaneous speech practice consists of the patient:
  - giving short replies to questions having planned the answers, and applying principles of good voice production in a controlled situation
  - describing objects or events
  - giving prepared talks on any subject (if the patient is a lecturer or teacher, for example, sections from teaching material can be given to an imaginary audience); if possible, this can be carried out in group treatment
  - if a patient's profession requires speaking against a high level of background noise it is useful for this to be part of the practice in the final stages of treatment. A tape recording of traffic, factory noise, children or whatever is appropriate can be used. Played loudly, it assists the individual to cope with the situation and to increase vocal volume without becoming tense and reverting to forcing the voice.

Pharmacological influences

Medication may significantly affect vocal function and must be taken into account in the management of the voice-disordered patient. Some patients may be prescribed drugs as part of the treatment regimen for their vocal dysfunction. Others may be taking medication coincidentally, the possible effects of which should be considered by the voice therapist.

When a voice disorder is produced by a pathophysiological process, the voice may be improved by pharmacological treatment of the pathology or its associated symptoms (Harris, 1992). Examples include anti-tussives for suppressing coughing and antihistamines for reducing allergic symptoms in the respiratory tract. In some instances, however, there may be adverse side effects to drugs prescribed to help vocal function. Antihistamines, for example, can cause dryness with reduction and thickening of mucosal secretions. As a result, the prescription of mucolytic agents which increase and thin secretions, thus improving lubrication, may be necessary (Sataloff, 1991). In cases where gastric reflux appears to be an important factor in laryngeal inflammation, anti-reflux medication is prescribed together with the introduction of lifestyle changes aimed at reducing reflux.

Ongoing medication that might have adverse effects on the voice should be taken into account during treatment. Patients whose voice disorders are associated with a sore throat, whether or not they have an upper respiratory tract infection, may have been gargling with soluble aspirin in order to reduce the discomfort. As aspirin tends to cause haemorrhages, this practice should be stopped and aspirin products should be avoided, particularly when there is hyperfunctional phonation that might precipitate submucosal bleeds. Bronchodilators, which are used in the treatment of asthma to expand the diameter of the bronchioles, are known to affect the vocal folds adversely when used for long periods and steps must be taken to minimise these effects (see page 348).

Summary

- Voice therapy is a complex process influenced by the patient, the clinician and the chosen treatment programme.
- Evidence-based practice does not exclude the use of non-proven techniques, but involves critical evaluation rather than popular appeal.
- Evidence that a technique *can* work does not mean that it *will* work, particularly if it is not carried out well.
- Most treatment programmes employ a combination of techniques and pedagogic strategies.
- Voice pathologists must be able to model target vocal behaviours for patients. It is unreasonable and theoretically unsound not to be able to demonstrate vocal behaviours that are required of the patient.
- Effective treatment depends on changing vocal behaviour and the generalisation of these changes to everyday life.
- The effects of other medical intervention should be taken into account during the voice therapy treatment programme.

15 CHAPTER

Specific techniques

The overall process of voice therapy and techniques that can be used in treatment have been described and discussed in the preceding chapters. Dysphonia caused by vocal misuse and abuse is the most common problem referred to the voice pathologist. The preceding chapters provide a framework of treatment for that aetiological group which is also applicable as a foundation for the treatment of other types of dysphonia. The basic principles pertain whether the voice disorder is the result of vocal fold paralysis, vocal fold nodules or psychogenic factors. The aim of treatment is to restore normal voice if possible but, when the voice disorder cannot be resolved, as in some neurological or structural anomalies, compensatory strategies have to be developed which help the patient to achieve maximum vocal potential. This chapter deals with treatment approaches and specific remediation procedures for voice disorders other than those where hyperfunctional phonation is the primary problem. It should be remembered that hyperfunction frequently develops as a secondary feature of most voice disorders as the speaker struggles to overcome the primary problem. Consequently, an integrated treatment programme that deals with this aspect of vocal behaviour, as well as the specific intervention strategies, is essential.

Psychogenic disorders

CONVERSION SYMPTOM APHONIA

It is generally agreed that, in cases of conversion symptom aphonia, the voice should be recovered as quickly as possible. Ideally, the voice pathologist should see the patient immediately after the diagnosis has been made. Tucker (1987c) advocates that the laryngologist and speech pathologist should 'consider the treatment of the conversion disordered patient a near emergency and initiate the voice evaluation immediately after the laryngological examination whenever possible'. When time elapses between diagnosis and the first interview with the speech–language pathologist, the patient has a complex situation to deal with which can consolidate the problem. The patient is voiceless, but is told that there is no significant laryngeal abnormality and is having to deal with daily life without a voice. There may also be the reaction that pathology has perhaps been overlooked: how is it possible to have no voice and yet have a normal larynx? The aim is to restore voice at the first interview, if possible. Damsté (1983) cautioned against being drawn into 'playing the patient's game' and advocated firm handling. Linford Rees (1982) advised concentrating on improvement rather than dwelling on the patient's symptoms.

The manner in which the clinician handles this important session is crucial to the eventual outcome. A quietly confident demeanour which remains positive and unperturbed by the patient's account of the problem, and any initially unsuccessful attempts at regaining voice, is an essential element of treatment. This does not mean that the patient's fears and concerns should be insensitively disregarded but that a professional distance should be retained which also allows for sensitivity to the patient's predicament. Patients with a conversion symptom aphonia are suggestible and this factor will affect their response to the speech–language pathologist. Negative behaviour by the clinician in the form of comments that 'This is a difficult case' or 'Sometimes this sort of problem can take a long time to resolve' will delay recovery. Positive remarks such as 'We know your larynx is healthy' and 'When your voice has returned . . .' help the patient to accept that there is an assumption that voice will be restored. It may also be helpful to mention during explanations that this type of voice loss is a well-known phenomenon which responds well to treatment. The longer patients perceive that their 'difficult' problem is confounding all treatment, the more entrenched the symptom will become. As these patients are so suggestible, it is important that particular care is taken when giving the usual explanations of normal voice production and the reasons for their symptoms. Some patients will ask an obstructive question or query an explanation at every opportunity, in an unconscious attempt to deflect direct treatment and confirm the severity of their symptoms.

Many patients, although not necessarily unduly concerned by their conversion aphonia, are very distressed to learn that the larynx is normal and that the symptom is therefore psychological. Patients sometimes say that they would have preferred that an organic abnormality, even cancer, had been found rather than this dramatic psychogenic symptom.

Treatment strategies

Explanation

Most patients find it acceptable to be told, quite truthfully, that the vocal tract and vocal fold movement are particularly responsive to emotional changes. In some individuals this is more marked than in others who may succumb to headaches or abdominal pain. It can be pointed out that, even when under stress, most individuals have to continue with the routine of daily life. To do so true feelings are repressed and, as a result, in this instance, the vocal folds have become so tense that they will not fully adduct. Further discussion about the psychodynamics of the problem are usually less important at this time than voice recovery. The patient is reassured that there is no physical reason why voice cannot be produced, apart from an element of habit, and the therapist introduces strategies for eliciting voice.

Facilitating techniques

- Before attempts are made to elicit voice, it is helpful to ensure that the vocal tract musculature is sufficiently relaxed to produce a vocal note. This patient group appears to respond well to **manual techniques to reduce tension of the laryngeal musculature** (see page 498). It is probable that this results partly from the direct benefits of the procedure, but also from the fact that this 'hands-on' approach is perceived as a very positive intervention. The speech–language pathologist can take the opportunity at this time to provide a positive running commentary, which feeds back to the patient the fact that muscles can be felt to be relaxing and that the larynx is becoming increasingly mobile. As a result of the physical contact and encouraging commentary, the patient can be helped to trust and have confidence in the speech–language pathologist. This is the basis for success for the next stage of treatment.
- **Vegetative techniques** provide a route to achieving voice which is removed from using the voice for communication. After the relaxation of the laryngeal musculature, the patient can be asked to throat clear in readiness for the next stage of treatment. Occasionally, voice can be heard at this point and this should be pointed out to the patient with some enthusiasm as evidence that the vocal folds are 'coming together', and that this will be the basis of regaining voice. If voice is not heard spontaneously in this way, most patients with conversion symptom aphonia respond well to a confident and relaxed approach which involves the speech–language pathologist therapist firmly but

gently depressing the larynx. The patient is then asked to cough or clear the throat. Immediately phonation is heard, however brief or 'croaky', the patient is encouraged to extend the sound on to 'mmm' and then on to vowels, e.g. cough – mm – ah, etc. It is important to keep up a degree of momentum at this stage and to give the patient a great deal of encouragement and reassurance. When definite voicing has been heard it should be extended to automatic and serial speech, e.g. counting, days of the week, etc. Patients who say that their voices sound strange at this point should be reassured that they have not used their voices for some time and are 'out of practice', but that the voice will steadily return to normal as the session progresses.

Patients vary in the time that they take to respond to this stage of treatment in the first session. Some will produce voice almost immediately after the laryngeal musculature has been relaxed, whereas others respond more slowly over a period of 30–45 minutes. In most cases, patients leave the first session using voice in conversation; occasionally voice is not achieved but will generally return before or during the next treatment session. It is important that the speech–language pathologist does not appear to be disconcerted if voice does not return quickly, and that treatment does not become a succession of frantic attempts using a succession of increasingly desperate techniques. It should be explained calmly to the patient that individuals respond differently to various strategies and that a number of approaches will be tried to ascertain which will be most beneficial. It can be helpful for the voice pathologist to remember that these cases involve dealing with a normal vocal tract, which is therefore capable of producing normal voice. Even if the problem appears to be resistant initially, it is rarely insurmountable.

As the voice returns, many patients become tearful as tensions are released. They may feel overwhelmed by a range of emotions and must be given sufficient time to come to terms with the restoration of voice, to discuss their reactions, and to become calm and more composed before leaving the clinic. Unresolved issues and the stabilisation of voice will usually be addressed in subsequent sessions.

Historical note

A survey of the literature describing the various methods recommended in the past for the recovery of voice in conversion aphonia patients demonstrates forcibly that practically any tactics will succeed if put into effect with sufficient aplomb during the first session with the patient. Smurthwaite (1919) recommended groaning or coughing after deep inspiration, or the application of a laryngeal probe to produce a paroxysm of coughing. Pulling the tongue out with the instruction to say 'ah' was also found to be efficacious. Lell (1941) advocated provoking the gag reflex by probing with the laryngoscopic mirror. This use of the 'surprise attack' was supported by Sokolowsky and Junkermann (1944) who found that strong verbal suggestion and a confident authoritative manner led to a cure in the great majority of their cases at the first session. The administration of systematic voice training techniques, which they tried at the outset, took time and produced only 60% recovery of voice. Jackson (1949) recommended encouraging the patient to bring the elbows down to the sides with a thump coincident with a phonatory cough or grunt. Some patients are helped by the use of white noise through head-phones. The patient is asked to sing or talk against this noise. With auditory control of the voice removed, the voice returns and convinces the patient that it is not irrevocably lost (Labarraque, 1952). This procedure will not be successful with those patients who do not vocalise while wearing the headphones. Although patients often do produce voice while 'deafened' in this way, many do not. In the past, application of a strong faradic current to the larynx was used. This method generally produced a scream which was convincing to the patient. If there were an associated anaesthesia – and this is pos-sible – the patient remained impervious to the electric shock.

Vocal function exercises

It can be argued that vocal function exercises are superfluous in treatment of conversion aphonia and dysphonia. However, the regimen advocated in Chapter 14 is helpful, particularly in long-standing cases, in establish-ing normal phonation after a vocal note has been elicited. Although the aetiology is psychogenic, phonation patterns and their associated kinaes-thetic feedback have been abnormal and patients frequently feel that they have 'forgotten' how to produce normal voice. A programme of voice therapy stabilises the restored voice and provides a focus for the interac-tion between speech–language pathologist and patient as support is grad-ually withdrawn. The fact that the patient has unconsciously selected a vocal symptom may be caused entirely by a failure to communicate in a traumatic social encounter, but it may also be the result of the fact that phonation is poorly produced habitually and that there is an element of vocal strain which engenders laryngeal and pharyngeal discomfort. Therefore direct therapy for improving phonation will establish confi-dence in the voice and reduce the factors that predispose the patient to dysphonia.

This patient group can benefit from relaxation techniques as described in Chapter 14. Tension can be reduced further by slowing and regulating the breathing rate while concentrating on diaphragmatic inter-costal breathing patterns. Attention to central breathing also diverts preoc-cupation with the throat and sensations of pressure or a lump.

Counselling

Recovery of the voice is not the sole aim in these cases; a patient needs to gain insight into the reason for the voice loss and to be helped to cope with the difficulties from which it originated. There is always a possibility of recurrence of the aphonia or development of another conversion symptom if the mental conflict is not resolved. Clinical experience indicates that, in most cases, this can be dealt with by the speech–language pathologist. Linford Rees (1982), presenting the analytical approach, cautioned against taking a particular stance on the patient's problems, of taking sides in reported conflicts and, above all, of giving advice on how to act. It is advisable to avoid becoming involved in the patient's personal relationships, especially when this is the scenario that the patient is skilled in manipulating. On the other hand, the patient needs support and counselling which encourages a positive outlook. Subsequently, the patient is guided through ways of handling the situations that provoked the conversion symptom.

If the patient's voice does not recover after a few sessions, it is advisable for the speech–language pathologist to recommend that the patient should be referred for a psychological assessment.

Note

Conversion symptom **dysphonia** (see page 205) can present a greater problem with regard to treatment than conversion aphonia because of the need to modify vocal behaviours arising from the underlying psychodynamics rather than elicit the dramatic change of behaviour from aphonia to voice, a less subtle change. A similar treatment protocol is appropriate in both conditions.

Case history

Mrs C (36 years) was referred for speech therapy with aphonia which started with an upper respiratory tract infection. On indirect laryngoscopy there was no laryngeal abnormality. She had been aphonic for 16 months, during which time she had visited her general practitioner repeatedly for advice and medication without improvement. Eventually she was referred to a laryngologist.

During the interview with the speech–language pathologist, she was vivacious and verbose, all conversation being conducted in a forced whisper. She was not unduly concerned by her lack of voice. Having reassured her that there was no reason why the voice should not recover completely, the therapist gently manipulated the larynx and encouraged relaxation of the neck muscles. She was encouraged to cough and then to give a cough immediately followed by various vowels. Within 5 minutes she was counting, saying the days of the week, etc. and after 10 minutes was phonating throughout conversation. The patient was tearful and amazed that her voice had returned so quickly after its long absence. As a result of the explanations given to her concerning the reasons for such symptoms, she was soon able to identify the precipitating factor. She had two children, a girl of 14 years and a boy of 10 years. She felt that there had been constant conflict with her daughter over everything, from homework to the time she should come home and the suitability of her clothes. The arguments between mother and daughter were disrupting the whole family, with her husband blaming her for not being able to control their daughter. It was significant that the family had been more cooperative since the mother had been voiceless, and that the father fulfilled a more positive role in relation to his daughter since his wife had been unable to shout. Two further appointments directed at establishing a secure voice through traditional voice therapy in combination with counselling ensured the stable return of the voice.

PUBERPHONIA

Despite the possible psychopathology of puberphonia, the results of voice therapy are excellent. Most patients are highly motivated to achieve an appropriate post-pubertal voice because they have been made painfully aware of the social and career disadvantages of the 'unbroken' voice. Treatment is unlikely to be successful if the individual has no real desire to change the voice but has responded to the pressure of others who think that treatment should be sought. Normal laryngeal growth and length of vocal folds ensure that mature male voice can be produced as long as the patient is cooperative.

Patients with puberphonia tend to present themselves for treatment in their mid to late teens, when the ridicule of fellow students and the prospect of starting work or university with this problem causes considerable distress. Some patients, still with 'unbroken' voice long past the normal mutation period, appear to have adjusted satisfactorily to their problems in the process of growing up and obtaining economic independence after leaving school, but find that their voices cause social and occupational difficulties. Van Riper and Irwin (1958) stressed the force of vocal habits in dysphonia; even if the voice symptoms start as a psychogenic symptom and the expression of emotional conflicts, they may become purely reflex and habitual. Shyness at switching over to a new and more appropriate voice may ensure the perpetuation of an undesirable vocal habit. Sometimes a deeper pitch can be produced quite easily, but the patient lacks the confidence to use this in public, knowing that it will cause comment and possible ridicule. A laryngologist's report confirming normality of laryngeal growth and structure (see Chapter 8) is essential. A careful case history is necessary so that comprehensive information regarding the patient's childhood, home background and personality is obtained.

It is also necessary to gain the patient's full cooperation at the initial interview to ensure that he has a sincere desire to improve his voice. Frequently, the patient complains of vocal 'weakness' and he seems unaware of the unsuitable pitch of the voice. When the failure in voice mutation is largely a question of habit and the patient has adjusted psychologically, and especially when voice 'breaks' are present, the mature male voice is established at first interview. The longer the high-pitched voice has persisted past adolescence and into maturity, the more difficult it may be to induce the required change of pitch.

Treatment strategies

Biofeedback

An **audio recording** of his voice in conversation should be played back to the young man in the initial session and his reaction to it discussed. It is unusual for the teenager not to know what his voice sounds like because many own tape-recorders and have been video-recorded. Dislike of the pre-pubertal voice should be apparent. Audio recording is also an essential tool when mature voice has been elicited so that the patient can hear objectively that the 'new' voice is acceptable, although it initially sounds and feels strange as he speaks. Recordings of tenor, baritone and bass voices humming, played loudly, and asking the patient to imitate or join in these vocal notes may produce results. If sound can be relayed through earphones as a masking device, the self-conscious individual may succeed in lowering pitch (Van Riper and Irwin, 1958).

Patients can also benefit from visual feedback about speaking fundamental frequency and pitch range, and from electroglottography (Carlson, 1995a).

Counselling

If there is resentment towards parents or teachers who have persuaded him to attend the voice clinic against his will, the conflict has to be sorted out as soon as possible. Willing cooperation on the part of the boy must be gained and there must be no resistance to therapy if it is to be successful (Weiss, 1955). The attendance of a parent who is sympathetic and not critical of the boy, but encouraging, can be a great inducement and relieve the domestic situation of embarrassment when the boy uses his mature male voice at home. The father's involvement in treatment can be helpful. Many boys and young men, however, prefer to deal with the situation alone in the early stages.

Facilitating techniques

The authoritative manner and strong suggestion on the part of the therapist are potent influences in therapy. It has been suggested that a male voice
pathologist is more suitable than a female and will achieve the necessary
voice mutation more easily (Hildernesse, 1956), although most female
voice pathologists appear to elicit and restore the mature voice satisfactorily. Although a female, she can demonstrate that she can produce a much
lower voice than the adolescent boy and that, therefore, this is possible for
him.

Manual reduction of laryngeal muscle tension

The vocal fold musculature is inevitably tense and the larynx is held high
in the vocal tract as the young man produces a high-pitched voice with a
post-pubertal vocal tract. To obtain falsetto voice, the larynx is elevated by
the suprahyoid musculature while the cricothyroid muscles approximate
the cartilages anteriorly and the arytenoids are pulled back by the cricoarytenoids. The vocal folds are thinned and stretched and the voice is raised in
pitch (see Chapter 4). This is the habitual vocal tract gesture for phonation
which reasserts itself every time he speaks. When the laryngeal musculature
has been relaxed manually, the vocal tract posture has been modified and
the kinaesthetic image changed. This facilitates phonation at a lower
frequency.

Vegetative techniques

Vegetative techniques to elicit a post-pubertal voice are effective most
easily when the patient's deep voice can be heard in spontaneous vegetative
behaviours such as coughing and laughing. It is important that the clinician
should present any therapeutic method with calm confidence and persist
with it for a reasonable time before giving up. Any suggestion from the
voice pathologist, either explicitly or in attitude, that there is a desperate
search for an approach that works will only confirm to the patient that he
or she is attempting a difficult or impossible task.

- The patient is asked to cough, clear his throat, laugh or sing down the
  scale in order to produce low notes. The prime aim is to discover a
  vowel an octave lower than the habitual pitch. This provides the
  starting point from which normal voice can be developed through
  exercises in humming and vowel prolongation. Luchsinger and
  Arnold (1965) described the Gutzman pressure test. If pressure can
  be exerted on the thyroid cartilage by pressing on the laminae with

finger and thumb, while the patient hums and drops the chin over the therapist's hand, the necessary relaxation of the intrinsic laryngeal muscles may be obtained.

- If an electrolarynx is placed against the thyroid cartilage as the patient is asked to phonate, the sensation and the low pitch can produce a change in phonation. This approach appears to be successful because there is an element of the 'surprise attack' in using equipment apparently designed to change the voice.

- Using a tongue depressor, the speech–language pathologist depresses the posterior part of the patient's tongue as the patient emits a groan. This results in descent of the hyoid bone and therefore of the larynx, with associated lowering of the pitch of the vocal note. For this exercise to be effective, the patient must be relaxed. The back of the tongue should not be rigid and thus resist the tongue depressor.

- With head slightly tipped forward and neck and shoulders relaxed, the patient phonates on 'hm' while placing thumb and forefinger on the thyroid laminae, so that any tendency to elevate the larynx on phonation can be monitored and corrected.

- The patient holds the arms up horizontally and drops them heavily to his sides while saying 'ah'. The arms must drop through force of gravity and not be brought down to the sides by the patient.

- After a period of relaxed diaphragmatic breathing, the patient vocalises on a deep sigh on the expiratory airstream.

- Some patients are able to produce a different, and mature, male voice if they are impersonating another man when they have the protection of assuming another identity (Greene, 1955).

- Froeschels (1948) advocated chewing therapy and voluntary jaw and chin wagging when vocalising.

Establishment of mature male voice

Immediately normal vocal pitch is achieved and seized upon with enthusiasm by the clinician, it can be developed in the usual ways. The deep voice should be practised assiduously in meaningless mechanical exercises that will establish the auditory and kinaesthetic patterns desired and enable their effortless recall. Intoning meaningless vowels and nonsense syllables when using the 'new' voice will be found easier at first than connected speech. In most cases, the voice is strong and resonant immediately a pitch appropriate to the adult resonators is used. The contrast in the vocal expression of personality is startling and dramatic for the therapist, and highly rewarding. The first audio recording should be played and the contrast with the new voice evaluated and praised.

Very great difficulty is often encountered in persuading the patient to use the mature male voice outside the clinic, because he is frequently convinced that it is more conspicuous than the habitual mutational falsetto. This is so at first and the 'new' voice does provoke comment. If parent, sibling, friend or work colleague can be taken into the patient's confidence, perhaps accompanying him to the clinic, confidence may be increased. Assignments with hospital staff who understand the problem and give appropriate encouragement and praise extend the situations in which the patient feels sufficiently confident to speak normally.

If speech therapy does prove to be unsuccessful in eliciting or establishing the mature voice, referral to a psychiatrist is advisable if the patient consents.

Case note

A married man of 47 years, with three young daughters, repeatedly sought help but had been told by a succession of doctors that there was no treatment for his high-pitched voice. He owned a small general store and was constantly ridiculed by local youths who imitated his voice and made abusive remarks about his sexuality. By speaking as little as possible in his shop, he managed to tolerate the situation while maintaining his income. His wife and daughters were angry and distressed and the patient became quietly depressed. In desperation he asked for yet another medical opinion. Laryngoscopy confirmed a normal larynx and he was referred for voice therapy. Normal voice was elicited within the first 20 minutes of the initial consultation and he left the clinic using his new voice in spontaneous conversation. At his next appointment a week later, he confirmed that he had not returned to using his high-pitched voice. The expressions of gratitude from the patient and his family bore witness to the distress that they had been experiencing because appropriate referrals had not been made for treatment that was essentially straightforward.

TRANS-SEXUAL VOICE

This section discusses voice therapy with male-to-female trans-sexual patients (see Chapter 8). (Female-to-male trans-sexuals develop deeper voices as a result of the male hormones that they are prescribed. The vocal folds of the male-to-female trans-sexual do not reduce in mass as the result of the oestrogens that are taken, so the voice remains deep.) The treatment approach in this area has two important elements. First, voice therapy is only one aspect of management and treatment which includes psychiatric, hormonal and surgical intervention as the individual progresses towards the goal of living as a woman. Second, this is the only condition that the speech pathologist deals with in the area of voice pathology where a normal vocal tract is functioning normally but the clinician's aim has to be to elicit abnormal voice.

Treatment of male trans-sexuality

The male trans-sexual frequently decides to seek medical help during his late teens or early 20s. The most logical treatment would appear to be directed at changing the individual's conviction that he is a man in a woman's body. However, psychotherapy is unsuccessful and the professional approach is for a multidisciplinary team to manage and support these individuals (Bralley et al., 1978; Oates and Dacakis, 1983). The team is composed of psychiatrists, surgeons, medical social workers, speech–language pathologists and others because of the complexity of the medical, psychological and surgical issues that must be considered in each case. Treatment is conducted on the basis of attempting to satisfy the individual's aims of taking on a woman's appearance, living as a woman and changing the body to resemble that of a woman.

Presurgical phase

The individual's involvement with the team is long term. Surgical change of sex, known as gender reassignment surgery, is undertaken only when it has been established that the man is able to adjust to living daily as a member of the opposite sex. It is also essential that the man fully appreciates the problems that accompany such surgery. Sim (1981) stresses the importance of thorough psychiatric examination because of the mutilating nature of the operation, which leaves the individual sterile and incapable of orgasm. In England, even after surgery, the male trans-sexual is still legally regarded as male. This pre-surgical period usually lasts for about 2 years and during this time female hormones are prescribed.

For medical, psychological and social reasons, it is important that the change should be gradual. In response to the female hormones, breasts and female distribution of body fat develop. Hormones may produce unpleasant side effects such as nausea and dizziness or more serious risks, including thrombosis and malignant breast tumours (Gelder, Gath and Mayou, 1983). The lengthy process of electrolysis for the removal of facial hair is started and breast enlargement may be further enhanced by mammoplasty. It is during this transition period that the speech–language pathologist usually becomes involved in the patient's treatment.

Adjustment difficulties

Although there is a compelling desire to become a woman, the onset of femininity brings enormous problems. There is fear that family, friends and strangers will discover the situation if attempts are made to conceal what is happening, but complete honesty may result in rejection and isolation. In some instances, the unwanted attention of curious males has to be dealt with. The individual needs encouragement for a considerable time and depression is a common feature. When sex change surgery, which involves castration, penectomy and the creation of an artificial vagina (Oates and Dacakis, 1983), is eventually performed, the postoperative period may produce severe depression (Sim, 1981). Linford Rees (1982) questioned the legality of such surgery. Moreover, it is extremely expensive and time-consuming, and the person, after much suffering, is never normal and rarely completely satisfied.

Having undergone this prolonged pursuit of femininity and assuming female dress, hairstyle and make-up, the visual result is frequently convincingly female, but the mature masculine voice is a major factor in not being accepted as a woman.

Voice and communication modification

Treatment procedures have as their basis a vocal tract that is anatomically and physiologically normal for a male, not a female. In addition, established patterns of verbal and non-verbal communication are essentially masculine. Possible treatment for these communication problems may be divided into **surgery** and **speech therapy**.

Surgery

Cosmetic surgery

Surgical reduction of the thyroid cartilage (Adam's apple), also known as laryngeal shaving, may be performed in order to give the much flatter appearance of the female larynx. This is a cosmetic operation which allows the neck to resemble the female neck more closely. It does not affect the quality of the voice (Isshiki, 1980).

Phonosurgery

Phonosurgery (surgery involving the vocal folds) for trans-sexuals is still relatively experimental and does not always produce satisfactory results. Various procedures are advocated to raise vocal pitch by changing the mass, length and tension (or stiffness) of the vocal folds. Isshiki (1980) notes that stiffness is the most important factor. Bralley et al. (1978)

describe restriction of the anterior third of the vibrating segment of the vocal folds. These authors also note the work of Donald (1982) who describes a procedure in which a laryngeal web is created in order to obtain raised vocal pitch. A procedure that involves removing the anterior third of the vocal folds and then stretching them and reattaching them to the thyroid cartilage is described by Oates and Dacakis (1983). This has the effect of increasing vocal fold tension and decreasing vocal fold mass, so that higher fundamental frequency is produced.

Isshiki (1980) regards three types of intervention as possible in these cases:

- increasing vocal fold tension by cricothyroid approximation
- a longitudinal incision of the vocal folds
- steroid injection into the vocal folds in order to reduce mass. The rationale of the steroid injection is that steroids cause local atrophy but the author reports that the results are unsatisfactory.

Surgical intervention in these cases is still experimental. Maintaining an unobstructed airway and avoiding marked deterioration in voice quality are major considerations.

Speech therapy

Voice therapy is only one aspect of a speech therapy programme concerned with many aspects of verbal and non-verbal communication, including a careful analysis of the individual's communicative behaviour. The programme is based on the following factors.

Treatment goals

The patient and the speech–language pathologist should be agreed on the goals of treatment. Unrealistic expectations of treatment will eventually cause distress; the clinician must make every effort to understand the trans-sexual's expectations and to clarify the limitations that are placed on the possibility of acquiring a female voice by the size of the larynx and vocal tract.

Discussion concerning well-known trans-sexuals and the patient's view of the degree of their success in presenting as a female may give further insight into the individual's perception of a 'successful' voice. A male trans-sexual was most impressed by the television appearance of a well-known trans-sexual and indicated that it would be a considerable achievement to acquire such a voice. This response was surprising as the voice was definitely male; it was significant that the non-verbal communication and dress were convincingly female.

Most trans-sexuals embarking on therapy are highly motivated to cooperate, but this may be the first time that such active involvement in the achievement of goals has been required. Hormonal treatment and surgery require a more passive role. The clinician may need to make it clear that therapy will not consist of a programme of speech exercises alone, which will subsequently result in a suitable voice. Reassurance should be given that the clinician is fully aware that both voice and non-verbal communication should avoid creating a caricature of a female.

Male/female speech and language features

Voice pitch is generally regarded as the most important factor in identifying the sex of a speaker (Bralley et al., 1978; Oates and Dacakis, 1983), but there are other important vocal features that also contribute to the impression of masculinity or femininity. Several studies indicate, for example, that females may use a greater variety of intonational patterns than males, whereas males tend to speak more loudly than females (Yanagihara, Koike and Von Leden, 1966). In addition, the differing dimensions of male and female resonators result in identifiable differences in the quality of vocal resonance. These suprasegmental aspects of voice give some of the most important clues about the sex of the speaker (Smith, 1979). Various studies cited by Oates and Dacakis describe female speech as generally having more accurate articulation than that of males, who tend to articulate with less mouth opening and greater degrees of lip-rounding than females.

Sex markers in speech also extend to conversational topics and type of vocabulary used. Speech therapy should therefore include discussion of topics with a feminine bias so that the trans-sexual develops this aspect of communication.

Increasing the individual's awareness of paralinguistic behaviours

Postures adopted may remain essentially masculine in some individuals, although the regular wearing of female clothes tends to encourage more feminine movements. It will be necessary for the therapist to give guidance about appropriate postures and gestures as part of a programme in which the trans-sexual learns to communicate femininity. Video recordings are essential for monitoring all aspects of appearance, including hairstyle, make-up and clothes. More subtle aspects of posture that directly affect voice may also have to be considered. For example, if the habitual head posture is for the head to be tipped forward and the chin tucked in, the larynx will be depressed in the vocal tract and the pitch of the voice lowered.

Habitual articulation may enhance an impression of masculinity but hearing training, in conjunction with analysis of video recordings, can be successful in eradicating this problem. The tense jaw with little mouth opening, and flexing of the masseter muscles and clenched teeth when at rest, may result in an aggressive appearance which is perceived as masculine. Similarly, emphatic and explosive articulation is less likely to indicate a female speaker than softer and more gentle contacts.

The individual must be aware of the habitual voice quality. The tendency to use hard glottal attack, harshness, roughness and creak will have to be guarded against if the more female voice quality is to be convincing. It is not that females do not produce these voice features, but that distinctively male voice pitch is used when these features are produced by the mature male larynx. A similar, and difficult, problem is the use of vegetative behaviours such as laughing and coughing. These can be dealt with satisfactorily if performed gently under voluntary control, but the natural male voice remains apparent if voluntary control is lost.

All aspects of speech, language and content of conversation must be considered.

Psychological support from the voice pathologist

The trans-sexual's difficulties in acquiring and maintaining the new behaviours related to voice and communication should not be underestimated. Although highly motivated, translating these new skills into daily life and dealing with responses that are not always favourable may be discouraging and consequently depressing. The speech–language pathologist may be the only member of the team who sees the patient regularly and frequently, and realistic encouragement and support are an intrinsic element of the treatment programme.

The therapy programme will incorporate the points outlined above and its implementation will include the following treatment strategies.

- **Vocal skills strategies** (see page 477), which will encourage voluntary control over the various elements of voice production with increased kinaesthetic and auditory awareness as a basis for changing habitual patterns.
- **Facilitating techniques** and **vocal function exercises** directed at comfortably raising vocal pitch and subsequently increasing the vocal range within the pitch range. It is essential that any voice therapy does not allow vocal abuse and that the therapist should notice any signs of voice fatigue or strain.

- **Hierarchical tasks** in which the newly acquired intonation patterns and prosody are developed.

Studies indicate that, although the vocal pitch is raised by therapy, it is likely to be distinguishable from the female voice on account of the larger resonating spaces in the male. Bralley et al. (1978) found that both the trans-sexual and voice pathologist overestimated the extent to which pitch had been raised, and they suggest that objective assessment is probably required. However, if the general appearance of the male trans-sexual is feminine the voice tends to be perceived as female. This was highlighted by a patient in the early stages of therapy who was engaged in conversation by a male who commented on the 'lovely deep voice'; there was no recognition of a male voice. Responses will vary according to the listener and the situational context of the conversation. When the voice is the only indication of sex, e.g. on the telephone, it is particularly important for the speaker to give the name immediately so that the listener will be encouraged to accept that the caller is female. Signalling femininity affects the listener's set of expectancy, so that the voice is more likely to be perceived as that of a woman.

Structural abnormalities

CLEFT PALATE (HYPERNASALITY)

Treatment of the speech problems associated with cleft palate is ideally treated by the specialist speech–language pathologist working within a cleft palate team, but children may also receive treatment from a generalist speech–language pathologist if ongoing treatment is necessary. If pharyngoplasty is successful, little or no speech rehabilitation will be necessary but, when cleft palate speech persists, therapeutic intervention is required. Theoretically, although cleft palate speech is not generally regarded as falling within the domain of voice disorders, the patient's voice may be affected by **hypernasality** and, in some cases, by a higher incidence of **vocal abuse** than in the rest of the population (see page 233). It is appropriate, therefore, to include here the main tenets of treating these problems in the cleft palate patient. These principles are summarised in Table 15.1.

Reduction of hypernasality

Therapy to reduce hypernasality will be fully integrated with strategies to normalise articulation and eliminate audible nasal escape. After hearing training, the therapist should encourage relaxation of the patient's mandible, tongue, faucial pillars and pharynx, for the production of vowel sounds with normal resonance. This ensures an increase in the total volume of the oral and pharyngeal resonators. Some vowels are more nasalised than others. For instance, /u:/ and /i:/ are often markedly hypernasal because the back of the tongue is necessarily moved upwards and forwards in order to produce these vowels. This creates a large pharyngeal resonator with a small oropharyngeal opening which favours nasal resonance. The vowel

Table 15.1 Hypernasality associated with cleft palate: main tenets of treatment

Auditory training	Hearing training precedes therapy
	Hearing test before treatment
	Therapist demonstrates hypernasal and normal vowels and speech samples until patient can reliably differentiate between the two qualities
Imitation	Patient imitates normal vowels/phrases.
	Negative practice to reinforce reduced hypernasality
Reduction of articulatory tension (excessive vocal tract tension exacerbates hypernasality)	Importance of relaxed speech mechanism is emphasised (facilitating strategies may be used [see page 495])
	It might be necessary to reduce loudness and to slow speech rate if these factors appear to be contributing to excessive vocal tract tension
Biofeedback	Audio recording of clinician and patient in order to provide feedback re: matching the model of normal resonance

/a:/, in contrast, may not be nasalised because the tongue is relatively flat, the pharyngeal space small and the oropharyngeal orifice wide. The non-nasal vowels can be used to decontaminate the nasalised vowels in exercises such as the following:

- The vowel with a greater tendency to hypernasality is preceded and followed by the vowel with more normal resonance. When the hypernasal vowel (in this case /i:/) has been produced with normal resonance in this context by the patient, it is articulated in isolation,

    e.g. /a:i:a:/, /a:i:a:/, then isolate /i:/
    /a:u:a:/, /a:u:a:/, isolate /u:/

- Non-nasalised consonants may also be used with the same purpose of reducing nasality in vowels. If /p/ and /t/, for example, are produced normally by the patient, it can be helpful to practise exercises such as:

    /pu:p/, /tu:p/, /tu:t/, /tu:tu:/, etc.

When /u:/ is produced without hypernasality, the patient produces it in isolation and then in words.

Voice therapy for hyperfunctional phonation associated with cleft palate

As has been previously discussed, an individual with a cleft palate may develop hyperfunctional phonation as a direct result of attempts to increase intelligibility and vocal loudness. A voice disorder might also develop as a result of all the factors that affect other individuals and possible contributory factors should be investigated in the usual way. In either case, the treatment programme incorporates previously described strategies for reducing hyperfunction and developing vocal skills.

Psychological factors

Although cleft palate is an organic condition and the speech problems that arise are organically based, it is important that psychological problems are not overlooked. The response of the vocal tract to emotion and the effects on voice in all individuals have been discussed earlier and should not be disregarded in those with obvious structural anomalies. Although maladjustment may not be present, there is frequently great sensitivity about speech and especially facial appearance in adolescence.

NASAL OBSTRUCTION (HYPONASALITY)

Cases of hyponasality should be fully investigated by an ENT specialist in order to determine the aetiology of the obstruction. Speech therapy should not be attempted until appropriate medical or surgical treatment has been initiated.

Nasal hygiene

As a large number of cases of hyponasality involve nasal congestion, even after adenoidectomy and tonsillectomy, it is important to ensure that the nasal passages are clear of mucus, particularly at the beginning of therapy sessions. Decongestant nasal drops, antibiotics and steam inhalations with appropriate medication may be prescribed by the family doctor or laryngologist, but it may be necessary for the speech–language pathologist to teach the child how to blow the nose efficiently.

Nose blowing

The child's ability to nose blow should be tested at the start of treatment; many children only sniff or wipe the nose even when using a handkerchief.

The sound effects may be convincing but it is necessary to check that the blow has been productive. In some instances, the inability to nose blow efficiently may be the result of lack of early training, but it seems that some children have coordination problems or dyspraxia which make it a genuinely difficult task. For this reason, it is not easy to teach but perseverance usually results in success and greatly improves the health of the nasal mucosa.

Method

- Tell the child to keep the mouth closed. Close one nostril by applying pressure to the lateral wall. With a tissue ready at the other nostril, encourage the child to breathe out or to sniff in and puff out. Only one nostril should be blown at a time as this avoids excessive air pressure accumulating in the nasopharynx and consequently driving mucus into the Eustachian tube.
- Working with one nostril at a time, ask the child to sniff in three times, then to puff out three times. The child begins to feel and hear air circulating.
- The child holds the handkerchief and practises the above exercises independently with the mouth closed.
- A nasal manometer can be used in practice once the child has learned to nose breathe.

Mouth–breathing correction

Breathing through the mouth can persist by habit after adenoidectomy and also because of persisting congestion. After carrying out the above procedures for removal of nasal obstruction, habitual nasal breathing can be established in the following way.

Method

- With the child seated before a mirror, contrast the appearance when mouth breathing and when breathing with the mouth closed.
- The child practises sniffing and puffing with the mouth shut, with a finger over the lips as a tactile reinforcer.
- Seated in front of a mirror, the child aims to keep the mouth shut while being read a story. A score is kept of the time for which the closure can be maintained and the number of mouth openings.
- Games of any sort are played while the child endeavours to keep the mouth closed throughout; any mouth opening is monitored and a system of marks, rewards and penalties can be used.
- Parents and teachers are asked to remind the child.

Remediation strategies

Hearing training

The principles and methods of application are similar to those described in the treatment of hypernasality. The patient is encouraged to discriminate between nasal and denasalised phonemes by identifying those sounds that 'come down the nose' and those that 'come out of the mouth':

- /m/, /n/, /ŋ/ contrasted with /p, b, t, d, k, g/
- contrast in syllables, e.g. /ma:, pa:, ba:/
- contrast in words and sentences, e.g. mad–bad, not–dot.

Development of nasal resonance:

- Humming on /m/, /n/ and /ŋ/, feeling the lips tingle when relaxed and feeling vibrations when hands are placed on either side of the nose. Cup palms of hands over ears and hum, listening to increased resonance.
- Practise singing syllables starting with /m/.
- Sentences and verse, and with children composing nonsense verse, containing as many nasal continuants as possible.

Case note

A boy of 8 years from a neglectful family attended a speech and language unit. His speech was unintelligible and his educational development was severely delayed, although he was of average intelligence. His voice was hoarse and speech denasalised as a result of constant nasal congestion. When tested, he was unable to blow his nose. Under instruction several times a day from the speech–language pathologist, he learned to blow his nose and to clear the nasal airways. At first, he removed large quantities of mucus; paper kitchen towels were used because tissues were inadequate. He cooperated well after a while because he said his nose felt better and his ears 'didn't pop'. His general alertness improved. He had been referred to the hospital ENT department originally by the school doctor, but when he was given an appointment 2 months later his ears, nose and throat were clear and hearing was normal.

Case history

CZ, a girl of 9 years, exhibited severe hyponasality as a result of chronic rhinitis since the age of 2 years. /b/, /d/and /g/ were substituted for /m/, /n/ and /ŋ/. Adenoidectomy at 6 years had not improved the condition or her speech. Extensive examinations had been made without revealing the cause of the rhinitis, and the speech–language pathologist was the last in a long line of specialists who had endeavoured to help the child. The oral structure was normal, but the nose and cheek bones were flattened, exhibiting the typical skeletal structure of the adenoidal facies. The soft palate surprisingly showed no movement at all during the articulation of vowels. The child kept her nose clear by constant blowing and did not breathe through her mouth. She was tense, holding her shoulders high, and her breathing involved the upper thorax almost entirely. She was nervous and so conscious of her speech that she was unable to read aloud in class without stumbling over every word, although in clinic she could read adult material fluently. She was unusually well behaved and polite, and so quaintly old fashioned that the school staff referred to her as 'great-grandmother'. Her speech, which was precise and clipped, was in keeping with her personality.

Despite the rhinitis, which did not improve during treatment, she was able to hum with normal nasality and to produce normal nasal consonants in isolation from the beginning of treatment. She enjoyed humming tunes and practising 'playing on her trumpet', as we called it, with hands over the nose or ears. Great difficulty was experienced in obtaining normal nasal sounds in nonsense syllables and speech. Her auditory discrimination was good and she was able to discriminate correct and incorrect resonance accurately, and was distressed by hearing a recording of her speech. Speech suddenly improved when it was suggested that she should relax and not try so hard with nonsense syllable exercises but speak lazily and easily, drawling and prolonging the nasal continuants instead of producing them briskly so that plosives resulted. Not only did nasal consonants now become normal, but resonance and voice quality improved to her great pleasure.

Neurogenic voice disorders

CENTRAL NERVOUS SYSTEM

Speech and voice therapy for patients with neurological damage is primarily based on the standard principles of voice therapy as described in Chapter 14. Treatment approaches are directed at respiratory, laryngeal, velopharyngeal and orofacial movements designed to counteract the underlying neuromuscular cause of the perceptual deficits (Kearns and Simmons, 1990). After careful assessment of a patient's voice, articulation, respiration, health and motivation, specific difficulties will emerge and realistic targets for improvement in communication can be envisaged. In the complex spectrum of dysfunction associated with neurological damage inflicted by the diseases already described, vocal pathology is usually only one aspect of the patient's disordered communication which, in turn, may be only one element of a spectrum of physical and cognitive deficits. Consequently, an holistic approach is necessary. Whatever the objective dysfunction on assessment, progress is influenced by the attitude and motivation of the patient. In addition to direct therapeutic strategies, the speech–language pathologist can help to alleviate anxiety and depression in both patient and carers. Whether by speech and voice exercises, or use of speech aids, any improvement is worth while because it improves the quality of life. Studies are emerging regarding the efficacy and effectiveness of voice therapy in neurological voice disorders (Table 15.2).

General principles

Compensatory techniques

The primary aim in therapy is to achieve intelligibility of speech by improving function or sustaining it by means of compensatory mechanisms. Therapy cannot reverse the underlying neuropathology. There is the possibility of some spontaneous recovery of function in certain cases, but the compensatory functions remaining in less impaired pathways are usually the basis of treatment. In degenerative disease, strategies and techniques can be learned in the early stages in order to deal with increasing

Table 15.2 Efficacy and effectiveness studies of voice therapy in the treatment of neurological voice disorders

Disorder	Study	Treatment
Parkinson's disease	Scott and Caird (1983)	Prosodic exercises/traditional group treatment. At 3-month review post-treatment, improvement maintained or if deterioration had taken place, not to baseline
	Ramig et al. (1995)	LSVT[a]
	Smith et al. (1995)	LSVT
	Ramig and Dromey (1996)	LSVT
Glottal incompetence	Yamaguchi et al. (1993)	Pushing exercises
Spasmodic dysphonia	Murry and Woodson (1995)	Botox in combination with voice therapy produced better results than voice therapy alone

[a]LSVT, Lee Silverman Voice Treatment Programme (see Chapter 14 and below).

difficulties as effectively as possible. Techniques can include behavioural, prosthetic, instrumental and pragmatic techniques (Kearns and Simmons, 1990).

Holistic approach

In many instances of neurogenic dysphonia, other speech parameters are involved; effective treatment must integrate all relevant features of communication. In addition, a particular aspect of dysphonia may predominate, in which case treatment will naturally have its bias, but this one symptom is never an isolated entity.

Psychological encouragement

Early treatment is advisable for both psychological and physiological reasons. The morale of patients and carers is helped by having clear treatment goals and the acquisition of appropriate compensatory behaviours as soon as possible. Patients need considerable encouragement after neurological trauma or the onset of neurological disease. A well-structured multidisciplinary treatment programme can help to promote a positive attitude and counteract understandable negative feelings. It is also important to prevent inappropriate speech and voice patterns from developing because of a deterioration in self-perception and self-monitoring.

Practice

The reinforcement of motor, proprioceptive and kinaesthetic patterns achieved in exercises during therapy should continue with practice outside the treatment session. If patients can be motivated to carry out regular practice, alone or with those who care for them, more benefit is derived from therapy than if it is forgotten once away from the clinic.

Biofeedback

The importance of biofeedback is discussed in relation to certain disorders in this chapter and this technique should be used whenever possible, unless there is any danger of the patient being distressed by its use. Audio and video-recorders, Visi-pitch and VisiSpeech, amplifiers and loudness indicators are helpful.

Organisation of treatment sessions

Neuromuscular disorders are particularly susceptible to the effects of fatigue. For this reason, the length of treatment and time of day it is given should be considered. The success of an exhausted patient is low and very discouraging. Cooperation with other professionals is essential in order to facilitate a coordinated approach without conflicting elements.

Drug regimen

The therapist should be aware of the effects of medication on each patient and arrange treatments to avoid periods of the day when adverse reactions make maximum cooperation difficult.

Augmentative and alternative communication aids

Patients should be given the opportunity to use such equipment if functional communication is enhanced. Carefully considered introduction of alternative communication aids to patients with degenerative diseases before they really need them can be reassuring. Before such equipment becomes necessary, familiarity and proficiency are established.

Assessment

Assessment has been fully described in Chapter 13. Instrumental and informal and formal perceptual assessments of voice are appropriate. In addition, evaluation of linguistic skills and the general effectiveness of communication is essential. Where there is involvement of the articulators, in addition to laryngeal involvement, a dysarthria profile can be compiled using a formal perceptual assessment such as the Frenchay Dysarthria Assessment (Enderby, 1983) or the Robertson Dysarthria Profile (Robertson, 1982). These profiles indicate the relative severity of deficits affecting various speech parameters, in addition to the areas of phonatory inefficiency.

Treatment

Voice therapy in neurological voice disorders is directed at the biomechanical deficits that give rise to the vocal profile, rather than at a particular condition. The speech–language pathologist's understanding of laryngeal function and the way it relates to the acoustic features is fundamental to treatment.

Respiratory and laryngeal deficits

These, and problems of incoordination, are treated using strategies described in Chapter 14, but it is the identification of the underlying laryngeal behaviour that is the basis of therapy. The categories of vocal features as described by Ramig and Scherer (1992) (see page 265) indicate the appropriate treatment strategies (Table 15.3).

Table 15.3 Categories of vocal strategies for central nervous system dysphonias

Vocal feature in CNS dysphonia	Treatment strategy
Hypoadducted vocal folds (associated with LMN[a] and brain-stem lesions – flaccid musculature)	Laryngeal valving/pushing exercises to adduct vocal folds Raised pitch to increase vocal fold tension Medial compression of thyroid lamina to facilitate vocal fold adduction Diaphragmatic breathing to improve subglottal air pressure
Hyperadducted vocal folds (associated with UMN[b] and extrapyramidal lesions: spastic musculature)	Easy onset Increase transglottal airflow with attempted breathy voice Lower vocal pitch with the aim of encouraging the vocal folds to be more relaxed Manual therapy to relax extrinsic laryngeal musculature General relaxation
Phonatory instability	Reduce excessive vocal tract tension as above Practise maintaining consistent, steady air flow with phonation Practise regulating speech rate Extend maximum phonation time on steady vowel
Phonatory incoordination	Tasks to coordinate expiratory airflow with voice onset Visual feedback of intonation patterns

Robertson and Thomson (1986) list useful exercises for all aspects of dysarthria, including dysphonia.
[a]LMN, lower motor neuron; UMN[b], upper motor neuron.

Hypernasality

Neurogenic hypernasality, resulting from the inability of the soft palate to maintain appropriate closure with the posterior pharyngeal wall, can be treated with **exercises** and **prostheses**. Surgical intervention in neurogenic palatopharyngeal incompetency is not successful (Johns and Salyer, 1978) and should be avoided.

* *Articulation and phonation exercises*

   These are directed at strengthening muscle movement initially, if necessary, with non-speech strategies aimed at increasing intraoral air pressure, e.g. closing the lips and puffing up the cheeks. Coordination of palatal movement is encouraged by practising consonant–vowel (CV) syllables using plosives, and gradually progressing to words and phrases. Hypernasality resulting from incoordination of palatopharyngeal closure is frequently the result of sluggish movement of the velum. Consequently, a slightly slower speech rate, allowing time for closure, in combination with increased mouth opening, reduces the impression of hypernasality. When incompetent velopharyngeal closure is the result of spasticity of the orofacial musculature, strengthening exercises can exacerbate the problem. Reducing phonatory and speech effort while concentrating on articulatory accuracy, increased subglottic air pressure and mouth opening can reduce the perception of hypernasality.

- *Palatal prostheses*

Palatal lift prostheses are widely reported to reduce hypernasality (Massengil, 1972; Wedin, 1972; Enderby, Hathorn and Servant, 1984; Rosenbek and LaPointe, 1985). Aten et al. (1984) reviewed the reported efficacy of palatal lifts in the improvement of resonance and carried out their own investigation. A group of 16 dysarthric patients with severe articulation, respiratory and voice problems were given palatal prostheses and then evaluated perceptually by a panel of judges. There was considerable disparity of opinion about the improvement of speech intelligibility, but general agreement that there was a reduction in nasality. These authors considered that palatal prostheses with wire connectors were better than the traditional solid acrylic bulb prosthesis.

Tudor and Selley (1974) described a palatal training aid (PTA) and a visual speech aid for use in the treatment of hypernasality. The palatal device is a simple removable intraoral appliance not to be confused with a palatal lift prosthesis. It is made for the individual patient by a dental surgeon. It consists of a 'U'-shaped wire with the open ends embedded in an acrylic dental plate. The wire has to be adjusted so that it only just touches the palate (Selley, 1979, 1985). This palatal training device is worn throughout the day and removed at night.

The Exeter Visual Speech Aid (VSA) allows rapid visual feedback of soft palate movements. The patient can confirm visually that the soft palate is moving when phonating vowels, and thus bring movement under voluntary control. The VSA, like the PTA, consists of a removable dental plate carrying a pair of insulated electrodes, which just touch the soft palate in the region of the maximum lift. The wires from the VSA are connected to a control box with a small lamp which lights up when the palate is lowered and touches the wires, and goes out when the palate is raised. The VSA is used for periods of practice only and under the supervision of the speech–language pathologist, but the PTA is worn continuously during the day. The PTA and VSA provide very successful treatment for isolated cases of velopharyngeal malfunction (Curle, 1979; Selley, 1985).

After swallowing assessment, the patient is given advice regarding correct posture, lip closure, chewing and tongue movements, with advice about suitable diet and food consistency. This specialised management comes outside the treatment of dysphonia.

Note

Many patients with dysphonia arising from CNS lesions also have swallowing difficulties. This neurological dysphagia is comprehensively assessed with videofluoroscopy. In some cases, bedside examination using FEESS (fibreoptic examination for the evaluation of safe swallowing) is carried out initially (see page 429). 'Wet' vocal quality can reflect pooling of laryngeal secretions and indicate that the patient is at risk of aspirating fluids into the lungs.

Parkinson's disease

In the past, it was observed that patients with Parkinson's disease could imitate and execute speech exercises during therapy, but were unable to generalise these improvements (Greene and Watson, 1968). As a result, doctors and neurologists regarded speech therapy as ineffective and failed to refer patients for assessment. Subsequently, research has shown the value of therapy, resulting in a more positive attitude (Robertson and Thomson, 1984; Johnson and Pring, 1990; Ramig et al., 1995, 1996; Ramig and Dromey, 1996). Scott and Caird (1983) concluded that phonation is a particular requisite for intelligible, effective speech in Parkinson's disease and that, as voice production improves, so also do other aspects of speech. Treatment appears to be most beneficial when it is carried out on an intensive group basis, when biofeedback is employed and when specific vocal function exercises are used.

Intensive group therapy

Efficacy studies (Table 15.2) of the treatment of the speech and voice problems of patients with Parkinson's disease have been based on intensive group treatment for a fixed period. As Parkinson's disease is a steadily deteriorating condition, it would be unrealistic in most situations for treatment to be open-ended. Studies have been designed not only to evaluate the efficacy of various treatment techniques, but also to assess whether any improvements following treatment are subsequently maintained. The long-term benefits of instruction appear to depend on intensive courses of speech therapy. Robertson and Thomson (1984) and Stones and Drake (1984) reported the success of intensive 2-week courses on a daily hospital outpatient basis. Robertson and Thomson noted that, in addition to the therapeutic strategies employed, benefits of treatment were derived from the fact that patients became motivated as a result of group activity, which was a strong determinant in their improvement. Most encouraging was the fact that improvement after this course lasted for 3 months and, in some cases, speech continued to improve without further speech therapy. Johnson and Pring (1990) also reported the benefits of 10 treatment session over 4 weeks, with patients showing significant improvement on baseline measures, whereas a control group receiving traditional therapy deteriorated or did not improve on any measure over the same period. More recently, Ramig and her colleagues (1996) have reported on two studies each with courses of 4 weeks' duration consisting of 16 treatment sessions, using the Lee Silverman Voice Treatment (LSVT) programme (see Chapter 14 and below), where improvements were maintained when patients were reassessed 12 months later.

Feedback

Delivery of treatment must take into account the self-monitoring difficulties associated with parkinsonism. Proprioceptive, kinaesthetic and auditory feedback are impaired so that the patient has difficulty in perceiving inadequacies of speech and voice, and in modifying these behaviours during treatment.

• Kinaesthetic feedback

The observations of Liberman (1957), in his research into how the individual perceives and discriminates speech signals, are pertinent. Liberman found that individuals learn new and unfamiliar speech patterns by constant repetition. He stated:

> Speech is perceived by reference to articulation, that is, that the articulatory movements and their sensory effects mediate between the acoustic stimulus and the event we call perception.

The individual mimes orally what is heard, then responds to the articulatory movements and the proprioceptive and tactile stimulus. Liberman reversed the long-accepted view regarding the primary importance of acoustic stimuli in recognition of speech, and suggested that perception is actually more closely related to articulation than is the acoustic stimulus itself. Consequently, the repetitive nature of the speech and vocal function exercises discussed below address the issue of kinaesthetic and proprioceptive feedback while simultaneously improving motor performance.

• Auditory feedback

Greene and Watson (1968) found that patients' auditory feedback was enhanced by amplification. Many patients have extremely quiet voices and as a result they frequently have difficulty in monitoring their voices and articulation. Scott and Caird (1981, 1983) reported substantial improvement in vocal volume, quality and rate using the Vocalite training device, although prosody was little improved. The Vocalite lights up only when the voice is loud enough. It can be used for improvement of vocal strength and monitoring of rhythm and speed of vocalisation, but not pitch change. The Voice Loudness Indicator (see Chapter 14) serves a similar purpose. Methods that succeed in causing the patient with Parkinson's disease to self-monitor speech are a fundamental element of all treatment approaches.

• *Delayed auditory feedback*

Delayed auditory feedback (DAF) in selected cases was found to be efficacious in slowing festinant speech by two patients in a sample of 11 patients with Parkinson's disease (Downie, Low and Lindsay, 1981). The constant use of a portable body-worn DAF device was necessary to sustain speech improvement and intelligibility.

• *Video feedback*

Video-recording to help patients monitor their communication patterns and their performance in therapeutic tasks stimulates discussion and group interaction as well as providing feedback. Robertson and Thomson (1984) found that facial expression improved as a result of videos being played back to their group and that social awareness was enhanced.

Speech and voice skills

Therapeutic strategies address the various parameters of speech and voice which are commonly seen in patients with Parkinson's disease.

• *Speech festination and dysprosody*

Rapid speech rate and the disturbance of rhythm, stress and intonation resulting in dysprosody considerably reduce intelligibility. The voice makes a significant contribution to prosody and, if it can be improved in conjunction with slowing the rate of speech, intelligibility is increased (Mueller, 1971; Scott and Caird, 1981, 1983; Scott, Caird and Williams, 1984). Strategies to reduce rate and to retrieve prosody are reinforced by visual and auditory biofeedback.

• *Breathy voice, reduced loudness and loudness decay.*

Patients' voices are generally quiet because of inadequate vocal fold closure and shallow breathing patterns (see Chapter 10) and there is also a tendency for loudness to deteriorate over the duration of a phrase or sentence. Ramig and colleagues (1995, 1996) hypothesised, therefore, that vocal loudness could not be improved until glottal closure was more efficient. They conjectured that improving respiratory function alone would not be successful because air leakage would still occur if vocal fold adduction was not competent, whatever air was available for phonation. Studies were designed using the LSVT programme, which focuses on developing glottal efficiency. A group treated using LSVT in conjunction with respiratory exercises over 1 month of intensive treatment showed considerable improvement in vocal loudness and general intelligibility, whereas treatment in the group undergoing respiratory exercises alone was less successful. Vocal function exercises such as laryngeal valving can provide a straightforward and easily practised method of increasing glottal efficiency. Subsequently, vocal loudness can be increased with the integration of breathing exercises. Table 15.4 outlines the possible laryngeal and respiratory pathophysiology of the vocal characteristics in Parkinson's disease and the goals and strategies of voice therapy.

Table 15.4 Summary of treatment strategies in Parkinson's disease

Laryngeal/respiratory pathophysiology	Goals and strategies	
• Bowed vocal folds	• **Goal:**	To increase efficiency of vocal fold adduction
	Strategy:	laryngeal valving and pushing exercises
• Rigidity/hypokinesia in laryngeal and/or respiratory muscles	• **Goal:**	to increase maximum phonation time
	Strategy:	sustained, loud phonation on a steady vowel
	Goal:	to increase pitch range
	Strategies:	(i) rising/falling glides
		(ii) sustained phonation at highest and lowest pitches
• Reduced inspiratory and expiratory volumes	• **Goal:**	to increase subglottal air pressure
	Strategies:	(i) deep breath before phonation
		(ii) more frequent breaths in connected speech
		(iii) improve posture

Based on Dromey, Ramig and Johnson, 1995

• *Monotone*

Reduced pitch range, and its effect on the flexibility of intonation, can be addressed initially by using fall–rise and rise–fall vocal glides on individual vowels. Visual feedback is helpful. Subsequently, exaggerated stress on words in practice sentences, e.g. 'It's **my** turn to go', 'It's my turn to **go**', etc., results in marked intonation changes.

• *Reduced clarity of articulation*

An integrated approach to improving voice and articulation benefits both parameters and contributes to intelligibility. Increased mouth opening, in association with greater range and accuracy of articulatory placement, improves resonance of the fundamental vocal note. Tongue and lip exercises provide proprioceptive feedback and increase motor skills. There is also some evidence that increasing vocal loudness improves articulation because of the greater jaw opening and exaggerated articulatory patterns that usually accompany talking more loudly (Schulman, 1989).

Maintaining facial communication and correcting the mask-like expression of the patient with Parkinson's disease is an important element of treatment. Greater facial mobility enhances the verbal message and so increases intelligibility, as well as encouraging a more favourable response from the listener. Scott, Caird and Williams (1985) have described the beneficial effect of proprioceptive neuromuscular facilitation (PNF) in this respect (see below).

Cerebral palsy

The diffuse damage of cerebral palsy produces composite forms of motor disorder, including dysarthria. As a result, phonation is frequently impaired together with other elements of speech and language. Children with cerebral palsy are not routinely treated by voice pathologists but by those working in this particular area of paediatric speech pathology. These clinicians treat a child's abnormal phonation in parallel with the associated communication problems.

Although spasticity or athetosis may predominate, for example, a general approach to therapy based on assessment of each child's difficulties is advisable rather than an attempt to treat refined neurological symptoms of flaccidity, spasticity, hypo- and hyperkinesia, ataxia, etc. Treatment of dysarthria in children differs radically from that of the adult with acquired neurological damage who has had established motor speech patterns premorbidly. The adult has experience of the necessary speech movements, but the child has to learn from the beginning by imitation in order to overcome motor deficiencies. The child has the advantage of a developing nervous system, however, and improvements also occur with maturation. There are certain basic tenets of intervention (Table 15.5).

General progress depends on a number of factors, including the severity of the condition, intelligence, hearing, stimulation and encouragement.

Table 15.5 Cerebral palsy: treatment principles

Multidisciplinary approach	Team consists of neurologist, paediatrician, psychologist, audiologist, physiotherapist, speech–language pathologist and child's parents Speech-language pathologist and physiotherapist work closely together
Realistic aims	To achieve optimal function rather than unattainable normalcy To give the child encouragement and the opportunity to experience success
Encouragement of vocalisation and babbling in infancy	The parents or those caring for the infant must be made aware of the importance of the early developmental stages of vocalisation and that it is dependent on speaking and singing to the child

There are various schools of thought regarding the best method of treatment for cerebral palsy. These approaches include therapy to improve phonation.

Bobath method: reflex inhibition

The Bobath method based on reflex inhibition for eliciting speech has been described by Marland (1953) and Mysak (1959a):

- To facilitate phonation, the child is placed in a supine position with flexed abducted knees and shoulders supported on the therapist's arm to prevent the head from falling back. Voicing is elicited by vibrating the child's chest with the therapist's other hand, while the therapist vocalises the desired sound for the child to imitate.
- Reverse breathing and inspiratory phonation can be corrected in the stages summarised in Table 15.6.

Peto method: conductive education

Conductive education for cerebral palsied children was devised by Professor Peto of Budapest who founded the Institute for Conductive Education of the Motor Disabled and Conductors' College in 1945. This approach is based on the importance of a Conductor who acts as physiotherapist, occupational therapist and speech–language therapist to a small group of children, as well as being their teacher and nurse. All activities are taught by the highly trained graduate Conductor, so that no conflicting therapies are applied. Phonation is worked on together with other aspects of speech and language.

Table 15.6 Cerebral palsy: modifying inspiratory phonation

- Roll the child onto his or her back. Neck and shoulders supported on therapist's arm
- As knees are brought up to chest, expiration takes place under tensed and compressed abdominal muscles
- Child inhales as therapist extends the child's legs
- The two preceding stages are repeated until breathing is synchronised with the body movements in a slow, easy rhythm
- When this is established, the therapist encourages the child to vocalise on the expiratory phase of the movement
- Vowels, glides and rhythmic babbling, with the therapist's hands on the lower chest to guide respiratory movements

From Young and Hawk (1955).

Proprioceptive neuromuscular facilitation

The basic principle of PNF is that of increasing the excitability of neurons by bombarding them with impulses which facilitate movement of paralysed muscles (Kabat and Knott, 1953; Knott and Voss, 1963; Mysak, 1968; Voss, Ionta and Myers, 1985). Stimulation is achieved by icing, brushing and manipulation of muscle stretch and resistance. 'Slow' icing uses a slow, rhythmic stroking of lips and tongue to reduce spasticity. Sucking an ice cube before eating can facilitate swallowing (Langley, 1988). Ice packs applied to the thyroid prominence can facilitate voice, the subject being exhorted to cough, to produce vowel sounds and to count. 'Fast' icing, in which flicks with an ice cube are administered, can be applied to the lips or cheeks and is helpful in flaccid paralysis. The treatment may help parkinsonian patients (Scott, Caird and Williams, 1985).

PNF techniques should be instituted by the speech–language pathologist only after discussion with medical and nursing staff. Ideally, treatment should be in collaboration with physiotherapists.

Spasmodic dysphonia

In view of the difficulties of differential diagnosis between conversion spastic dysphonia and adductor spasmodic dysphonia, a trial course of voice therapy is essential initially. The aim of therapy is to reduce phonatory effort so that the adductor spasm is minimised at the onset of phonation. The respiratory muscles are generally involved with laryngeal spasm, not necessarily as part of the neurological involvement, but as a result of the endeavour to force air between the forcefully adducted vocal folds. This intervention frequently has a diagnostic role as well as providing treatment. If there is no significant improvement which is also being generalised to daily life after a short course of treatment, the case should be discussed with the laryngologist and the opinions of a neurologist and psychiatrist sought in an attempt to clarify the aetiology of the voice disorder. If it is decided that the patient should be given Botox injections (see page 298), voice therapy is essential after this procedure, in order to help adjustment to the changed laryngeal status and to ensure best vocal function.

The treatment programme and the strategies used are similar to those for hyperfunctional dysphonia. Treatment techniques commonly used are listed in Table 15.7.

Counselling is an important aspect of therapy for this conspicuous condition, which can affect communication so dramatically and inevitably draws unwanted attention to the speaker. Some patients, especially those who do not depend on speech in their professions, will be satisfied with the improvement in the voice following a course of therapy. Rehabilitation appears to arrest vocal deterioration, but it is arguable that only those patients with a mild and stable form of adductor spasm benefit from voice therapy. If treatment results of voice therapy are unsatisfactory, Botox injections will be considered. Some patients reject this procedure and may continue to need voice therapy. For those who progress to Botox treatment, the decision tends to be made with some desperation, because this is the only remaining route with the possibility of alleviating the problem. The relief at having agreed to the decision is tempered by anxiety in anticipation of the injection procedure (Epstein, Stygall and Newman, 1996). The role

Table 15.7 Spasmodic dysphonia: treatment techniques

Musculoskeletal tension reduction	• reciprocal muscle relaxation (Wolpe) • yawn/sigh • chanting • chewing • manual laryngeal muscle tension reduction
Speech–breathing modification	• increasing airflow • reduced, but adequate subglottal air pressure • easy, relaxed, rhythmic
Voice modification	• easy onset • breathy voice • reduced loudness • pitch elevation • elimination of vocal creak • 'light' voice: develop from CV combinations using sibilants, fricatives, plosives • changing the place of the voice', i.e. 'from throat to mouth'
Counselling	

of the speech–language pathologist is to support the patient with appropriate advice and voice therapy pre- and postoperatively. It has to be remembered that, as the effects of Botox are temporary, the patient will go through
this process every few months if the improved voice is to be maintained.

Immediately after the Botox injection, when the voice is weak and
breathy (see page 299), treatment strategies are exactly contrary to those
for the untreated larynx. The voice improves spontaneously about 72
hours after the injection, but patients welcome vocal strategies to improve
voice and reduce coughing, when this is a problem. Laryngeal valving exercises (see Chapter 14) facilitate vocal fold adduction while reducing the
likelihood of excessive effort and supraglottal activity.

Apraxic aphonia/dysphonia

Laryngeal dysfunction is only one aspect of oral apraxia in which purpose-
ful movements of tongue, lips, pharynx and cheeks may be affected. The
patient is unable to execute learned, skilled movement, although motor
strength and coordination are adequate. Therapy is, therefore, based on a
hierarchy ranging from reflexive laryngeal function, such as a cough or
laugh, to exercises involving increasing laryngeal control (Halpern, 1981)
(Table 15.8). Voluntary phonation is stabilised only gradually and treatment sessions should be frequent, possibly two or three times a day in the
first days of treatment, for maximum effectiveness.

Even when voice has been achieved and is increasingly under voluntary control, voicing is not always consistent. At this stage, it is frequently
sufficient for the speech–language pathologist merely to point to the larynx
in order to elicit sound. As therapy continues, the presentation of target
sounds should also have a hierarchical structure. A suggested pattern might
be as follows:

- The therapist says the sound or word; patient and therapist repeat
  the sound in unison. When there is a high success rate, the next step
  can be taken.
- The therapist says the sound or word; the patient repeats it alone.
- Following high achievement, the target is presented in written form.
  The clinician and patient say the target together and with progress the
  therapist withdraws. Audio tapes are helpful and allow the patient to
  work alone. In the early stages of treatment particularly, the patient
  will benefit from seeing the therapist's lip movement for articulatory
  placement. Articulograms (diagrams of articulatory positions)
  provide useful guidance.

Table 15.8 Apraxic aphonia/dysphonia: treatment techniques

Vegetative phonation	• Use for apraxic aphonia when patient unable to initiate voice voluntarily • Prolong cough/laugh
Biofeedback	• Clinician says /a:/ when facing patient, providing clear visual and auditory models. Patient feels clinician's laryngeal vibrations with finger-tips and then places hand on own larynx • Target is repeated several times but care should be taken to minimise failure and patient's frustration • Nasal consonants: place patient's fingers on side of nose • Fricatives/plosives: patient feels clinician's and own oral airstream
Automatic/serial speech	• Some patients phonate more readily when attempting familiar songs, rhymes, counting, etc.
Generalisation of voice	• With increased voluntary control, voice is integrated into syllables and practised in structured progression (Dabul and Bollier, 1976; Halpern, 1981)
Melodic Intonation Therapy	See text

Melodic Intonation Therapy (Sparks and Holland, 1976; Sparks, 1981) is another approach used successfully in the treatment of apraxia and for improving the prosodic aspects of speech. It is also used successfully in the treatment of cerebral palsied children (Alvin, 1961). A hierarchy of four levels, beginning with humming the melodies of phrases and sentences accompanied by hand tapping, is clearly defined by Sparks. Dysprosody is improved by various strategies using musical instruments, especially drums, and audio tapes of rhythms and chants.

The complexities and divergence of opinion about apraxia of speech and the theoretical basis of treatment are too complex for extended discussion in a text on voice disorders. It is sufficient to say that apraxia, with or without laryngeal involvement, may occur and that for further information the reader should refer to the work of authorities such as Dabul and Bollier (1976), Halpern (1981) and Rosenbek and LaPointe (1985).

PERIPHERAL NERVOUS SYSTEM

Unilateral vocal fold paralysis

Voice therapy for voice disorders resulting from unilateral vocal fold paralysis has three main elements:

1. Improving glottal closure either by encouraging compensatory movement of the healthy vocal fold or early movement of the affected fold in cases of neuropraxia (see Chapter 10).
2. Improving speech–breathing patterns.
3. Preventing or eliminating inappropriate compensatory behaviours.

The use of pushing and laryngeal valving strategies have been discussed in Chapter 14 as means of achieving glottal closure. Table 15.9 includes some specific strategies.

These exercises should be practised at frequent intervals throughout the day, but for short periods only. When the vocal note has been improved in short controlled utterances, vocalisation and control of the expiratory air stream can be extended by the following activities:

- Singing vowels or humming and feeling the laryngeal vibrations with the finger tips.
- Phonating a string of vowels, attempting a glottal plosive on the initiation of each sound.
- Counting or reciting the alphabet starting with one or two numbers of letters and gradually increasing.
- Speaking phrases of gradually increasing length, e.g. 'a blue sky', 'a bright blue sky', 'a bright blue clear sky', etc., while aiming to maintain phonation throughout.

Voice disorders associated with asthma

The potential effects on phonation of asthma and asthma medication are discussed in Chapter 11. Voice therapy is directed at the phonatory features in Table 15.10.

Voice disorders associated with hearing impairment

Abnormal voice in speakers with impaired hearing is the result of the disturbance in their perception of speech. It is only one aspect of speech that is affected by the inability to hear normal speech patterns, although the vocal tract is normal. All aspects of voice can be affected by deafness, including the quality of the fundamental vocal note, speaking fundamental frequency, pitch range, loudness and nasality. It is therefore inevitable, given their subtle nature, that the paralinguistic and prosodic aspects of voice are also disturbed. There are a number of factors that can influence the quality of speech and voice of a hearing-impaired person:

Table 15.9 Voice therapy for unilateral vocal fold paralysis

Target vocal behaviour	Treatment task

Vocal fold approximation	• Laryngeal valving (see page 496) plus:
	  – vegetative vocal behaviours, e.g. laugh
	  – cough, prolonged on to vowel
	  – swallow and phonate /i:/ (Pollack, 1952)
	  – link fingers, lift arms to shoulder level, pull while voicing /i:/
	• Pushing (see page 496):
	  – push hands against table and phonate on a vowel
	  – while sitting on chair, push down firmly with hands holding seat of chair on either side
	• CV syllables with firmly articulated plosive initially, e.g. /ba:/ (Van Thal, 1961)
	• Medial compression of the thyroid cartilage laminae by the voice pathologist can be a useful facilitating method to improve the fundamental laryngeal note initially
	• Head rotation to the affected side on phonation

Reduction of transglottal airflow; improve subglottal air pressure	• Encourage diaphragmatic breathing • Reduce upper chest breathing • Reduce attempts at vocal loudness and aim for improved quality of vocal note (There is a strong tendency to try to increase loudness. As a result of glottal incompetency this results in high transglottal airflow which reduces HNR[a]) • Reduce phrase length in spontaneous speech initially while glottal insufficiency results in air leakage
Eliminate/prevent supraglottal activity, i.e. false vocal fold adduction during phonation	• Patient learns to discriminate between true vocal fold adduction and false vocal fold activity via negative practice (see page 493) • Accurate, firm vocal fold closure encouraged via laryngeal valving strategies • Quietly articulated words with initial vowels to encourage true vocal fold closure only
Eliminate inappropriate compensatory vocal behaviours	• Vegetative vocal behaviours to establish natural pitch (which is lowered in cases of unilateral vocal fold paralysis) • Negative practice with inappropriate high pitch vowels, words, phrases on natural pitch

Froeschels (1948) appears to have been the originator of pushing exercises. He stressed that the push must be perfectly synchronised with phonation, so that voice is attempted simultaneously with the maximum sphincteric action of the glottis. It is essential that this is a firm, accurate manoeuvre and does not involve excessive effort which can result in false vocal fold approximation and mucosal damage. Moolenaar-Bijl (1956) recommended fast repetition of CV syllables with initial /f/ and /s/ as 'useful laryngeal gymnastic'. Casper, Colton and Brewer (1986) have reviewed various therapy techniques. If an inappropriately high pitch is being used in connected speech, this must be resolved before other therapeutic strategies are used.

[a]HNR, harmonics-to-noise ratio.

Table 15.10 Voice therapy for voice disorders associated with asthma

Therapeutic goal	Therapeutic strategy

Improve speech breathing patterns:
    increase air volume
    increase maximum phonation time
    encourage effortless speech–breathing
	Diaphragmatic breathing
	Reduction of upper chest breathing
	Prolonged /ʃ/ (timed in 1-second intervals)
	Prolong vowel or hum
	Counting aloud at 1-second intervals,
	increasing by one at each attempt

Ensure good vocal tract hygiene	Voice care advice (see leaflet page 473) Patient must rinse mouth with water after each use of inhaler
Improve glottal closure in order to improve vocal note quality and vocal intensity (Poor glottal closure may be the result of steroid myopathy or of excessive laryngeal tension)	Myopathy: laryngeal valving strategies Muscle tension dysphonia: reduce hyperfunction via manual therapy, modelling relaxed voice, etc.

- degree and type of hearing loss
- age of the speaker at the onset of hearing impairment
- type of education
- method of communication used (speech or sign)
- type and effectiveness of hearing aids, including cochlear implants.

It is generally acknowledged that there are typical characteristics of the voice of a deaf speaker and that most listeners recognise a 'deaf voice' (studies quoted by Abberton, 2000). These are likely to be more apparent in those who are congenitally deaf who have neither heard normal voices nor had the benefit of auditory feedback of their own vocalisation. The individual who acquires a hearing loss will have developed normal voice, although the loss of auditory feedback may affect the voice after prolonged, severe hearing loss.

Vocal characteristics that are related to congenital deafness can be analysed in terms of both laryngeal and supraglottic features, as described by the source-filter theory of vowels (see page 72). Wirz (1986), in a study using the Vocal Profile Analysis (VPA) system (see page 420), reported the differences between vocal profiles of deaf and hearing speakers. These are summarised in Table 15.11.

The laryngeal and pharyngeal tension in deaf speakers can contribute to perceived **hypernasality**. This is possibly the result of the formation of a cul-de-sac resonator by the elevated back of the tongue and excessive pharyngeal tension. Palatal movement is normal and there is no audible nasal escape. More generally, high levels of vocal tract tension can cause **hyper-**

Table 15.11 Characteristics of voice in deaf speakers (after Wirz 1986)

Speech parameter	Hearing-impaired speech/voice pattern
Range of movements	Articulatory movements may be less or more extensive than in hearing speakers
Pitch	Narrow pitch range Low pitch variation
Loudness	Low loudness mean Narrow loudness range Low loudness variability
Tension	Laryngeal and pharyngeal tension may be marked features, but some hearing-impaired speakers exhibit 'laryngeal laxness', a feature not present in hearing speakers
Laryngeal factors	Harshness and falsetto. Raised laryngeal position

Wirz comments on the surprising fact that the pitch means of the deaf and hearing groups in this study were not significantly different. Some deaf speakers speak excessively loudly.

functional voice disorders to develop and, in addition, clinicians dealing with this patient group must not overlook the possibility of other vocal tract conditions unrelated to deafness. It is also relevant that living with profound deafness is stressful and that voice changes and vocal tract discomfort might result from psychogenic factors. Delayed pubertal voice change (see Chapter 8) is a problem in some male adolescents and appears to be the result of laryngeal and vocal tract tension, which maintains a raised vocal pitch and, presumably, a strong kinaesthetic model for falsetto phonation which is not altered by hearing mature male voices.

Treatment directed at improving vocal quality in deaf speakers requires a multidisciplinary approach with the ENT surgeon, teacher of the deaf and speech–language pathologist working closely together. Amplification provided by appropriate hearing aids and cochlear implants (Cowie, Douglas-Cowie and Kerr, 1982; Fraser, 1987; Fourcin, 1990) is the basis of providing improved speech perception, but the deaf speaker needs further help from a teacher of the deaf or speech–language pathologist to improve vocal patterns.

Improved phonation is achieved by various methods, many of which depend on visual display instrumentation for developing self-perceptual and, subsequently, self-monitoring skills.

Pitch

• The **Voiscope** and **VisiSpeech**, by displaying frequency traces, enable the patient to observe pitch, intonation, improved vocal flexibility and prosodic patterns (Parker, 1974; Pronovost, 1977; Wirz, 1986). Once imitation of prosodic visual patterns can be done using biofeedback, new vocal skills can be developed by producing target responses without visual feedback.

• **Spectrographic displays** may be used because there are distinct differences between normal and deaf speakers, with the latter showing a greater proportion of higher frequencies in connected speech (Wirz, Subtelny and Whitehead, 1980).

• The **Laryngograph** provides a real-time frequency display as well as information about vocal fold contact, which enables the deaf speaker to receive feedback of pitch and vocal quality throughout the pitch range.

Loudness

As excessive or insufficient vocal volume is a common characteristic of deaf speech, **intensity meters** with a digital display or light display can be used for feedback.

Comprehensive instrumentation such as the Kay CSL provides feedback for all speech characteristics. Individual vowels and diphthongs are presented with clearly distinct differences in harmonic structure, enabling the speaker to match their production. Vowels are more difficult to produce than consonants because of their less distinct tactile, kinaesthetic and visual sensory feedback. Prosody and the linking of segments, and their separation and timing in short phrases, can also be monitored.

Tension (laryngeal, supraglottic, general)

Speech and voice therapy should not rely entirely on biofeedback instrumentation. Relaxation of the articulatory and laryngeal muscles may be necessary to improve vocal quality and reduce nasality. Breathing patterns may also need attention (Parker, 1974). As with all patients with voice disorders, stress-related factors must be dealt with appropriately.

Many deaf and deafened individuals do not receive treatment for their speech and voice as adults, although help is frequently intensive in childhood. The development of cochlear implants has stimulated interest in improving communication skills in adults who are deaf, and speech–language pathologists can make an important contribution in this field.

Summary

■ Specific therapeutic techniques are required for certain voice disorders but they are frequently combined with strategies for dealing with hyperfunctional phonation, which may be a secondary feature.

■ Voice disorders requiring specific techniques are also likely to have a multifactorial aetiology which must be taken into account during planning and treatment.

Specific intervention: children, elderly people and singers

'Sing again, with your dear voice revealing a tone of some world far from ours, where music and moonlight and feeling are one.'

Shelley.

Voice therapy for children, elderly people and singers is based on the principles and techniques described in earlier chapters, but with consideration for the particular requirements of these groups. In many cases, for example, children have very few concerns about their voice problems. As long as phonation is not painful and they are understood by their friends, there may be little motivation for complying with treatment. The clinician has the responsibility for making the assessment and treatment sessions inherently interesting and enjoyable in order to bring about a change in the child's vocal behaviour. In contrast, singers and performers are acutely aware of their voices, anxious about their voice problems and sometimes have entrenched vocal behaviours associated with performance which are difficult to discard. Elderly patients may be exhibiting the degenerative changes associated with normal ageing, but which give rise to vocal dysfunction, so affecting their quality of life. This chapter addresses some of the issues that are specific to these groups, but it does not stand alone; it is an addendum to earlier chapters on the aetiology, assessment and treatment of voice disorders that apply to all voice-disordered individuals.

Voice disorders in children

Voice disorders in children may be congenital or acquired and can be organised into the same categories as dysphonia in adults (see Chapter 6). In addition, there are certain problems that are particularly associated with childhood. They differ in their presentation and management because they occur within a developing and changing vocal tract. Some of the conditions that involve increased vocal fold mass are of minor physiological significance to an adult, for example, but may restrict the airway of a small child. When significant congenital structural abnormalities of the vocal tract cause aphonia or severe dysphonia, the small child's developing oral communication is adversely affected because self-monitoring of speech output is impaired, and the way in which listeners react to the child's communication may differ from the norm.

ASSESSMENT

Analysis and evaluation of paediatric voice disorders follow the same format as those for adults but, in order to obtain accurate information and data, the process should be as relaxed, informal, unthreatening and as much fun as possible. It is helpful if parents, or another adult who is close to the child, attends the initial session. Many children are less intimidated by clinical instrumentation than adults; they are familiar with visual displays that respond to their input and are intrigued by seeing images of their fingers, hair and teeth conveyed through an endoscope before laryngeal examination. The ease with which laryngoscopy can be carried out is greatly affected by the surroundings and atmosphere in the clinic, as well as the clinician's manner. If the accompanying adult is anxious about the procedure, this is inevitably conveyed to the child, so it is important that everyone is put at ease from the start of the session.

The onset of the voice disorder is of fundamental importance. It should be established whether or not the child has had an abnormal voice from birth in order to ascertain whether the presenting symptoms are congenital or acquired. Obtaining this information frequently requires careful questioning, particularly if the voice disorder has a long history. The situation may be clarified by asking about the child's cry at birth and vocal quality during the early days of life. When the cry has been abnormal mothers frequently report that 'everyone' commented on the baby's voice, that the baby sounded different from all the other babies in the nursery or that this baby's cry did not sound like that of an older sibling. This suggests that there may be a congenital abnormality such as a web or a congenital vocal fold cyst; there has not been time for the neonate to abuse the larynx before the cry sounded abnormal. In other cases, it becomes clear that, although the voice may have been abnormal from when the child was very young, initially the voice was unremarkable. Subsequently, vocal fold pathology may have arisen from prolonged temper tantrums and long periods of crying as well as shouting within the family and with friends. The speech–language pathologist's close observation of the parents' vocal behaviour can be revealing. Clinical experience suggests that children who abuse their voices may be reared in a very noisy family and, in some cases, the mother exhibits signs of vocal abuse. As with all voice disorders, however, the laryngopathology should be carefully evaluated because other abnormalities also occur and accurate information concerning laryngeal status is the essential basis for remediation.

Laryngoscopic examination most commonly reveals vocal fold nodules or other vocal fold changes related to vocal abuse. As with all voice disorders, however, it is essential never to presume that vocal abuse is the basis of voice problems in children. In cases where it is not possible to obtain a satisfactory view of the larynx, a short period of trial therapy on the presumption of vocal abuse is reasonable but, if there is no improvement within about 4 weeks, further laryngoscopic examination, if necessary under general anaesthetic, should be considered.

The dysphonia resulting from changes in the laryngeal mucosa caused by vocal abuse is usually well established by the time the child is seen by the laryngologist, because it is not an inconvenience until the late, severe stages. A common history in cases of vocal abuse is of either a voice problem that did not resolve after an upper respiratory tract infection, or of episodes of hoarseness after periods of shouting which have eventually become more established. The dysphonic child with symptoms of vocal misuse or abuse probably talks loudly, shouts frequently, uses hard glottal attack and talks incessantly. Talking may continue regardless of the level of background noise, and there may be no awareness that effort is increased in an attempt to counteract the competition. The voice is frequently misused in games and when imitating mechanical noises. These phonation patterns can be part of the speech pattern of an exuberant, extrovert child who is involved and integrated in the peer group, is a leader of activities and directs with enthusiasm. The same vocal patterns can be heard in the tense, angry, frustrated child who uses the voice as a means of expressing his or her negative feelings. The habitual level of vocal loudness used in the family will also affect the child's vocal volume. The dynamics of family relationships can contribute significantly to vocal abuse or be its prime cause. For example, a mother with vocal nodules had three children, all of whom had the same condition. In most cases, a parent has become concerned by the increasing problem but, occasionally, children complain of laryngeal soreness or embarrassment at not being able to sing, read aloud or shout. Speech–breathing patterns in children with dysphonia have been observed to have certain characteristics (Table 16.1).

Table 16.1 Speech–breathing patterns in children with dysphonia

Airflow studies in dysphonic children	Speech–breathing patterns in children with dysphonia resulting from vocal abuse
Sedlackova (1960)	Rapid drop in thoracic pressure at the end of phonation
	Exaggerated contraction of abdominal muscles
	Expiratory movement far exceeding the normal
	Arrests in expiration during speech
	Inverse breathing movement
Gordon, Morton and Simpson (1978) (noted two predominant breathing types)	An exceptionally high flow rate with short phonation time resulting from poor glottal closure
	Exceptionally low flow rate with prolonged phonation time but considerable laryngeal tension and glottal resistance

In view of the fact that most children shout during play, it is perhaps surprising that more do not suffer from chronic hoarseness. Seth and Guthrie (1953) reported that in Germany 40% of school children had hoarse voices. Boys are more commonly afflicted than girls, and the incidence is high below the age of 10 and diminishes considerably as children grow older (Curry 1949). Baynes (1966) found 7.1% of children suffering from chronic hoarseness with the highest incidence in children in the first grade at school. Silverman and Zimmer (1975) found 23.4% of children with similar symptoms in their study.

CONTRIBUTORY HEALTH PROBLEMS

General health can be a primary factor in paediatric vocal abuse or can make a significant contribution to the problem.

Frequent upper respiratory tract infections

These may give rise to an acute laryngitis from which the child has little time to recover between episodes. These infections also lead to mouth-breathing so that dry air is drawn over the vocal folds and has an irritant effect. In addition, an infected postnasal discharge may aggravate the situation.

Laryngitis

A mild laryngitis is often associated with enlarged tonsils and adenoids.

Hearing loss

There may be an intermittent or long-term hearing loss with this condition and others of the upper respiratory tract, which results in children speaking more loudly in an attempt to hear themselves. Seeman (1959) observed that many children with hearing loss develop vocal nodes for this reason. Conductive hearing loss is a common symptom in cleft palate children in whom vocal nodules also occur frequently. McWilliams, Bluestone and Musgrove (1969) found that 27 children with repaired clefts and hoarseness had developed vocal nodules. The follow-up 5 years later showed that 70% of these children still had some abnormality of the vocal folds. It is not clear whether these children had incompetent palatopharyngeal sphincters and therefore used excessive laryngeal effort in compensation, or suffered from emotional disturbance. Renfrew (1988), in a personal communication, confirmed the high incidence of vocal nodules in cleft palate children with incompetent palatopharyngeal sphincters. Surgery to improve the sphincter can contribute to reduction of the nodules.

Allergic reactions

In children, allergic reactions are common; the allergen may be airborne or ingested. Wilson (1987) cited a study by Senturia and Wilson who found a family history of allergy present in about 25% of children with laryngeal dysfunction. Dust (the house dust mite), fur, feathers and many other substances can cause a perennial rhinitis which gives rise to well-recognised symptoms. There are dark circles under the eyes and the child constantly performs the 'allergic salute', which consists of rubbing the nose with the finger, hand and even the arm, in one action, in an attempt to deal with the ever-present moisture and itching. Pollens and moulds give rise to seasonal rhinitis (hay fever). In both types of rhinitis, there will be sneezing, running nose, watering eyes and congested mucous membranes. The voice lacks nasal resonance and is breathy.

Asthma

This may also be linked with vocal abuse because of incessant coughing during attacks and respiratory involvement. In any condition of the upper respiratory tract that produces excessive secretions, resultant coughing and throat clearing predispose the child to vocal abuse because of the vigorous approximation of the vocal folds. The throat clearing may also become an habitual element of the vocal abuse pattern (see psychosomatic aspect in anxiety state and disorders of nasal resonance, page 188). Wilson (1987) also noted that allergies to certain foods, especially dairy products, may produce mild-to-severe oedema of the laryngeal structures. Any portion of the larynx that looks pale and glistening may be indicative of an allergic reaction. Whatever the organic basis, there is also a psychogenic aspect in allergic reactions (Linford Rees, 1982). If the mother is obviously anxious and over-protective symptoms are exacerbated.

INTERVENTION

In cases of benign mass lesions resulting from vocal abuse, voice therapy is the preferred course of treatment. The aims of therapy are:

- to change vocal behaviour in order to reduce or eliminate the vocal fold nodules or other mucosal changes
- to improve all aspects of voice
- to prevent recurrence of the problem.

Even if there are vocal nodules, most laryngologists prefer not to operate but to refer the child for voice therapy. Others prefer to do no more than reassure the parents that the trouble is not serious and that their children will grow out of the symptoms, because as they mature shouting and screaming reduce. Moreover, as the larynx grows in puberty, especially in boys, the pitch drops and the point of maximum excursion of the vocal folds alters position so the original site of mechanical trauma is no longer affected. Phonosurgery is appropriate only if there are marked fibrotic changes. When vocal nodules are soft, even if very large, they should respond to voice therapy. If nodules are so large that a child becomes permanently aphonic they will need surgical removal.

The following factors are important in resolving the voice problem.

• Identification of vocally abusive vocal behaviours and when they occur

By careful questioning of parents, teachers and the child, the behaviours can be identified. It may be reported that the child is noisy and excitable in the playground or yells at football matches or baseball games. Arguments with siblings are a common cause of fierce bouts of shouting and many children shout from room to room.

• Family involvement

Involving the whole family can be an important way of giving each member some insight into how loudly everyone in the household speaks and awareness of high noise levels. Resting the voice cannot be imposed on the child in most cases, and rigid rules for the avoidance of vocal abuse may only create frustration which results in shouting. Various strategies for encouraging voice conservation require the commitment of a parent if motivation is to be maintained (see below). If parents understand the underlying aetiology, the problem resolves with their help and the laryngeal symptoms disappear. Reassurance for the mother that the condition is not serious or harmful helps to allay anxiety.

• Motivating the child to comply with voice conservation

It is much more effective to give the child positive goals to achieve rather than constant instruction not to shout. For example, each member of the family can keep a daily chart on which they score vocal behaviour for each day out of 10. These charts can be pinned up in the kitchen as a reminder of the 'game'. Stars or 'smiley faces' can be given for each occasion on which they might have shouted but restrained themselves. Some older children enjoy producing computer-generated graphs which are brought to each visit to the speech–language pathologist. If it is appropriate for the child to have seen the initial laryngoscopic video of the vocal fold nodules, a sense of purpose can be achieved if the aim is to reduce the size of vocal fold nodules by the time of the next laryngeal examination.

• Improving vocal technique

When the initial inflammation and oedema have subsided, recurrence of the problem can be prevented and further improvement achieved if the child is shown how to produce loud voice with minimal effort. This involves developing vocal skills as described in Chapter 14. Therapy is initially directed at relaxed breathing patterns and phonation. Computerised visual feedback is invaluable for modelling and changing vocal behaviour in the early stages. As the laryngeal status improves, the increased loudness can be encouraged while ensuring that this is carried out safely with excellent breath support and minimal laryngeal tension. The child's cooperation is essential in order to obtain carry-over of new patterns of voice conservation and production into everyday situations. Wilson (1987) describes suitable treatment procedures in detail.

• Group treatment

This can be structured to motivate children of a roughly similar age who have similar voice problems. This approach can also be used to involve parents in a suitable programme to encourage good voice care.

• Other professionals

In certain cases where the vocal abuse appears to be only one symptom of a behavioural disorder or emotional disturbance, referral to a child guidance clinic or enlisting the help of a social worker or health visitor may be more beneficial than direct voice therapy.

Case histories

Case 1

A 13-year-old boy was referred by his general practitioner to the ENT department following his teacher's concern about his permanently husky voice, which occasionally became aphonic. Bilateral vocal nodules were diagnosed and he was referred to the speech therapist. The boy was unconcerned by the 'problem'. When he was interviewed with his mother, it gradually became clear that his academic abilities were limited and he had little interest in school work, but he had a wide circle of friends with whom he was popular and who regarded him as the initiator and leader of their games. The boy lived on an open-plan housing development with extensive open spaces and the games involved a great deal of running, chasing and shouting instructions to different groups. He was an out-going, communicative individual at home, school and in the clinic, with a boisterous sense of humour. The family, consisting of mother, father and sister, was happy and supportive. Management of the case without surgical intervention was based on helping the boy to understand the functioning of the larynx and the aetiology of the nodules. It was pointed out to him and his mother that the condition would not remain static, but that with his cooperation the nodules would completely recede; the alternative was steady deterioration. Voice therapy chiefly consisted of creating awareness of his damaging vocal behaviours and giving advice on more appropriate phonation. As his voice improved, he was shown that, by ensuring adequate subglottal air pressure and suitable pitch, it was possible to produce loud voice without effort. Biofeedback using VisiSpeech was fun and effective. He responded particularly well to the competitive idea of aiming to reduce the size of the nodules significantly by the date of his next laryngological examination. He was shown the video after the first examination and had a clear image of what his aims were. Apart from minor transgressions he maintained the suggested regimen and subsequent laryngoscopy 4 months later revealed normal vocal folds.

Case 2

A 2-year-old girl was referred because of her hoarse and breathy voice; it did not worry her but her mother's concern had initiated the referral to the ENT department. Initial discussion revealed that the child had the expected tantrums of this age group which involved shouting and screaming; her vocal behaviour was apparently not exceptional. However, bearing in mind that some degree of vocal abuse had played a part in her symptoms and that all 2 year olds do not have dysphonia, further information was necessary. It transpired that there were five older children in the family and that the little girl was frequently driven to a fury of frustration when she was ignored or unable to take part in the general conversation. The only way in which she ensured attention was by shouting more loudly than her brothers and sisters or screaming in uncontrollable rage. Management of this case could take place only with the mother's understanding and cooperation. A year later her voice was within normal limits.

> **Case 3**
>
> A woman of 27 years was receiving treatment for a unilateral vocal nodule. She was a vivacious and assertive individual who always spoke extremely loudly. On one occasion she brought her 3 year old son to the clinic. He also spoke excessively loudly and his voice was hoarse and breathy and showed vocal behaviours similar to those of his mother.

Note

A comprehensive overview of the aetiologies of paediatric voice disorders can be found in Maddern, Campbell and Stool (1991). Wilson (1987) and Andrews (1991) provide comprehensive information regarding paediatric voice disorders and their management.

Presbyphonia

Age-related changes of the vocal tract have been described in Chapter 5. Most individuals accept the changes in the quality of the vocal note, the speaking fundamental frequency and timing as inevitable consequences of increasing age. Increasingly, however, a relatively small but concerned group seek help for what they perceive as significant vocal changes. They find that their voices are functionally inefficient for certain tasks, such as singing to grandchildren or sustaining adequate volume in noisy social settings. Others are concerned that 'my voice doesn't sound like me', with complaints of rough vocal quality common in men and women. The changes are sufficiently obvious in some elderly people for them to be concerned that there is laryngeal pathology, particularly carcinoma. All complaints of voice change in elderly patients, as in all other groups, must be fully investigated by the laryngologist. After assessment, even when the larynx shows no abnormality and there are only signs of presbylaryngis (ageing larynx), voice therapy should be instituted with the patient's agreement. Some individuals wish to be reassured only that there is no disease, but there are a significant number who are highly motivated to achieve optimal laryngeal function. The role of voice therapy in this age group is not only to improve the voice but to prevent misuse in an attempt to overcome the primary vocal deficiencies (Shindo and Hanson, 1990).

Individuals with presbyphonia are usually very rewarding for voice pathologists to treat. They are highly motivated, carry out home practice tasks conscientiously and recognise when they have achieved their goal of improved vocal function. Clinical experience indicates that the course of treatment is usually short, with approximately four sessions resulting in vocal improvement. Treatment rationale and possible tasks are summarised in Table 16.2.

Table 16.2 Presbyphonia: voice therapy tasks

Phonatory/laryngeal feature	Vocal task
Anteroposterior glottal chink (poor vocal fold adduction)	laryngeal valving (see page 496) articulation of individual vowels with firm, gentle glottal attack initially phrases beginning with word with initial vowel, using firm glottal attack
Atrophic vocal folds	as above. frequent practice, i.e. 5–6 times daily for 5 minutes
Reduced air volume due to weakened respiratory muscles	breathing exercises: • diaphragmatic breathing • increasing extent of thoracic expansion • increasing period of rib elevation • increasing period of expiratory airflow on voiceless phoneme /S/ • increasing maximum phonation time
Rough fundamental vocal note	coordination of onset of expiratory airstream and phonation on sung, steady vowels, aiming at clear vocal note
Limited pitch range	vocal glides on vowels, starting at mid-pitch and gradually extending to higher and lower notes sung arpeggios of extending range (in combination with improved breathing patterns)
Reduced loudness	phrases of increasing loudness incorporating earlier skills

Laryngeal framework surgery to reduce vocal fold flaccidity is of limited value in elderly people because the improvement only lasts for a few months before the tissue returns to its flaccid state (Tucker, 1988).

Frequent practice five to six times daily for 5 minutes appears to improve voices exhibiting age-related changes. Patients commonly remark that their voices are improving within a week or 10 days of the start of treatment. Improvement is probably the result of a combination of muscle strengthening, increasing the repertoire of vocal behaviours of which the speaker was unaware and increasing confidence in vocal ability. General voice care and vocal tract hygiene should be given: elderly patients may not be adequately hydrated and many also have a tendency to phonate on residual air.

It is essential that the vocal strategies to improve laryngeal approximation are carried out correctly, without excessive effort, so that the vocal fold mucosa is not damaged. Patients should be advised that, if they notice any soreness or discomfort of the vocal tract after a practice session, they are attempting the tasks with too much force. As very elderly people may have difficulty remembering advice and vocal tasks, it is particularly important for the voice pathologist to provide clear, printed information.

Patients' personal circumstances have to be taken into account when planning and carrying out treatment. There may be factors exacerbating the presbyphonia which need to be addressed in addition to the treatment programme outlined in Table 16.2:

- Elderly people who live alone may not speak to anyone for several days at a time and should be encouraged to use their voices as much as possible through singing and using the telephone, or being helped to increase social contact.
- If one partner is hearing impaired, the spouse may be suffering from muscle tension dysphonia or vocal strain in an attempt to produce a sufficiently loud voice, rather than straightforward presbyphonia. In these circumstances, the voice pathologist can also make suggestions about face-to-face contact and the need for improved hearing aids, in addition to advice about voice care and improved vocal skills.
- There may be a an emotional component to voice problems in elderly people, as in all cases of dysphonia. The death of a partner of many years and the resulting loneliness can cause grief and depression that last for months or years. The elderly person may feel, quite justifiably, that younger people do not understand that the emotional effects of such events can be just as devastating in old age. Even when old age and poor health are obvious predictors that an individual may not have long to live, the feelings of loss by the remaining partner are not necessarily lessened. Family members may give considerable support, but the very elderly person can feel isolated as friends of the same age gradually die. Presbylaryngis will still require direct treatment, but the clinician must also take the patient's emotional status into account as an aetiological factor and in the treatment approach.
- Hearing loss in elderly people affects auditory feedback and the speaker with age-related vocal changes finds it difficult to monitor loudness and vocal quality. At an early stage of treatment, the hearing aid should be checked to ensure that it is working satisfactorily. Visual feedback can be helpful in establishing a useful kinaesthetic model of appropriate vocal volume and a fundamental vocal note of greater clarity.

Vocal dysfunction commonly occurs with ageing, but it is essential that any voice disorder is fully evaluated laryngoscopically and within a multidisciplinary team. The vocal symptoms may be caused entirely by age-related changes within the vocal tract or compounded by attempts to compensate for these deficiencies, but the patient's complete medical history and emotional status must form the basis of treatment.

Voice problems in singers

Singers are at particular risk of trauma to the vocal folds because of the increased vocal loading that is involved in many types of singing. It is generally accepted that singers who are properly trained and who use the techniques of good voice production are less likely to damage the vocal folds (Zilstorff, 1968; Bunch, 1982) and that there is a correlation between training and the level of vocal skills for singing (Teachey, Kahane and Beckford, 1991). Even so, an excellent singer may have some vocal strain after lengthy rehearsals or a demanding performance. A tiny vocal fold haemorrhage can occur but will gradually disappear when the exertion is over. However, if the voice is poorly produced and excessive effort is being used in an attempt to 'project' it or to achieve notes above or below the natural range, the long-term result will be damage to the laryngeal mucosa and, eventually, traumatic vocal fold lesions such as polyps or nodules. Even extremely competent singers, who have had vocally trouble-free careers for many years, can develop these problems if they sing during an upper respiratory tract infection or if other factors that put them at risk occur concurrently (see below).

Even the most successful singers are anxious before performances and may be generally volatile and temperamental. Their anxiety aggravates the vocal symptoms and they need sympathy and understanding as Punt (1968, 1983) emphasised. A laryngologist is often present in the opera house when major performances are in progress, ready to administer medication and reassurance behind the scenes. Although trained singers can, in emergencies, sing with a cold and infective laryngitis (Zilstorff, 1968), the untrained or poorly trained singer with signs of vocal abuse and chronic laryngitis should never do so. The performance will be disastrous and this will not only aggravate the condition but be psychologically traumatic. It should be a general rule that, if laryngitis is sufficiently painful to warrant analgesics, the performance should be cancelled (Sataloff, 1991). Masking the pain allows the singer to perpetuate further damage. In particular, aspirin is contraindicated because of its tendency to cause haemorrhage of the vocal folds in singers. Sataloff (1991) warns that singers should take particular care to ensure that they are not taking aspirin in cold remedies and similar preparations. In addition, singers should avoid self-medication. It is evident that some singers use various remedies recommended by other performers (such as gargling with port or taking inappropriate over-the-counter preparations) which can exacerbate their vocal problems. Laryngoscopy is essential to determine the aetiology of their voice problems (see Pharmacological influences on voice, page 510).

Vocal fold nodules are most likely to occur in untrained or poorly trained singers, members of amateur choirs and groups, nightclub, pop, country and western singers, and rock band singers. The classical singer who is badly trained and has an unscrupulously ambitious singing teacher who concentrates on the aria at the expense of technique will inevitably develop symptoms of vocal abuse. Non-classical singers fall into various categories such as musical theatre, pop, country and western, and rock. Excessive vocal tension may arise from the style of singing and, in cases of the singer who does 'cover' versions, the requirement to sing outside the natural pitch range. In singing styles such as country and western, pharyngeal tension eliminates the singer's formant (see Chapter 4 and Sundberg, 1974, 1977) and the singer may increase laryngeal effort to increase loudness. In a study of 100 healthy singers, Koufman et al. (1995) concluded that various levels of laryngeal muscle tension are associated with different styles of singing. Choral singing appeared to have the lowest level of muscle tension, followed by operatic and barbershop singing. Tension levels increased in popular, jazz and musical theatre, with the highest levels of laryngeal tension observed in country and western, and rock/gospel singing. These results indicate that muscle tension is generally higher in non-classical than in classical singing. Tension levels were lower in singers with formal training and those who warmed-up before singing. Unexpected findings included the fact that muscle tension scores were not significantly different for professional and amateur singers, and that the use of alcohol and tobacco, previous voice problems and regular exercise did not appear to influence the muscle tension scores.

In addition to the style of singing, there are a number of other factors that may increase the risk of mucosal damage in singers:

- The particular sound of the voice that is produced and that is admired by the audience may be the antithesis of well-produced voice. An aggressive, forceful, harsh quality may reflect the anarchic quality of the music, but it may be extremely difficult to produce this sound without causing impact trauma to the vocal folds. This is a dilemma for the speech–language pathologist and the singer who will be reluctant to alter a mode of singing that is commercially successful and by which he or she is identified.

- The non-classical singer frequently performs in surroundings that are noisy, dusty and smoky.
- Singers of all styles may be required to sing while moving vigorously, dancing or lying in one position for a long period. All these activities affect the capacity and control of air and, as a result, interfere with the steady subglottal air pressure that is required to maintain the singing voice.
- Some performers admit to drinking alcohol and taking illegal drugs before and after a 'gig' in order to give an uninhibited and confident performance. These substances exacerbate the effects of vocal abuse.
- As many singers avoid eating a heavy meal before an evening performance, they then eat late at night with the possibility of aggravating gastric reflux.
- Travelling from one venue to another is an inevitable part of a professional singer's schedule. Air travel, in particular, has certain factors that put the singer at risk. The atmosphere is dry and the individual can become dehydrated systemically. There is ready access to alcohol, with its dehydrating effects, and the temptation to talk against the high ambient noise level (about 90 dB). As a result, the singer may use considerable vocal loading during conversation while the vocal fold mucosa is relatively dry and vulnerable to abuse.
- Performance anxiety and the general stresses associated with the life of a performer, such as auditions and concerns about the availability of work, help to maintain a level of tension in many performers that affects vocal function and that must be taken into account during the treatment of voice problems.

The precursor to changes in the vocal fold mucosa may be vocal fatigue, when singing becomes increasingly effortful and performance deteriorates. Vocal fatigue is experienced by the singer as changes in the kinaesthetic and proprioceptive sensations of singing, including soreness, and changes in vocal dynamics (Kitch and Oates, 1994). Reduced pitch range and flexibility, a decrease in the ability to produce notes at the desired pitch, a deterioration in vocal quality, a need to 'push' the voice and, in some cases, hoarseness are all associated with vocal fatigue. During these episodes, increased muscle tension, most obvious in the throat, neck and jaw (Sataloff, 1981), is required to maintain the voice and can contribute to the symptoms, thus putting the singer at risk of damaging the vocal fold mucosa. There is some indication that training reduces the susceptibility to vocal fatigue (Scherer et al., 1986), presumably because vocal skills are improved (Teachey, Kahane and Beckford, 1991) and the singer is able to achieve the full range of pitch and loudness without resorting to hyper-functional phonation. When singers are generally fatigued or stressed, whether emotionally or physically, there is a greater tendency to vocal fatigue and to causing vocal fold damage (Harris, 1998).

ASSESSMENT

Some singers seek help at a very early stage of the vocal problem because of their acute awareness of sensory changes associated with singing, as well as any deterioration in vocal function. Others 'sing round' the problem for some time, making various laryngeal adjustments to minimise the effect of a developing vocal fold lesion on the singing voice. It is essential that the clinicians involved in the initial examination take the singer's concerns seriously, even when there is no obvious laryngeal abnormality and the voice appears to be well within normal limits. Symptoms may be revealed only by the vocal loading required by performance, in the early stages, but are an indication that intervention is necessary if future damage and vocal deterioration are to be prevented. Small unilateral mass lesions, such as a polyp, may affect the voice only at certain frequencies, but this can represent a significant problem for a singer. In busy general ENT clinics, clinicians may regard the complaints of a professional singer with an apparently normal voice and larynx as trivial, in comparison with obvious pathologies, but careful examination is required to ensure that the problem is fully evaluated. A combined voice clinic examination using videostroboscopy is the gold standard for assessing singers' larynges so that the subtleties of laryngeal structure and function can be viewed repeatedly until an accurate assessment and diagnosis are made. It is important that evaluation of vocal function and subsequent voice therapy is not confined to the singing voice. Even singers spend much more time speaking than singing and, in many instances, it is abuse of the speaking voice that subsequently leads to problems with the singing voice.

As with all voice disorders, intervention can include voice therapy and, in some cases, phonosurgery. Voice therapy is the preferred treatment for muscle tension dysphonia and benign vocal fold lesions in singers, whenever this is a realistic course of action. The various elements of voice therapy relevant to hyperfunctional voice disorders, as described in described in previous chapters, are also used with singers. A short course of treatment can help to prevent unemployment and avoid damage to the vocal fold mucosa, if the problem is in its early stages. Even when it seems that phonosurgery will probably be necessary, a trial course of treatment is advisable, so that surgical intervention can be avoided if possible. This is because excision of a lesion may leave scar tissue which will interfere with the mucosal wave. Although this may

Case histories

Case 4

A 35-year-old woman had sung without training in amateur choirs for many years. Her choral activities ceased for 2 years during which time she had two children. When she resumed her singing, she frequently found that her throat was uncomfortable after choir practice. As time progressed, her voice became breathy and the upper singing range was lowered, although she reported no problems when speaking. Her vocal folds were mildly inflamed. It transpired that there were two main contributory factors to her vocal abuse. She had always sung as a soprano and had associated feelings of exertion and effort with singing; it was found that she sang the alto part much more comfortably. Although this was an important factor, it did not produce difficulties until she had her two boisterous, noisy children with whom she used a loud speaking voice. The laryngeal misuse that she perpetrated during the day was fully realised in the evening when she attempted to sing the soprano part which was not ideal for her particular voice.

Case 5

A quietly spoken solo singer with a rock band was transformed during concerts into a yelling, frenetic performer whose voice was heard, albeit with a microphone, above the accompanying instruments and the screaming audience. He frequently 'snorted' cocaine before performances and drank spirits afterwards. The vocal folds were hyperaemic and 'thickened'. The voice was hoarse and breathy and was beginning to reflect the excessive effort he used during performance. His dilemma was that the sound he produced was the sound his fans wanted and which made him such a marketable commodity, but to continue to produce it in this way would also ensure its complete loss. After the appropriate explanations, he continued to give his usual stage performance but was able to maintain the voice by attention to vocal hygiene and voice conservation when not performing.

Case 6

A professional soprano who was a soloist and teacher had sung for 20 years without any voice problems. After a severe flu-like illness, during which she was coughing a great deal, she took great care of her voice. A month later she performed at a concert, but was aware of some 'tightness' in the throat and the next day she had a raised temperature and her infection had returned. As the symptoms resolved, she complained of vocal tract discomfort. On examination, laryngeal structure and function were unremarkable, but there was considerable tenderness on palpation of the extrinsic laryngeal muscles.

She was extremely anxious and very concerned that any attempt at singing might do irreparable damage. As a result, she had lost confidence in her ability to sing and was bracing the extrinsic laryngeal musculature as if to 'protect' her larynx. Manual therapy (see Chapter 14) rapidly eliminated this discomfort and was the foundation of re-establishing her singing voice. Voice therapy followed and it became clear that, because she was so concerned that she might harm her larynx, she needed the reassurance of being led through a range of vocal strategies by the speech–language pathologist. It was as if she wanted 'permission' to use her voice again. Two treatment sessions restored her normal singing voice and she returned to her engagements.

have little impact on the voices of most people, it can cause problems for the production of certain notes by the singer. When phonosurgery proves to be unavoidable, the patient should be seen by the voice pathologist routinely pre- and postoperatively (see Chapter 14). Careful video and audio recording of the speaking and singing voice preoperatively is advisable as a precaution in cases of litigation, besides being essential to the vocal rehabilitation pro- gramme (Kleinsasser, 1968).

After excision of a vocal fold lesion, the singer must comply with voice rest and voice-conservation advice. Although the folds appear to heal very quickly, the complex vibratory patterns of the mucous membrane take some time to become re-established and it may take up to 3 months before full vocal loading at 'concert pitch' should be attempted. Singers become anxious to sing again during this interval, and it is necessary to warn them that there will be a delay in full vocal recovery if they do not comply with the advice, even when vocal patterns are less hyperfunctional.

Professional singers rely on their voices for their income. When the 'instrument' becomes defective, it is understandable that they become extremely anxious and may be depressed. It is not only the loss of income caused by cancelled performances that causes great concern, it is the adverse effect on their reputations and the fact that future engagements might not be forthcoming if it becomes known that they have been having problems. The clinician should also appreciate that, for all singers, amateur and professional, the ability to sing well without discomfort makes a signif- icant contribution to their feelings of well-being and quality of life. Patients who are no longer able to sing feel deprived of an important element of their existence and their self-image.

Many singers know very little about vocal anatomy and physiology, although this situation is changing. As a result, there is a great deal of misinformation among some groups of singers about voice problems, accompanied by dramatic stories of vocal disasters which are unfounded. Some anxiety can be allayed by careful explanations of laryngeal structure and function, the aetiology of the voice problem, the planned treatment and expected outcome. Reassurance and explanation throughout treatment are fundamental aspects of the programme. If phonosurgery is necessary, patients' anxiety increases before surgery and continues to be at high levels until the voice is heard again in speech. There is a great temptation at this time to sing to 'see if the voice is still there'. This must be anticipated by the speech–language pathologist so that the patient is told that singing should not be attempted until an agreed stage of treatment.

DISCHARGE

The role of the voice pathologist in treating a singer with voice problems is to restore vocal function to within normal limits and to prevent further damaging vocal behaviour. All singers must be particularly aware of the importance of not using a hard glottal attack in place of a clear and con-trolled initiation of the vocal note. Appropriate diaphragmatic breathing, with optimum capacity and control, is essential if there is to be sufficient breath support for the vocal note at the end of phrases; without it, the vocal folds will be forcefully adducted in an attempt to continue to maintain phonation. Voice therapy alone is not, however, sufficient to enable the singer to return to full use of the voice at a superior level. It is essential that the voice pathologist coordinates the discharge process with a competent singing teacher who continues working with the singer until the voice is fully restored.

Note

The importance of a coordinated approach to the vocal health and treatment of voice disorders in singer has been recognised by the American Speech–Language–Hearing Association (ASHA) and the National Association of Teachers of Singing (NATS) in a joint statement (National Association of Teachers of Singing, 1992). The general guidelines recommend: '1. The preparation of the teacher of singing needs to be augmented by inclusion of training in anatomy and physiology and in clinical management of voice dis-orders. 2. The preparation of the speech–language pathologist who works with singers needs to be augmented in a parallel manner to include instruction in vocal pedagogy (the art and science of teaching voice) and vocal performance.'

Summary

■   The general principles of voice therapy apply to voice disorders in children, elderly people and singers, but consideration must be given to the particular circumstances and needs of these groups during treatment.

- Assumptions must not be made about the voice disorder because of the status of the patient, i.e. not all paediatric voice disorders are caused by vocal abuse; vocal deterioration in old age is not necessarily the result of age-related changes; singers do not necessarily have voice disorders because they sing.

Laryngeal cancer: treatment and management

Laryngeal cancer is a relatively rare cause of dysphonia but it must always be considered as a possible reason for abnormal voice. It is mandatory that any patient who is hoarse for more than 2 weeks, in the absence of an upper respiratory tract infection, should be examined by a laryngologist. Assumptions must not be made about the reasons for a voice disorder, even when heavy demands on the voice suggest that vocal misuse or abuse is the probable reason for the vocal changes. Similarly, patients who appear to be 'low risk' must not be managed with less urgency than heavy smokers as there is evidence that life-long non-smokers can and do develop upper aerodigestive tract cancers (British Association of Otorhinolaryngologists, 1998). Early detection of laryngeal cancer is critical for the patient's survival, for the best potential outcome of treatment and for post-treatment quality of life.

Incidence

The incidence of laryngeal cancer varies in different parts of the world and even from one region of a country to another. Variations are probably the result of a combination of environmental factors and genetic predisposition (BAO, 1998). It is acknowledged that it is on the increase. In 1980, the American Cancer Society estimated that about 10,000 new cases of laryngeal cancer would be diagnosed each year in the USA. By 1990, this estimate was adjusted to 13,000 cases per year. In the UK, of the 50,000 new referrals to otolaryngology clinics annually, 5% (2,500) are new laryngeal cancers. Berry (1983) reported that approximately 1.5% of new patients with cancer have cancer of the larynx. The regional incidence of head and neck cancer in the UK varies from 7.7 to 15.3 cases per 100,000 of the population with the larynx being the most common site (BAO, 1998). The comparative rarity of the condition is highlighted in the British Association of Otorhinolaryngologists' report (1998) which notes that the 39,000 general practice principals in the UK will each encounter only one new case of laryngeal cancer in 13 years.

Laryngeal carcinoma occurs most frequently in middle-aged or elderly men who smoke, with the peak incidence occurring in the fifth and sixth decades. The ratio of men to women, 25 years ago, was 7:1 (Leonard, Holt and Maran, 1972), but there is some evidence that it is increasing among women as their years of smoking increase. Doyle (1994) cites a number of studies confirming this trend. The general increase in the numbers of patients with a diagnosis of laryngeal cancer, and other carcinomas, is thought to be related to increased life expectancy. Cancer is a disease of old age and, as people live longer, the likelihood of developing a carcinoma increases. The increased figures are also related to improved detection techniques and the possibility of diagnosis being made at a much earlier stage of the disease.

Although rare under 30 years of age, there is evidence that the incidence is increasing in younger individuals (Doyle, 1994) and a number of much younger cases are reported in the literature. Recognition of this possibility by professionals is important in relation to early diagnosis and treatment. One of the youngest cases quoted is that of a 20-month-old boy (Peterson, 1973) whose malignant tumour required total laryngectomy. Figi and New (1929) reported on two of their patients – a boy (15 years) and a young woman (24 years) – both of whom had squamous cell epithelioma. Total laryngectomy was considered to be the only possible procedure because of the extent of the growths. A fibrosarcoma of the larynx in a girl of 15 years, described by Garfield Davies (1969), was initially arrested by radiotherapy but necessitated total laryngectomy 15 months later after recurrence. Early cases used to be related to papillomas treated by radiotherapy in childhood (Rabbett, 1965; Vermeuling, 1966), but the danger of this treatment of papillomas is now appreciated.

Aetiology

The chief causes of cancer of the larynx are cigarette smoking and the consumption of alcohol. The synergistic effect of tobacco and alcohol greatly increases the risk (BAO, 1998). Doyle (1994) cites a study by Wynder et al. (1976) which indicated that, for individuals who smoked more than 35 cigarettes per day, the 'relative risk' of developing a laryngeal carcinoma was seven times greater than for non-smokers. When the smoker of 35 cigarettes per day also consumed 7 fluid ounces of alcohol per day, the relative risk became 22 times greater when compared with those who did not smoke or drink. Environmental factors such as exposure to asbestos and other substances may also be implicated in laryngeal cancer, but the evidence is not as substantial. It is unclear what levels of exposure are required to initiate malignant changes in the squamous cell epithelium and more information has to be acquired about the interaction of these elements. It is perturbing, but encouraging, to consider that most cases of laryngeal cancer are preventable (BAO, 1998).

Classification of malignant laryngeal tumours

Tumours can occur at any site in the larynx; they may be glottic (Figure 17.1), supraglottic or subglottic, with various structures within each area being involved. Glottic carcinoma is the most common form of intralaryngeal growth (Ballantyne and Groves, 1982) (Table 17.1). Direct extension of a laryngeal tumour in the early stages is confined to the membranes and muscular tissues of the larynx and is limited by the cartilaginous structures. Prognosis for intrinsic laryngeal cancer is better than for any other site in the body. Primary cancer may spread by direct penetration into the surrounding tissue, but a more serious risk of secondary growth arises with involvement of the lymphatic glands, because cancer may then occur widely throughout the body by lymphatic metastases. As there are practically no lymphatic vessels in the vocal folds, lymphatic metastases will occur only when considerable invasion of the larynx has taken place.

Laryngeal cancer is classified by a system that includes information about the site and extent of the **tumour**, lymph **node** involvement and whether or not there is **metastatic** disease. This is known as the TNM system (Table 17.2).

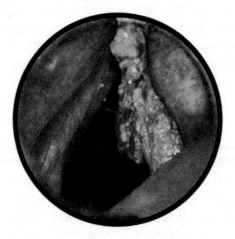

Figure 17.1 Glottic carcinoma.

Table 17.1 Sites of laryngeal tumours

Site	Subsites	Common symptoms	Management

supraglottis	Epiglottis
	Pyriform fossae
	Aryepiglottic folds
	Arytenoids
	False vocal folds
	(ventricular bands)
	Ventricles
		• few/no symptoms
		  until well advanced
		• throat discomfort
		  followed by radiating
		  pain to ear on
		  swallowing
		• voice changes and
		  increasing dysphagia
		  as carcinoma extends
		• dysphagia
		• respiratory problems
		• metastatic lymph
		  node
			• radiotherapy to primary
			  site and neck nodes
			• total laryngectomy and
			  neck dissection for
			  recurrent disease
			• supraglottic laryngectomy
			  in a small minority of
			  cases

**glottis (most
common site of
malignant
laryngeal tumour)**
	Vocal folds (usually
	free edge)
	Can spread
	throughout vocal
	fold
		• hoarseness,
		  increasing in severity
		  as carcinoma extends
		• stridor and increasing
		  airway obstruction
			• radiotherapy (95% cure
			  rate for T1 lesions[a])
			• surgery for
			  advanced disease
			• total laryngectomy
			  for recurrent disease
			• partial laryngectomy for a
			  few patients[b]

**subglottis (least
common site of
laryngeal cancer)**
	Inferior surface of
	vocal folds
		• symptoms not
		  apparent until
		  carcinoma well
		  advanced
		• respiratory distress/
		  obstruction
		• dysphonia as late
		  feature as vocal folds
		  become involved
			• radiotherapy if no
			  metastatic lymph nodes
			• surgery when disease
			  has extended

Ballantyne and Groves (1982); Dhillon and East (1994); Doyle (1994); BAO (1998).
[a]See TNM classification (page 576).
[b]See surgery (page 583).

Signs and symptoms

DYSPHONIA

Dysphonia is the first presenting sign when the vocal folds are involved, but it is usually a late symptom in supraglottic and subglottic laryngeal cancer. The severity of the dysphonia may correlate with the size of the lesion, but many patients will evolve vocal behaviours to deal with the problem which might compound the primary voice disorder. As Doyle (1994) points out,

Table 17.2 Primary laryngeal tumours: summary of staging system (BAO, 1998)

T1S	• carcinoma in situ: a stage of laryngeal cancer with the histological changes of carcinoma, but which is not invasive; may become invasive
T1	• tumour limited to one subsite • normal vocal fold mobility
T2	• tumour extends to more than one subsite with normal or impaired vocal fold mobility
T3	• tumour limited to larynx with vocal fold fixation
T4	• tumour invades through thyroid cartilage and extends to other tissue beyond larynx (e.g. thyroid gland, oesophagus, trachea, pharynx, soft tissues of neck)

Nodes and metastatic disease are similarly classified in order to stage the progress of the spread of the disease.

changes in the voice might be subtle and long term, and only noticed when the patient goes to his or her doctor with frequent coughing, throat clearing, shortness of breath and a 'catch' in the voice. It is of clinical importance that the vocal changes arising from laryngeal carcinoma do not differ significantly in most cases from those caused by benign mass lesions of the vocal folds. In advanced cases the patient is extremely hoarse and, as the airway becomes obstructed by the tumour, inspiratory stridor and respiratory distress are apparent.

DYSPHAGIA

As the tumour increases in size, swallowing is affected in cases of both glottic and supraglottic tumours.

RESPIRATORY PROBLEMS

Similarly, as glottic and subglottic malignancies enlarge, the airway is gradually obstructed. As a result, the patient becomes stridulous and in advanced cases an emergency tracheotomy may have to be performed.

NECK LUMPS

Palpable lymph nodes in the neck occur as the result of the spread of metastatic disease. They occur most commonly in cases of supraglottic carcinoma (Dhillon and East, 1994).

SENSORY SYMPTOMS

Sensory symptoms, such as discomfort, pain on swallowing and the need for throat clearing, cannot be distinguished from those associated with other voice disorders in many cases. Complaints of discomfort or changes of sensation in the throat must never be minimised or disregarded. These symptoms, particularly if they coexist with a dysphonia of 2–3 weeks in the absence of upper respiratory tract infection, require immediate and careful examination by a laryngologist.

Diagnosis

Laryngeal carcinoma is diagnosed after biopsy of the tumour at direct laryngoscopy and histological confirmation of the disease. Before treatment can be decided upon, further information is required about the volume of the tumour and the dimensions of both primary and nodal disease (BAO, 1998). This information is acquired through various imaging techniques. The British Association of Otorhinolaryngologists, Head and Neck Surgeons (BAO, 1998) recommends the following procedures:

- **Spiral computed tomography (CT) scan** as the best modality for assessing laryngeal cartilage invasion with mediastinal computed tomography when there is significant subglottic extension. Chest computed tomography is also recommended.
- **Magnetic resonance imaging (MRI)** for assessing pre-epiglottic space and tongue-base invasion. This procedure also indicates spread of the tumour into cartilage.
- **Videofluoroscopy** and **pulmonary function testing** may be used before supraglottic laryngectomy.

PATIENT REACTION TO DIAGNOSIS

Some patients with voice disorders are anxious that their symptoms are the result of laryngeal cancer, perhaps because they have known someone with the condition. Others have not considered the possibility of malignancy. In both instances, patients react with a range of emotions from the moment they are informed that a biopsy is necessary. Many maintain high levels of anxiety and distress throughout the process of anticipating hospital admission, during the inpatient period, and while waiting for and receiving the results of the biopsy. Confirmation of their fears is, therefore, the start of a second stage of concerns. Reactions range from disbelief (such as 'This can't be happening to me') through wanting to know what can be done or, in some instances, indications that the patient thinks that death is almost inevitable. The way in which explanations are given and the integrated working of the multidisciplinary team are fundamental in helping patients, and their partners and families, to come to terms with the situation. Apart from attempting to reduce the patient's distress, constructive and sympathetic support from the start facilitates good relationships as a basis for subsequent therapeutic intervention.

THE CLINICAL TEAM

It is mandatory in the UK that all patients with a diagnosis of cancer of the head and neck be seen in a combined oncology clinic at which the minimum staffing level should be a head and neck surgeon and a clinical oncologist. The British Association of Otorhinolaryngologists (1998) recommend that staffing should be as shown in Table 17.3. The head and neck surgeon is the leader of the team. The combined expertise helps to ensure that all aspects of the patient's condition are addressed and that various members of the team can be fully informed of issues that could affect their intervention. It should be remembered that, although there are many advantages in providing integrated care, the combined clinic can be an intimidating experience for the patient because of the number of personnel involved. For many patients, the seriousness of their condition is confirmed by the need for so many professionals.

Table 17.3 Recommended staffing for combined oncology clinic (head and neck)

Present in clinic	Available throughout clinic	Affiliated to clinic
Head and neck surgeon	Speech pathologist (dysphagia)	Pathologist
Clinical oncologist	Dental surgeon	Prosthodontist
Nurse counsellor	Physiotherapist	Cytologist
Dietitian		Radiologist
Speech pathologist (voice)		Gastrointestinal surgeon
		Social worker

Source: The British Association of Otorhinolaryngologists, Head & Neck Surgeons 'Effective Head and Neck Cancer Management' Consensus Document, 1998.

Treatment of laryngeal cancer

The paramount aim of all treatment of laryngeal carcinoma is to save life. Untreated, the tumour will gradually occlude the airway and result in a distressing death. Preservation of a method of phonation is also considered when making decisions concerning management of the tumour. The range of possible treatments for laryngeal carcinoma is listed in Table 17.4. Radiotherapy and partial laryngectomy are more likely to preserve vocal fold phonation, but if total laryngectomy is necessary the preservation or construction of suitable structures for production of pseudo-voice are essential whenever possible. Surgical voice restoration is increasingly carried out as a primary procedure at the time of total laryngectomy.

Table 17.4 Possible treatments for laryngeal carcinoma

• Laser or microsurgical excision	• Used for treatment of T1S (carcinoma in situ)[a]
• cordectomy	
• radiotherapy	• Treatment of choice in UK
• partial laryngectomy	• Possible surgical approach in some cases so that voice can be preserved
• total laryngectomy	• Usually confined to: – treatment of advanced cases – disease that has not been eradicated by radiotherapy – recurrent disease
• chemotherapy	

[a]See Table 17.2.

RADIOTHERAPY

In the UK, the treatment of choice is radiotherapy in order to destroy or arrest active tumour growth. The permanent cure rate is 80–90% and only a small percentage of patients, under 10%, have a recurrence that requires laryngectomy. There is a 95% cure rate for T1 glottic tumours. Ballantyne and Groves (1982) noted that there was a slightly higher rate of cure in early cordal growths treated by radiotherapy than by surgery and that there are minimal adverse effects on the voice (see below).

In the past there have been differences in approach between British and American surgeons, the former usually being more conservative (Shaw, 1966; Cheesman, 1983). In the USA surgery has usually been the initial treatment of choice. Some American laryngologists, however, do favour the use of radiotherapy initially when treating certain types of laryngeal carcinoma (Fisher et al., 1986). In Britain, it is the convention to perform a total laryngectomy when radiation has failed, although in theory it may have been possible to carry out a partial laryngectomy. A cordectomy can be carried out if the recurrence involves the same vocal fold to a similar and minimal extent. A simple laryngectomy may be considered safer in the long term especially if there is some extension of laryngeal malignancy.

On referral for radiotherapy, the patient is under the joint care of the radiotherapist and otolaryngologist. Attendance for treatment will vary according to the treatment regimen, but will usually be daily for several weeks, depending on the size of the irradiation doses being administered. This is a stressful time for the patient who is anxious about the diagnosis of cancer and the possible outcome of treatment. Tissue reaction is usually mild with some reddening of the skin externally. Reaction to radio-therapy within the larynx includes vocal fold stiffness, oedema and mucosal dryness, during and after the course of treatment. These changes result in discomfort and dysphonia (see below) so that patients often talk as little as possible during the course of treatment. The dry, sore throat usually improves in the early weeks after the end of treatment. Rarely, radiotherapy produces acute oedema and emergency laryngectomy is necessary.

Radiotherapy may be used postoperatively if it is found that a tumour has not been completely removed during surgery when this been the first choice of treatment. The patient is not regarded as having been cured of laryngeal carcinoma until 3 years after completion of radiotherapy without recurrence. Some authorities take a 5-year period. During this time, the patient is regularly and frequently reviewed by the otolaryngolo-gist and radiotherapist to ensure that there is no evidence of recurrence. After this period reviews continue less frequently.

Radiotherapy: effects on voice

Oedema and mucosal dryness resulting from radiotherapy inevitably affect the voice. Speaking fundamental frequency is reduced because of the increase in vocal fold mass. The quality of the vocal note may become rough as the vibratory characteristics of the vocal fold mucosa are affected by oedema and dryness. Patients also notice that vocal fatigue occurs after prolonged talking. As changes in the laryngeal mucosa persist after radiotherapy has been con-cluded, vocal changes do not resolve immediately, but most have been over-come within about 2 months of the end of successful treatment. Quiet voice presents few problems, although extremes of pitch and loudness may be dif-ficult to achieve (Carlson, 1995b). Where a degree of dysphonia persists, it may be the result of permanent changes in the vocal fold caused by the radio-therapy or by vocal abuse because the patient has attempted to overcome vocal limitations by using excessive effort. Changes in the vocal fold mucosa not seen on indirect laryngoscopy may be established by stroboscopic exami-nation. In some instances, persisting dysphonia will be organically and psy-chogenically based. In her study of voice quality in irradiated laryngeal cancer patients, Carlson (1995b) found that patients did not consider that their voices had been a significant problem and in general their evaluation of their own voice quality was more positive than that of the clinician.

CHEMOTHERAPY

In some advanced cases of laryngeal carcinoma, when cancer also involves the lymphatic system, cytotoxic drugs are administered intravenously.

There are unpleasant side effects such as severe nausea, vomiting and hair loss.

SURGERY

In the UK, laryngeal surgery is usually a salvage operation after unsuccessful radiotherapy or when a tumour has recurred some time after completion of a course of radiotherapy. Occasionally it is carried out as an urgent procedure in cases of advanced disease. Total laryngectomy is carried out more frequently than partial laryngectomy. However, for various reasons, in America surgery has been the preferred treatment for certain types of laryngeal carcinoma, although radiotherapy is the treatment of choice for early glottic cancer (Doyle, 1994).

Partial laryngectomy

Partial laryngectomy is far less traumatic than total laryngectomy because the respiratory, phonatory and sphincteric functions of the larynx can be retained (Leonard, Holt and Maran, 1972). It is a relatively uncommon procedure in the UK, however, because most of the carcinomas suitable for this procedure respond well to primary radiotherapy. Recurrence of cancer, of which there is a higher risk than with other procedures, can be treated by radiotherapy or total laryngectomy without any increased hazard to the patient. Postoperative chest infections occur more frequently than after total laryngectomy because of the risk of aspiration (Ballantyne and Groves, 1982).

Pressman and Bailey (1968) related the surgery for partial laryngectomy to knowledge of embryonic development and laryngeal anatomy as a basis for understanding the spread of cancer via the lymphatic system. The embryological development of the larynx in two halves and the significance of superficial and deep lymph routes are of prime importance in these surgical techniques. Whereas a superficial tumour in the mucosa of the larynx may freely travel across the anterior commissure and invade the other half of the larynx, the deeper structures and lymph routes do not readily communicate with each other. The interior of the larynx being divided, as it were, into a number of compartments anatomically segregated from each other, allows a wide variety of surgical procedures. These may be vertical, horizontal and frontolateral procedures, besides supraglottic horizontal procedures combined with radical neck dissection for removal of involved nodes (Shaw, 1966). All methods involve the airway and the voice to a greater or lesser extent. With supraglottic procedures the vocal folds are not involved and the patient's voice may remain unimpaired despite possible difficulties in swallowing.

Lateral partial laryngectomy (laryngofissure with cordectomy)

Cordectomy is performed only in cases of a very small, early, localised tumour in the anterior part of the vocal fold and on the extreme edge. The interior of the larynx is reached by laryngofissure (also called thyrotomy and thyrochondrotomy) which entails making a vertical medial incision through the anterior angle of the thyroid cartilage. The vocal fold alone is excised in one piece with a surrounding margin of 1 cm of healthy tissue.

Hemilaryngectomy (verticofrontolateral laryngectomy)

In most cases, however, it is considered safer to remove the vocal fold, the ventricular band and the thyroid ala of the affected side. The larynx is left lined with the external perichondrium which heals more readily than if stripped cartilage is left exposed, and the wound heals with the formation of a fibrous band of cicatricial tissue. Thus, in the place of the thyroarytenoid muscle a substitute vocal fold conveniently forms. In time, the healthy fold may pass across the midline to meet the adventitious fold and a serviceable voice can be acquired. Teflon injection may be used to improve closure (Dedo, Urrea and Lawson, 1973; Biller and Lawson, 1986).

Sessions, Maness and McSwain (1965) reviewed the literature and 40 cases of laryngofissure performed between 1938 and 1963, on 34 males and 6 females. They drew attention to the fact that the resultant voice is dependent on the position of the substitute cicatricial cord. The voice is strong if the healthy fold does not have to pass over the midline. The voice depends on the degree of approximation achieved between cicatricial and true cords. Eighteen patients in this series had good voices and 18 only fair voices (four were not followed up). Kennedy and Krause (1974) reported excellent results in conservative hemilaryngectomy and a 95% 5-year survival rate.

A later study by Mohr, Quenelle and Shumrick (1983) also reported good results when patients are carefully selected. They stressed the importance of considerable expertise in relation to preoperative and postoperative patient management, endoscopy and surgical skills.

Standard hemilaryngectomy is not appropriate if the subglottic extension of the tumour is 5 mm or more. In such cases extended hemilaryngectomy with cricoid resection can be performed but has a greater complication rate (Biller and Lawson, 1986).

Hemilaryngectomy and skin-graft

Figi (1953) described hemilaryngectomy and skin graft in reconstruction of one vocal fold. Conley (1961, 1962) devised a single-stage operation after partial laryngectomy and removal of both vocal folds, whereby regional flaps are transposed to form imitation vocal folds. Brodnitz and Conley (1967) described the vocal rehabilitation necessary after this procedure. The voice is deep but strong and gentle pushing exercises with great circumspection are advised.

After the work of Conley (1961) in performing hemilaryngectomy and reconstruction of a substitute vocal cord from a unilateral pedicled skin flap from the neck, Maran, Haast and Leonard (1968) described a vertical hemilaryngectomy operation with vocal fold reconstruction. The sternohyoid and thyrohyoid muscles are cut close to their insertions and a bipedicled muscle transposition is carried out to replace the excised cord. The voice is strong immediately after operation, then deteriorates but improves with healing of the wound. Leonard, Holt and Maran (1972) reported long-term results of this operation on 75 patients operated on during the period 1963–1970. They emphasised the need for careful selection of patients; the cancer must be localised and the vocal fold mobile.

Supraglottic laryngectomy

This procedure may be used for treatment of some cases in which carcinoma involves one arytenoid, the medial wall of the pyriform fossa, the aryepiglottic fold or the epiglottis. It allows voice to be unaffected (Burstein and Calcaterra, 1985), but aspiration of fluids may be a complication.

Total laryngectomy

Total laryngectomy is necessary when carcinoma is not cured by radiotherapy or partial laryngectomy. If the tumour is causing dyspnoea, a tracheotomy may be performed before the main operation but generally this is done at the time of the operation, before removal of the larynx. The new airway ensures freedom from breathing complications as far as possible and gives the surgeon freedom of action in the laryngeal field above.

A U-shaped flap is raised to expose the larynx which is removed in its entirety and the resulting defect in the pharyngeal wall is carefully closed. The hyoid bone is usually excised with the larynx (Cheesman, 1983); this is particularly important when the anterior commissure is involved in the carcinoma and there is danger of the pre-epiglottic space being invaded (Ballantyne and Groves, 1982). However, preservation of the hyoid bone has been advocated, and Vrticka and Svoboda (1961) reported that an intact hyoid bone was found much more frequently in their good speakers. They pointed out that preservation of the hyoid often signifies preservation of the strap muscles; their importance in facilitating aspiration of air into the oesophagus for production of pseudo-voice was

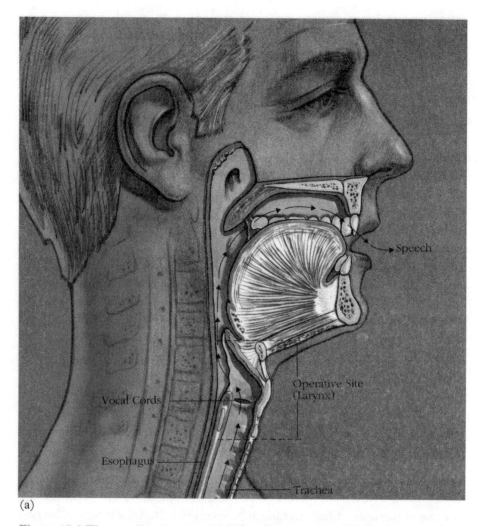

(a)

Figure 17.2 The aerodigestive tract (a) before laryngectomy (b) after laryngectomy. (Reproduced by permission of International Healthcare Technologies, 1110 Mark Avenue, Carpinteria, CA 93013-2918, USA. Blom–Singer is a registered trademark of Hansa Medical Products, Inc.)

emphasised as early as 1922 by Seeman. Of course, removal of all malignant cells must have priority.

The trachea and oesophagus are now entirely separate, with respiration and expectoration taking place via the permanent tracheal stoma (Figure 17.2). The patient wears a tracheostomy tube in the early stages of recovery until there is no danger of the stoma stenosing. In normal recovery, the feeding tube, which is inserted during surgery, remains in situ for approximately 10–14 days.

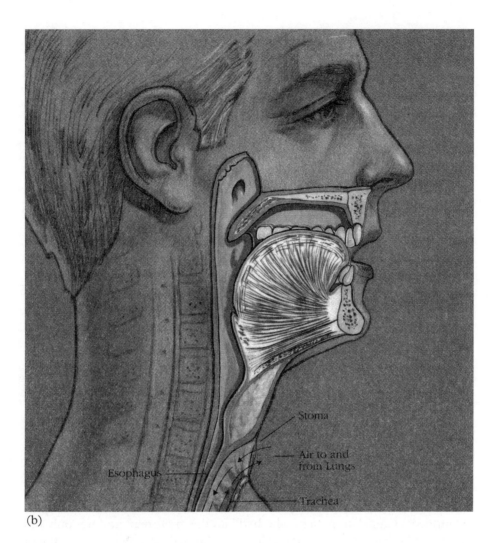

(b)

Note

In rare cases, laryngectomy is performed on victims of road traffic accidents, when the larynx and trachea are so severely damaged that this surgical procedure is the only method of ensuring a competent airway. Children may also occasionally undergo laryngectomy as the result of laryngeal trauma from ingesting corrosive substances (Jacobs and Abramson, 1980), from penetrating wounds (Gardner, Hill and Carano, 1962) or because of congenital tracheo-oesophageal malformation.

Radical neck dissection (block dissection)

Metastases of malignant cells in the lymph glands of the neck necessitate radical surgery if the patient has previously had radiotherapy. The throat will be flatter and tighter than after simple laryngectomy because additional tissue has been removed. An uncomfortable consequence of the unavoidable removal of the spinal accessory nerve in this procedure results in a 'dropped' shoulder. In addition to experiencing discomfort, the patient's arm movements on the affected side become restricted, so that the hand and arm cannot easily be raised above shoulder level. As a result, many tasks, such as combing the hair and driving, are affected. Carrying any weight on the affected side, e.g. shopping, is possible only for short periods. A course of physiotherapy may be helpful.

Pharyngolaryngectomy

Radiotherapy has a low success rate in cases of carcinoma in the hypopharynx and the post-cricoid and cervical oesophagus. Consequently, surgical removal of the larynx, pharynx and variable amounts of the oesophagus is necessary. In addition, most cases will need a unilateral or bilateral block dissection. Repair presents many problems and sacrifice of the cricopharyngeal sphincter means that acquisition of pseudo-voice will be difficult.

In repair of the cervical oesophagus, a single-stage operation and Thiersch graft round a Portex tube may be used in reconstruction and was first described by Negus. This procedure is fraught with difficulties (Harrison, 1964). Stenosis of the pharynx and oesophagus resulting in dysphagia may occur, the patient having to be admitted to hospital for bougienage and stretching of the reconstructed tube under general anaesthetic. Plastic surgery for reconstruction of the pharynx and oesophagus is possible from thoracic flaps, but this multi-stage operation necessitates long hospitalisation. Recurrence is anticipated within 2–3 years. Greene examined a Canadian patient who had had this treatment and not only did her throat appear normal externally, but she had an excellent and fluent voice.

Stuart (1966), because of the difficulties of reconstruction and hazards of operation and of the short life expectancy, advocated insertion of a plastic tube prosthesis. These patients obtain characteristically hollow and sometimes quite strong voices with great ease and without speech instruction.

Stomach and colon transplants

Lewis (1965) drew attention to the formidable procedures in bringing up stomach or colon through the thorax to the neck. A major abdominal operation is added to extensive neck surgery. He advocated reconstruction of the pharynx by local cervical skin flaps or tubed pedicle flaps that have migrated from the chest wall. Pectoralis major myocutaneous flaps

(Murakami et al., 1982) and quilted, skin-grafted, pectoralis major flaps (Robertson and Robinson, 1984) continue to be used and researched in relation to reconstructing the cervical oesophagus after laryngopharyngectomy. Studies have also been carried out using a posteriorly based tongue flap for reconstructing the hypopharynx after total laryngectomy with subtotal pharyngectomy (Calcaterra, 1983). Rehabilitation was rapid and articulation unaffected.

A good pseudo-voice can develop after repair by skin flaps. This operation is not, however, suitable after irradiation therapy, so the numbers who can benefit are few in the UK. All these procedures of reconstruction, whether partial or total, are vulnerable to fistula, stricture and the death of the patient (Fee, 1984). The survival rate in total reconstruction is poor. The priority of surgery in these cases is to use the most straightforward procedure in order to achieve acceptable swallowing without subjecting the patient to endless surgery in the last months of life (Fee, 1984).

Pharyngo-laryngo-oesophagectomy

Extensive involvement of the oesophagus in addition to the larynx and pharynx presents even greater difficulties than those already described in connection with laryngectomy. Stomach pull-up and colon transplant are used in reconstruction of the oesophagus. Ranger (1964, 1983) and Le Quesne (1964) carried out immediate repair after pharyngolaryngectomy and oesophagectomy by creating a pharyngogastric anastomosis. Stomach and duodenum are mobilised and transplanted into the neck to form a continuous tract between pharynx and stomach. There is no difficulty in swallowing postoperatively and this surgical procedure is suitable in irradiated cases. Pseudo-voice can be as satisfactory as oesophageal speech.

The operation is hazardous and even if the patient survives the prognosis is not good. The balance of prolonging life and the quality of that life has to be considered by the surgeon. Harrison (1964) remarked that the surgeon has both 'moral and technical responsibilities' and quoted Gardham:

How often by prolonging life do we really add to its sum of happiness and how often do we prolong the quantity of life at the expense of its quality?

Although these decisions are not made by the speech pathologist, an awareness of them helps to maintain perspective and to plan the rehabilitation programme. As Ranger (1983) realistically pointed out, even those patients who die of the disease before the 3-year stage of survival can be helped by alleviating their swallowing problems and prevented from death as a result of dysphagia.

The voice will be weak but some patients do develop good voice. Voice results are similar with stomach and colon transplants. Lall and Evison (1966) reported on the performance of four patients: one developed excellent speech and another a reasonable voice. Radiographs showed narrowing of the transplant. The patient who showed no narrowing of the reconstructed oesophagus had only a strong whisper as did the last patient who was unable to shift air in the tube transplant. We have treated patients who produced satisfactory functional voice.

The pharyngo-oesophageal segment (Figure 17.3)

The acquisition of an acceptable voice is a secondary aim of laryngectomy surgery. If survival is a realistic goal, the subsequent quality of life is a major consideration and satisfactory communication must be considered in making surgical decisions. The pharyngo-oesophageal (P-E) segment is the upper oesophageal sphincter at the level of cervical vertebrae 5–7 (C5–C7) and is composed of fibres of the inferior pharyngeal constrictor muscle, the cricopharyngeal muscle and the upper fibres of the oesophagus. At rest, the sphincter is in a tonic state and relaxes only on swallowing to allow entry of the bolus into the oesophagus. The P-E segment is innervated by the recurrent laryngeal nerve. Oesophageal and tracheo-oesophageal voice are dependent on the P-E segment, which is vibrated by air introduced into the oesophagus by the alaryngeal speaker and acts as a substitute vibrator or pseudo-glottis. Appropriate tonicity of the P-E segment is fundamental for it to function as an adequate pseudo-glottis. In normal individuals, the sphincter is tightly closed to prevent the entry of air into the stomach during the respiratory cycle and during speech (Batemen and Negus, 1954). The sectioning of the constrictor muscles during laryngectomy reduces the tonicity of the P-E segment and can thus impair its effectiveness for pseudo-voice (Singer, Blom and Hamaker, 1986). Repair of the sphincteric muscles may also affect acquisition of pseudo-voice if it results in a hypertonic segment. The appropriate tonicity of the P-E segment and its site, width and length are important factors affecting the acquisition of oesophageal voice.

Bentzen, Guld and Rasmussen (1976) made a distinction between high and low positioned pseudo-glottis in a videoradiographic study of 41 patients. The high situation was at the level of C4–C5 and the low situation at C6–C7. The high pseudo-glottis, especially with posterior muscular rigidity, produced the best voice. These findings can be related to Simpson's surgical techniques which aimed to provide an optimally functioning P-E segment (Simpson, Smith and Gordon, 1972). Although it may vary widely, there are certain irregularities of the P-E segment which operate against good functional control over the vicarious lung, glottis and

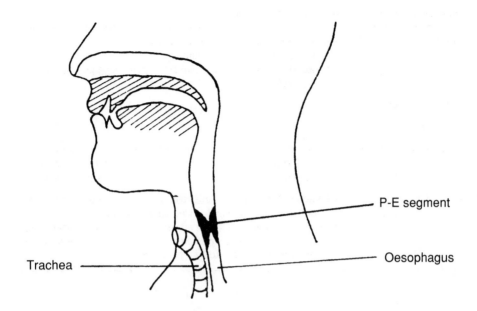

Figure 17.3 Pharyngo-oesophageal segment.

resonator (Singer and Blom, 1980; Perry and Edels, 1985). Inability to produce voice because of an inadequate P-E segment is discussed below.

Post-laryngectomy complications

Uncomplicated recovery from total laryngectomy allows removal of the feeding tube within 10–14 days of surgery and the early stages of acquiring voice can be initiated. A number of complications may prolong this stage of recovery, however. The incidence of problems increases when more radical and extensive surgery is necessary and if the patient has had radiotherapy preoperatively. The irradiated tissue is ischaemic and this results in slower and less satisfactory healing. Complications that can occur after laryngectomy are listed in Table 17.5.

LIFE EXPECTANCY AFTER TREATMENT FOR LARYNGEAL CANCER

UK survival rates for patients undergoing treatment for laryngeal cancer is 50–60% 5-year survival – a statistic that has not changed for at least 20 years (BAO, 1998). Berry (1983) stated that patients who have had no recurrence 3 years after surgery can be regarded as cured. In tumours that are confined to the larynx without vocal fold immobility, the cure rate is 90–100% by radiotherapy. When the cervical nodes are involved, the outlook is less sanguine.

Table 17.5 Complications that can occur after laryngectomy

Fistula	• If surgical repair fails to heal or breaks down • May heal spontaneously if small • Large fistulae may require plastic surgery using pedicle of non-irradiated skin
Postoperative bleeding	
Wound infection	
Thyroid and parathyroid deficiencies	• Removal of these glands disrupts the endocrine system • Thyroxine and calcium supplements must be taken by the patient as a result
Dysphagia	• Postoperative difficulties in swallowing caused by discomfort and constriction, usually resolves spontaneously • Later dysphagia can occur at any time if the site of the pharyngeal repair fibroses, causing narrowing. Dilatation of the area can be performed repeatedly if necessary

Pharyngolaryngectomy and radical neck dissection may have results as good as simple laryngectomy as far as longevity is concerned, if combined with radiotherapy. Ranger (1983) was of the opinion that 20–25% of patients who have undergone pharyngo-laryngo-oesophagectomy and immediate stomach pull-up or colon transplant will have prolonged survival, with normal swallowing and the possibility of pseudo-voice.

Some individuals in the laryngofissure and laryngectomy categories live to normal old age and eventually die from other causes. Guthrie (1966) reported the case of a man who underwent laryngectomy when aged 35 years and was still alive 42 years later. Usually, the outlook is more optimistic for elderly than for young people because carcinoma tends to be more ebullient in youth than in old age, when the rate of cell replacement is slowed down.

Surgical voice restoration (tracheo-oesophageal puncture)

In addition to improving techniques for prolonging life, surgeons have sought to develop surgical procedures that provide the patient with voice. By diverting expired lung air into the oesophagus, air is subsequently vibrated as it passes into the pharyngeal cavity and phonation is generated. Fistula voice is similar to oesophageal voice, but is much less arduous to acquire if surgery is successful. It is of higher pitch and greater fluency. The pitch is more acceptable to women laryngectomees than oesophageal voice (Snidecor, 1968; Edwards, 1976).

In 1980, Singer and Blom first reported on their prosthesis by which air is introduced into the oesophagus via the tracheostoma through a fistula in the posterior tracheal wall. Pulmonary air enters the prosthesis and is directed by the prosthesis into the oesophagus, where it vibrates the P-E segment for production of pseudo-voice. When first developed, the tracheo-oesophageal (T-E) puncture was performed some time after laryngectomy (secondary voice restoration). Primary restoration is also now undertaken at the time of the laryngectomy (Hamaker et al., 1985; Trudeau, Hirsch and Schuller, 1986). The procedure is easily reversible because the fistula closes spontaneously if the prosthesis is not inserted. Originally, it was necessary for the patient to use finger occlusion of the tracheostoma, but a suitable tracheostoma valve was developed to eliminate manual occlusion (Blom, Singer and Hamaker, 1982). Voice prostheses, incorporating variations of insertion procedures and design are available from a number of manufacturers. Constant improvements of prostheses and valves continue. (See below about acquisition of pseudo-voice after T-E puncture.)

PATIENT SELECTION FOR T-E PUNCTURE

Suitable candidates are carefully selected for both primary or secondary procedures. The criteria for selection are listed in Table 17.6. Although successful speech rehabilitation is reported to be as high as 80–90%, this procedure is not suitable for all laryngectomees.

A suitable P-E segment is of paramount importance in the criteria for patient selection. This is investigated by an air insufflation test (Taub test). A catheter is introduced into the oesophagus through the nose to just below the P-E segment, approximately to the level of the tracheostoma. The patient is at rest as air is insufflated. Air subsequently leaving the

Table 17.6 Selection criteria for T-E puncture candidates

Manual dexterity	To clean and insert prosthesis
Motivation	
Adequate vision	
Adequate pulmonary support	To provide sufficient air pressure through prosthesis and into oesophagus in order to vibrate P-E segment
Stoma of adequate depth and diameter	To accommodate prosthesis without obstructing airway
Suitable P-E segment	As demonstrated by air insufflation test (Taub test)
Mental stability	

Singer and Blom (1980); Singer, Blom and Hamaker (1983).

oesophagus vibrates the P-E segment, producing oesophageal voice. The patient speaks on the egressive airstream so that quality and duration of the pseudo-voice can be assessed (Singer and Blom, 1980). If there is no oesophageal sound or if it is unsatisfactory, this may be the result of a hyper-tonic or hypotonic P-E segment or P-E spasm. Reflexive spasm is confirmed by the effectiveness of a parapharyngeal injection of local anaesthetic, which allows the P-E segment to relax and oesophageal voice to be produced. It can be relieved surgically by pharyngeal constrictor myotomy (Singer, Blom and Hamaker, 1983) or pharyngeal plexus neurectomy. Various studies report improvements on the air insufflation test (Blom, Singer and Hamaker, 1985), which has relied on subjective evaluation of the sound produced. It is argued that objective assessment of oesophageal insufflation, which provides intraoesophageal pressure measurements, is essential for effectively identify-ing patients who would benefit from pharyngeal myotomy at the time of T-E puncture (Baugh, Lewin and Baker, 1987).

Complications associated with T-E puncture

Although widely adopted because it can provide excellent pseudo-voice rapidly after surgery, this procedure can give rise to major postoperative complications at early and late stages (Silver, Gluckman and Donegan, 1985; Andrews et al., 1987) (Table 17.7).

Table 17.7 Complications associated with T-E puncture

Early complications

- oesophageal perforation during creation of T-E fistula
- severe allergic reaction to the prosthesis
- severe cellulitis in the peristomal area
- leakage of saliva and food through the puncture resulting in aspiration

Later complications

- enlargement of the T-E fistula
- pneumonia as a result of recurring aspiration
- aspiration of the prosthesis
- fistula migration
- tracheal stoma stenosis
- oesophageal stenosis
- fungal colonisation of prosthesis

Avoidable problems occur if the prosthesis is not kept scrupulously clean. The oesophageal end is vul-nerable to food deposits. Colonisation by fungi must be constantly removed if health and voice quality and efficiency are to be maintained (Izdebski, Ross and Lee, 1987).

The incidence of problems has been found to be similar whether or not the patient has had radiotherapy, but when complications occur in the irradiated patient they are more severe. The surgeons reporting these problems consider that, when benefits are weighed against the risks, it is worth while continuing with the procedure (Silver, Gluckman and Donegan, 1985). Some patients prefer to remain voiceless after complications rather than risk encountering further difficulties.

Historical note

External fistula speech (prosthesis and air shunt; reed–fistula speech)

The first artificial larynges consisted of a membrane or reed vibrator activated by lung air from a tube fitted into the tracheal stoma. The 'voice' thus created was piped into the mouth and shaped by articulation into intelligible speech (Hunt, 1964; Holinger, 1975). The reed type of vibrator was still in use in the Netherlands, Spain and Japan in the 1980s. A further development in fistula speech was the adaptation of the reed vibrator for use together with a constructed skin tube in the neck. This piped vibrated air into the pharynx produced more natural speech and a less conspicuous speech aid.

Taub's voice

Taub (1975) devised this valved prosthesis, which fits into a fistula opening into the trachea above the tracheostoma. It is activated by air shunted upwards from the usual tracheal opening. The superior fistula can be created at any time after laryngectomy. The voice created was claimed to be good and the patient could laugh, shout, whisper and even sing. Healing difficulties made this an unsuitable procedure for patients who had had radiotherapy, and the equipment was expensive and awkward, and required regular maintenance.

Weinberg, Shedd and Horii – reed–fistula speech

Weinberg, Shedd and Horii (1978) used a modified form of the Tokyo external pneumatic artificial larynx and a surgically created pharyngeal fistula. These researchers reported promising progress with four patients but noted that the procedure does not merit consideration as a routine method in pharyngolaryngectomy. They also mentioned the need for a speech pathologist to help the patient with management of the prosthesis and fistula speech after the operation.

Internal fistula speech

This category includes procedures where a fistula is constructed so that pulmonary air is directed into the vocal tract at some point. Various techniques were used, but the success achieved by the originator of these techniques was frequently not duplicated by others.

The Asai technique

In 1972, Asai of the University of Kobe, Japan first reported his now famous three-stage operation, which constructed a dermal tube from the tracheostoma to a pharyngeal fistula at about the level of the hyoid bone. The first stage was performed at the time of the laryngectomy and the next two followed at intervals of a month later. Digital closure of the stoma while speaking enabled a moving column of air from the lungs to be directed through the tube into the pharynx. Miller (1967, 1968) performed operations of this type in the USA and found that only 20% of patients achieved good voice and that there was a high proportion of patients in whom saliva entered the trachea. Asai (1972) reported good speech results of surgery in 72 patients. This operation was not adopted universally because good surgical and speech results were difficult to achieve. Some patients had to exert digital pressure on the neck at the level of the internal pharyngeal exit; others had difficulty in swallowing. Healing presented difficulties and strictures commonly developed in the dermal tube. It was not a viable procedure after radiotherapy.

Serafini operation

Arslan and Serafini (1972) reported success with an operation that involved raising the trachea and suturing it to the hyoid, so that it was continuous with the hypopharynx. This maintained respiration through the mouth and nose in addition to phonation. The editor of *Laryngoscope*, in which this report was published, commented on the problems arising from this operation. Pulling up the trachea created swallowing difficulties; two-thirds of the patients had breathing difficulties and required tracheostomy tubes in situ.

Staffieri technique

Staffieri's operation designed in the early 1970s to construct a neoglottis did produce some good voice results and was adopted by many surgeons, but aspiration and stenosis were ongoing problems (Singer, Blom and Hamaker, 1983).

Tanabe, Honjo and Isshiki neoglottic construction

A new technique for neoglottic construction was evolved by Tanabe, Honjo and Isshiki (1985) using the upper tracheal rings in an attempt to overcome the complications of postoperative stenosis and aspiration. After tracheotomy and laryngectomy, the upper three tracheal rings are used to create a neoglottis, with the first ring being sutured to the oesophageal wall. Seven of the eight patients in the study were reported to use voice that was superior to oesophageal voice when judged on the basis of duration and intelligibility. The neoglottis in the eighth patient was closed as a result of aspiration.

Tracheo-oesophageal flap

In a technique performed on 19 patients in China (Li, 1985), a tongue-like T-E flap is transposed into the oesophageal lumen in a downwards direction through the T-E fistula. Li reported that voice is produced effortlessly when the stoma is occluded with the finger and that speech therapy is not required. During swallowing, food and liquids are prevented from entering the trachea by the flap covering the fistula.

Note

Edwards (1983) and Singer, Blom and Hamaker (1983) have given succinct accounts of the history of surgical speech rehabilitation.

Physiological effects of laryngectomy

In addition to complete loss of voice after laryngectomy, there are various physiological sequelae resulting from the changes in the configuration of the aerodigestive tract, to which the patient has to adjust.

RESPIRATORY COMPLICATIONS

Immediately after surgery, the radical change in the anatomy of the breathing mechanism no longer allows air to be warmed and filtered before entering the lungs. A humidifier is used in the early days postoperatively in order to avoid crusting around the tracheostoma and the accumulation of tenacious mucus.

The most common and troublesome postoperative complication is bronchitis induced by the aspiration of secretions into the bronchi during surgery. The patient is distressed by the difficulty in breathing and becomes exhausted by the effort to expectorate mucus. A cannula is inserted into the tracheal opening at first; this cannula consists of two tubes fitting one within the other. The outer tube is left in position until the wound is healed, but the inner tube can be removed, cleaned and sterilised frequently by a nurse. Suction apparatus is also used to extract mucus via the tracheostoma. This provides temporary relief for the patient and prevents the formation of bronchial plugs of mucus which can cause asphyxia. In most patients, these problems resolve in the early days and weeks of recovery and suction apparatus will not be necessary for long. If patients have had chronic respiratory problems preoperatively, however, or if they are asthmatic their management will present a greater problem.

Persistent post-laryngectomy bronchial mucus may delay the patient's recovery and discharge from hospital for several weeks. Breathing exercises may be prescribed by the surgeon, as well as postural drainage of the lungs, which is undertaken by the physiotherapist. If this is the case and the speech–language pathologist wishes to give instruction in breathing for speech, liaison with the physiotherapist is essential to avoid possible conflict of exercises and instructions. If the breathing technique taught by the physiotherapist is different from that of the speech–language pathologist, and it may be, then it must be explained to the patient that one set of instructions is for chest health and the other relates to the acquisition of pseudo-voice.

Management

It is important that bronchial infection should be eliminated as soon as possible because, quite apart from the considerations of health, it interferes with the acquisition of pseudo-voice. Unfortunately, congestion cannot be cured in heavy smokers who develop emphysema and the mucus may be too viscid to remove from the upper trachea by coughing. Some patients always carry a pair of tweezers or forceps in order to extract particularly 'stringy' mucus near the tracheostoma; a small mirror completes the equipment required and they are able to ensure a patent airway. Patients should be advised to take care if using a paper tissue to clear mucus around the rim of the stoma or just inside, because this can result in irritation which triggers the cough reflex. Rapid inspiration of air can suck the tissue into the trachea and result in asphyxiation.

Tracheostoma protection

Even when the laryngectomee has recovered from the immediate effects of surgery and has been discharged home, inspired air should be warmed and moistened so that tracheal and lung secretions are easily removed. The trachea should not be exposed to sudden temperature changes. Stoma protectors of various types are available.

Laryngectomy bibs (Buchanan laryngectomy protector, Mediquip laryngectomy bib)

These are made of a lightweight material which absorbs mucus and so protects clothing while also warming inspired air. The bib is either tied round the neck or has Velcro tabs; it is washable.

Foam squares (Laryngofoam)

These disposable foam filters are held in place over the stoma by a hypoallergenic adhesive strip. They are not suitable for patients with a very forceful or productive cough unless worn with a laryngectomy bib. Patients who need the square only for warming, filtering and moisturising air, wear them under normal clothing.

Romet filters

This protector is worn inside the open neck of a blouse or shirt and looks like the neck of a lightweight sweater. It is bib-shaped with a ribbed neck band with Velcro fasteners and comes in several colours. It can be worn without additional stoma protection, although many patients prefer to wear either a foam square or bib immediately over the stoma. These filters are washable.

Humidification filter systems

Some patients with a T-E prosthesis wear a baseplate around the stoma which is attached to the skin with adhesive. Into this can be fitted a valve (so that finger occlusion of the stoma is not required) or a humidification system.

Note

Patients are advised to stop smoking but some continue to do so. It is possible to use the buccinator muscles for suction and aspiration of air through the nose as with smelling.

LOSS OF NASAL BREATHING

Laryngectomees cannot blow their noses and are therefore unable to clear the nose of mucus. Although this is no longer the airway, patients report that a blocked nose is particularly unpleasant during a head cold.

LOSS OF OLFACTION

Loss of smell is often noticed, as a result of the inability to inhale through the nose and stimulate the olfactory nerve endings. The sense of taste is also impaired because we scent flavours and taste salt, sweet, sour and bitter. The laryngectomee will complain that food no longer tastes so good and that appetite is lost. Inhalation of air into the oesophagus as for oesophageal voice production by change in thoracic pressure, when mastered, can be used to inhale air in through the nose. Explanation of cause and effect and practice in sniffing will help in restoration of olfaction. Movements of the back of the tongue making contact with the soft palate can agitate nasal air.

INEFFICIENT EXPECTORATION

Without closure of the vocal folds, the patient is unable to increase subglottic air pressure in the normal way in order to clear obstructions from the airway. Although the glottis is usually considered a necessary part of the mechanism of coughing, the laryngectomee is able to increase the efficiency of the cough by using the abdominal muscles and diaphragm for raising intrathoracic pressure.

The most difficult and unacceptable aspect for the patient to tolerate, if a normally sensitive individual, is the tracheal opening and airway. In some patients, this takes precedence in importance over loss of voice. It is particularly difficult to cope with coughed up mucus discreetly and excessive coughing may be an affliction for many weeks after leaving hospital. Although blowing the nose and wiping the mouth with a handkerchief are socially permissible, wiping mucus from the stoma and placing the hand under the blouse, shirt or 'bib' draw attention to the action. Embarrassment may at first prevent a patient from leaving the house and this may contribute substantially to depression. The speech–language pathologist can give patients guidance on the type of clothes that make the task of clearing mucus easier.

Violent coughing can render a patient incontinent. One patient with a persistent irritating cough could not go back to work for 18 months for this reason despite acquiring excellent speech early. In these cases, physiotherapists may be able to help with exercises for incontinence.

SWALLOWING ADJUSTMENTS

Most patients are aware of changes in the efficiency of their swallow mechanism even when there are no marked problems. Food and liquid usually need to be taken rather more slowly than preoperatively if accumulation of solids in the pharynx and nasal regurgitation of fluids are to be avoided. The patient can be encouraged to perceive the pharynx as a funnel that empties rather more slowly than preoperatively. The practice of taking slightly smaller mouthfuls of food, chewing it carefully and not taking another mouthful until the previous bolus is swallowed soon becomes established. The inability to speak and eat at the same time presents obvious social difficulties. Many patients will eat only with members of the family and avoid eating in restaurants.

DYSPHAGIA

Dysphagia will occur in some patients as a result of the surgery required. Although there is no danger of food being aspirated (except after certain surgical speech restoration procedures), the pharyngeal phase of swallowing may present problems for a number of reasons.

• Scar tissue

In some patients a band of scar tissue at the base of the tongue occurs as a result of the surgical closure of the defect in the pharyngeal wall. During swallowing, this scar tissue band is pulled posteriorly so that a pouch develops at the base of the tongue in which food collects, simultaneously occluding the pharynx so that the bolus cannot enter the oesophagus (Logemann, 1983a).

• Stenosing of the hypopharynx and oesophagus

This may result from a necessarily tight closure when pharyngolaryngectomy has been carried out. Swallowing will be slow and restricted because of the narrow lumen and loss of pharyngeal peristalsis. The narrowing may be corrected by dilatation or further surgery. Careful consideration and experimentation will be necessary to determine which foods can be eaten most easily. Apparently obvious substances such as mashed potato and minced meat are often far from ideal because of the way in which they accumulate and clog the pharynx. The dietitian will give advice to ensure that nutrition is balanced when a diet of suitable texture has been decided on.

• Regurgitation

This may occur if the patient has eaten a particularly large meal or bends over too soon after eating when the cricopharyngeal muscle has been removed in extensive surgery together with the cardiac sphincter. Ranger (1983) also noted that, in some of these patients, food drains into the duodenum from the stomach too rapidly. This gives the patient a feeling of fullness, faintness, tachycardia and nausea, accompanied by sweating for an hour or two after a heavy meal. This condition is known as 'dumping'.

It is interesting to consider the study conducted by Mendelsohn and McConnel (1987) which demonstrated the importance of laryngeal elevation as a major factor in controlling sphincter function in the P-E segment, in addition to the cricopharyngeal muscle. As described elsewhere, the cricopharyngeal muscle acts as a sphincter which relaxes to allow the bolus to pass into the oesophagus. Using manofluoroscopy, a technique combining manometry and videofluoroscopy, it can be seen that rapid elevation of the larynx produces the drop in pressure and transient negative pressure observed in the P-E segment as the bolus passes through. Mendelsohn and McConnel also established that, if laryngeal elevation is impaired, the pressure drop during deglutition is slower and the fleeting negative pressure does not occur. It can, therefore, be concluded that, if the larynx is so crucial to the function of the P-E segment during deglutition, all laryngectomees will almost certainly have less efficient patterns of swallowing than preoperatively, even if more obvious problems are not apparent. If dysphagia develops after satisfactory swallowing has been established, it is possibly the result of recurrence of the disease and must be fully investigated.

DEFAECATION

The loss of the glottis, which closes during exertion, may make effortful defaecation a problem. It is important, therefore, that the laryngectomee maintains a diet that reduces the possibility of constipation.

WATER PENETRATION INTO THE AIRWAY

Care has to be taken not to inhale water into the tracheostoma when taking a bath or shower or washing the hair. A plastic stoma apron should be worn tied round the neck for protection. Swimming is not normally possible unless special apparatus is worn and instruction given by an experienced instructor.

LIFTING

The maintenance of thoracic pressure to provide prolonged fixation of the thorax, and to meet the demands of manual work, is difficult to achieve. Despite this, many patients are able to continue employment involving lifting and other physical exertion. Their previously well-developed muscles in the back, shoulders, arms and elsewhere appear to compensate for the loss of the glottis in this respect. If the patient has a dropped shoulder, of course, lifting weights will not be possible and even turning the steering wheel of a heavy goods vehicle will be difficult.

RESUSCITATION REQUIREMENTS

It is essential that everyone working in the emergency services or involved in first aid is aware that laryngectomees are neck breathers. This means that resuscitation is mouth to tracheostoma (Figures 17.4 and 17.5).

Psychological effects of laryngeal cancer and its treatment

It can be argued that the psychological effects of laryngeal cancer are felt by many patients even before diagnosis. There may have been a significant period of anxiety before a patient presents to the doctor, during which vocal changes or throat discomfort has signalled that all is not well. In the UK, patients have to visit their family doctors before being referred to the otorhinolaryngologist so that the waiting period until diagnosis can be protracted over several weeks. Laryngological examination and hospital admission, however brief, for biopsy of the lesion inevitably maintain the level of anxiety. The positive diagnosis elicits a range of reactions which have been discussed above (see page 579). It is in this context, therefore, that the patient has to deal with the effects of treatment. Of all patients who undergo treatment for laryngeal carcinoma, the greatest psychosocial effects are experienced by those who undergo laryngectomy. However excellent the surgical result and speech therapy, progress will not be made if the patient's emotional reaction to the situation is not taken into consideration. The operation of laryngectomy is one of the most traumatic and mutilating procedures. Emotional trauma is unavoidable, but can be alleviated by good management.

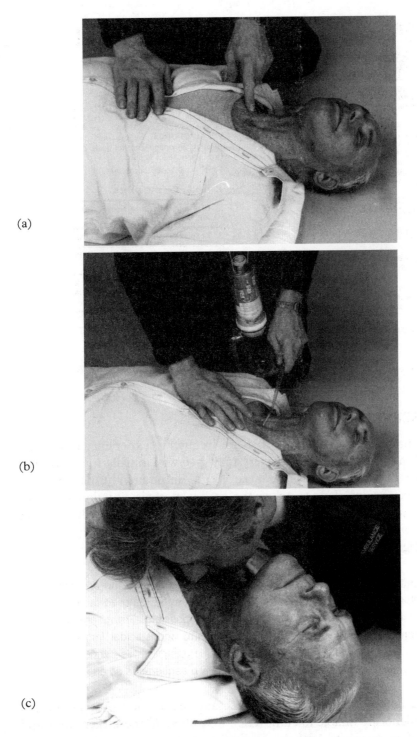

Figure 17.4 Mouth-to-neck resuscitation: (a) tracheostoma, (b) suction is used to remove secretions and (c) mouth-to-stoma resuscitation.

EMERGENCY!

I am a
Partial Neck Breather
(LARYNGECTOMEE)

I breathe MAINLY through an opening in my neck, very little through my nose or mouth.

If I have stopped breathing:
1. Expose my entire neck. Pinch my nose between the middle two fingers of your hand, and cover my lips with the palm of same hand. Press thumb on upper neck under chin.

2. Give me **mouth to neck breathing only.**

3. Keep my head straight-chin up.

4. Keep neck opening clear with clean CLOTH (not tissue)

5. Use oxygen supply to neck opening, ONLY, when I start to breathe again.

BE PROMPT-SECONDS COUNT
I NEED AIR NOW!

EMERGENCY!

One or more occupants of this car is a Total Neck Breather. He (or she) is a Laryngectomee and has **NO VOCAL CHORDS!** He breathes only through an opening in his neck. Not through nose or mouth.

If he has stopped breathing:

1. **Expose the Entire Neck.**

2. **Give Him Mouth to Neck Breathing Only.**

3. **Keep His Head Straight - Chin Up.**

4. **Keep Neck Opening Clear With Clean Cloth (Not Tissue).**

5. **Use Oxygen Supply To Neck Opening, Only, When He Starts to Breathe Again.**

BE PROMPT — SECONDS COUNT
HE NEEDS AIR NOW!

Figure 17.5 Laryngectomy emergency cards.

DEPRESSION

The intense negative emotions that are frequently experienced after the diagnosis and anticipation of surgery may give way initially to a period of relief that the operation has been survived. Subsequently, patients frequently experience depression as the reality of their situation becomes apparent and adjustments to daily life have to be made in the early days and weeks after leaving hospital. Heaver and Arnold (1962), as psychiatrist and laryngologist working together, summarised this emotional route:

> A pathologic reactive depression is the usual sequel to the doctor's dictum that the larynx is cancerous, that it must be removed at once, and that natural speech no longer will be possible. Fright, anxiety, insomnia, confusion, self-pity, fear of death, and suicidal impulses pervade and devitalise the patient's psychic energy. It also should be remembered that a depression occasionally masquerades as euphoria.

Euphoria before surgery frequently presages depression postoperatively. Some patients are unable to comprehend the effect of the surgery fully and are therefore unrealistic in their expectations, whereas others can only deal with such a serious situation by becoming euphoric.

Acute depression can interfere with speech progress. Fontaine and Mitchell (1960) emphasised the need for cooperation between medical social worker and speech therapist in the alleviation of anxiety, and of obtaining adjustment of interpersonal relationships within the patient's family before oesophageal voice could be expected to develop. The classic symptoms of depression are listed in Table 17.8.

Many of these symptoms are normal in the circumstances after laryngectomy and resolve spontaneously. Real depression is characterised by the persistence for months of a cluster of these symptoms. Murphy, Bosna and Ogura (1964) emphasise that this needs psychotherapy, discussion and support, combined with antidepressant drug therapy. These authors noted significant details related to their group of 24 laryngectomised patients, of whom four were suffering from depression and three had not returned to work: age, education, employment history, marital relations, alcohol abuse, psychiatric history, and the estimated importance of speech in the patient's usual employment. None of these factors or group of factors was predictive of the patient's final adjustment, mastery of oesophageal speech or return to work. Depression in the absence of other psychiatric illness can be treated effectively.

FEAR OF CANCER

The laryngectomee has to deal with the fears experienced normally by anyone suffering from cancer in addition to the specific anxieties of disfigurement, communication problems, and eating and breathing difficulties (Harris, Vogtsberger and Mattox, 1985). When cancer is diagnosed, the victim feels helpless to control the course of the illness and may withdraw

Table 17.8 Symptoms of depression

- Sustained mood of dejection, sadness and joylessness
- Insomnia
- Undue fatigue
- Reduced appetite
- Lack of interest
- Social withdrawal
- Feelings of hopelessness
- Crying
- Impaired concentration
- Indecisiveness
- Neglect of personal cleanliness or grooming
- Either a passive wish for death or thoughts of suicide

Murphy, Bosna and Ogura (1964).

emotionally from others while experiencing anger, isolation and loneliness. There will also be considerable fear of various treatments such as surgery, radiation and medication. The severity of these reactions may be reduced by the doctor's and surgeon's sympathetic discussion preoperatively. The psychosocial implications of laryngectomy are frequently not discussed (Berkowitz and Lucente, 1985). The laryngologist's ability to establish rapport with the patient and family preoperatively is crucial in helping the patient to deal with fear of the disease and its treatment. If the patient has complete confidence in the surgeon, anxiety can be markedly reduced. Barton (1965) examined the adjustment of 50 patients to total laryngectomy (among whom there were five suicides) and of 50 patients to partial laryngectomy. He concluded that the individual's adjustment to the disease and operation should be of primary concern to the surgeon. Many patients are ill before the operation and are overwhelmed by the catastrophe. Instability in a patient in the past is an indication for extra care and vigilance in rehabilitation, and psychotherapy may be advisable. Inability to speak and express fears causes acute anxiety. Lack of motivation in learning to speak is a danger signal.

PSYCHOSEXUAL PROBLEMS

The understanding and forbearance of partner and family are essential to the patient's rehabilitation, but they need the support and explanations of the clinical team to be able to deal with their own concerns. Sleeping together is a haunting experience; the patient's coughing may alarm the partner who becomes tired and over-wrought. Many spouses describe the hours they spend awake at night, particularly in the early stages, as they listen for their partner's breathing and periodically check that blankets are not covering the stoma. Even when the patient has fully recovered from surgery, the spouse can be so repulsed by the tracheostoma and noisy breathing that the couple's sexual relationship is seriously affected. This, in combination with the communication difficulties, can have a devastating effect on the relationship and referral to appropriate counselling services will be necessary.

ALTERED SELF-IMAGE

The operation is an amputation and many patients will go through a long period of grieving for the loss of this part of themselves and its significance. Some men mourn the lost laryngeal voice which was part of their masculinity while women may find the deeper pseudo-voice unfeminine and regret the loss of a beautiful voice. Even when voice is excellent, paralinguistic features cannot be produced with the same degree of subtlety (see Chapter 1).

EMOTIONAL EXPRESSION

Without the larynx the normal routes of catharsis for emotional relief are also curtailed. The inability to shout or sob is frequently mentioned by patients as an added frustration at times of stress. Similarly, enjoyment of humour is reduced with the inability to laugh aloud.

IMPAIRED SOCIAL INTERACTION

Communication difficulties can lead to reduced social contact and to isolation. This is not the case with all patients. Many with good communication skills preoperatively and a positive attitude to their recovery rapidly overcome the primary hurdles of making themselves understood. It is more difficult, however, to deal with the subtle aspects of voice and communication and the inferences that others make about us from these aspects of social interaction. Good communication skills, rightly or wrongly, are equated with intelligence. The opposite is also true and many laryngectomees feel socially devalued. They may have to contend with the 'Does he take sugar?' syndrome, when enquiries are directed to companions of the laryngectomee, in addition to other social indignities. Rehabilitation must take into account all these distressing features. There is no doubt that the effects of laryngectomy are psychologically far more traumatic than the operation itself. There is a need for weeks and often months of reassurance to the patient and family. The misery of being unable to communicate effectively must be recognised and, from the start, the patient must be helped to communicate as effectively as possible by the most efficient means.

The role of the speech–language pathologist

As a result of the effects of laryngeal cancer on phonation and swallowing, the speech–language pathologist is an essential member of the clinical team (see Table 17.3 on page 580). For patients whose carcinoma is effectively treated by radiotherapy, or excision or laser biopsy, the treatment approach will be similar to that for other conditions where vocal pathology is multifactorial. The psychological effects of disease, and medical and surgical treatment, are taken into account in the treatment programme. This section, therefore, is concerned with patient care pre- and post-partial laryngectomy and total laryngectomy.

PARTIAL LARYNGECTOMY: VOICE THERAPY

Before partial laryngectomy, a preoperative session with the speech–language pathologist is essential to explain the mechanism of phonation, to answer questions and to give reassurance. Postoperatively, speech therapy plays an important role in vocal rehabilitation with or without reconstructive vocal fold surgery. The substitute vocal fold on the excised side does not project so far towards the midline as the normal vocal fold and it is also immobile. The contralateral healthy fold must be trained to pass over the midline and compensate for the deficiency of its fellow in the same way as in a case of total unilateral vocal fold paralysis. Pushing exercises (page 496) are generally recommended, but often equally good results may be obtained, without the danger of building up laryngeal and pharyngeal tension, by raising the volume of the voice with good breath support. It may assist to press the wings of the thyroid cartilage between thumb and finger (medial compression) to emphasise tactile and kinaesthetic cues. Relaxation and correct diaphragmatic breathing are vital preliminaries to the vocal exercises because there is considerable air wastage. The practice of strong vowel sounds with hard glottal attack is another useful exercise.

Granulomatous tissue on the healing surfaces may interfere with phonation at first and, if it does not disperse spontaneously in the course of 2 or 3 months, it may be removed surgically during direct laryngoscopy. The speech pathologist needs to know that this is not a case of local recurrence of tumour, in order to reinforce the reassurances given by the surgeon and allay the patient's anxiety.

The voice may become comparatively good but is never quite normal and is generally rather deep and hoarse. As a result of the amount of breath wasted in phonation and the precipitate emptying of the lungs, there is always a strong tendency to continue speech in a forced whisper. This involves considerable tension in an attempt to achieve the previous length of phrase despite inadequate breath pressure. The patient must be taught first to increase his or her usual breath capacity and then to obtain better control over expiration. When approximation of the adventitious cord and the vocal fold is poor, there is sometimes a tendency to attempt vocalisation on inspiration. The patient must be taught to inspire more frequently and to use shorter phrases. A pocket amplifier can be used very successfully to increase vocal volume.

Some improvement in tone can be obtained by the usual vocal exercises. Increased range may also be achieved by practising scales, attempting to sing and speaking phrases with various intonation patterns. Many patients thus acquire surprisingly serviceable voices in a very short time. On the whole the vocal results with elderly people are disappointing. Levin (1962a) made the following observations based on wide experience:

> Following healing, repeated observations of these patients indicates
> that there is a partial or complete replacement of the removed fold by

> a scar tissue band. Since approximation is only partial or non-existent, the voice is very harsh and seriously impaired. The outgoing air cannot be interrupted properly. There are extraneous harsh noises as a result of the more or less continuous flow of air.

The exceptional case of a reasonably satisfactory voice can, however, occur.

TOTAL LARYNGECTOMY: MANAGEMENT AND TREATMENT

The patient who is about to undergo laryngectomy may not see the speech–language pathologist until the traumatic period of diagnosis and failure of radiotherapy is over and surgery is essential. As a member of a team consisting of ENT surgeon, oncologist, radiotherapist, nurse, physiotherapist, medical social worker and other professionals, the speech–language pathologist's involvement begins at a relatively late stage. The patient and family are contending with distress resulting from unsuccessful intervention and the anticipation of surgery. The goals of speech therapy can be broadly divided into those related to the acquisition of an acceptable and efficient method of communication, and those concerned with the patient's adjustment to the consequences of laryngectomy.

PREOPERATIVE CONTACT

In ideal circumstances, the speech–language pathologist should see the patient and, if possible, the patient's partner during the days before laryngectomy. The interview must be tailored to the needs of each patient and for this reason may be brief or, in some cases, very lengthy indeed. It will be relaxed and unhurried and will take place where there is privacy and little chance of interruption. Although it is carried out in a conversational setting, the therapist will incorporate specific goals into what should be a dialogue, not an outpouring of factual information. This encounter can be one of the most challenging that a speech–language pathologist can have in clinical practice (Doyle, 1994). The clinical skills employed can have a significant effect on the patient's attitude to the forthcoming surgery and subsequent rehabilitation. Whatever assessment protocols have to be carried out, the patient's emotional well-being and need for information must have priority. If it is apparent that all the goals of the preoperative session are unlikely to be achieved in one visit, it can be counterproductive to overload the session. It is a matter of clinical judgement that meetings are arranged where necessary. It is also helpful to see patient and partner together, so that the family is involved in treatment from an early stage and domestic relationships can be observed. The partner can provide essential support for the laryngectomee after hospitalisation but will also need considerable support to deal with a potentially frightening and distressing situation from the early stages. For this reason, the therapist may also arrange an interview with the spouse alone so that the family's fears and concerns may be discussed freely.

Goals

• Establish patient/therapist relationship and understanding

As with all therapy for voice disorders, it is essential that the patient has confidence in the speech–language pathologist if progress is to be made. By the end of preoperative contact, whether on one or more occasions, the patient should be confident that treatment will be with a clinician who will ensure a satisfactory means of communication postoperatively. The clinician's manner is an important factor which is difficult to quantify objectively, but which can negate the usefulness of meticulous assessment procedures and comprehensive explanations if it is unsatisfactory. Essentially, the speech–language pathologist has to convey some understanding of the patient's predicament while calmly and positively indicating that everything possible will be done to improve the situation. Considered answers to each question asked by the patient enhance the feeling of individual care. The relationship between clinician and patient is also helped by the speech–language pathologist being prepared to listen to fears and concerns, whether the patient wants to talk about the previous history of the disease or what the future holds.

• Provide reassurance and information

Throughout the interview, the therapist will provide information about the changed postoperative anatomy, postoperative communication and other issues as they arise. This should be simple and straightforward and patients should be observed carefully for signs that they are being overwhelmed. Individuals vary enormously in what they want to know and in what they have understood and remembered of the explanations given to them by other team members. The speech–language pathologist is only one member of a team, which should coordinate the areas of advice that each member is providing. In addition to keeping each other informed, all professionals involved should know what the surgeon has told the patient so that conflicting information and terminology relating to the disease are avoided. In the USA, surgeons have discussed cancer openly with their patients for many years and this is increasingly the case elsewhere. Some surgeons still tend to use ambiguous terminology and only tell patients that they have cancer if asked directly. It is not the speech–language pathologist's task to inform the patient that the condition is cancer.

Reassurance must have a realistic basis and is most effective when the facts are regarded positively. For example, many patients are reassured by the explanation that it is the voice alone that will be lost. As the terms 'speech', 'language' and 'articulation' are used interchangeably in general conversation, some patients are surprised and heartened to learn that they will not be like the stroke victim who has lost his 'voice', but that it will be possible to mouth words clearly in structured sentences. A demonstration of clear speech without voice by the therapist can be reassuring.

• Informally evaluate communication skills

Patients' preoperative communication skills have a significant bearing on postoperative intelligibility and general effectiveness of communication. The parameters listed in Table 17.9 can be observed in general conversation.

• Observe the patient's emotional status

As with all significant, traumatic experiences, different individuals cope with the situation in different ways. It is important to remember that the outward demeanour may be substantially different from what the patient is actually feeling. At this stage, it is not necessarily desirable that patients should be encouraged to reveal their true feelings. For example, individuals who adopt an outwardly stoical approach may feel that this is the only effective coping strategy they have. To reveal their inner thoughts and distress might be too overwhelming at this stage. The role of the speech–language pathologist is to monitor emotional status and to give patients time to talk at greater length if they wish. The nurse counsellor in the team

Table 17.9 Preoperative factors which indicate postoperative communicative progress

Positive	Negative
Outgoing, social individual	Withdrawn, isolated individual
Mobile facial expressions	Immobile facial muscles, particularly
Clear articulation	around the mouth
Moderate speech rate	Indistinct speech/low intelligibility
Moderate mouth opening	Very rapid speech rate
Moderate vocal volume without effort	High degree of mouth closing
	Forced, loud speaker/very quiet speech
	Edentulous and no false teeth

will also explore these issues. It is significant if the patient is euphoric or light-hearted about the forthcoming procedure (see above). At the other end of the scale, despair is dealt with by discussion and reassurance regarding how various aspects of immediate and long-term aftercare will be managed. It is never appropriate to give glib reassurances that all will be well.

Laryngectomee preoperative visit

In most cases, the patient will find it reassuring and encouraging to be visited by a laryngectomee with good speech and a tactful approach. This visit is usually organised by the speech–language pathologist whose responsibility it is to arrange an appropriate visitor for each laryngectomy candidate. Considerable harm can be done to a vulnerable patient by an unsuitable visitor, however efficient the pseudo-voice, and the effects may be long lasting and militate against successful therapy. If possible, a good speaker of the same sex and similar age should visit – someone who is able to empathise with the patient rather than embark on a detailed and horrendous account of his or her own operation. Generally, patient and partner do not react adversely to a less than ideal voice regarding quality and loudness, but they are dismayed by a speaker with noisy stoma blast which highlights for them the permanent tracheostoma.

Consideration must be given to the comparability of the necessary surgery in each case. It is cruel and pointless to introduce a visitor who has had 'simple' laryngectomy to the prospective laryngo-pharyngo-oesophagectomy patient, when the task of acquiring pseudo-voice may be very different. In these cases we do not arrange for a laryngectomised visitor to demonstrate, but we assure the patient that a loud whisper will be achieved quite easily and mention the various artificial larynges and amplifiers available (see page 647).

The speech–language pathologist should not arrange the visit until it has been discussed and agreed by the patient, whose wishes should be respected. Most patients welcome the opportunity. Others, understandably, feel that they cannot cope with yet another person and new experience when there can be no choice as to whether or not they undergo surgery. A visit may be more valuable postoperatively when the future and the need to develop new skills are a reality.

The visiting laryngectomee should be accompanied by the speech–language pathologist initially so that introductions can be made. If visitor and patient establish a good relationship, the therapist can leave them to talk freely. Visiting laryngectomees are usually fully rehabilitated and living life to the full. The opportunity to help others in this way can be fulfilling and a late stage in their own recovery. It is essential, however, to remember that they too may be coping with residual problems and must be treated with sensitivity.

IMMEDIATE POSTOPERATIVE MANAGEMENT

To maintain contact, the speech–language pathologist should visit the patient as soon after the operation as allowed, even if this visit is fleeting. Ideally, during the period of 10 days to a fortnight while the nasogastric tube remains in situ, daily visits should continue. In the first few days of recovery, swelling and stiffness around the neck and mandible will restrict movement. Strenuous attempts at speech may damage the wound so the patient is encouraged to articulate clearly but gently. This relaxed 'whisper' is intelligible and some voiceless consonants can be heard so that the patient is encouraged. An intraoral speech aid, such as the Cooper Rand oral vibrator, can be used effectively at this stage but patients usually write down what they want to say on a 'whiteboard' or use a notebook.

Clearly articulated speech is much less tedious and frustrating than writing if it can be achieved successfully. This depends not only on the patient, but on the motivation and skill at lip-reading of nurses and family. Other benefits of this approach include maintaining the mobility of articulatory muscles, especially the tongue, which may be paretic or stiff after surgery. Encouraging relaxed and accurate articulation is also an ideal basis for pseudo-voice. A realistic approach must be employed and some patients may prefer written communication. Their frustration should not be compounded by the feeling that the speech–language pathologist has 'forbidden' them to use writing. Any method of facilitating communication should be considered.

In patients where healing is delayed and the nasogastric tube is retained for some weeks because of a fistula, the surgeon should be consulted about the advisability of whispering and the possible danger of exaggerated articulatory movements of the tongue straining the wound. Much depends on the height of the fistula in the pharyngeal wall and also the manner of speech; some patients 'whisper' with excessive effort. Similarly, even when recovery has been straightforward and the nasogastic tube removed, therapy directed at achieving voice should not begin without the surgeon's agreement. In practice, it is usually possible after the patient has successfully taken two 'meals' by mouth. To inject air into the oesophagus before healing is complete may result in rupture of the sutures.

VOICE AND SPEECH REHABILITATION

There are three main types of alaryngeal phonation: **tracheo-oesophageal voice, oesophageal voice** and the **artificial (electronic) larynx**. The first two methods are similar in that they rely on air moving through the P-E segment, causing it to vibrate. These vibrations result in sound that can be used as pseudo-voice. The route by which air enters the oesophagus differs in each. In T-E voice, pulmonic air reaches the P-E segment via the prosthesis inserted in the T-E wall (Figure 17.7). Oesophageal voice, in contrast, depends on air being moved into the oesophagus from the oral cavity. Both methods depend on the competency of the P-E segment. The electronic larynx provides a sound source external to the vocal tract, but the sound generated is transmitted through the tissues of the neck into the vocal tract. The 'voice' is then modified by the articulators in the normal way (Figure 17.6(a), (b), (c)).

During the last decade, the rehabilitation of laryngectomees has been transformed by the development of surgical speech restoration (T-E voice). In the past, therapy was chiefly directed at achieving oesophageal voice and when this was successful the results were functionally satisfactory. Unfortunately, for various reasons (see below), this was not physiologically possible for every patient and, even for those for whom it was a possibility, treatment was frequently protracted over many months. Patients then used electronic larynges or remained voiceless. The British Association of Otorhinolaryngologists (1998) recommends that an active programme of surgical voice rehabilitation should be in place wherever laryngectomy is performed. In the final instance, the restoration of a satisfactory method of communication has to be based on pragmatic decisions for each individual depending on the extent of the disease, realistic possibilities, the patient's physiological and psychological status, and what the patient wants.

Tracheo-oesophageal voice

Tracheo-oesophageal voice is achieved by pulmonic air (air from the lungs) passing through a puncture in the T-E wall into the oesophagus. As the air leaves the oesophagus, sound is generated at the P-E segment and subsequently modified into speech in the usual way by the articulators. A prosthesis is inserted into the puncture from the tracheal wall and prevents spontaneous closure of the puncture while acting as a conduit for the air used during speech. Air is directed through the prosthesis by the speaker occluding the tracheostoma either with the fingers (or thumb) or a purpose-made flap valve which closes automatically as the patient speaks. Various prostheses are produced by a number of manufacturers and they

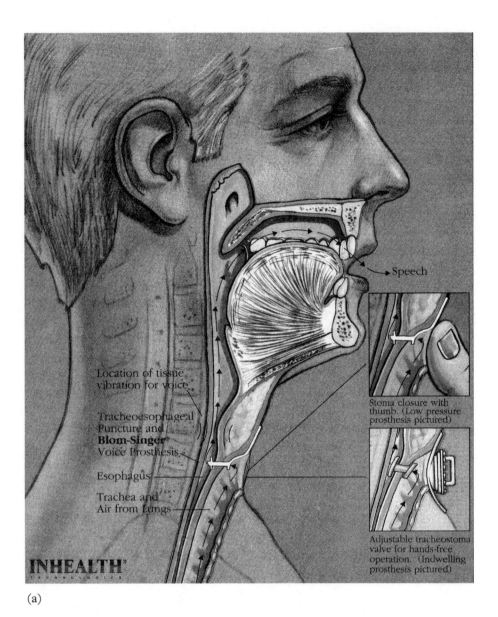

(a)

Figure 17.6 Sound production: (a) in tracheo-oesophageal voice, (b) in oesophageal voice and (c) with an artificial larynx. (Reproduced by permission of International Healthcare Technologies, 1110 Mark Avenue, Carpinteria, CA 93013-2918, USA. Blom–Singer is a registered trademark of Hansa Medical Products, Inc.)

(contd)

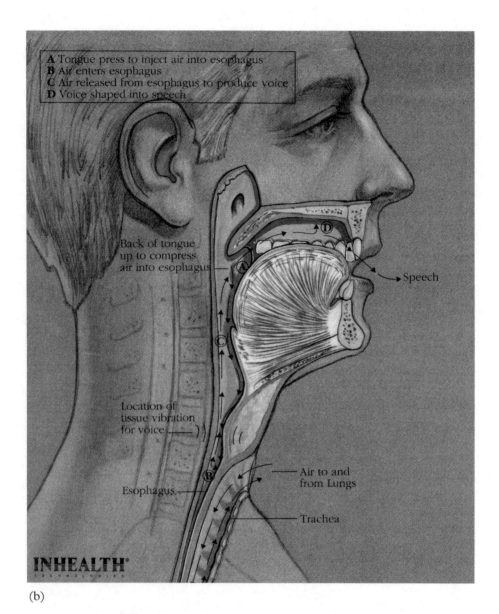

A Tongue press to inject air into esophagus
B Air enters esophagus
C Air released from esophagus to produce voice
D Voice shaped into speech

Back of tongue up to compress air into esophagus

Speech

Location of tissue vibration for voice

Esophagus

Air to and from Lungs

Trachea

INHEALTH

(b)

can be put in place as a primary procedure at the time of laryngectomy or as a secondary procedure, after laryngectomy. Some examples of the types of prostheses are described in Table 17.10 and Figure 17.8.

When prostheses are inserted during total laryngectomy, insertion is carried out by the surgeon while the patient is under general anaesthetic. Speech–language pathologists are frequently responsible for the sizing and insertion of a voice prosthesis in the outpatient clinic as well as showing the patient how to look after it and produce satisfactory voice. Table 17.11 shows the insertion and supplementary equipment for a voice prosthesis.

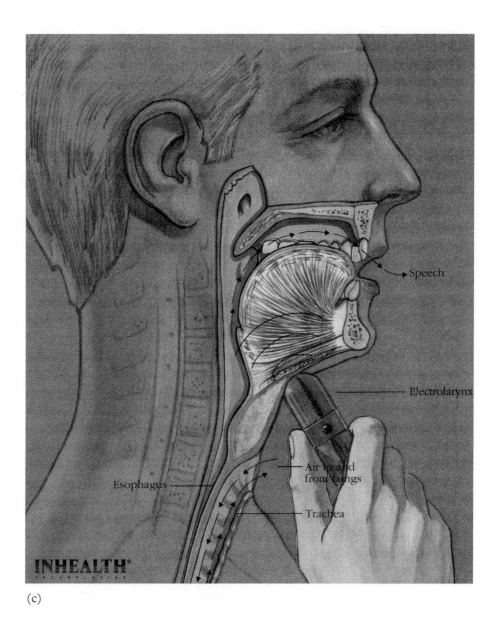

Speech

Electrolarynx

Air to and from lungs

Esophagus

Trachea

INHEALTH®

(c)

An extensive range of items is available for all aspects of prosthesis insertion and maintenance (Figures 17.9 and 17.10).

There are four stages in establishing T-E voice as a secondary procedure.

• Establishing that the patient can produce voice via the T-E puncture

The puncture is maintained by a catheter initially and closes rapidly without this or a voice prosthesis in place. The catheter is removed, the patient is asked to inspire, and the clinician occludes the stoma with a thumb as the

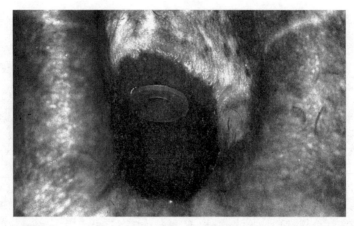

Figure 17.7 Voice prosthesis in place. (Reproduced by permission of International Healthcare Technologies, 1110 Mark Avenue, Carpinteria, CA 93013-2918, USA.)

Table 17.10 Types of tracheo-oesophageal prostheses

Duckbill voice prosthesis	A slit in the oesophageal end of the prosthesis allows air to pass from the trachea into the oesophagus. Two flanges, or collars, one below the slit and one at the other end of the prosthesis retain it in place. They are positioned on either side of the tracheo-oesophageal wall. A plastic tag attached to the tracheal end of the prosthesis allows the clinician to test that it is securely in position (and that the flange on the oesophageal side has passed through the puncture) by tugging the tag firmly (Figure 17.8). The tag is also used for removing the prosthesis
Low-pressure voice prosthesis	A one-way flapper valve in this prosthesis allows air to pass from the trachea to the oesophagus, but prevents contents of the oesophagus penetrating the trachea (Figure 17.8)
Indwelling low pressure prosthesis	Can be inserted as a primary or secondary procedure. Can remain in place for long periods without being removed for cleaning (Figure 17.8)

patient exhales. If sustained voice is produced on a single vowel, the voice prosthesis can be inserted (Table 17.12 for problem-solving).

• Correct sizing of the voice prosthesis

The clinician measures the depth of the puncture from the trachea to the oesophagus with a purpose-made sizer, similar to the prosthesis, on which measurements are marked (see Table 17.11). The prosthesis must be long enough to protrude into the oesophagus but, if it is too long, it may be obstructed by the posterior oesophageal wall. Measurements taken in the

Table 17.11 Tracheo-oesophageal voice: insertion and supplementary equipment

Sizer	Similar to a prosthesis, this device is used to measure the length of the oesophageal puncture between the trachea and the oesophagus to establish the size of the prosthesis required
Lubricants	To facilitate insertion of the prosthesis
Inserter	The prosthesis is loaded on to the inserter which guides it into place and is then detached
Tracheostoma valve	Allows patient to speak without using digital occlusion of stoma (Figure 17.9)
Personal humidification systems	Similar to the tracheostoma valve in appearance, a foam filter is placed in its holder onto a self-adhesive baseplate and covers the stoma. Warmth and humidification of the tracheal air are maintained.
Pipettes	Specially designed pipettes can be used to flush water through the prosthesis for cleaning while in place

early postoperative period may need to be revised periodically. After the trauma of the puncture procedure, the tissues of the T-E wall are frequently thicker than they will be at a later stage of recovery.

• Insertion

The voice prosthesis is introduced into the puncture site with an inserter. Lubrication of various types is used to ease its passage from trachea to oesophagus, but some bleeding may occur during this manoeuvre. Insertion is complete when the retention collar at the oesophageal end of the prosthesis has passed into the oesophagus. This is confirmed when the prosthesis stays securely in position as the strap at the tracheal end (see Figure 17.8) is pulled firmly.

• Eliciting voice

When the clinician is satisfied that the prosthesis is correctly in place, the patient is asked to produce voice on a single vowel, occluding the stoma with a thumb or fingers. A relaxed approach is likely to be most successful; this can be a tense moment for the patient and increased effort is usually counterproductive. Forceful inspiration and expiration accompanied by excessive digital pressure to occlude the stoma prevent air from passing through the prosthesis. The use of a prosthesis to achieve alaryngeal voice does not obviate the need for the clinician to take the patient's emotional status into account as an element of achieving successful communication. If the patient is tense and over-anxious, voicing potential will be adversely affected, even if the prosthesis has been correctly sized and inserted. After achieving voice on a single vowel, patients frequently progress to phrases

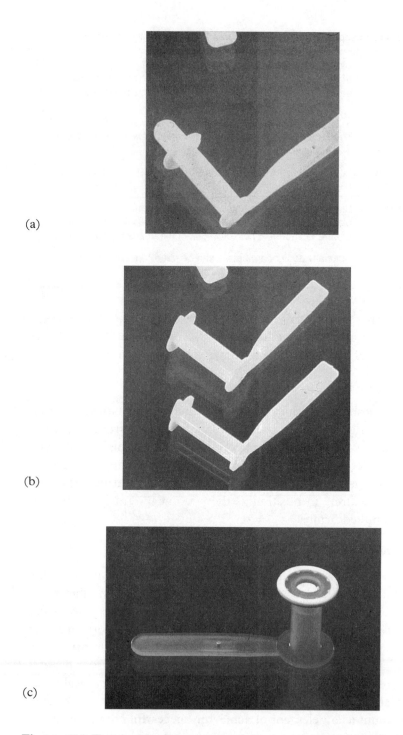

(a)

(b)

(c)

Figure 17.8 Types of tracheo-oesophageal voice prosthesis: (a) duckbill; (b) low pressure; (c) indwelling low pressure. (Reproduced by permission of International Healthcare Technologies, 1110 Mark Avenue, Carpinteria, CA 93013-2918, USA.)

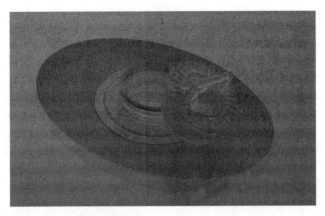

Figure 17.9 Tracheostoma valve and baseplate. (Reproduced by permission of International Healthcare Technologies, 1110 Mark Avenue, Carpinteria, CA 93013-2918, USA.)

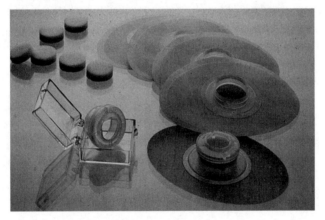

Figure 17.10 Personal humidification system. (Reproduced by permission of International Healthcare Technologies, 1110 Mark Avenue, Carpinteria, CA 93013-2918, USA.)

and continuous speech by the end of the session in which the prosthesis has been fitted. Coordination of stoma occlusion, appropriate air-pressure levels and voicing improve with practice. As with any method of alaryngeal speech, intelligibility ultimately depends on clarity of articulation and appropriate speech rate together with a satisfactory voice, not voice alone. The speech pathologist's role is, therefore, to give the patient insight into all aspects of communication and to develop these skills evenly, rather than to allow the production of voice to override other important elements of the process. When voice is not achieved on insertion of the voice prosthesis, or fails subsequently, there are a number of common causes that the clinician has to investigate. Some of these are outlined in Table 17.12.

Table 17.12 Failure to produce satisfactory tracheo-oesophageal voice: problem solving

Cause	Action
P-E spasm	Investigate competency of P-E segment using air insufflation test. Spasm of the P-E segment causes intermittent voicing and can be relieved surgically by myotomy or pharyngeal plexus neurectomy (see page 594)
Voice prosthesis too long and making contact with the posterior oesophageal wall	Voice prosthesis should be resized and replaced
Large or tilted stoma which makes competent digital occlusion difficult to achieve	Patients may be helped by using two fingers instead of a thumb. In some cases, the valve which allows hands-free voice may be helpful (Table 17.11 and Figure 17.9)
Patient using excessive digital pressure to occlude stoma which prevents pulmonic air from entering the prosthesis	The speech–language pathologist can demonstrate the appropriate pressure required to occlude the stoma competently
Insufficient air pressure to vibrate the P-E segment	The patient should be encouraged to inspire more deeply, but not excessively, to provide adequate air pressure
Prosthesis blocked with food debris or mucus	Prosthesis must be cleaned. In an established user of a voice prosthesis, blockage can be reduced and eliminated by regular cleaning with purpose-made equipment
Fungal infestation of prosthesis	Fungal infestation can be avoided or reduced by the careful use of fungicidal preparations

Singer and Blom (1980) reported fluent voices in 90% of their first 60 patients who underwent T-E puncture. There are reports that the percentage of patients continuing to use T-E fistula voice in the long term is less than this (Wetmore et al., 1985). It appears that careful patient selection and a well-trained team whose members are well integrated will maintain a high long-term percentage of successful users. The speech pathologist has a key role in the assessment and treatment of these patients (Perry, 1983).

Studies of the effectiveness of T-E voice demonstrate the advantages of T-E voice over oesophageal voice. T-E and oesophageal voice are compared in Table 17.13.

The development of the Blom–Singer prosthesis has been a major contribution to the process of providing voice for the laryngectomee and other prostheses have been developed using the same concept. The speech–language pathologist's role in evaluating suitable candidates for T-E voice

Table 17.13 Tracheo-oesophageal and oesophageal voice: comparisons

Tracheo-oesophageal voice	Oesophageal voice
Speech rate and prosody well-preserved because of pulmonic air stream	Speech rate markedly slower than normal and prosody disturbed because of air injection
Relatively long voice duration because of pulmonic air source	Voice duration reduced by limited amount of injected air in oesophagus
Approximately 10 dB louder than normal voice (acoustic parameters generally more similar to laryngeal speech than traditional oesophageal speech)	Approximately 6–10 dB quieter than normal voice. Low intensity is a common problem for the oesophageal speaker
Pseudo-voice can be achieved rapidly without prolonged speech therapy	Prolonged speech therapy usually required to elicit and develop voice
Prosthesis cleaning, maintenance and changing	If successful, oesophageal voice requires no equipment

Robbins et al. (1984); Merwin, Goldstein and Rothman (1985); Tardy-Mitzell, Andrews and Bowman (1985); Williams and Watson (1985, 1987).
According to some studies, both types of speech have been rated as comparable in intelligibility and overall communicative effectiveness (Bridges, 1991). The quality of voice in both methods of laryngeal phonation is similar but in many aspects, tracheo-oesophageal voice is regarded as superior (Max, de Bruyn and Steurs, 1997).

procedures, sizing and fitting prostheses, and applying appropriate therapeutic skills may vary from one multidisciplinary team to another. It must be remembered that, although voice may be excellent in appropriately selected patients in whom there are no surgical complications, the procedure is not without its problems even when performed by the most competent surgeons. It is the combined expertise of an integrated clinical team involved with a large number of laryngectomee patients that is likely to achieve the best result.

Oesophageal voice

Oesophageal voice depends on air that has been introduced into the oesophagus vibrating the P-E segment as it returns to the oral cavity. Kallen (1934) reviewed vicarious vocal mechanisms and, subsequently, Seeman (1959) claimed to have been the first to determine by lateral radiography that the oesophagus acts as a vicarious or substitute 'lung' and the oesophageal sphincter as a pseudo-glottis. Seeman drew attention to the fact that:

> The cervical and upper portions of the oesophagus contain transverse striated muscle fibres; the muscles of the lower part are smooth. As the recurrent laryngeal nerve gives off branches some of which (the

so-called rami oesophagi nervi recurrentis) are distributed to the oesophagus, the phenomenon associated with phonation is probably the result of an irradiation to the musculature of the oesophagus of the nerve impulses attending phonation.

Seeman sought to prove that phonatory contractions in the cervical and upper portions of the thoracic oesophagus were genuinely active and not dependent on respiratory movements. Only in the middle and lower thoracic oesophageal sections did he observe changes in the lumen effected by thoracic movement. In skilful laryngectomised speakers, it seems possible that there is extension to the oesophageal sphincter of the nerve impulses for normal laryngeal phonation. Voluntary relaxation and tension of the sphincter can be acquired for oesophageal voice production (Levin, 1962a).

The adaptation of the upper oesophagus to function as a vicarious lung can be seen clearly in xeroradiographs (Figures 17.11 and 17.12). It is obvious that the volume of air available for voice production is far less than when a pulmonic air supply is available. Stetson (1937) thought that the oesophageal air reservoir consisted of only 2.5 ml. Snidecor and Isshiki (1965) discovered, however, that airflow is considerably higher than this and volume per syllable ranged from 5–16 to 27–72 ml/second in good speakers. There are three main methods of charging the oesophagus with air: **injection**, **inhalation** and **swallowing**. The last is not suitable for oesophageal speech.

Injection method

Standard injection

Standard injection consists of compressing air in the oral cavity by sealing the lips, closing the palatopharyngeal sphincter and compressing the cheeks, while the tongue pumps the air posteriorly into the pharynx. As the compressed air descends to the hypopharynx, the fibres of the P-E segment either relax to allow air into the oesophagus or the air pressure is sufficient to pass through the sphincter (Edels, 1983).

Diedrich and Youngstrom (1966), by means of lateral radiographic studies, examined tongue movements during air intake in 20 laryngectomees. They noted that these movements are different from a swallow movement and that rapid air intake facilitates more fluent speech. Standard injection revealed two types of tongue movement:

- Glossal press consists of contact by the tongue with the alveolus, and frequently middle of the tongue contact with the hard palate. At the same time the posterior portion moves backward but fails to touch the pharyngeal wall. The lips may be opened or closed.

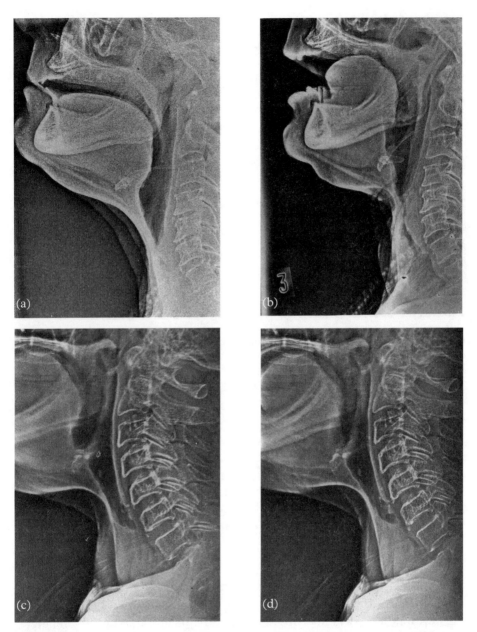

Figure 17.11 Post-laryngectomy xerographs: (a) Patient 1: total laryngectomy, fluent speaker (male). At rest: the P-E segment is at the level of the junction of C5 and C6; the posterior wall of the pharynx bulges forwards. (b) Patient 1: producing /iː/. The P-E segment is vibrating as air returns from the capacious 'vicarious lung' (oesophagus). (c) Patient 2: total laryngectomy, fluent speaker (female). At rest: the P-E segment is at the level of the junction of C6 and C7. The anterior wall of the pharynx bulges to meet the posterior wall. (d) Patient 2: producing /iː/. The shallow P-E segment vibrates on the returning air. Note the small air reservoir in comparison with patient 1. Although she is a fluent speaker, patient 2 needs to charge the oesophagus with air frequently in order to maintain fluent speech. (Reproduced by permission of Dr Frances MacCurtain, London, UK.)

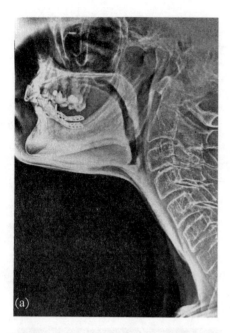 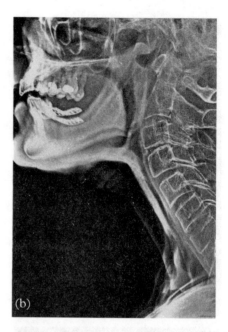

Figure 17.12 Post-pharyngolaryngectomy xerographs. (a) Patient 3: pharyngola-ryngectomy, no pseudo-voice (male). At rest: there is no P-E segment. (b) Patient 3: attempting to produce /iː/. Oesophageal voice can be produced only in single sylla-bles with great effort. There are swallowing difficulties because of the tight, narrow tract. He uses an electronic larynx very successfully. (Reproduced by permission of Dr Frances MacCurtain, London, UK.)

• Glossopharyngeal press occurs when the tip and middle of the tongue contact the alveolus and hard palate, and posterior tongue moves back to make contact with the posterior pharyngeal wall. The hypopharyngeal cavity may be completely obliterated. There is palatopharyngeal closure and the lips may be open or closed.

Consonant injection

This term is used to describe the method whereby air injection occurs together with articulation of consonants, particularly voiceless plosives. This technique always involves closure of the palatopharyngeal sphincter, but approximation of the lips and the tongue-tip with the alveolar ridge, or posterior tongue with the velum, will vary according to the consonant being produced. Articulation assists injection.

Inhalation method (insufflation or aspiration)

At rest the oesophagus below the P-E segment is closed. On inspiration, the drop in thoracic pressure also results in a fall in pressure in the oesophagus. Air then flows into the oesophagus from the pharynx in order to equalise pressure. (This transfer of air may not occur if the P-E segment is tense or hypertonic.) The air is then held in the oesophagus by closure of the P-E segment once the air pressure is equalised, and will subsequently be used for oesophageal voice. During 'inhalation' the tongue never occludes the oral cavity (Diedrich and Youngstrom, 1966), and there is little or no movement of the dorsum of the tongue. The lips are open, there is no velopharyngeal closure and the airway from lips to pharyngo-oesophageal junction is open.

Air swallowing

This is not a viable method of air intake for speech because of the time delay between air intake and return which disrupts fluency. It may also result in discomfort as air accumulates in the stomach. Nevertheless, occasional instances of air swallowing in the early stages of treatment may help the patient to identify the sound and sensation of air passing through the P-E segment as air from the stomach is released.

The various methods used by oesophageal speakers were highlighted by Isshiki (1965, 1968). Six speakers of variable proficiency were assessed. It was found that air intake and use, in conjunction with respiration and vocalisation, varied greatly with individual speakers. Some speakers injected air while speaking and as they exhaled, which is what other researchers had found. All speakers apparently 'inhaled' air into the oesophagus synchronous with lung inspiration, whereas some speakers relied more on injection than inhalation. Negative pressure in the oesophagus during lung inhalation assists injection of the air by the injection method. The more effective and larger the air intake, the better the speech. Lung expiration and speech are synchronised. There is some agreement that fluent oesophageal speech is synchronised with the normal respiratory cycle. Bateman and Negus (1954), Di Carlo, Amster and Herer (1955), Robe et al. (1956c), Hodson and Oswald (1958), Vrticka and Svoboda (1961, 1963) and Isshiki (1965, 1968) were unanimous that fluent oesophageal speech occurs only during lung expiration and that it is always prefaced by lung inspiration as in normal speech. A slow and normal deep breathing movement alone did not insufflate air into the oesophagus. This is important and confirms the observation that a quick diaphragmatic pant is necessary for sucking air into the oesophagus and needs to be developed by the patient.

Diaphragmatic action

Samuel and Adams (1976) examined the role of oesophageal and diaphragmatic movements in successful speakers. The neoglottis relaxes as the diaphragm descends and near the end of the diaphragm's descent the oesophagus suddenly dilates like an inflated sausage-shaped balloon. As the diaphragm ascends, the lower end of the oesophagus collapses and the upper segment increases slightly in diameter with increased air pressure. The neoglottis opens and the neck of the balloon undergoes controlled release until emptied as the diaphragm reaches maximum ascent. There is good coordination between movements of neoglottis and diaphragm. The quality of speech is related to the length of the oesophageal dilatation. (These authors note that emphysema [see page 346] will interfere with air-flow from the lung and expiratory control.)

Combined approach

Traditionally, various advocates of either injection or inhalation have stressed the advantages of their preferred approaches to air intake and these are discussed on pages 629–631. It is advisable for the therapist to be flexible, however, and to use the approach that appears to be easiest for the patient. In the early stages, an exploratory and empirical approach is appropriate. The rigidity of one fixed approach may exclude potentially successful routes to achieving oesophageal voice. It is obviously unwise to confine speech therapy to teaching one method, but advisable to introduce a combination of methods, because this is actually what takes place when fluent speech is mastered.

Eliciting oesophageal voice

The speech–language pathologist knows that this is likely to be a tense and anxious time for the laryngectomee; voice is desperately desired and yet thoughts of failure intrude. With some patients, the therapist's task is easier if relaxed, firm patterns of clear articulation have been established while the nasogastric tube is in place. Also, if there is an ideal P-E segment, vibration of the segment will occur spontaneously with the articulation of certain plosive consonants. Therapeutic intervention is directed at maintaining relaxed speech, slightly slower than normal, so that maximum benefit may be derived from injection of air into the oesophagus. These patients progress rapidly with appropriate support. The laryngectomee whom we treated and who was speaking with fluent oesophageal voice 2 weeks after removal of the nasogastric tube is an exception, unfortunately. Such patients owe their success to the surgeon's skill and their own determination rather than to the attentions of the speech–language pathologist.

It is important that any attempts at producing voice are not introduced in a pass/fail setting. The patient and therapist should perceive this as an exploratory situation in which the therapist is experimenting with various strategies in order to ascertain the most promising route for treatment.

The first aim is production of a sound; it does not matter how this is achieved, but it should be achieved as soon as possible. This is chiefly for psychological reasons because one of the patient's greatest concerns is remaining silent. Failure to achieve voice after laryngectomy has a depressing effect on the patient and may delay speech for many months, even when it is physically possible. Some patients find that the analogy of learning to swim is an everyday example that puts the task ahead of them into perspective. Once the 'knack' of keeping afloat for one or two strokes has been acquired, it is only a matter of time and practice before longer distances can be swum in style. Once a sound has been produced, by whatever method, accidentally or intentionally, the rest is practice and refinement.

Exploration of the patient's voice potential is based on the three ways in which the oesophagus may be charged with air.

● Injection

Experimentation should be tried using consonant/vowel (CV) combinations with voiceless plosives, e.g. p, t, k, st, sk, sp, skr, followed by vowels, preferably those requiring marked mouth opening, e.g. /pa:/, /ta:/, /ka:/. The patient should be relaxed, especially in the shoulder, neck and jaw muscles. No more effort should be put into articulation than for the normal articulation of these consonants. If the therapist can produce these sounds with pseudo-voice and demonstrate what is desired, this is helpful. It gives the patient something to imitate and also does much to remove embarrassment at what the patient may regard as 'belching'. However, if the therapist is unable to produce oesophageal voice, a passable imitation can be achieved by using excessively creaky voice.

Many patients will use a combination of standard injection and consonant injection spontaneously even at this early stage. Most find it helpful if the therapist acts as a visual model so that the degree of pressure and timing of articulation can be seen. This is a technique for ensuring that excessive effort is not used. Our experience is that it is equally, if not more, important for the laryngectomee to see what has to be done and how to do it, as it is to hear pseudo-voice. Practice before a mirror and with another laryngectomee is helpful.

The image of having a bubble of air in the mouth (Diedrich and Youngstrom, 1977), which is firmly compressed and squeezed into the pharynx and then released on saying /pa:/, is frequently successful. From the beginning, it is important that on all CV combinations voicing is encouraged without delay after injection of air. Patients frequently equate effort with probable success, but forceful injection will drive air down to the stomach or the P-E segment will tighten and prevent injection.

Although it would appear logical to instruct the patient in breathing, drawing attention to the fact that quick, brief inspiration should preface speech may possibly cause confusion. Some say it provides too many things to concentrate on at once. By the time the patient has mastered easy injection in successive syllables, it is generally found that chest expansion takes place before speech unconsciously as it did preoperatively. This is one reason why the naturally good speaker before laryngectomy is often the naturally good speaker afterwards. The possession of good kinaesthetic sense and naturally good habits of breathing and articulation appear to be important factors influencing the speech progress of the laryngectomee. Tongue exercises may be necessary to improve speech clarity, especially with a lingual paresis after block dissection with laryngectomy.

● Inhalation

The patient may be able to produce voice easily by 'inhaling' air through open lips, with tongue relaxed, and then phonating on prolonged vowels as the air returns simultaneously with expiration. If not, and this is more probable, various methods can be experimented with:

- Simulate a long relaxed yawn in which air may enter the oesophagus and then be expelled.
- Sniff air in through the nose, lips closed, tongue flat with slight forward thrust of the mandible, which enlarges the pharyngeal cavity and is a method often used by laryngectomees for recharging of air. Placing the hand on the throat under the chin checks excessive jaw thrust.
- A four-step procedure for trapping air in the oesophagus may be used (Gately, 1971):
  - open mouth wide, flatten tongue
  - close lips with little or no elevation of the mandible, puckering lips
  - bring teeth together
  - hold nose.
- Blow bubbles through a straw into water.

When an individual is tense and breathing is shallow, and preoperative speech patterns were poor, proper instruction in relaxation and central breathing is essential. The slightly exaggerated and rapid descent of the diaphragm is an obvious feature of every proficient oesophageal speaker. If a patient is unable to achieve coordination of respiratory and articulatory muscles, speech will lack fluency, and injection and inhalation of air into the oesophagus will not be synchronised.

It is advisable to instruct the patient in relaxation and correct breathing technique as soon as possible and this should form part of every treatment session. Initially, exercises need not be linked to phonation. The patient may learn to produce voice by the injection method independently as previously described and, if the oesophageal voice is effortless, attention may need to be drawn to the connection between voice and respiration only at a later stage. Some patients never work on relaxation and breathing and produce excellent results, but most need help in these areas early in treatment in order to increase the air reservoir and so obtain greater duration and volume of voice.

Di Carlo, Amster and Herer (1955) found that abdominal expansion in breathing occurred in their poor speakers and thoracic expansion in their better speakers. Abdominal breathing is to be discouraged and the intercostal diaphragmatic method emphasised. The quick, pant-like intake essential for drawing air into the oesophagus (Isshiki, 1968) can be encouraged by panting exercises for toning up the muscles and by sitting upright, abdominal muscles firm, not sagging.

● Injection and inhalation

The danger of confusing the patient with 'breathing exercises' and encouraging increased blowing from the stoma is not so great as the antagonists of the inhalation method believe. The patient has nothing to learn; inspiration and expiration coincide with the preparatory and active phases of speech in exactly the same way as they did preoperatively. There is, on the other hand, a real danger in concentrating exclusively on air injection. This is an unnatural process quite foreign to the reflex habit patterns of the individual, and as difficult to acquire as any other new skill demanding muscular coordination invariably is in adult life. It is quite common to find patients concentrating on injection to the complete cessation of respiration. The breath is held while injection and ejection of air take place and the abdomen and thorax are held rigid. Attention must be paid to the necessity of relaxing and coordinating respiration with inhalation of air into the oesophagus and production of voice. As stated earlier, negative pressure in the thorax aids inhalation of air into the oesophagus, hence the need to synchronise exactly inhalation with the quick inspiration of lung air. In fluent speakers consonant injection plays an important role in re-charge of air and voice duration.

Aberrant patterns of oesophageal voice

In some cases, if voice does not develop easily, the speaker's attempts to produce oesophageal voice can result in sound being produced at sites in the tract other than at the P-E segment. These techniques usually derive from excessive tension and should be discouraged because they tend to be less acceptable socially and less efficient than true oesophageal voice.

Pharyngeal voice

The injection method alone may encourage the undesirable pharyngeal voice with its Donald Duck quality. The P-E segment tends to be tightly closed when this method of air charging is used, and air is trapped in the hypopharynx and is vibrated at a site between the base of the tongue and the posterior pharyngeal wall of the oropharynx. Patients with a tense, hypertonic or spasmodic P-E segment are particularly liable to develop pharyngeal voice.

Pharyngeal voice should not be allowed to become established because it is extremely difficult to unlearn and unpleasant to listen to. Relaxation and a firm but gentle approach to articulation and air charging, while learning the injection method, reduce possible development of this distinctive and unpleasant form of voicing. The inhalation method counteracts pharyngeal voice. If in doubt as to whether the initial sounds made by the patient are pharyngeal or oesophageal, patient and therapist can verify vibration of the P-E segment (rather than a higher and unsuitable pseudo-glottis) by placing the finger-tips on the front of the neck at the level of the previous site of the larynx. Vibrations will be felt here if the P-E segment is acting as the pseudo-glottis.

Buccal speech

When the P-E segment is hypertonic and does not allow inhalation, turbulent air can be used in the mouth to produce a quasi-whisper. Tense articulation while attempting to achieve oesophageal speech may also give rise to buccal whisper. Air is vibrated orally by vigorous movements of the tongue and is also pushed between the constricted cheek muscles and the lateral dental arch. If buccal whisper develops, it should be discouraged immediately and speech therapy must concentrate on relaxed articulation.

Air swallowing

Although not viable as a method of air intake for oesophageal speech, swallowing air and vibration of the P-E segment as the air is expelled may be a useful start to therapy. If the patient has not lost the facility for 'burping', it may be possible for air to be eructated from the oesophagus immediately.

The necessary kinaesthetic and tactile sensations will be familiar and control can be readily obtained over relaxation and dilatation of the cricopharyngeal sphincter.

Many patients find it difficult to overcome their dislike of oesophageal speech because of its similarity to belching, against which there are strong taboos in Western society. This is, of course, a strong argument against advocating air swallowing and belching as the first method of instruction. Another objection is the long latency period between air intake and sound production. This technique, aided by aerated drinks, may serve a temporary purpose if other methods do not produce results but, as it has to be unlearned at some stage, it is wasteful of effort if another method can be readily mastered. No proficient oesophageal speaker uses air swallowing for charging the vicarious lung.

Establishing oesophageal voice

Voluntary control

Once oesophageal voice has been obtained, the next task is to bring CV production under voluntary control so that there is consistency of performance. Relaxed and effortless repetition of syllables reinforces kinaesthetic feedback. Progress from this level should not be made until syllables are consistently being produced successfully. Edels (1983) recommends a 90% success rate before a more ambitious step is taken.

It is essential that, from the earliest stages of therapy, bad habits of voice production (discussed on pages 636–9) are not allowed to develop. The temptation to progress in the face of these faults may be great, but will be disastrous eventually. It is extremely difficult to unlearn them and they detract from, or delay, the acquisition of good oesophageal voice. The faults may arise purely as a result of the patient's poor technique. More significantly, the P-E segment may be hyper- or hypotonic and, as a result, the patient is forced to use inappropriate manoeuvres in an attempt to produce voice.

Monosyllables

Different syllables beginning and ending with voiced and voiceless plosives and containing different vowels can now be practised. It is generally found that some consonant combinations are more helpful than others with individual patients. These assist in the acquisition of the skill of flattening the tongue to the roof of the mouth, forcing compressed air from the oral cavity into the pharynx and so into the oesophagus. Consonant combinations such as /sk/, /ch/, /skr/ may be found helpful, and words beginning with these sounds can be practised. Treatment should be adapted to individual needs. Gradually all consonants and vowels are worked on with the aim of obtaining clear and effortless phonation.

In most cases, it is advisable to leave the nasals /m/ and /n/ till late because they allow the escape of air through the nose and render air compression difficult. The speaker learns, however, to overcome the difficulty by using insufflated air only or by putting an unreleased plosive equivalent before the nasal in order to compress the air silently, e. g. (b)man; (d)no. The consonant /h/ is very difficult because its normal mode of articulation by laryngeal whisper is, of course, no longer possible, and it should be taught last, if at all. A good imitation can be produced by lifting the back of the tongue as for the voiceless palatal fricative in 'loch', as suggested by Paget (1930) and Oswald (Hodson and Oswald, 1958). A slight pause before the following vowel is also an effective substitute for /h/.

The aim of a short latency period (Edels, 1983) is added to the goal of consistency in voice production in these exercises. The latency period is the time between injection of air into the oesophagus and sound being produced at the P-E segment. It is fundamental to fluent oesophageal speech that this should be as short as possible. As in other aspects, this is enhanced by a relaxed and effortless technique.

Monosyllabic and polysyllabic words leading to phrases

These build on the early achievements of phoneme production. All tasks are directed at duration of the sound for continuous fluent speech. Breathing technique can now be positively linked with speech as the length of phrases is extended, e.g.

Part – party – part-time
Don't – don't go – don't go back
Scratch – scratch it – scratch it off
Try – try to – try to go
Pack – pack it – pack it up.

In this way the laryngectomee also learns to use the consonant at the end of a word to air charge for a subsequent word beginning with a vowel.

Easy mechanical exercises such as saying 'chapter 1, chapter 2, chapter 3', etc. are helpful as are counting, days of the week, etc. Duration of voice is also encouraged by practising strings of CVC syllables where the consonants are plosives, e.g. /cap–cap–cap/; /tut–tut–tut/.

The next stage is to use short sentences or phrases, omitting 'difficult' consonants, e.g.

bake a cake	pint of bitter
cup of coffee	take it back
kick the cat	go to bed

Loudness

Direct work on increased loudness is not appropriate in the early stages of treatment. Effort is counterproductive and causes tightening of the P-E segment and reduction in volume. An amplifier enables the patient to relax and volume frequently increases spontaneously, continuing when the amplifier is switched off.

When pseudo-voice is well established, increase in volume of oesophageal voice can be achieved by stronger inspiration and expiration and slightly exaggerated articulation which increases the air reservoir and assists in more forceful ejection. Care must be taken to avoid forcing the voice and the development of tension and stoma blast. As the voice improves, volume improves spontaneously in many patients and, in all cases, it is related to relaxation.

Increase of range and flexibility of the vocal note

This is important if oesophageal voice is to emulate laryngeal intonation:

- Syllables with rising and falling intonation are practised.
- Short phrases and sentences said by the therapist with varying intonation and stress patterns are imitated by the patient.
- The patient places the forefinger and thumb on either side of the throat at the level of the pseudoglottis and experiments with varying pressures and changing note and pitch. This is repeated without external pressure while endeavouring to reproduce the necessary muscular adjustment by ear alone (Stetson, 1937).
- As the patient becomes more accomplished, singing familiar tunes can be attempted. Although the whole melody will not be possible, the mental concept of melody results in pitch changes. The attempt at singing also develops breathing technique and inhalation.
- Rhymes with emphasised rhythm can be used to encourage the normal rhythms of speech. These give an impression of improved intonation in connected utterance.

Development of intelligibility

The truly proficient speaker can be understood without being seen. This is essential if the telephone is to be used. A hierarchy of tasks helps to minimise failure:

- Ten easily produced words are listed which the patient reads aloud clearly while the speech–language pathologist watches. The clinician then looks away from the patient who says the words at random for repetition by the therapist. A score of identifiable words is kept for future comparison. This is repeated with different lists of words and phrases, until there is a consistently high achievement level, with the therapist identifying and helping to correct behaviours that reduce intelligibility.
- The patient lists words and phrases that are unknown to the therapist. It is advisable to confine the list to five words initially until reasonable success is assured. Gradually the lists and length of phrases can be increased until the patient reads from text, with the therapist repeating each phrase.
- Finally, telephone practice should be preceded by demonstrating the importance of holding the mouthpiece to the mouth so that the sound of air from the stoma is not amplified. Increased effort will reduce effectiveness. Ideally, the patient should have telephone practice from an adjacent room so that problems can be immediately analysed and discussed.

Common faults in oesophageal speech

The faults and difficulties that commonly arise in learning oesophageal speech are frequently the result of generalised tension, which interferes with the rhythmic coordination of articulation and respiration. It arises out of the excessive effort that the individual uses in the attempt to vocalise. The therapist must be able recognise these faults as soon as they show signs of developing, so that they are not allowed to become established.

Air swallowing

An excessive amount of air may be directed into the oesophagus and then enter the stomach, causing distension of the gas cap. This will cause considerable discomfort and the accidental eructation of air interrupts speech, to the embarrassment of the speaker, or causes uncontrolled voicing. Patients complain of indigestion and need explanation. This difficulty arises in patients who have been allowed to develop air swallowing or very forceful injection. Both faults must be eliminated as methods of air intake. The individual generally manages to make this adjustment after a few weeks and so prevent air from entering the stomach. It will be necessary to inspire less forcibly before speaking and also to reduce the over-forceful movements of the back of the tongue, which are nearly always found to accompany the intake of air in these patients.

Accumulation of air in the stomach may also be the result of poor diaphragmatic intercostal breathing. It is possible to hold the abdominal wall rigid and use upper thoracic breathing so that, in a fluent speaker, air enters the stomach inadvertently. Concentration on using the abdominal muscles to expel air during speech using the normal intercostal diaphragmatic method will correct this fault.

Stoma blast

Noisy exhalation of air from the stoma can be troublesome and the noise of exhaled air so loud that it masks the voice. This is generally the result of excessive effort in an attempt to eject air from the oesophagus and acquire a louder voice. Tension in the throat and upper thorax is evident, and as muscular tonicity increases the voice fades. Relaxation, central breathing, lack of effort and further drills in the easy injection and expulsion of air from the oesophagus must be practised. Practice with an amplifier is generally successful as the patient no longer strives to increase volume and, as a result, relaxes.

Bubbling in the trachea is of course difficult to avoid when mucus is present. It occurs in heavy smokers. The treatment of the chest condition is the only remedy. Patients who have learned to speak well often lose their voices with a respiratory infection as a result of excessive mucus. This can be readily understood in relation to the importance of breathing in the production of oesophageal voice. When speech deterioration takes place in these circumstances, the patient should be reassured by an explanation of its cause and be assured of its temporary nature.

Noisy air intake (klunk)

A gulping sound, rather like a noisy swallow, often precedes voice in the initial stages of voice acquisition. It is caused by air being forced under pressure through a tense P-E segment on air intake. The gulp occurs if over-forceful injection is employed. Air charging will also be noisy in patients using the inhalation method, when there is excessive glossopharyngeal tension. If 'klunk' becomes part of the kinaesthetic pattern of air charging and is not corrected immediately, it is extremely difficult to unlearn.

At the first signs of this problem, it is advisable to go back to the initial stages of the treatment programme with general relaxation and diaphragmatic breathing. Emphasis should be placed on the importance of a relaxed technique and less pharyngeal tension. Air intake with mouth shut and tongue-tip pressed behind the front teeth will help correction of the exaggerated posterior movement of the tongue when 'klunk' occurs with glossopharyngeal press.

Perseverance in improving the method of air intake is worth a temporary set-back in speech performance. This problem highlights the importance of ensuring maximum performance with minimal faults at each stage of treatment before progressing with the therapeutic plan. Use of an amplifier is recommended.

Double pump

This problem occurs in patients using the injection method. Instead of making one firm contact for air intake, a double or multiple 'munching' action is used. This inevitably impairs normal speech rhythms and is visually intrusive and confusing for the listener. It arises in the early stages when the laryngectomee lacks confidence in the newly learned skill of charging the oesophagus with air; the 'insurance policy' of a double pump is employed. If it appears as an emergent fault at the start of treatment, higher stages of the treatment plan should not be attempted until the patient is consistently achieving voice easily on syllables without the fault. If the behaviour pattern is established, a return to earlier stages of treatment is necessary.

Grimacing and 'button-holing'

Grimacing caused by over-exaggerated articulation is a minor problem that develops through the anxiety to be understood when the voice is weak. An inclination to 'button-hole' the listener and to stand too close for comfort may also develop for the same reasons. It is sufficient just to draw the individual's attention to these quite unconscious speech habits for them to be corrected. Video-recording will be useful at this stage with these patients.

Lack of fluency

Proficiency in the ability to obtain and maintain a sufficient air reservoir for phrases of more than a few words is mainly a matter of time. Poor coordination and poor breathing are the prime causes of limited phrase length, unless there is an inadequate P-E segment. The inveterate talker is the one who finds the limits imposed by laryngectomy the most frustrating; tense, rapid speech accompanied by gesticulation overrides the newly acquired technique of oesophageal voice. Insistence on slower speech, the need for patience and the reassurance that with correct technique voice duration will gradually be extended will improve the situation.

Even a slight and transient pharyngeal tension will render a proficient speaker speechless. The cricopharyngeal sphincter is as vulnerable to emotional changes in the laryngectomee as it is in the laryngeal speaker, and patients will lose their voices if embarrassed, angry or in any state of emotional upheaval. The voice may also be lost if attempts are made to shout in emotion, to call someone or to overcome background noise. Any increase in tension, however caused, will reduce the potential phrase length.

Progress assessment (oesophageal voice)

Assessment of the laryngectomee's progress can be divided into evaluation of pseudo-voice, communication skills and general rehabilitation (Perry, 1983). Rating scales are useful in providing objective measurements of progress and motivate therapist and patient to raise their aims and achieve more ambitious targets. Some scales are qualitative – as, for example, the seven-point scale devised by Wepman et al. (1953). Others, like Berlin's four-skills measurement (1963) are quantitative.

Wepman's oesophageal speech rating scale

This scale is based on the fact that, when developing oesophageal voice, most laryngectomees pass through recognised stages of development in a natural progression. The levels of the scale can be briefly described as follows.

Level Description

7   No oesophageal sound production; no speech. There is neither involuntary nor voluntary audible air movement through the P-E segment. At this level, the patient may not attempt to speak or is only 'mouthing' words.

6   Involuntary oesophageal sound production; no speech. Involuntary oesophageal sound occurs during speech and/or at rest. It indicates that although pseudo-voice is uncontrolled, the patient has the potential for oesophageal voice.

5   Voluntary sound production part of the time; no speech. The patient is able to produce some oesophageal sound at will, but in the early stages this is infrequent. Wepman et al. (1953) stress the importance of this level which demonstrates that voluntary control is possible in addition to confirming the suitability of the P-E segment for oesophageal sound production.

4   Voluntary sound production most of the time; vowel sounds differ-
     entiated; monosyllabic speech.
3   Oesophageal sound produced at will; single-word speech. Although
     there is no continuity, single words are produced with pseudo-voice.
2   Oesophageal sound produced at will with continuity; word grouping.
     Oesophageal speech is not automatic and the patient is conscious of
     careful production of pseudo-voice. Short phrases are voiced but
     oesophageal sound fails if the patient hurries in an attempt to
     increase phrase length.
1   Automatic oesophageal speech which is rapid, continuous, auto-
     matic and effortless.

Berlin's measurement of four skills

Berlin (1963) stressed that this scale is designed to chart progress in acquiring pseudo-voice in the early stages. It is not adequate for assessing the
overall efficiency of communication using oesophageal voice. Berlin's
patients were seen for half-hour treatments, two or three times daily. The
four skills are:

1   Ability to phonate reliably on demand. The patient is asked to inflate
     the oesophagus and to phonate /a:/. Twenty attempts are made. Only
     vocalisations lasting longer than 0.4 second are considered success-
     ful. A success rate of almost 100% after 10–14 days occurred in
     Berlin's patients who developed into good speakers.
2   Short latency between inflation of the oesophagus and vocalisation.
     Potentially good speakers can have an average latency of 0.5 second
     by day 18.
3   Adequate duration of phonation. The patient produces /a:/ for as
     long as possible after one inflation. This can be sustained for approx-
     imately 3 seconds by day 24 in good speakers.
4   Ability to sustain phonation during articulation. Eight to ten CV syl-
     lables on one inflation can be expected from a potentially good
     speaker by day 25.

Failure to achieve functionally useful oesophageal voice

There is general recognition that a substantial number of laryngectomees do
not achieve successful oesophageal voice. The incidence of failure is difficult
to establish because of the variability in standards of what constitutes good,
bad and indifferent. The basis for selection of cases varies between assessors
and the standards of assessment. Diedrich and Youngstrom (1966)

estimated that a third fail and Edwards (1976) agrees. Goode (1975) at the Stanford Medical Center placed failure rate as high as 50% and made the point that it takes 12 months of arduous endeavour to attain real proficiency. Blom, Singer and Hamaker (1986) also state that, although traditionally considered to be the method of choice, oesophageal voice cannot be achieved by more than half those patients who try to acquire it. They also qualify this statement by adding that the standard of oesophageal speech when acquired is very variable. Schaeffer and Johns (1982) note reports of success ranging from 98% to 25%, and conclude that it is reasonable to assume that at least one-third of laryngectomees fail to achieve satisfactory oesophageal communication. The reasons for failure are summarised in Table 17.14.

A videofluoroscopic study of eight good oesophageal speakers and 42 'failed' oesophageal speakers, carried out by Perry and Edels (1985), helped to clarify the various insufficiencies of the P-E segment which occur as a direct result of the type and extent of surgery. They concluded that the 'failed' oesophageal speakers could be divided into four groups, each with a clearly identifiable inadequacy of the P-E segment (Table 17.15).

Table 17.14 Reasons for failure to develop functionally useful oesophageal voice

Inadequate P-E segment	Hypotonic Hypertonic Spasmodic Stricture
Neurological damage	Damage to the pharyngeal and lingual nerve supply produces muscular weakness, especially of the tongue, which impedes air injection and articulation. Swallowing difficulties can also result from neurological damage
Amount and timing of radiotherapy	
Frailty and lack of motivation	
Deafness and inability to monitor speech	
Inability to initiate and develop the new skill	
Rejection of oesophageal speech	These patients may prefer to use 'whispered' speech or an electronic larynx
Previously inadequate speech	
Unsympathetic partner	
Partner with hearing loss	
Depression	
Quality and quantity of therapy	

Table 17.15 Insufficiencies of the P-E segment which occur as a direct result of the type and extent of surgery

P-E segment status	Description	Possible intervention
Group 1: hypotonic	P-E segment does not close and is functionally ineffective	Digital or neck band pressure may improve pseudo-voice by closing the P-E segment (Logemann, 1983b)
Group 2: hypertonic	P-E segment is constantly tense	The tightness of the P-E segment in both hypertonic and spasmodic groups can affect both air intake and expulsion. These groups may benefit from pharyngo-oesophageal myotomy (Henley and Souliere, 1986) or pharyngeal plexus neurectomy (Singer, Blom and Hamaker, 1986)
Group 3: spasmodic	Increase in oesophageal air pressure required for generating oesophageal voice causes spasm of the P-E segment	
Group 4: stricture	Fibrous tissue which does not dilate during swallowing. Some patients exhibit a pouch at the base of the tongue (Logemann, 1983b)	Surgical intervention may be necessary

After Perry and Edels (1985).

• Hypotonic (group 1)

In the hypotonic group, the P-E segment does not close and is functionally ineffective, resulting in a weak voice which may be improved by exerting digital pressure (Logemann, 1983b).

• Hypertonic (group 2) and spasmodic (group 3)

In the hypertonic group, the P-E segment is constantly tense whereas in the spasmodic group the increased air pressure occurring in attempted oesophageal speech causes the P-E segment to go into spasm. The tightness of the hypertonic and spasmodic groups can affect both air intake and expulsion, and it is this group that might benefit from P-E myotomy (Henley and Souliere, 1986) or pharyngeal plexus neurectomy (Singer, Blom and Hamaker, 1986).

• Stricture (group 4)

This was defined as fibrous tissue that did not dilate during swallowing; some of these patients exhibited the pouch at the base of the tongue described by Logemann (1983a) and discussed on page 600.

It is significant that all the patients in this study who failed to develop oesophageal speech had anatomical or physiological problems to account for their failure. Previously, failure to achieve voice had frequently been attributed to lack of motivation. The importance of motivation should not be undervalued, but this study highlights appropriate assessment of the P-E segment when voice is not developing satisfactorily. Videofluoroscopy can be an important tool in evaluation of the status of the P-E segment.

Insufficiencies of the P-E segment can be compounded by the other reasons for failure to develop oesophageal voice listed in Table 17.14.

Superior oesophageal voice

The good oesophageal speaker can become so fluent that strangers do not realise the true nature of the disability and may ask whether the speaker has a cold or laryngitis. The vocal profile in these cases relates relatively favourably to normal voice, but there are significant differences between oesophageal and laryngeal speakers. Table 17.16 lists the key features of superior oesophageal voice.

Pitch

Studies indicate that pitch and quality in oesophageal speech appear to be interdependent (Williams and Watson, 1985) as are pitch and intensity (Snidecor and Curry, 1959). Variations of intensity on the same frequency may induce impression of pitch change. To raise the pitch, greater volume has to be employed, necessitating replenishment of the oesophageal reservoir. For a drop in pitch, less intensity must be used. The accomplished speaker may have a range of an octave, but the fundamental pitch is an octave lower than normal voice. Damsté (1958), in a study of 20 male patients, found a median pitch of 67.5 Hz and Snidecor and Curry (1959) 63.3 Hz. Kallen (1934) noted that movements of the head and neck could contribute to pitch change and this aspect might be utilised for emphasis and expressiveness in speech. Understandably, oesophageal speakers with pitch levels and inflection variations approximating those of a laryngeal speaker are considered most acceptable (Hyman, 1979).

Table 17.16 Superior oesophageal voice

pitch	may have range of 1 octave (but fundamental pitch is an octave lower than normal voice)
duration	11–12 syllables per breath intake
speech rate	80–120 words per minute (laryngeal speakers 166 wpm)
short latency period second (i.e. time from start of injection or inhalation of air into oesophagus until pseudo-voice produced)	0.5 second
excellent articulation	

Snidecor and Curry (1960).

Duration

Length of phrase varies considerably. Snidecor and Curry (1960) measured the number of syllables per breath intake of superior laryngeal speakers. They found that the mean lowest consecutive sequence consisted of 3.8 syllables and the highest 8.7, with an overall average of 4.98 syllables. The extreme value in these subjects was 22 syllables in one speaker, but Snidecor (1968) considered that 11–12 syllables is a very satisfactory number for superior speakers.

Speech rate

Snidecor and Isshiki (1965) thought that the number of syllables per air charge was not of critical importance and that the speed of utterance is a preferable indicator of similarity to normal speech. A good average rate is between 80 and 120 words per minute (wpm), although a very superior speaker was found to achieve 153 wpm (laryngeal speakers have a rate of 166 wpm).

Latency period

Speech rate depends on the efficiency of the air charge. The latency period, from the start of injection or inhalation of air into the oesophagus until pseudo-voice is produced, is approximately 0.5 second in superior oesophageal speakers. Snidecor concluded:

> There is no magic in a long phrase. Clearness, ease of speech and reasonable rate of words per minute should take precedence over any struggle to break records in regard to words per air charge.

Articulation

Superior oesophageal speech is not attainable without excellent articulation, however good the oesophageal voice itself. Hyman (1979) noted that oesophageal speakers considered to be intelligible have articulation that is correctly identified 90% of the time.

Even in superior oesophageal speakers, the rough quality of the vocal note and the lack of vocal volume are inevitable problems. Although the quality of vowels may be improved by carefully adjusted articulation, much improvement of the partials is not feasible on account of the poor quality of the fundamental note (Snidecor, 1968). All speakers have difficulty making themselves heard against background noise. Clarke and Hoops (1970) found that laryngectomees' speech deteriorated with increased speech-type background noise as they tried to increase vocal volume. Although intelligibility was not reduced, there was a reduction in general speech proficiency, with a decrease in phrase length and increase in lung airflow. An amplifier can help to counteract this problem.

Pseudo-voice in the absence of a P-E segment

In pharyngolaryngectomy, as the upper portion of the oesophagus and the hypopharyngeal muscular tissue have been excised, the P-E segment is lost. Without the pseudo-glottis, fluent speech is much more difficult to acquire but voice is possible, with air being aspirated rather than injected. If there is sufficient narrowing of the reconstructed tube, vibration may be obtained for weak voice as the air is expelled. The air charge is under very little control during speech and is quickly lost, generally after one or two syllables. Consequently, air intake has to take place very frequently and, as a result, over-breathing and dizziness can develop. Pseudo-voice is tiring for the individual to maintain and, initially, the throat muscles tend to fatigue and ache. The voice may be deeper than oesophageal voice after simple laryngectomy.

Very rarely, the reconstructed oesophagus, without causing difficulty in swallowing, presents sufficient narrowing at some point to offer resistance to the outgoing air. Then the voice is produced as loudly and as fluently as that obtained by the patient who has undergone simple laryngectomy. Only one of our patients has obtained speech of such high standard, but Dornhurst and Negus (1954) stated that the difficulty in producing the necessary narrowing of the oesophagus should not be insuperable. Where no such narrowing exists, digital pressure on the front of the neck, a specially designed band or even a collar worn moderately tightly, may be sufficient to create an adequate pseudo-glottis.

Some patients develop the skill of vibrating air in the reconstructed pharynx on both ingoing and outgoing air. Air is moved in the new tract as the result of pressure changes achieved by rapid inspiration and expiration. No air injection takes place. This method of voice production can be a great advantage because it doubles the number of syllables for each air charge and speech can be fluent and rapid as a result, although the voice is weak. In these patients, the method frequently develops naturally and spontaneously and can be encouraged because of its effectiveness. It is not an appropriate method for acquiring oesophageal voice after simple laryngectomy.

General principles of therapy

Frequency and duration of therapy

Ideally, in the early stages of treatment, patients should be seen daily. If this is not possible, a minimum of two or three treatments per week is essential. The length of each treatment should be governed by the patient's recovery from the operation, the amount of direct work that can be tolerated, and the amount of counselling and supportive discussion necessary.

Some oesophageal sound should be achieved as early as possible and, by 3 months postoperatively, a substantial amount of oesophageal voice should be in use. A patient who is progressing satisfactorily can often be discharged or placed on less frequent appointments at this stage. If there is no functionally useful voice by 3 months, further investigation of the P-E segment should be considered if all other aspects of the treatment situation are satisfactory (Perry and Edels, 1985). Frequently, patients are still without voice at this stage, but subsequently develop satisfactory voice while persevering with therapy without any other intervention. It seems probable that these patients have a less than ideal P-E segment postoperatively, although not grossly abnormal, and that necessary adaptations of the hypopharynx occur which enable voice to be produced as the cut muscles recover function.

Less frequent visits may continue for about a year. In many instances, the oesophageal voice continues to improve during the 2 or 4 years after completion of formal therapy, before finally stabilising.

Practice

Regular practice of exercises achieved successfully in the clinic is essential reinforcement of the new behaviour patterns. Patients can practise for 5 minutes each hour in the early stages of treatment. Longer than this is inadvisable because muscle fatigue may cause deterioration in performance, which leads to discouragement and excessive effort in compensation. The therapist should clearly indicate the material to be practised. It is unwise for the patient to attempt tasks that have been unsuccessful in the clinical situation and where faulty technique may develop without guidance.

Group treatment

Most patients require individual attention from the speech–language pathologist during treatment, but group therapy can be a valuable supplement. The great difficulty, once voice is achieved, is in overcoming self-consciousness. The beginner feels oesophageal voice is conspicuous and socially unacceptable. Women especially may dislike the deep voice, which is harder to accept in the female than the male patient. Working in a group in a sympathetic atmosphere where everyone is in the same predicament breeds confidence, and gives the patient the courage eventually to speak freely at home and in the outside world. The congratulations and obvious pleasure of more experienced members of the group, when a newer member achieves and uses voice, is valuable encouragement and reinforcement. Laryngectomee teachers have been used in the USA.

Artificial (electronic) larynx voice (Figure 17.6(c) and 17.13)

The artificial larynx enables many patients to have audible speech if they are not using the P-E segment to produce sound. It can be used either before tracheo-oesophageal or oesophageal voice has been developed, in situations where the P-E segment voice is inefficient or as a permanent means of communication, if necessary. It provides a sound source external to the neck (Figures 17.13 and 17.6c). At one time, it was thought that patients would lose the motivation to produce oesophageal voice if allowed to use an artificial larynx in the early stages of recovery. As a result, artificial larynges were not supplied as a temporary expedient, but tended to be given to patients only when therapy to establish voice had failed, although authorities such as Diedrich and Youngstrom (1966), Gardner (1978) and Salmon (1978) strongly advocated their use in the early stages. As indwelling voice prostheses are used increasingly as a primary procedure, there may be less need for an artificial larynx in the early postoperative stage. Significant numbers of patients may not have effective P-E segment voice in all situations, however, and a pragmatic view is generally taken by laryngologists and speech–language pathologists now, with the patient's needs for an effective means of communication taking priority at any time

(Greene, Atkinson and Watson, 1974). Lauder (1968), himself a laryn-gectomee and speech pathologist, commented that the use of one mode of communication does not exclude another.

Most models consist of a hand-held sound generator with a vibrating diaphragm at one end which is held to the neck (or cheek in some cases) during speech. There are controls for adjusting volume, pitch and quality, although some models provide the possibility of intonation (e.g. Servox Intone). An intraoral speech aid, such as the Cooper Rand, delivers sound through a plastic tube, the tip of which is positioned in the mouth. Some of the 'neck' vibrators also have an oral adapter. This enables the patient to use an artificial larynx immediately after surgery or when the neck is unsuit-able for conventional artificial larynxes.

It should be remembered that the speech–language pathologist's train-ing and skill at interpreting speech of poor intelligibility can lead to overly optimistic judgements about laryngectomees' communicative effectiveness. McCroskey and Mulligan (1963), in rating the relative intelligibility of oesophageal and artificial larynx speech, discovered that naive listeners rated the artificial larynx as having higher intelligibility, whereas students and speech therapists rated oesophageal speech higher. Williams and Watson (1985) found that naive judges did not rate oesophageal speakers as being significantly more intelligible than electrolarynx speakers in their study

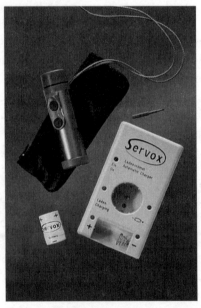

Figure 17.13 Artificial larynx. (Reproduced by permission of International Healthcare Technologies, 1110 Mark Avenue, Carpinteria, CA 93013-2918, USA.)

comparing oesophageal, tracheo-oesophageal and electrolarynx speakers. This study also produced the surprising result that the three laryngectomee groups were not rated differently on pitch and quality by naive or expert listeners. In fact, oesophageal and electrolarynx speakers were not rated significantly different in overall communication effectiveness.

In addition, the speech clinic is usually quiet and patients can be understood relatively easily in a relaxed one-to-one situation. Patients can find that, in the general noise of daily life, it is much more difficult to be easily understood even if voice is relatively well developed. In these circumstances, an artificial larynx can be a useful aid if it is not rejected by the patient on aesthetic and social grounds. Situations when an artificial larynx can be helpful are listed in Table 17.17.

Learning to use an artificial larynx

The speech–language pathologist should take as much care in introducing an artificial larynx, demonstrating its use and helping the patient to use it effectively, as in other sensitive therapeutic situations. Occasionally, patients readily accept the idea of the instrument and quickly adapt to this method of voicing. More frequently, there are concerns about being conspicuous in public and disliking the sound generated which are accompanied by feelings of embarrassment. The following stages are suggested to develop patients' skills with the artificial larynx:

Table 17.17 Rationale for providing an artificial larynx

Early postoperative stage when patient has not acquired pseudo-voice	particularly important if patient lives alone and needs to summon help by telephone
Pseudo-voice is ineffective in certain situations	e.g. on telephone, against background noise (particularly speech noise)
Enables patient to return to work	
Patient very tense	some patients are helped to relax as they receive auditory feedback and they know they can be heard. This can subsequently lead to easier acquisition of P-E voice
Partner with hearing impairment	
Advantages over P-E segment voice	no latency period: voicing is immediately available no physical effort
Failure to achieve P-E segment voice	
Patient prefers artificial larynx	some patients reject the 'belching' quality of oesophageal voice

- It should be explained that the vibrator only provides the sound source for speech and that the clarity and rate of utterance are provided by the speaker in the usual way.
- The speech–language pathologist demonstrates how it is used. This enables the patient to start to become accustomed to the mechanical sound. Patients are frequently surprised and disconcerted by the loudness of the artificial larynx when they use it themselves. Any steps that can be taken to desensitise a patient to the volume, before placing the instrument on the neck, are necessary in order to reduce the possibility of rejection.
- The patient can be given the opportunity to become familiar with the vibrator by handling it, getting used to the amount of pressure required on the button and trying it out on the palm of the hand. In this way, the importance of placing the whole of the vibrating diaphragm on to the skin surface becomes clear. If complete contact is not maintained unpleasant ambient noise occurs.
- In some patients, the area of the neck to be used for placement of the head of the artificial larynx is obvious. A flat area, near the original site of the larynx, which can be reached without changing head posture unnaturally, is ideal. Where surgery has been extensive, finding a suitable area may take some time. It is helpful to experiment with different artificial larynxes with varying head sizes. Occasionally, if considerable amounts of tissue have been removed, a patient will experience nausea if the vibrator is positioned too anteriorly. Some patients are able to use the vibrator on the cheek successfully. The optimal position for use is obvious when the patient is asked to articulate vowels, words, phrases and eventually connected speech.
- Having found the ideal position, it may be necessary to mark the patient's skin in some way, e.g. with a marker pen, until the movement of correct placement is automatic. The neck often lacks normal sensation and, as a result, it is difficult to find the right spot quickly which is essential for conversation. It can be helpful for certain patients to sit in front of a mirror and just practise placing the vibrator correctly. When this movement is established, the same task is carried out without visual monitoring.
- Practice is required in timing the onset and cut-off of 'voice' with articulation. Routine drills may be used initially such as counting, days of the week, etc. until conversational standard is reached.
- Some patients frequently need reminding that they only have to articulate, not attempt to produce voice. Other problems include the tendency to articulate silently and a demonstration of the sound of

articulation without voice is useful. Patients also try to separate syllables so that normal prosody is disrupted. Work on articulation and the preservation of normal prosody are essential elements of learning how to use an artificial larynx successfully.

There are several reasons why some patients cannot use an artificial larynx successfully (Table 17.18).

Attempts to introduce a vibrator should not be abandoned if they are unsuccessful initially. A patient may be able to use a vibrator efficiently, as neck anaesthesia resolves or attitude changes, even if there has been earlier failure. With patience and determination initial difficulties can frequently be overcome. Studies analysing the acoustic features and differences in speaking proficiencies of laryngeal, oesophageal, electronic larynx and tracheo-oesophageal speakers may be of interest to the reader (Robbins et al., 1984; Merwin, Goldstein and Rothman, 1985; Williams and Watson, 1985, 1987).

Common problems arising during rehabilitation

By the very nature of the major surgery that the laryngectomee has undergone, there will be various problems in most cases. The speech pathologist must be alert to the fact that the difficulties described by the patient may signal a serious underlying aetiology and that the otolaryngologist's

---

Table 17.18 Reasons for failure to use an artificial larynx

- inadequate pharyngeal air-filled space for conducting vibrations from the artificial larynx
- lack of sensation in the skin of the neck
- 'neck hardness' which does not conduct the vibrations
- inadequate or no flat sites of sufficient area (to accommodate head of artificial larynx)
- highly sensitive neck surface after radiotherapy
- hearing impairment
- reactions too slow or incoordinated to manipulate on–off button in synchrony with phrases
- nervousness dealing with a noisy item of equipment
- poor articulation and relatively closed oral cavity
- poor motivation
- preference for alternative methods of communication, even 'whisper'
- rejection of artificial larynx because, among other reasons, it signals the speaker's disability

---

opinion is necessary. Reassurance and advice outlining the appropriate strategies for dealing with the problem are generally sufficient.

Swallowing difficulties

In the early stages of recovery, the patient may need to adjust the rate at which food and drink are taken. If there is narrowing of the pharynx/oesophagus, a build-up of food may accumulate. Similarly, very rapid drinking, particularly of gassy drinks, may cause nasal regurgitation. It is usually sufficient to eat and drink more slowly. If the problem is severe and the dysphagia shows no sign of improving, further investigation will be necessary (see Swallowing page 600).

Throat tightening: 4–6 weeks postoperatively

Some patients are very perturbed that the throat tightens and swallowing may become more difficult in the early postoperative weeks. This appears to be related to healing processes and, in most cases, this sensation resolves in subsequent weeks but will need attention if it persists. Swallowing problems are common after extensive surgery and the dietitian's advice will be sought.

Debris from the stoma

Debris is sometimes expelled from the tracheostoma after surgery, and patients may be frightened by scabs that they expectorate. Examination by the otolaryngologist is advised.

Neck hardness

After radiotherapy and surgery, the neck and surrounding area may be extremely hard as a result of post-radiotherapy fibrosis and oedema. Although it does not entirely resolve, the stiffness becomes less obvious.

Leakage at the site of voice prosthesis in T-E puncture patients

Leakage through or round a voice prosthesis indicates that it needs changing (Doyle, 1994). Prostheses can usually be used for about 3 months; beyond this, leakage through the prosthesis is more likely to occur. When leakage occurs round the prosthesis, it might be caused by movement of the prosthesis which has enlarged the puncture. Expansion of the puncture might also be the result of more serious causes, such as migration of the puncture site, and should therefore be discussed with the surgeon.

Adverse listener reaction

People do not intend to be hurtful, but are often unintentionally tactless through simple embarrassment in the face of a misfortune that they do not understand. Instead of treating the patient normally, they may be over-sympathetic or apparently callous. It helps the patient to discuss listener reactions.

> **Case note**
>
> A transport driver who was excellently adjusted and spoke well before going back to work was infinitely depressed by his reception when he resumed his duties. He did not know, he said, which was the harder to bear: the men teasing him over his oesophageal voice, or the tender sympathy of the girl in the canteen whose eyes filled with tears whenever he asked for a cup of tea.

Laryngectomees frequently complain of the following reactions:

- The tendency to shout at the laryngectomee 'as if I were deaf and daft'.
- Whispering in reply to the patient.
- Not looking at the patient. Some listeners cannot make eye contact because of their embarrassment, while others turn their ear to the laryngectomee in an attempt to hear more successfully, when 'lip-reading' is much more effective.
- Cutting conversations short. This is perhaps understandable on the part of the listener who is having difficulty in understanding an inexperienced speaker, but it is still hurtful.
- The 'Does he take sugar?' syndrome of speaking to the laryngectomee through a companion.
- The listener who pretends to understand what is being said, when asking for clarification would be the less complicated and kinder course.
- The listener writing down the response to the laryngectomee when the patient is using written communication.
- Adverse reactions on the telephone. These occur when the patient is telephoning a stranger and fall into two broad categories. The listener may think that the laryngectomee is joking and putting on a funny voice, in which case he laughs or becomes angry. Alternatively, the listener thinks that he is answering an obscene call so he subjects the caller to abuse or slams down the handset. These reactions on the telephone can be reduced if laryngectomees state immediately that they have had a throat operation that has affected the voice. If a laryngectomee is anxious about using the telephone, voice may be slow in starting or fail when the call is answered so that the recipient puts down the receiver. Some people find it helpful to have an

introductory sentence pre-recorded which clarifies the situation and allows the patient to relax before speaking. A telephone with an integral amplifier is useful for the patient with quiet oesophageal voice.

Frustration with reactions such as these are frequently greatest in the home. The family can be advised not to expect too much at first, to watch the patient's lips, to listen without interruption and to make every endeavour to understand. The partner should be advised not to pursue everyday tasks when being addressed, but to encourage speech in every way possible. The use of a self-erasing pad is better than the patient suffering the exasperation of not being understood in the early stages of acquiring voice.

Stoma management

Practical management of the tracheostoma is discussed on page 598. Adverse reactions to the patient can be reduced by careful management of the stoma. Laryngectomy protectors fulfil a practical and aesthetic function, of which some patients will need to be made aware if they are to be successfully rehabilitated. It is not socially acceptable for the laryngectomee to leave the stoma unprotected and most patients take care to dress suitably. Some patients do not appear to be sensitive about their appearance or perhaps wish to obtain sympathy by drawing attention to their disability, leaving the stoma uncovered. A man can wear a collar and tie if he wishes, or a cravat. The Romet filter is popular with men and women because it looks like a sweater but the stoma remains accessible after coughing for wiping away mucus. If a shirt or blouse is buttoned up to the neck the second button can be removed from the shirt edge and sewn to the site of the button hole so that the shirt looks properly buttoned but the opening provides access for cleaning the stoma. Blouses with high necklines or bows look attractive, and scarves and jewellery can also be used without impairing breathing.

Laryngectomy clubs

Counselling and emotional support from the speech–language pathologist is an integral part of vocal rehabilitation, but membership of a laryngectomy club is invaluable as a source of additional support and information for laryngectomees and their families. No one can give more sincere and realistic help in adjustment to all the physical changes in a laryngectomee that are to have widespread repercussions in everyday life than another laryngectomee. This fact is clearly illustrated in the book *Laryngectomy is Not a Tragedy* by Norgate (1984), himself a laryngectomee and founder of the Cancer Laryngectomy Trust.

Anxieties and questions about breathing, speaking, coughing, nose blowing and other aspects of changes that may be embarrassing or infuriating can be discussed with others who have encountered these problems. Horror may be felt at the prospect of permanently breathing through a 'hole in the neck' and fears concerning loss of sexual attractiveness torment both men and women. These issues can be explained by professional staff, but relaxing with other laryngectomees, sharing the same problems and visiting a club where partners can meet makes the stressful early days easier for both patient and family (Parkes, 1975).

In Britain, the National Association of Laryngectomee Clubs (NALC), affiliated to the International Association of Laryngectomees founded by Warren Gardner in the USA, promotes rehabilitation through clubs run by laryngectomees, usually with the support of a speech–language pathologist. These associations provide up-to-date information about speech aids for laryngectomees, emergency cards and stickers identifying their condition in case of accident, and regular newsletters. In the USA, the American Cancer Society also provides support for laryngectomees. Many clubs also seek to publicise the existence of this patient group and its problems by arranging meetings with members of police, fire, ambulance and medical services. In particular, the importance of mouth-to-neck resuscitation and the necessity for emergency services to be on the alert for neck breathers is emphasised.

The traditional objection to laryngectomee clubs is that deaths are depressing for the remaining members, but our experience is that patients in these groups are generally realistic about their situation. When a member is ill, the support the group gives is encouraging for all concerned and, if death occurs, the partner derives comfort from being able to talk to club members who have become understanding friends. Inevitably, a death causes grief but, on balance, the benefits of a club outweigh the potential disadvantages.

Quality of life

Patients' effective communication and postoperative quality of life, in combination with their health and safety, are the overriding considerations in rehabilitation after laryngectomy. The individual's preferences must be taken into account as the range of possible methods of communication are explained and demonstrated. The acknowledgement by the professionals involved in the treatment of patients with laryngeal carcinoma that quality of life is of prime importance, as opposed to survival alone, is demonstrated by the proliferation of papers on this subject in recent years (Antonio et al., 1996; Finizia et al., 1998; Young et al., 1998; Wax et al., 1999).

Summary

- Laryngeal carcinoma in its early stages responds well to treatment.
- In advanced cases, total laryngectomy is carried out as a life-saving procedure.
- There are three methods by which oral communication can become audible after total laryngectomy: surgical voice restoration (T-E puncture); oesophageal voice; and the use of an artificial larynx.
- The speech–language pathologist, working as a member of a coordinated team, assesses and treats the patient whichever method of communication is instituted.
- Care of the patient involves more than making speech audible. The role of the speech–language pathologist is also to explain, support and encourage pre- and postoperatively, while enabling the patient to achieve optimal oral communication.
- Enabling the patient to develop suitable pseudo-voice is one aspect of rehabilitation towards an acceptable quality of life, which is the aim of the clinical team.

Appendices

Appendix A Fairbanks' 'Rainbow Passage'

When the sunlight strikes raindrops in the air, they act like a prism and form a rainbow. The rainbow is a division of white light into many beautiful colours. These take the shape of a long round arch, with its path high above and its end apparently beyond the horizon. There is, according to legend, a boiling pot of gold at one end. People look, but no one ever finds it. When a man looks for something beyond his reach his friends say he is looking for the pot of gold at the end of the rainbow.

Throughout the centuries men have explained the rainbow in various ways. Some have accepted it as a miracle without physical explanation. To the Hebrews it was a token that there would be no more universal floods. The Greeks used to imagine that it was a sign from the gods to fortell war or heavy rain. The Norsemen considered the rainbow as a bridge over which the gods passed from the earth to their home in the sky.

Other men have tried to explain the phenomenon physically. Aristotle thought that the rainbow was caused by the reflection of the sun's rays by the rain. Since then physicists have found that is not reflection, but refraction by the raindrops which causes the rainbow. Many complicated ideas about the rainbow have been formed. The difference in the rainbow depends considerably upon the size of the water drops, and the width of the colored band increases as the size of the drops increases. The actual primary rainbow observed is said to be the effect of superposition of a number of bows. If the red of the second bow falls upon the green of the first, the result is to give a bow with an abnormally wide yellow band, since red and green lights when mixed form yellow. This is a very common type of bow, one showing mainly red and yellow, with little or no green or blue.

(Fairbanks,G. [1960] Voice and Articulation Drill Book (2nd edn.) New York: Harper)

Appendix B Vocal Profile Analysis Protocol

Speaker: _____   Sex: _____   Age: _____

I VOCAL QUALITY FEATURES

CATEGORY	FIRST PASS			SECOND PASS						
	Neutral	Non-neutral		SETTING	Scalar Degrees					
					1	2	3	4	5	6
Vocal Tract										
1. Labia				Lip Rounding/Protrusion						
				Lip Spreading						
				Labiodentalization						
				Extensive Range						
				Minimised Range						
2. Mandibular				Close Jaw						
				Open Jaw						
				Protruded Jaw						
				Extensive Range						
				Minimised Range						
3. Lingual Tip/Blade				Advanced						
				Retracted						
4. Lingual Body				Fronted Body						
				Backed Body						
				Raised Body						
				Lowered Body						
				Extensive Range						
				Minimised Range						
5. Velopharyngeal				Nasal						
				Audible Nasal Escape						
				Denasal						
6. Pharyngeal				Constriction						
7. Larynx Position				Raised						
				Lowered						
Phonation Type										
				Harshness						
				Whisper(y)						
				Creak(y)						
				Falsetto						
				Modal Voice						
Tension										
8. Supralaryngeal				Tense						
				Lax						
9. Laryngeal				Tense						
				Lax						

"VOCAL PROFILES OF SPEECH DISORDERS" Research Project. (M.R.C. Grant No. G978/1192)
Phonetics Laboratory, Department of Linguistics, University of Edinburgh.
© 1981 revised 1988.

Date of Analysis: _____ Tape: _____ Judge: _____

II PROSODIC FEATURES

CATEGORY	Neutral	SETTING	MILD	MOD	EXTREME
1. Pitch		High Mean			
		Low Mean			
		Wide Range			
		Narrow Range			
		High Variability			
		Low Variabaility			
2. Loudness		High Mean			
		Low Mean			
		Wide Range			
		Narrow Range			
		High Variability			
		Low Variability			
3. Tremor		Present			

III COMMENTS

CATEGORY	FIRST PASS		SECOND PASS		
	Appropriate	Inappropriate	Scalar Degree Inappropriate		
			1		3
1. Breath Support					
2. Continuity		Interrupted			
3. Rate		Fast			
		Slow			
4. Rhythmicality					
5. Other (including posture, diplophonia, etc.)					

SPECIMEN

Reproduced by permission of Professor John Laver, Dr S. Wirz, Dr J. Mackenzie-Beck and Dr S.M. Hiller.

Appendix C Manufacturers' addresses (equipment referred to in the text)

InHealth
International Healthcare Technologies
1110 Mark Avenue
Carpinteria
CA 93013-2918
USA
Tel: 800-477-5969   Fax: 805-684-8594
http://www.inhealth.com
(Products for laryngectomees)

UK distributor of InHealth products:
Forth Medical Limited
Forth House
42 Kingfisher Court
Hambridge Road
Newbury, Berkshire RG14 5SJ
UK
Tel: 01635-550100   Fax: 01635-550050

Kay Elemetrics Corporation
2 Bridgewater Lane
Lincoln Park, NJ 07035-1488
USA
Tel: 1-800-289-5297
e-mail: sales@kayelemetrics.com   www.kayelemetrics.com

UK Suppliers of Kay products:
Wessex Electronics Ltd
114 -118 North Street
Downend
Bristol BS16 5SE
UK
Tel: 0117-957-1404   e-mail: Sales@wessexm.freeserve.co.uk

Karl Storz Endoscopy (UK) Ltd
392 Edinburgh Avenue
Slough
Berkshire SL1 4UF
UK
Tel: 01753-503500   Fax: 01753-578124

The 3Ears Company Ltd
PO Box 3461
London NW8 0AF
UK
Fax: (44) 20 7372 1788
and
PO Box 34 S - 193 21 Sigtuna
Sweden
Fax: + 46 8 592 512 70

(Video Textbook: Assessing Dysphonia: The Role of Videostroboscopy by Drs Guy Cornut and Marc Bouchayer)

Appendix D Organisations

The British Voice Association (BVA)
at The Royal College of Surgeons
35/43 Lincoln's Inn Fields
London WC2A 3PN
UK
Tel: +44(0)20 7831 1060
e-mail: bva@dircon.co.uk   www.bva.dircon.co.uk/

The Voice Foundation
1721 Pine Street
Philadelphia
PA 19103
USA
Tel: (215) 735-7999   Fax: (215)735-9293
http.//www.voicefoundation.org/

The International Association of Laryngectomees (IAL)
7440 North Shadeland Avenue
Suite 100
Indianapolis
IN 46250
USA
Tel: 317-570-4568   Fax: 317-570-4570

The American Cancer Society
Tel: 1-800-ACS-2345 (In USA)
http://www.cancer.org

Motor Neurone Disease Association
David Niven House
10-15 Notre Dame Mews
Northampton
NN1 2PR
UK
Tel: 01604-250505   Fax: 01604-624726
Helpline: 08457-626262 (Monday-Friday 9.00am - 10.30pm)

The Multiple Sclerosis National Centre
372 Edgware Road
London NW2 6ND
UK
Tel: 020 8438 0700   Fax: 020 8438 0701
http://www.mssociety.org.uk/

Royal National Institute for Deaf People (RNID)
PO Box 16464
London EClY 8TT
UK
Tel: 0808 808 9000   Fax: 020 7296 8199
e-mail: helpline@rnid.org.uk

National Association of Laryngectomee Clubs (NALC, UK)
Ground Floor
6 Rickett Street
London SW6 1 RU
UK
Tel: 020 7381 9993   www.members.aol.com/nalcuk.index.htm

The Parkinson's Disease Society
215 Vauxhall Bridge Road
London SW1V 1EJ
UK
Tel: 020 7931 8080

The American Parkinson Disease Association, Inc.
1250 Hylan Boulevard, Suite 4B
Staten Island, NY 10305-1946
USA
Tel: 718-981-8001   Fax: 718-981-4399
http://apdaparkinson.com/newlogo.htm

References

ABBERTON E (1987) An introduction to voice research within phonetics departments within the UK. Voice Research Society Newsletter 2(3).

ABBERTON E (2000) Voice quality of deaf speakers. In: Voice Quality Measurement. Kent RD, Ball MJ, eds. San Diego: Singular.

ABBERTON E, FOURCIN A (1984) Electro-laryngography in Clinical Phonetics, Code C, Ball M, eds. London: Croom Helm.

ABBERTON ERM, HOWARD DM, FOURCIN AJ (1989) Laryngographic assessment of normal voice: a tutorial. Clinical Linguistics and Phonetics 3: 281-296.

ABERCROMBIE D (1967) Elements of General Phonetics. Edinburgh: Edinburgh University Press.

ABITBOL J, de BRUX J, MILLOT G et al. (1989) Does a hormonal vocal cord cycle exist in women? Study of vocal premenstrual syndrome in voice performers by videostroboscopy-glottography and cytology on 38 women. Journal of Voice 3: 157-162.

ABRAMSON AL, STEINBERG BM, WINKLER B (1987) Laryngeal papillomatosis: clinical, histopathologic and molecular studies. Laryngoscope 97: 678.

ADDINGTON DW (1968) The relationship of selected vocal characteristics to personality perception. Speech Monographs 35: 429.

AGGER WA, SEAGER GM (1985) Granulomas of the vocal cords caused by Sporothrix schenkii. Laryngoscope 95: 595.

AKERLUND L, GRAMMING P (1994) Average loudness level, mean fundamental frequency and subglottal pressure: Comparison between female singers and non-singers. Journal of Voice 8: 263-270.

ALEXANDER FM (1942) The Universal Constant in Living. London: Chaterson.

ALLAN CM (1970) Treatment of non-fluent speech resulting from neurological disease - treatment of dysarthria. British Journal of Disorders of Communication 5: 3-5.

ALLEN GW (1984) Neoplasms of the thyroid gland. In: Otolaryngology, Vol. 5. English GM, ed. New York: Harper & Row.

ALLEN KD, BERNSTEIN B, CHAIT DH (1991) EMG biofeedback treatment of pediatric hyperfunction dysphonia. Journal of Behavioural Therapy and Experimental Psychiatry 22: 97-101.

ALVIN J (1961) Music therapy and the cerebral palsied child. Cerebral Palsy Bulletin 3: 255.

AMADO JH (1953) Tableau général des problèmes posés par l'action des hormones sur le développement du larynx. Annales d'Otolaryngologie (Paris) 70: 117.

ANDERSSON K, SCHALEN L (1998) Etiology and treatment of psychogenic voice disorders. Journal of Voice 12 No 1: 96-106.

ANDREWS AH, MOSS HW (1974) Experience with carbon dioxide laser in the larynx. Annals of Otology 83: 462.

ANDREWS JC, MICKEL RA, HANSON DG, MONAHAN GP, WARD PH (1987) Major complications following tracheoesophageal puncture for voice rehabilitation. Laryngoscope 97: 562.

ANDREWS ML (1991) Voice Therapy for Children. San Diego: Singular Publishing.

ANDREWS ML (1995) Manual of Voice Treatment: Pediatrics through geriatrics. San Diego: Singular.

ANDREWS ML, SCHMIDT CP (1995) Congruence in personality between clinician and client: relationship to ratings of voice treatment. Journal of Voice 9: 261-269.

ANDREWS S, WARNER J, STEWART R (1986) EMG biofeedback and relaxation in the treatment of hyperfunctional dysphonia. British Journal of Disorders of Communication 21: 353.

ANTONIO LL, ZIMMERMAN GJ, CELLA DF, LONG S (1996) Quality of life and functional status measures in patients with head and neck cancer. Archives of Otolaryngology Head and Neck Surgery 122: 482-487.

ARGYLE M (1970) The Psychology of Interpersonal Behaviour. Harmondsworth: Penguin.

ARNOLD GE (1957) Vocal rehabilitation of paralytic dysphonia III. Present concepts of laryngeal paralysis. Archives of Otolaryngology 65: 317.

ARNOLD GE (1958) Dysplastic dysphonia. Laryngoscope 68: 142.

ARNOLD GE (1962) Vocal nodules and polyps: Laryngeal tissue reaction to habitual hyperkinetic dysphonia. Journal of Speech Disorders 27, 205.

ARNOLD GE, HEAVER L (1959) Spastic dysphonia. Logos 2, 3.

ARONSON AE (1971) Early motor neurone disease masquerading as psychogenic breathy dysphonia - a clinical case presentation. Journal of Speech and Hearing Disorders 36: 115.

ARONSON AE (1980) Clinical Voice Disorders. New York: Thième.

ARONSON AE (1990) Clinical Voice Disorders, 3rd edn. New York: Thième.

ARONSON AE, DE SANTO LW (1983) Adductor spastic dysphonia: three years after recurrent laryngeal nerve re-section. Laryngoscope 93: 1.

ARONSON AE, HARTMAN DE (1981) Adductor spastic dysphonia: a sign of essential (voice) tremor. Journal of Speech and Hearing Disorders 46: 52-58.

ARONSON AE, BROWN JR, LITIN EM, PEARSON JS (1968a) Spastic dysphonia 1. Voice, neurologic and psychiatric aspects. Journal of Speech Disorders 33: 203.

ARONSON AE, BROWN JR, LITIN EM, PEARSON JS (1968b) Spastic dysphonia 2. Comparison with essential (voice) tremor and other neurologic and psychogenic disorders. Journal of Speech Disorders 33: 219.

ARONSON A, McCAFFREY T, LICHY W, LIPTON R (1993) Botulinum toxin injection for adductor spastic dysphonia: patient self-ratings of voice and phonatory effort after three successive injections. Laryngoscope 103:683-692.

ARSLAN M, SERAFINI I (1972) Restoration of laryngeal functions after total laryngectomy in the first 25 cases. Laryngoscope 82: 1319.

ASAI R (1972) Laryngoplasty after total laryngectomy. Archives of Otolaryngology 95: 114.

ATEN JL, McDONALD A, SIMPSON M, GUTTIERREZ R (1984) In: The Dysarthrias: Physiology, acoustics, perception, management. McNeil MR, Rosenbek JC, Aronson AE, eds. College Hill Press.

ATKINSON J (1978) Correlation analysis of the physiological factors controlling fundamental voice frequency. Journal of the Acoustical Society of America 63: 211-222.

AVIV JE (1997) Effects of aging on sensitivity of the pharyngeal and supraglottic areas. American Journal of Medicine 103: 74S-76S.

AWAN SN, FRENKEL ML (1994) Improvements in estimating the harmonics-to-noise ratio of the voice. Journal of Voice 8: 255-262.

BACHYNSKI JE, VYAS US (1976) A radiological and clinical correlative study of laryngeal abnormalities seen in Northern Alberta. Journal of Otolaryngology 5: 213-220.

BAER T, SASAKI C, HARRIS K, eds (1991). Laryngeal Function in Phonation and Respiration. San Diego: Singular Publishing Group Inc.

BAKEN RJ (1977) Estimation of lung volume change from torso hemicircumference. Journal of Speech and Hearing Research 20: 808.

BAKEN RJ (1987) Clinical Measurement of Speech and Voice. London: Taylor & Francis.

BAKEN RJ (1994) The aged voice: a new hypothesis. Voice 3(2): 57-73.

BAKEN RJ (1995) Into a chaotic future. In: Diagnosis and Treatment of Voice Disorders, Rubin JS, Sataloff RT, Korovin GS, Gould WJ, eds. New York: Igaku-Shoin.

BAKEN RJ, ORLIKOFF RF (1991) Phonatory response to step-function changes in supraglottal pressure. In: Laryngeal Function in Phonation and Respiration, Baer T, Saski C, Harris KS, eds. San Diego: Singular Publishing Group Inc.

BAKEN RJ, ORLIKOFF RE (1992) Acoustic assessment of vocal function. In: Neurologic Disorders of the Larynx, Blitzer A, Brin MF, Sasaki CT, Fahn S, Harris KS, eds. New York: Thième.

BAKEN RJ, ORLIKOFF RF (2000) Clinical Measurement of Speech and Voice, 2nd edn. San Diego: Singular.

BAKER DC, SAVETSKY L (1966) Congenital partial atresia of the larynx. Laryngoscope 77: 616.

BALL MJ (1996) Describing voice quality: transcription and instrumentation. Logopedics Phoniatrics Vocology 21: 59-63.

BALL MJ, ESLING J, DICKSON C (2000) Transcription of voice quality. In: Voice Quality Measurement, Kent RD, Ball MJ, eds. San Diego: Singular.

BALLANTYNE JC, GROVES J (1982) A Synopsis of Otolaryngology, 3rd edn. Bristol: John Wright & Sons.

BARIMO JP, HUBAL MB, SCHEUERLE J, RITTERMAN SJ (1987) Postnatal palatoplasty: implications for normal speech articulation. Scandinavian Journal of Plastic and Reconstructive Surgery 21: 139.

BARLOW W (1959) Anxiety and muscle tension pain. British Journal of Clinical Practice 13: 339.

BARON A, JOURNEY W (1989) Age differences in manual versus vocal reaction times: further evidence. Journal of Gerontology: Psychological Services 44: 157-159.

BARTELLI TE, FORD CN, BLESS DM (1986) Teflon injection of vocal folds: an analysis of poor results. IALP 20th Congress Report, Vol 2, Abstract 17: 283.

BARTON RT (1965) Life after laryngectomy. Laryngoscope 75: 1408.

BASSICH CJ, LUDLOW C (1986) The use of perceptual methods by new clinicians for assessing voice quality. Journal of Speech and Hearing Disorders 51: 125.

BASTIAN RW, NAGORSKY MJ (1987) Laryngeal image biofeedback. Laryngoscope 97: 1346-1349.

BATEMEN GH, NEGUS VE (1954) Speech after Laryngectomy. British Surgical Progress. London: Butterworth.

BAUGH RF, LEWIN JS, BAKER SR (1987) Preoperative assessment of tracheoesophageal speech. Laryngoscope 97: 461-466.

BAYNES RA (1966) An incidence study of chronic hoarseness in children. Journal of Speech Disorders 31: 172-176.

BENNET S, BISHOP S, LUMPKIN SMM (1987) Phonatory characteristics associated with bilateral diffuse polypoid degeneration. Laryngoscope 97: 446-450.

BENNINGER MS, AHUJA AS, GARDNER G, GRYWALSKI C (1998) Assessing outcomes for dysphonic patients. Journal of Voice 12: 540-550.

BENTZEN N, GULD A, RASMUSSEN H (1976) X-ray videotape studies of laryngectomised patients. Journal of Laryngology 90: 655.

BERKOWITZ JF, LUCENTE FE (1985)

Counselling before laryngectomy. Laryngoscope 95: 1332.

BERLIN CI (1963) Clinical measurement of esophageal speech: I. Methodology and curves of skill acquisition. Journal of Speech and Hearing Disorders 28: 42.

BERNSTEIN L (1979) Cleft Lip and Palate in Otolaryngology, 4th edn, English GM, ed. New York: Harper & Row,

BERRY DA, HERZEL H, TITZE IR, KRISCHER K (1994) Interpretation of biomechanical simulations of normal and chaotic vocal fold oscillations with empirical eigen-functions. Journal of the Acoustical Society of America 95: 3595-3604.

BERRY RJ (1983) Radiotherapy and chemotherapy. In: Laryngectomy: Diagnosis to rehabilitation. Edels Y, ed. London: Croom Helm.

BERRY R, EPSTEIN R, FOURCIN A, FREEMAN M, MacCURTAIN F, NOSCOE N (1982) An objective analysis of voice disorders (Part 1 and 2). British Journal of Disorders of Communication 17: 67.

BHATNAGAR SC, ANDY OJ (1995) Neuroscience for the Study of Communicative Disorders. Baltimore: Williams & Wilkins.

BIEVER DM, BLESS DM (1989) Vibratory characteristics of the vocal folds in young adult and geriatric women. Journal of Voice 3: 120-131.

BILLER HF, LAWSON W (1986) Partial laryngectomy for vocal cord cancer with marked limitation or fixation of the vocal cord. Laryngoscope 96: 61-64.

BIRRELL JF (1986) Paediatric Otolaryngology, 2nd edn. Bristol: Wright.

BLESS DM (1991a) Assessment of laryngeal function. Phonosurgery: Assessment and Surgical Management of Voice Disorders 95-122.

BLESS DM (1991b) Measurement of vocal function. Otolaryngologic Clinics of North America 24: 1023-1033.

BLESS DM, ABBS JH, eds (1983) Vocal Fold Physiology. San Diego: College Hill Press.

BLESS D, HIRANO M, FEDER RJ (1987) Videostroboscopic examination of the

larynx. Ear, Nose and Throat Journal 66: 289-296.

BLITZER A, BRIN M (1991) Laryngeal dystonia: a series with botulinum toxin therapy. Annals of Otology, Rhinology and Laryngology 100: 85-89.

BLITZER A, LOVELACE RE, BRIN MF, FAHN S, FINK ME (1985) Electromyographic findings in focal laryngeal dystonia (spastic dysphonia). Annals of Otology, Rhinology and Laryngology 94: 591-594.

BLITZER A, BRIN MK, FAHN S, LOVELACE RE (1988) Localized injections of botulinum toxin for treatment of focal laryngeal dysphonia (spasmodic dysphonia). Laryngoscope 98: 193-197.

BLOM ED, SINGER MI, HAMAKER RC (1982) Tracheostoma valve for postlaryngectomy voice rehabilitation. Annals of Otology 91: 576.

BLOM ED, SINGER MI, HAMAKER RC (1985) An improved esophageal insufflation test. Archives of Otolaryngology 111: 211.

BLOM ED, SINGER MI, HAMAKER RC (1986) A prospective study of tracheoesophageal speech. Archives of Otolaryngology, Head and Neck Surgery 112: 440.

BLOOD GW (1994) Efficacy of computer-assisted treatment protocol. American Journal of Speech Pathology 3: 57-66.

BONE RC (1986) Laryngeal papillomatosis. In: Otolaryngology, Vol 3. English GM, ed. New York: Harper & Row.

BONE RC, FEREN AP, NAHUM AM (1976) Laryngeal papillomatosis: immunologic and viral basis of therapy. Laryngoscope 86: 341.

BOONE DR (1977) The Voice and Voice Therapy, 2nd edn. New Jersey: Prentice Hall.

BOONE DR, McFARLANE SC (1988) The Voice and Voice Therapy, 4th edn. New Jersey: Prentice Hall.

BORNHOLT A (1983) Interferon therapy for laryngeal papillomatosis in adults. Archives of Otolaryngology 109: 550.

BOSMA JF (1953) Studies of disabilities of the pharynx resultant from poliomyelitis. Annals of Otology (St Louis) 62: 529.

BOUCHAYER M, CORNUT G, LOIRE R, WITZIG E, ROCH JB (1985) Epidermoid cysts, sulci, and mucosal bridges of the true vocal cord: a report of 157 cases. Laryngoscope 95: 1087-1093.

BOULET MJ, ODDENS BJ (1996) Female voice changes around and after the menopause - an initial investigation. Maturitas. Journal of the Climacteric and Postmenopause 23: 15-21.

BOWDEN REM (1972) Innervation of intrinsic laryngeal muscles. In: Ventilatory and Phonatory Control Systems, Wyke B, ed. Oxford: Oxford University Press.

BRADLEY PJ, NARULA A (1987) Clinical aspects of pseudodysphagia. Journal of Laryngology and Otology 101: 689.

BRAIN WR (1969) Brain's Clinical Neurology, 6th edn (revised by R Bannister). Oxford: Oxford University Press.

BRALLEY RC, BULL GL, GORE CH, EDGERTON MT (1978) Evaluation of vocal pitch in male transsexuals. Journal of Communication Disorders 11: 443-449.

BRANDWEIN M, ABRAMSON AL, SHIKOWITZ MJ (1986) Bilateral vocal cord paralysis following endotracheal intubation. Archives of Otolarynology Head and Neck Surgery 112: 877.

BRIDGEMAN E, SNOWLING M (1988) The perception of phonemic sequence: a comparison of dyspraxic and normal children. British Journal of Disorders of Communication 23: 245.

BRIDGER, MW, EPSTEIN R (1983) Functional voice disorders; a review of 109 patients. Journal of Laryngology and Otology 97: 1145-1148.

BRIDGES A (1991) Acceptability ratings and intelligibility scores of alaryngeal speakers by three listener groups. British Journal of Disorders of Communication 26: 325-335.

BRITISH ASSOCIATION OF OTORHINOLARYN-GOLOGISTS, HEAD AND NECK SURGEONS (1998) Effective Head and Neck Cancer Management: Consensus Document. London: Royal College of Surgeons.

BRODNITZ FS (1959) Vocal Rehabilitation. Rochester, MN: American Academy of Ophthalmology and Otolaryngology.

BRODNITZ FS (1961) Contact ulcer of the larynx. Annals of Otology 74: 90.

BRODNITZ FS (1971) Vocal Rehabilitation. Rochester, MN: American Academy of Ophthalmology and Otolaryngology.

BRODNITZ FS (1988) Keep your Voice Healthy. New York: Taylor & Francis.

BRODNITZ FS, CONLEY JJ (1967) Vocal rehabilitation after reconstructive surgery for laryngeal cancer. Folia Phoniatrica 19: 89.

BRONDBO K, ALBERTI PW, CROWSON N (1983) Adult recurrent multiple laryngeal papilloma. Acta Otolaryngologica 95: 431.

BROWN RG, MacCARTHY B, GOTHAM AM, DER GJ, MARSDEN CD (1988) Depression and disability in Parkinson's Disease: a follow-up study of 132 cases. Psychological Medicine 18: 49.

BUCKINGHAM H (1979) Explanation in apraxia with consequences for the concept of apraxia of speech. Brain and Language 8: 202.

BUMSTEAD RM (1982) Velopharyngeal incompetence. In: Otolaryngology, 4th edn. English GM, ed. New York: Harper & Row.

BUNCH MA (1976) A cephalometric study of structures of the head and neck during sustained phonation of covered and open qualities. Folia Phoniatrica 28: 321.

BUNCH MA (1982) Dynamics of the Singing Voice. Vienna: Springer-Verlag.

BURNS P (1986) Acoustical analysis of the underlying voice differences between two groups of professional singers: opera and country and western. Laryngoscope 96: 549.

BURSTEIN FD, CALCATERRA TC (1985) Supraglottic laryngectomy: series report and analysis of results. Laryngoscope 95: 833.

BUTCHER P, ELLIAS A, RAVEN R, YEATMAN J, LITTLEJOHNS D (1987) Psychogenic voice disorder unresponsive to speech therapy: psychological characteristics and cognitive-behaviour therapy. British Journal of Disorders of Communication 22: 81-92.

BZOCH KR (1989) Communicative Disorders Related to Cleft Lip and Palate, 3rd edn. Boston: College-Hill.

CALAS M, VERHULST J, LECOQ M, DALLEAS B, SEILHEAN M (1989) Vocal pathology of teachers [French]. Revue de Laryngologie, Otologie et Rhinologie 110: 397-406.

CALCATERRA, TC (1983) Tongue flap reconstruction of the hypopharynx. Archives of Otolaryngology 109: 750-752.

CALNAN J (1953) Movements of the soft palate. British Journal of Plastic and Reconstructive Surgery 13: 275.

CALNAN J (1955) Diagnosis, prognosis and treatment of palato-pharyngeal incompetence with special reference to radiographic investigations. British Journal of Plastic and Reconstructive Surgery 16: 352.

CAMPBELL EJM (1974) Muscular activity in normal and abnormal ventilation. In: Ventilatory and Phonatory Control Systems, Wyke B, ed. Oxford: Oxford University Press.

CAMPBELL EJM, AGOSTINI E, DAVIS JN (1970) The Respiratory Muscles: Mechanics and neural control, 2nd edn. London: Lloyd-Luke Medical Books.

CAMPBELL SM, MONTANARO A, BARDANA EJ (1983) Head and neck manifestations in autoimmune disease. American Journal of Otolarynology 4: 187-216.

CANTRELL RW (1983) Laryngeal trauma reviewed. Archives of Otolaryngology 109: 112.

CAPPELLA JN, STREET RL (1985) Introduction: a functional approach to the structure of communicative behaviour. In: Sequence and Pattern in Communicative Behaviour, Street RL Jr, Cappella JN, eds. London: Edward Arnold.

CAPPS FCW (1958) The Semon Lecture: Abductor paralysis in theory and practice since Semon. Journal of Laryngology and Otology 72: 1.

CARDING P, CARLSON E, EPSTEIN R, MATHIESON L, SHEWELL C. (2000) Formal perceptual evaluation of voice quality in the United Kingdom. Logopedics Phoniatrics Vocology 25: 133-138.

CARDING PN, HORSLEY IA (1992) An evaluation study of voice therapy in non-organic dysphonia. European Journal of Disorders of Communication 27: 137-158.

CARDING PN, HORSLEY IA, DOCHERTY GJ (1999) A study of the effectiveness of voice therapy in the treatment of 45 patients with non-organic dysphonia. Journal of Voice 13: 72-104.

CARLSON E (1995a) Electrolaryngography in the assessment and treatment of incomplete mutation (puberphonia) in adults. European Journal of Disorders of Communication 30: 140-148.

CARLSON E (1995b) A study of voice quality in a group of irradiated laryngeal cancer patients with tumour stages T1 and T2. Unpublished PhD thesis, University of London.

CARROLL LM, SATALOFF RT, HEUER RJ, SPIEGEL JR RADIONOFF SL, COHN JR (1996) Respiratory and glottal efficiency measures in normal classically trained singers. Journal of Voice 10: 139-145.

CARUSO AJ, MAX L (1997) Effects of aging on neuromotor processes of swallowing. Seminars in Speech and Language 18: 181-193.

CASE JL (1991) Clinical Management of Voice Disorders, 2nd edn. Austin, TX: Pro-Ed.

CASIANO RR, GOODWIN WJ (1991) Restoring function to the injured larynx. Otolaryngologic Clinics of North America 24: 1215-1226.

CASPER J, COLTON R, BREWER D (1986) Selected therapy techniques and laryngeal physiological changes in patients with vocal fold immobility. Folia Phoniatrica 38: XXth Congress of IALP.

CASSELMAN JW, LEMAHIEU SF, PEENE P, STOFFELS G (1988) Polychondritis affecting the laryngeal cartilages. AJR-American Journal of Roentgenology 150: 355-356.

CAVANAGH F (1955) Vocal palsies in children. Journal of Laryngology 69: 399.

CAVO JW (1985) True vocal cord paralysis following intubation. Laryngoscope 95: 1352.

CHAN RWK (1994) Does the voice improve with vocal hygiene education? A study of some instrumental voice measures in a group of kindergarten teachers. Journal of Voice 8: 279-291.

CHEESMAN AD (1983) Surgical management of the patient. In: Laryngectomy: Diagnosis to rehabilitation, Edels Y, ed. London: Croom-Helm.

CHERRY J, DELAHUNTY JE (1968) Experimentally produced vocal cord granulomas. Laryngoscope 78: 1941.

CHERRY J, MARGULIES SI (1968) Contact ulcer of the larynx. Laryngoscope 78: 1937.

CHIA SE, ONG CN, FOO SC, LEE HP (1992) Medical students' exposure to formaldehyde in a gross anatomy dissection laboratory. Journal of the American College of Health 41: 115-119.

CHILDERS DG, HICKS DM, MOORE GP, ESKENAZI L, LALWANI AL (1990) Electroglottography and vocal fold physiology. Journal of Speech and Hearing Research 33: 245-254.

CITARDI MJ, GRACCO CL, SASAKI CT (1995) The anatomy of the human larynx. In: Diagnosis and Treatment of Voice Disorders, Rubin J, Sataloff R, Korovin G, Gould W, eds. New York: Igaku-Shoin.

CLARKE PM, DURHAM SR, PERRY A, MACKAY IS (1992) Objective measurement of voice change caused by inhaled steroids. Voice 1: 63-66.

CLARKE WM, HOOPS HR (1970) The effect of speech-type background noise on oesophageal speech production. Annals of Otology (St Louis) 79: 653.

CLOSE LG, WOODSON GE (1989) Common upper airway disorders in the elderly and their management. Geriatrics 43 (Jan): 67-72.

COHEN LG, LUDLOW CL, WARDEN M et al. (1989) Blink reflex excitability recovery curves in patients with spasmodic dysphonia. Neurology 39: 572-577.

COHN AM, PEPPARD SB (1979) Laryngeal trauma. In: Otolaryngology, English GM, ed. New York: Harper & Row.

COLTON RH, CASPER JK (1990) Understanding Voice Problems. Baltimore: Williams & Wilkins.

COLTON RH, CONTURE EG (1990) Problems and pitfalls of electroglottography. Journal of Voice 4: 10-24.

COLTON RH, STEINSCHNEIDER A (1980) Acoustic relationships of infant cries to the Sudden Infant Death Syndrome. In: Infant Communication: Cry and early speech, Murry T, Murry J, eds. Houston, TX: College Hill Press.

COMELLA CL, TANNER CM, DeFOOR-HILL L, SMITH C (1992) Dysphagia after botulinum toxin injections for spasmodic torticollis: Clinical and radiologic findings. Neurology 42: 1307-1310.

CONLEY JJ (1961) Glottic reconstruction and wound rehabilitation. Archives of Otology 74: 21.

CONLEY JJ (1962) Rehabilitation of the airway system by neck flaps. Annals of Otology (St Louis) 71: 924.

COOK TA, BRUNSCHING JP, BUTEL JS, COHN AM, GOEPFERT H, ROWS WE (1973) Laryngeal papilloma: etiologic and therapeutic considerations. Annals of Otology 82: 649.

COOPER M (1971) Papilloma of the vocal folds: a review. Journal of Speech Disorders 36: 51.

COOPER M (1973) Modern Techniques of Vocal Rehabilitation. Springfield, IL: Charles C Thomas.

COOPER M (1974) Spectrographic analysis of fundamental frequency and hoarseness before and after therapy. Journal of Speech and Hearing Disorders 39: 286.

COOPER M, NAHUM AM (1967) Vocal rehabilitation for contact ulcer of the larynx. Archives of Otolaryngology 85: 41.

COTES JE (1979) Lung Function, 4th edn. Oxford: Blackwell Scientific Publications.

COWIE R, DOUGLAS-COWIE BA, KERR AG (1982) A study of speech deterioration in post-lingually deafened adults. Journal of Laryngology and Otology 96: 101.

CRITCHLEY M (1939a) Spastic dysphonia: inspiratory speech. Brain 62: 96.

CRITCHLEY M (1939b) The Language of Gesture. London: Edward Arnold.

CRITCHLEY M (1949) Observations on essential voice tremor. Brain 72: 113.

CROCKFORD MP, KERR IH (1988) Relapsing polychondritis. Clinical Radiology 39: 386-390.

CRUMLEY RL (1990) Teflon versus thyroplasty versus nerve transfer: a comparison. Annals of Otology, Rhinology and Laryngology 99: 759-763.

CRUMLEY RL, IZDEBSKI K (1986) Voice quality following laryngeal reinnervation by ansa hypoglossi transfer. Laryngoscope 96: 611-616.

CRYSTAL D (1976) Child Language, Learning and Linguistics: an overview for the teaching and therapeutic professions. London: Edward Arnold.

CRYSTAL D (1980) Introduction to Language Pathology. London: Edward Arnold.

CRYSTAL D (1981) Clinical Linguistics. London: Edward Arnold.

CRYSTAL D (1982) Profiling Linguistic Disability. London: Edward Arnold.

CURLE RJ (1979) Therapeutic methods for the incompetent soft palate. In: Diagnosis and Treatment of Palato-glossal Malfunction, Ellis RR, Flack FC, eds. College of Speech Therapists, London .

CURRY ET (1949) Hoarseness and voice change in male adolescents. Journal of Speech Disorders 14: 23.

DABUL B, BOLLIER B (1976) Therapeutic approaches to apraxia. Journal of Speech and Hearing Disorders 41: 268.

DAMSTÉ PH (1958) Oesophageal Speech. Groningen: Hoitsema.

DAMSTÉ PH (1962) Congenital short palate without cleft. Proceedings of the 12th International Speech and Voice Therapy Conference, Padua. Croatto L, Croatto-Martolini C, eds.

DAMSTÉ PH (1964) Virilisation of the voice due to anabolic steroids. Folia Phoniatrica 16: 10.

DAMSTÉ PH (1983) Diagnostic behaviour patterns with communicative abilities. In: Vocal Fold Physiology: Contemporary research and clinical issues. Bless DM, Abbs JH, eds. San Diego: College Hill Press.

DAMSTÉ PH, LERMAN JW (1975) An introduction to voice pathology. Functional and Organic. Springfield, IL: Thomas.

DARLEY FL, ARONSON AE, BROWN JR (1969) Differential diagnostic patterns of dysarthria. Journal of Speech and Hearing Research 12: 246.

DARLEY FL, ARONSON AE, BROWN JR (1975) Motor Speech Disorders. Philadelphia: WB Saunders.

DAVIS CB, DAVIS ML (1993) The effects of premenstrual syndrome (PMS) on the female singer. Journal of Voice 7: 337-353.

DAVIS PJ, ZHANG SP, BANDLER R (1993) Pulmonary and upper airway afferent influences on the motor pattern of vocalization evoked by excitation of the midbrain periaqueductal gray of the cat. Brain Research 607(1-2): 61-80.

DAVIS PJ, ZHANG SP, WINKWORTH A, BANDLER R (1996) Neural control of vocalization: respiratory and emotional influences. Journal of Voice 10(1): 23-38.

DAWSON J (1919) The Voice of the Boy. New York: Kellog.

De SOUZA F (1980) Thyroidectomy in Otolaryngology, Vol. 5, English G, ed. Philadelphia: Harper Row.

DEAL J, DARLEY F (1972) The influence of linguistic and situational variables on phonemic accuracy in apraxia of speech. Journal of Speech and Hearing Research 15: 639.

DEBRUYNE F, DECOSTER W (1999) Acoustic differences between sustained vowels perceived as young or old. Logopedics Phoniatrics Vocology 24: 1-5.

DEDO HH (1976) Recurrent laryngeal nerve section for spastic dysphonia. Annals of Otology (St Louis) 85: 451.

DEDO HH, IZDEBSKI K (1983a) Intermediate results of 306 recurrent laryngeal nerve sections for spastic dysphonia. Laryngoscope 93: 9.

DEDO HH, IZDEBSKI K (1983b) Problems with surgical (RLN section) treatment of spastic dysphonia. Laryngoscope 93: 268.

DEDO HH, SHIPP T (1980) Spastic Dysphonia: A surgical and voice therapy treatment program. Houston, TX: College Hill Press.

DEDO HH, TOWNSEND JJ, IZDEBSKI K (1978) Current evidence for the organic etiology of spastic dysphonia. Paper presented at the Eighty-second Annual Meeting of the American Academy of Ophthalmology, Dallas, October 2-6 1977.

DEDO HH, URREA RO, LAWSON L (1973) Intracordal injection of Teflon in the treatment of 135 patients with dysphonia. Annals of Otolaryngology 82: 1.

DEJONCKERE PH (1995) Principal components in voice pathology. Voice 4: 96-105.

DEJONCKERE PH, HIRANO M, SUNDBERG J (1995) Vibrato. San Diego: Singular Publishing Group.

DEJONCKERE PH, OBBENS C, DE MOOR G, WIENEKE G (1993) Perceptual evaluation of dysphonia: reliability and relevance. Folia Phoniatrica 45: 76-83.

DEJONCKERE PH, REMACLE M, FRESNEL-ELBAZ E, WOISARD W, CREVIER-BUSHMAN L, MILLET B (1996) Differentiated perceptual evaluation of pathological voice quality: reliability and correlations with acoustic measurements. Revue de Laryngologie, Otologie, Rhinologie 117: 219-224.

DELAHUNTY JE (1972) Acid laryngitis. Journal of Laryngology and Otology 86: 335.

DELAHUNTY JE, ARDRAN GM (1970) Globus hystericus - a manifestation of reflux oesophagitis. Journal of Laryngology 84: 1049.

DeVITA MA, SPIERER-RUNDBACK L (1990) Swallowing disorders in patients with prolonged orotracheal intubation of tracheostomy tubes. Critical Care Medicine 18: 1328-1330.

DHILLON RS, EAST CA (1994) Ear, Nose and Throat and Head and Neck Surgery. London: Churchill Livingstone.

Di CARLO LM, AMSTER WW, HERER GR (1955) Speech After Laryngectomy. Syracuse, CA: Syracuse University Press.

DIEDRICH WM, YOUNGSTROM KA (1966) Alaryngeal Speech. Springfield, IL: Charles C. Thomas.

DIEDRICH WM, YOUNGSTROM KA (1977) Alaryngeal Speech, 2nd edn. Springfield, IL: Charles C. Thomas.

DIKEMAN KJ, KAZANDJIAN MS (1995) Communication and Swallowing: Management of tracheostomized and ventilator dependent adults. San Diego: Singular Publishing Group Inc.

DONALD PJ (1982) Voice change surgery in the transsexual. Head and Neck Surgery 4: 433.

DORNHURST AC, NEGUS VE (1954) Speech after removal of the oesophagus and the larynx and part of the pharynx. British Medical Journal ii: 16.

DOWNIE AW, LOW JM, LINDSAY DD (1981) Speech disorders in Parkinsonism - usefulness of delayed auditory feedback in selected cases. British Journal of Disorders of Communication 16: 135.

DOYLE PC (1994) Foundations of Voice and Speech Rehabilitation Following Laryngeal Cancer. San Diego: Singular.

DROMEY C, RAMIG LO, JOHNSON AB (1995) Phonatory and articulatory changes associated with increased vocal intensity in Parkinson Disease: A case study. Journal of Speech and Hearing Research 38: 751-764.

DUFF J (1968) Laryngeal trauma. Journal of Laryngology 82: 825.

DWORKIN JP, MELECA RJ (1997) Vocal Pathologies. London: Singular Publishing Group Inc.

ECKEL FC, BOONE DR (1981) The s/z ratio as an indication of laryngeal pathology. Journal of Speech and Hearing Disorders 46: 147-150.

ECKEL HE, THUMFART M, VOSSING M, WASSERMAN K, THUMFART WF (1994) Cordectomy versus arytenoidectomy in the management of bilateral vocal cord paralysis. Annals of Otology, Rhinology and Laryngology 103: 852-857.

EDELS Y (1983) Pseudo-voice. In: Its Theory and Practice in Laryngectomy: Diagnosis to rehabilitation. Edels Y, ed. New York: Croom Helm.

EDWARDS CRW, BOUCHIER IAD, HASLETT C, CHILVERS ER, eds (1995) Davidson's Principles and Practice of Medicine. Edinburgh: Churchill Livingstone.

EDWARDS JR (1982) Language attitudes and their implications among English speakers. In: Sequence and Pattern in

Communicative Behaviour. Street RL Jr, Capella J, eds. London: Edward Arnold.

EDWARDS M (1984) Disorders of Articulation: Aspects of dysarthria and verbal dyspraxia. Vienna: Springer-Verlag.

EDWARDS N (1976) The artificial larynx. British Journal of Hospital Medicine 16: 145.

EDWARDS N (1983) The surgical approach to speech rehabilitation. In: Laryngectomy: Diagnosis to rehabilitation, Edels Y, ed. London: Croom Helm.

EIBLING DE, GROSS RD (1996) Subglottic air pressure: A key component of swallowing efficiency. Annals of Otology, Rhinology and Laryngology 105: 253-256.

EKBERG O, FEINBERG M J (1990) Altered swallowing function in elderly patients without dysphagia: radiologic findings in 56 cases. American Journal of Radiology 156: 1181-1184.

ELLIS PDM, BENNETT J (1977) Laryngeal trauma and prolonged endo-tracheal intubation. Journal of Laryngology 91: 69.

ELLIS PDM, PALLISTER WK (1975) Recurrent laryngeal nerve palsy and endotracheal intubation. Journal of Laryngology 89: 823.

ELLIS R (1979) The Exeter nasal anemometry system. In: Diagnosis and Treatment of Palatoglossal Malfunction, Ellis R, Flack FC, eds. London: College of Speech Therapists.

ELLIS RE, FLACK FC, CURLE HJ, SELLEY WG (1978) A system for the assessment of nasal airflow during speech. British Journal of Disorders of Communication 13: 31.

ELSHAMI AA, TINO G (1996) Coexistent asthma and functional upper airway obstruction. Case reports and review of the literature (abbrev. source). Chest 110: 1358-1361.

EMERICH K, HOOVER C, SATALOFF RT (1996) The effects of menopause on the singing voice. Laryngoscope March/April: 39-42.

ENDERBY P (1983) Frenchay Dysarthria Assessment. San Diego: College Hill Press.

ENDERBY P, ed. (1987) Assistive Communication Aids for the Speech Impaired. Edinburgh: Churchill Livingstone.

ENDERBY P, PHILIPP R (1986) Speech and Language Handicap: towards knowing the size of the problem. British Journal of Disorders of Communication 21: 151-165.

ENDERBY P, HATHORN IS, SERVANT S (1984) The use of intra-oral appliances in the management of acquired velopharyngeal disorders. British Dental Journal 157: 157.

EPSTEIN R, STYGALL J, NEWMAN S (1996) Anxiety associated with botox injections for adductor spasmodic dysphonia. Logopedic Phoniatrics Vocology 21: 131-136.

ESKENAZI L, CHILDERS DG, HICKS DM (1990) Acoustic correlates of vocal quality. Journal of Speech and Hearing Research 33: 298-306.

FAABORG-ANDERSON K, NYKOBING F (1965) Electromyography of laryngeal muscles: techniques and results. In: Aktuelle Probleme der Phoniatrie und Logopedie, Vol 3. Basel: Karger.

FAHMY M (1950) The theory of habit control and negative practice as a curative method in the treatment of stammering. Speech 14: 24.

FAIRBANKS G (1942) An acoustical study in the pitch of infant wails. Child Development 13: 227.

FAIRBANKS G (1960) Voice and Articulation Drill Book, 2nd edn. New York: Harper.

FAIRBANKS G, WILEY JH, LASSMAN FM (1949) An acoustical study of vocal pitch in seven- and eight-year-old boys. Child Development 20: 63.

FALK A, BIRKEN EA (1985) Hyperthyroidism: a surgeon's perspective. In: Otolaryngology, Vol 4, English GM, ed. Philadelphia: Harper, Row.

FARLEY GR, BARLOW SM (1994) Neurophysiology, biomechanics, and modeling of normal voice production. Current Opinion in Otolaryngology and Head and Neck Surgery 2: 233-239.

FAWCUS M (1986a) The causes and classification of voice disorders. In: Voice Disorders and their Management, Fawcus M, ed. New York: Croom Helm.

FAWCUS M (1986b) Hyperfunctional voice: the misuse and abuse syndrome. In: Voice Disorders and their Management, Fawcus M, ed. New York: Croom Helm.

FEE WE (1984) Hypopharyngeal reconstruction. Archives of Otolaryngology Head and Neck Surgery 110: 384.

FERGUSON BJ, HUDSON WR, McCARTY S Jr (1987) Sex Steroid Receptor Distribution in the Human Larynx and Laryngeal Carcinoma. Archives of Otolaryngology Head and Neck Surgery 113: 1311-1315.

FEX B, FEX S, SHIROMOTO O, HIRANO M (1994) Acoustic analysis of functional dysphonia; before and after voice therapy (accent method). Journal of Voice 2: 163-167.

FIGI FA (1953) Hemilaryngectomy with immediate skin graft for the removal of carcinoma of the larynx. Annals of Otology 62: 400.

FIGI FA, NEW GB (1929) Carcinoma of the larynx in the young. Archives of Otolaryngology 51: 386.

FINITZO T, POOL KD, FREEMAN FJ et al. (1987) Spasmodic dysphonia subsequent to head trauma. Archives of Otolaryngology Head and Neck Surgery 113: 1107-1109.

FINIZIA C, HAMMERLID E, WESTIN T, LINDSTROM J (1998) Quality of life in patients with laryngeal carcinoma: a post-treatment comparison of laryngectomy (salvage surgery) versus radiotherapy. Laryngoscope 108: 1566-73.

FISHER AJ, CALDARELLI DD, CHACKO DC, HOLINGER LD (1986) Glottic cancer - surgical salvage for radiation failure. Archives of Otolarynology Head and Neck Surgery 112: 519.

FISHER KW, SWANK PR (1997) Estimating phonation threshold pressure. Journal of Speech Language and Hearing Research 40: 1122-1129.

FLACH M, SCHWICKARDI H, SIMON R (1969) What influence do menstruation and pregnancy have on the trained singing voice? Folia Phoniatrica 21: 199.

FLETCHER SG (1970) Tonar. The oral nasal acoustic ratio. Cleft Palate Journal 7: 601.

FLETCHER SG (1972) Contingencies for bio-electric modification of nasality. Journal of Speech and Hearing Disorders 37: 329.

FOGH-ANDERSEN P (1980) Incidence and aetiology. In: Advances in the Management of Cleft Palate, Edwards M, Watson ACH, eds. Edinburgh: Churchill Livingstone.

FONTAINE A, MITCHELL JCE (1960) Oesophageal voice: a factor of readiness. Journal of Laryngology 74: 870.

FORD CN, BLESS DM (1987) Collagen injection in the scarred vocal fold. Journal of Voice 1: 116.

FORD CN, BLESS DM (1991) Adjunctive measures for optimal phonosurgical results: medical & other supportive measures. In: Phonosurgery: Assessment and surgical management of voice disorders, Ford CN, Bless DM, eds. New York: Raven Press.

FORD CN, BLESS DM, CAMPBELL DA (1986) Studies of injectable soluble collagen for vocal fold augmentation. XXth IALP Congress, Tokyo. Folia Phoniatrica 38: 283.

FORD CN, GILCHRIST KW, BARTELL TE (1987) Persistence of injectable collagen in the human larynx: a histopathologic study. Laryngoscope 97: 724.

FORD CN, INAGI K, KHIDR A, BLESS DM, GILCHRIST KW (1996) Sulcus vocalis: A rational analytical approach to diagnosis and management. Annals of Otology Rhinology and Laryngology 105: 189-200.

FORDER RJ (1983) Laryngeal granuloma as a complication of the CO2 laser. Laryngoscope 93: 944.

FORMBY D (1967) Maternal recognition of infants cry. Developmental Medicine and Child Neurology 9: 293.

FORREST LA, WEED H (1998) Candida laryngitis appearing as leukoplakia and GERD. Journal of Voice 12: 91-95.

FOURCIN AJ (1981) Laryngographic assessment of phonatory function. Asha Reports II. Rockville Pike, MD: The American Speech-Language-Hearing Association, pp. 116-127.

FOURCIN AJ (1990) Prospects for speech pattern element aids. Acta Otolaryngologica (Stockholm) Supplementum 469: 257-267.

FOURCIN A (2000) Voice quality and electrolaryngography. In: Voice Quality Measurement. Kent RD, Ball MJ, eds. San Diego: Singular.

FOURCIN AJ, ABBERTON E (1971) First applications of a new laryngograph. Medical and Biological Illustration 21: 172.

FOURCIN AJ, ABBERTON E (1974) The laryngograph and the Voiscope in speech therapy. Proceedings of the XVIth IALP Congress, Copenhagen, pp. 116-122.

FRASER G (1987) Cochlear implantation: more than just an operation. In: Adjustment to Acquired Hearing Loss: Analysis, change and learning, Kyle JG, ed. Proceedings of Conference, Centre of Deaf Studies, University of Bristol.

FREEMAN FJ, CANNITO MP, FINITZO-HIEBERT T (1984) Classification of spasmodic dysphonia by perceptual-acoustic-visual means. In: Spasmodic dysphonia: State of the Art 1984, Gates GA, ed. New York: The Voice Foundation, pp. 5-13.

FREEMAN FJ, SCHAEFFER S, CANNITO MP, FINITZO T (1987) Episodic reactive dysphonia: a case study. Journal of Communication Disorders 20: 259.

FRENCH P (1994) An overview of forensic phonetics. Forensic Linguistics: the International Journal of Speech, Language and the Law 1: 170-181.

FREUD S (1943) A General Introduction to Psycho-Analysis. New York: Garden City.

FRIEDMAN M, GRYBAUSKAS V, TORIUMI DM, APPLEBAUM EL (1987) Treatment of spastic dysphonia without nerve section. Annals of Otology, Rhinology and Laryngology 96: 590-595.

FRITZELL B (1969) The velopharyngeal muscles in speech. An electromyographic and cineradiographic study. Acta Otolaryngologica Supplementum 250.

FRITZELL B (1996) Voice disorders and occupations. Logopedics Phoniatrics Vocology 21: 7-12.

FRITZELL B, SUNDBERG J, STRANGE-EBBESEN A (1982) Pitch change after stripping oedematous vocal folds. Folia Phoniatrica 34: 29.

FRITZELL B, FEUER E, HAGHUND S, KNUTSSON E, SCHIRATZKI H (1982) Experience with recurrent laryngeal nerve section for spastic dysphonia. Folia Phoniatrica 34: 160.

FROESCHELS E (1948) Twentieth Century Voice Correction. New York: Philosophical Library.

FROESCHELS E, JELLINEK A (1941) Practice of Voice and Speech Therapy. Boston: Expression

FRY DB (1979) The Physics of Speech. Cambridge: Cambridge University Press.

FUKADA H, SAITO S, KITAHARA S et al. (1983) Vocal fold vibration in excised larynges viewed with an X-ray, stroboscope and an ultra-high-speed camera. In: Vocal Fold Physiology, Bless DM, Abbs JH, eds. San Diego: College Hill.

GACEK HR (1976) Hereditary abductor vocal cord paralysis. Annals of Otology 85: 90.

GALLIVAN GJ, LANDIS JN (1993) Sarcoidosis of the larynx: preserving and restoring airway and professional voice. Journal of Voice 7: 81-94.

GALLIVAN GJ, DAWSON JA, ROBBINS LD (1989) Videolaryngoscopy after endotracheal intubation: Implications for voice. Journal of Voice 3: 76-80.

GARDNER WH (1978) Laryngectomee Speech and Rehabilitation, 2nd edn. Springfield, IL: Thomas.

GARDNER WH, HILL SD, CARANO HN (1962) Oesophageal speech for a 12 year old boy: a case report. Journal of Speech and Hearing Disorders 27: 227.

GARFIELD DAVIES D (1969) Fibrosarcoma and pseudosarcoma of the larynx. Journal of Laryngology 83: 423.

GARRETT JD, LARSON CR (1991) Neurology of the laryngeal system. In: Phonosurgery: Assessment and surgical management of voice disorders. Ford CN, Bless DM, eds. New York: Raven Press.

GATELY G (1971) A technique for teaching the laryngectomised to trap air for the production of oesophageal speech. Journal of Speech Disorders 36: 485.

GATES GA, MONTALBO PJ (1987) The effect of low-dose B-blockade on performance anxiety in singers. Journal of Voice 1: 105.

GELDER M, GATH D, MAYOU R (1983) Oxford Textbook of Psychiatry. Oxford: Oxford University Press.

GELFER MP, BULTEMEYER DK (1990) Evaluation of vocal fold vibratory patterns in normal voices. Journal of Voice 4: 335-345.

GILES H, POWESLAND PF (1975) Speech Style and Social Evaluation. London: Academic Press.

GIMSON AC (1962) An Introduction to the Pronunciation of English. London: Arnold.

GINSBERG BI, WALLACK JJ, SRAIN JJ, BILLER HF (1988) Defining the psychiatric role in spastic dysphonia. General Hospital Psychiatry 10: 132-137.

GOLDBERG J, KOVARSKY J (1983) Beclomethasone dipropionate inhalation treatment for chronic hoarseness in rheumatic diseases. Arthritis and Rheumatology 26: 1412.

GOLDBERG M, NOYEK AM, PRITZKER PH (1978) Laryngeal granuloma secondary to gastroesophageal reflux. Journal of Otolarynology 7: 196.

GOLDEN LI, DEEB ZE, deFRIES H (1990) Atypical findings in cephalic herpes zoster polyneuritis: case reports and radiographic findings. Laryngoscope 100: 494-497.

GOODE RL (1975) Artificial laryngeal devices in post-laryngectomy rehabilitation. Laryngoscope 83: 677.

GORDON M (1977) Physical measurements in a clinically orientated voice pathology department. Proceedings of XVIIth IALP Congress 1: 401.

GORDON M (1986) Assessment of the dysphonic patient. In: Voice Disorders and Their Management, Fawcus M, ed. New York: Croom Helm.

GORDON MT, MORTON FM, SIMPSON JC (1978). Airflow measurements in diagnosis, assessment and treatment of mechanical dysphonia. Folia Phoniatrica 30: 161.

GORDON MT, PEARSON L, PATON F, MONTGOMERY R (1997) Predictive assessment of vocal efficacy (PAVE): A method for voice therapy outcome measurement. Journal of Laryngology and Otology 111: 129-133.

GOTAAS C, STARR CD (1993) Vocal fatigue among teachers. Folia Phoniatrica 45: 120-129.

GOULD WJ (1981) The Pulmonary-Laryngeal System in Vocal Fold Physiology, Stevens KN, Hirano M, eds. Tokyo: University of Tokyo Press.

GOULD WJ, KOROVIN GS (1994) Laboratory advances for voice measurements. Journal of Voice 8: 8-17.

GOULD WJ, OKAMURA H (1973) Status lung volumes in singers. Annals of Otology 82: 89.

GOULD WJ, SATALOFF RT, SPIEGEL JR (1993) Voice Surgery. St Louis: Mosby.

GRAY H (1949) Gray's Anatomy: Descriptive and applied, 30th edn, Johnston TB, Whillis J, eds. London: Longman, Green & Co.

GRAY RF, RUTKA JA (1988) Recent Advances in Otolaryngology. London: Longman Group Co. Ltd.

GRAY S, HIRANO M, SATO K (1993) Molecular and cellular structure of vocal fold tissue. In: Vocal Fold Physiology, Titze IR, ed. San Diego: Singular Publishing Group, Inc.

GREENE MCL (1955) Puberphonia. Proceedings of the Royal College of Speech Therapists, Oxford Conference. London: College of Speech Therapists.

GREENE MCL (1957) Speech of children before and after removal of tonsils and adenoids. Journal of Speech Disorders 22: 361.

GREENE MCL (1961) Symposium on Speech Defects. Part III. Speech therapy problems. Radiography 27: 338.

GREENE MCL (1962) Possible areas of cooperation between speech therapists and teachers of the deaf. Speech Pathology and Therapy 5: 57.

GREENE MCL (1982) Ageing of the voice: a review. In: Communicative Changes in Elderly People, Edwards M, ed. London: College of Speech Therapy.

GREENE MCL (1984) Functional dysphonia and the hyperventilation syndrome. British Journal of Disorders of Communication 19: 263.

GREENE MCL, CONWAY J (1963) Learning to talk: a study in sound of infant speech development. New York: Folkways Records, Fx 6271.

GREENE MCL, WATSON BW (1968) The value of speech amplification in Parkinson's Disease patients. Folia Phoniatrica 20: 250.

GREENE MCL, ATKINSON P, WATSON BW (1974) A substitute voice after surgical removal of the larynx. Journal of Laryngology 88: 1103.

GREENE MCL, TIMMONS BH, GLOVER JHM (1983) Anxiety state and chronic hyperventilation syndrome: relevance in speech and voice disorders. Proceedings of the XIXth IALP Congress, 2: 704.

GREENE MCL, TIMMONS BH, GLOVER JHM (1984) The significance of anxiety and breathing disorders in functional dysphonia. 3rd International workshop on respiratory psychophysiology, Bordeaux. Bulletin Européen de Physiopathologie Respiratoire 20: 94.

GREWEL F (1957a) Classification of dysarthrias. Acta Psychologica et Neurologica Scandinavica 32: 325.

GREWEL F (1957b) Dysarthria in post-encephalitic Parkinsonism. Acta Psychologica et Neurologica Scandinavica 32: 440.

GRUNWELL P (1982) Clinical Phonology. London: Croom Helm.

GUDYKUNST WB (1986) Intergroup communication. In: Social Psychology of Language and Communicative Studies, Giles H, ed. London: Edward Arnold.

GUSSAK GS, JUROVICH GJ, LATERMAN A (1986) Laryngeal trauma: a protocol approach to a rare injury. Laryngoscope 96: 660.

GUTHRIE D (1966) Forty-two years survival after laryngectomy. Journal of Laryngology 80: 851.

HABIB MA (1977) Intra-articular steroid injection in acute rheumatoid arthritis of the larynx. Journal of Laryngology and Otology 91: 909.

HACKI T (1996) Comparative speaking, shouting and singing voice range profile measurements: physiological and pathological aspects. Logopedics Phoniatrics Vocology 21: 123-129.

HAGHUND H, LUNDQUIST PG, CANTRELL K (1981) Interferon therapy in juvenile laryngeal papillomatosis. Archives of Otolaryngology 107: 327.

HAHN FW, MARTIN JI, LILLIE JC (1970) Vocal cord paralysis with endotracheal intubation. Archives of Otolaryngology 92: 226.

HALPERN H (1981) Therapy for agnosis, apraxia and dysarthria. In: Language Intervention Strategies in Adult Aphasia, Chapey R, ed. Baltimore, MA: Williams & Wilkins.

HAMAKER RC, SINGER MI, BLOM ED, DANIELS HA (1985) Primary voice restoration at laryngectomy. Archives of Otolaryngology 111: 182.

HAMMARBERG B (1986) Perceptual and acoustic analysis of dysphonia. Studies in Logopedics and Phoniatrics. No. 1. Huddinge University Hospital, Sweden.

HAMMARBERG B, GAUFFIN J (1995) Perceptual and acoustic characteristics of quality differences in pathological voices related to physiological aspects. In: Vocal Fold Physiology: Voice Quality Control, Fujimura O, Hirano M, eds. San Diego: Singular Publishing Inc.

HAMMOND TH, ZHOU R, HAMMOND EH, PAWLAK A, GRAY SD (1997) The intermediate layer: a morphologic study of the elastin and hyaluronic acid constituents of normal human vocal folds. Journal of Voice 11: 59-66.

HANSON DG (1991) Neuromuscular disorders of the larynx. Otolaryngologic Clinics of North America 24: 1035-1051.

HANSON DG, LOGEMANN JA, HAIN T (1992) Differential diagnosis of spasmodic dysphonia: a kinematic perspective. Journal of Voice 6: 325-337.

HARRIES M, HAWKINS S, HACKING J, HUGHES I (1998) Changes in the male voice at puberty: vocal fold length and its relationship to the fundamental frequency of the voice. Journal of Laryngology and Otology 112: 451-454.

HARRIS C, THOMPSON C (1999) Managing functional aphonia. Bulletin of the Royal College of Speech and Language Therapists 561: 10-11.

HARRIS D (1998) Singing and therapy. In: The Voice Clinic Handbook, Harris T, Harris S, Rubin JS, Howard D, eds. London: Whurr.

HARRIS HH, AINSWORTH JZ (1965) Immediate management of laryngeal and tracheal injuries. Laryngoscope 75: 1103.

HARRIS LL, VOGTSBERGER KN, MATTOX DE (1985) Group psychotherapy for head and neck cancer patients. Laryngoscope 95: 585.

HARRIS TM (1992) The pharmacological treatment of voice disorders. Folia Phoniatrica 44: 143-154.

HARRISON DFN (1964) Pharyngo-esophageal replacement in post-cricoid and esophageal carcinoma. Annals of Otology 73: 1026.

HARTMAN DE, ARONSON AE (1983) Psychogenic aphonia masking mutational falsetto. Archives of Otolaryngology 109: 415.

HARTMAN DE, VISHWANAT B (1984) Spastic dysphonia and essential (voice) tremor treated with Primidone. Archives of Otolaryngology 110: 394.

HARTMAN E, VON CRAMON D (1984a) Acoustic measurement of voice quality in dysphonia after severe closed head trauma: a follow-up study. British Journal of Disorders of Communication 19: 253.

HARTMAN E, VON CRAMON D (1984b) Acoustic measurement of voice quality in central dysphonia. Journal of Communication Disorders 17: 425.

HEAVER L (1958) Psychiatric observations on the personality structure of patients with habitual dysphonia. Logos 1: 21.

HEAVER L, ARNOLD GE (1962) Rehabilitation of alaryngeal aphonia. Postgraduate Medicine 32: 11.

HEIDEL SE, TORGERSON JK (1993) Vocal problems among aerobic instructors and aerobic participants. Journal of Communication Disorders 26: 179-91.

HEINEMANN M (1969) Myxoedem und Stimme. Folia Phoniatrica 21: 55.

HENDERSON R (1954) Kathleen Ferrier. London: Hamilton.

HENLEY J, SOULIERE C (1986) Tracheoesophageal speech failure in the laryngectomee: the role of the constrictor myotomy. Laryngoscope 96: 1016.

HERRINGTON-HALL BL, LEE L, STEMPLE JC, NIEMI KR, McHONE MM (1988) Descriptions of laryngeal pathologies by age, sex, and occupation in a treatment-seeking sample. Journal of Speech and Hearing Disorders 53: 57-64.

HERZEL H, BERRY D, TITZE I, SALEH M (1994) Analysis of voice disorders with methods from non-linear dynamics. Journal of Speech and Hearing Research 37: 1008-1019.

HEUER RJ (1992) Behavioral therapy for spasmodic dysphonia. Journal of Voice 6: 352-354.

HICKS DM (1999) The efficacy of voice treatment. Current Opinion in Otolaryngology and Head and Neck Surgery 7: 125-129.

HILDERNESSE LW (1956) Voice diagnosis. Acta Physiologica et Pharmacologica Neerlandica 5: 73.

HILDICK-SMITH M (1980) Management of Parkinson's Disease. Postgraduate Medical Centres Publications.

HIRANO M (1974) Morphological structure of the vocal cord as a vibrator and its variations. Folia Phoniatrica 26: 89.

HIRANO M (1981) Clinical Examination of Voice. Vienna: Springer-Verlag.

HIRANO M (1991) Phonosurgical Anatomy of the Larynx: Assessment and surgical management of voice disorders. New York: Raven Press.

HIRANO M, BLESS DM (1993) Videostroboscopic Examination of the Larynx. London: Whurr.

HIRANO M, KIMINORI S (1993) Histological Color Atlas of the Human Larynx. San Diego: Singular Publishing Group Inc.

HIRANO M, SATO K (1993). Histological Color Atlas of the Human Larynx. San Diego: Singular.

HIRANO M, KOIKE Y, VON LEDEN H (1968) Maximum phonation time and air usage during phonation. Folia Phoniatrica 20: 185.

HIRANO M, KURITA S, NAKASHIMA T (1983) Growth, development and aging of human vocal folds. In: Vocal Fold Physiology, Bless DM, Abbs JH, eds. San Diego: College Hill Press.

HIRANO M, KURITA S, SAKAGUCHI S (1989) Ageing of the vibratory tissue of human vocal folds. Acta Otolaryngologica (Stockholm) 107: 428-433.

HIRANO M, SHIGEJIRO K, TERASAWA R (1985) Difficulty in high-pitched phonation by laryngeal trauma. Archives of Otolaryngology 111: 59.

HIRANO M, SHIN T, NOZOE I (1977) Prognostic aspect of recurrent laryngeal nerve paralysis. Proceedings of the IALP Congress, Copenhagen. Phonia-Arthria 1: 95.

HIRANO M, YOSHIDA T, KURITA S, KIYOKAWA K, SATO K, TATEISHI O (1991) Anatomy and Behaviour of the Vocal Process in Laryngeal Function in Phonation and Respiration, Baer T, Sasaki C, Harris K, eds. San Diego: Singular Publishing Group Inc.

HIROSE H (1977) Electromyography of the larynx and other speech organs. In: Dynamic Aspects of Speech Production, Sawashima M, ed. Tokyo: University of Tokyo, pp. 49-70.

HIROSE H (1985) Laryngeal electromyography. In: Otolaryngology, Vol 3. English GM, ed. Philadelphia: Harper & Row.

HIROSE H, SAWASHIMA M (1981) Functions of the laryngeal muscles. In: Speech in Vocal Fold Physiology, Stevens KN, Hirano M, eds. Tokyo: University of Tokyo Press.

HIROTO I (1981) Introductory remarks. In: Vocal Fold Physiology, Stevens KN, Hirano M, eds. Tokyo: University of Tokyo Press.

HIROTO I, HIRANO M, TOMITA H (1968) Electromyographic investigation of human vocal cord paralysis. Annals of Otology 77: 296.

HIRSCHBERG J (1986) Velopharyngeal insufficiency (VPI). Folia Phoniatrica 38: 221.

HIRSON A, ROE S (1993) Stability of voice and periodic fluctuations in voice quality through the menstrual cycle. Voice 2: 77-88.

HIXON TJ (1987) Respiratory Function in Speech and Song. London: Taylor & Francis.

HIXON TJ, GOLDMAN MD, MEAD J (1973) Kinematics of the chest wall during speech production: volume displacements of the rib cage, abdomen and lung. Journal of Speech and Hearing Research 16: 78.

HIXON T, HAWLEY J, WILSON K (1982) An around the house device for the clinical determination of respiratory driving pressure. Journal of Speech and Hearing Disorders 47: 413.

HIXON TJ, MEAD J, GOLDMAN MD (1976) Dynamics of the chest wall during speech production: function of the thorax, rib cage and abdomen. Journal of Speech and Hearing Research 19: 297.

HODGE KM, GANZEL TM (1987) Diagnostic and therapeutic efficiency in croup and epiglottitis. Laryngoscope 97: 621.

HODSON CJ, OSWALD MVO (1958) Speech Recovery after Total Laryngectomy. Edinburgh: Churchill Livingstone.

HOLBROOK A, ROLNICK MI, BAILEY CW (1974) Treatment of vocal abuse disorders using a vocal intensity controller. Journal of Speech and Hearing Disorders 39: 298.

HOLINGER LD (1979) Congenital anomalies of the larynx. In: Otolaryngology, Vol 3. English GM, ed. Philadelphia: Harper & Row.

HOLINGER LD, WOLTER RK (1979) Neurologic disorders of the larynx. In:

Otolaryngology, Vol 3, English GM, ed. Philadelphia: Harper & Row.

HOLINGER LD, HOLINGER PC, HOLINGER PH (1976) Etiology of bilateral abductor vocal cord paralysis: a review of 389 cases. Annals of Otology 85: 428.

HOLINGER PH (1959) Treatment of Cancer and Allied Diseases, Vol 3. Packand GT, Ariel IM, eds. London : Pitman, Chap 34.

HOLINGER PH (1975) A century of progress of laryngotomies in the northern hemisphere. Laryngoscope 85: 322.

HOLINGER PH, SCHILD JA, MAURIZ DG (1968) Laryngeal papilloma. Review of etiology and therapy. Laryngoscope 78: 1462.

HOLLIEN H (1974) On vocal registers. Journal of Phonetics 2: 125-143.

HOLLIEN H (1980) Developmental aspects of neonatal vocalization. In: Infant Communication, Murry T, Murry J, eds. San Diego: College Hill Press.

HOLLIEN H (1983a) Control of vocal frequency. In: Vocal Fold Physiology, Bless DM, Abbs JH, eds. San Diego: College Hill Press.

HOLLIEN H (1983b) In search of vocal frequency control mechanisms. In: Vocal Fold Physiology, Bless DM, Abbs JH, eds. San Diego: College Hill Press.

HOLLIEN H, SHIPP T (1972) Speaking fundamental frequency and chronological age in males. Journal of Speech and Hearing Research 15: 155.

HONJO I, ISSHIKI N (1980) Laryngoscopic and voice characteristics of aged persons. Archives of Otolaryngology 106: 149.

HOSNY A, BHENDWAL S, HOSNI A (1995) Transection of cervical trachea following blunt trauma. Journal of Laryngology and Otology 109: 250-251.

HOWARD DM (1998) Instrumental Voice Measurement: uses and limitations. In: The Voice Clinic Handbook, Harris T, Harris S, Rubins JS, Howard DM, eds. London: Whurr.

HOWARD D, LINDSEY GA, ALLEN B (1990) Toward the quantification of vocal efficiency. Journal of Voice 4: 205-212.

HUGHES AJ, LEES A J (1991) The place of pergolide in treating Parkinson's disease. Care of the Elderly July: 311-312.

HUNT RB (1964) Rehabilitation of the laryngectomee. Laryngoscope 74: 382.

HUTZINGA E (1966) Historical vignette: Sir Felix Seman. Archives of Otolaryngology 84: 473.

HYMAN M (1979) Factors influencing intelligibility of alaryngeal speech. In: Laryngectomy Rehabilitation, Keith RL, Darley FL, eds. San Diego: College Hill Press.

ILLINGWORTH RS (1980) The development of communication in the first year and factors which affect it. In: Infant Communication Cry and Early Speech, Murry TM, Murry J, eds. San Diego: College Hill Press.

IMAM AP, HALPERN GM (1995) Pseudoasthma in a case of asthma (abbrev. source). Allergologia et Immunopathologia (Madrid) 23: 96-100.

INNOCENTI DM (1983) Chronic hyperventilation syndrome. In: Cash's Textbook of Chest, Heart and Vascular Disorders for Physiotherapists, 3rd edn, Downie PA, ed. New York: Faber & Faber.

ISSHIKI N (1964) Regulatory mechanism of voice intensity variation. Journal of Speech and Hearing Research 7: 17-29.

ISSHIKI N (1965) Vocal intensity and air flow rate. Folia Phoniatrica 17: 19.

ISSHIKI N (1968) Airflow in esophageal speech. In: Speech Rehabilitation of the Laryngectomised, 2nd edn, Snidecor JC, ed. Springfield, IL: Thomas.

ISSHIKI N (1980) Recent advances in phonosurgery. Folia Phoniatrica 32: 119.

ISSHIKI N, HONJO I, MOROMOTO M (1967) Cineradiographic analysis of movement of the lateral pharyngeal wall. Plastic Reconstructive Surgery 44: 357.

ISSHIKI N, MORITA H, OKAMURA H (1974) Thyroplasty as a new phonosurgical technique. Otolarynology 78: 451-457.

ISSHIKI N, OKAMURA H, ISHIKAWA T (1975) Thyroplasty Type 1. Lateral compression for dysphonia due to vocal cord paralysis and atrophy. Acta Otolaryngologica 80: 465.

ISSHIKI N, OKAMURA H, MORIMOTO M (1967) Maximum phonation time and air-flow rate during phonation. Simple clinical tests for vocal function. Annals of Otology 76: 998.

ISSHIKI N, TANABE M, SAWADA M (1978) Arytenoid adduction for unilateral vocal cord paralysis. Archives of Otolaryngology 104: 555.

IZDEBSKI K (1992) Symptomatology of adductor spasmodic dysphonia: a physiologic model. Journal of Voice 6: 306-319.

IZDEBSKI K, DEDO HH, SHIPP T (1981) Dysphonia patients treated by recurrent laryngeal nerve section. Otolarynology Head and Neck Surgery 89: 96.

IZDEBSKI K, ROSS JC, LEE S (1987) Fungal colonisation of tracheoesophageal voice prosthesis. Laryngoscope 97: 594.

IZDEBSKI K, SHIPP T, DEDO HH (1979) Predicting postoperative voice characteristics of spasmodic dysphonia patients. Otolaryngology Head and Neck Surgery 87: 428-434.

JACKSON C (1949) Psychosomatic aphonia and ephemeral adductor paralysis. Laryngoscope 59: 127.

JACKSON C, JACKSON CL (1935) Contact ulcer of the larynx. Archives of Otolaryngology 22: 1.

JACKSON MCA (1987) The high male voice. Folia Phoniatrica 39: 18.

JACOBS AH, ABRAMSON AL (1980) Speech therapy after total laryngectomy and esophageal replacement in a preschool patient: a case study. International journal of Pediatric Otorhinolaryngology 2: 21.

JACOBSON BH, JOHNSON A, GRYWALSKI C et al. (1997) The Voice Handicap Index (VHI): development and validation. American Journal of Speech-Language Pathology 6(3): 66-70.

JANET P (1920) The Major Symptoms of Hysteria. New York: Macmillan.

JANKOVIC J, BRIN M F (1991) Therapeutic Uses of Botulinum Toxin. New England Journal of Medicine 324: 1186-1194.

JAYSON MIV (1987) Back Pain: The facts, 2nd edn. Oxford: Oxford University Press.

JIANG JJ, TITZE IR (1994) Measurement of vocal fold intraglottal pressure and impact stress. Journal of Voice 8: 132-144.

JIANG J, OMARA T, CONLEY D, HANSON D (1999) Phonation threshold pressure measurements during phonation by air-flow interruption. Laryngoscope 109: 425-32.

JIU JB, SOBOL SM, GROZEA PN (1985) Vocal cord paralysis and recovery with thyroid lymphoma. Laryngoscope 95: 57.

JOHNS DF, SALYER KE (1978) Surgical and prosthetic management of neurogenic speech disorders. In: Clinical Management of Neurogenic Communicative Disorders, Johns DF, ed. Boston: Little Brown.

JOHNSON JA, PRING TR (1990) Speech therapy and Parkinson's disease: A review and further detail. British Journal of Disorders of Communication 25: 183-194.

JOHNSON N (1990) Respiratory Medicine. Oxford: Blackwell Scientific.

JULIAN W, MacCURTAIN F, NOSCOE N (1981) Anatomical factors influencing voice quality. Journal of Physiology 315: 10.

JURIK AG, PEDERSEN U, NORGARD A (1985) Rheumatoid arthritis of the cricoarytenoid joints: a case of laryngeal obstruction due to acute and chronic joint changes. Laryngoscope 95: 846.

KABAT H, KNOTT M (1953) Proprioceptive facilitation techniques for treatment of paralysis. Physical Therapy Review 2: 33.

KAHANE JC (1983) A survey of age-related changes in the connective tissues of the human larynx. In: Vocal Fold Physiology, Bless DM, Abbs JH, eds. San Diego: College Hill Press.

KAHANE JC (1986) Anatomy and physiology of the speech mechanism. In: Studies in Communication Disorders, Halpern H, ed. Austin, TX: Pro-Ed.

KAHANE JC (1987) Connective tissue changes in the larynx and their effects on voice. Journal of Voice 1: 27-30.

KALIN R (1982) The social significance of speech in medical, legal and occupational settings. In: Attitudes towards Language Variation, Ryan EB, Giles H, eds. London: Arnold.

KALLEN LA (1934) Vicarious vocal mechanisms. Archives of Otolaryngology 20: 460.

KARELITZ S, FISICHELLI VR (1962) The cry thresholds of normal infants and those with brain damage. Journal of Pediatrics 61: 679.

KARNELL MP (1989) Synchronized videostroboscopy and electroglottography. Journal of Voice 3: 68-75.

KARNELL MP (1994) Videoendoscopy: From velopharynx to larynx. San Diego: Singular Publishing Group Inc.

KARNELL MP, FINNEGAN EM (1994) Tools for voice measurement. Current Opinion in Otolaryngology and Head and Neck Surgery 2: 240-246.

KEARNS KP, SIMMONS NN (1988) Interobserver reliability and perceptual ratings: More than meets the ear. Journal of Speech and Hearing Research 31: 131-136.

KEARNS KP, SIMMONS NN (1990) The efficacy of speech-language pathology intervention: motor speech disorders. Seminars in Speech and Language 11: 273-293.

KELMAN AW, GORDON MT, SIMPSON IC, MORTON FM (1975) Assessment of vocal function by airflow measurements. Folia Phoniatrica 27: 250.

KENNEDY JT, KRAUSE CJ (1974) Survival rates in conservative surgery of the larynx. Archives of Otolaryngology 99: 274.

KENT R, READ C (1992) The Acoustic Analysis of Speech. San Diego: Singular Publishing Group, Inc.

KENT RD, ROSENBEK JC (1983) Acoustic patterns of apraxia of speech. Journal of Speech and Hearing Research 26: 231.

KERTESZ A (1983) Subcortical lesions and verbal apraxia. In: Apraxia of Speech: Physiology, acoustics, linguistics, management, Rosenbek JS, McNeil MR,

Aronson AE, eds. San Diego: College Hill Press.

KING AI, ASHBY J, NELSON C (1987) Laryngeal function in wind instrumentalists: the woodwinds. Journal of Voice 1: 365-367.

KIRCHNER JA (1966) Atrophy of laryngeal muscles in vagal paralysis. Laryngoscope 77: 1753.

KIRCHNER JA (1983) Factors influencing glottal aperture. In: Vocal Fold Physiology, Bless DM, Abbs JH, eds. San Diego: College Hill Press.

KIRIKAE I (1981) In discussion following WJ Goulds' paper on 'The pulmonary-laryngeal system'. In: Vocal Fold Physiology, Stevens KN, Hirano M, eds. Tokyo: University of Tokyo Press.

KITCH JA, OATES J (1994) Perceptual features of vocal fatigue as self-reported by a group of actors and singers. Journal of Voice 8: 207-214.

KITZING P (1985) Stroboscopy - a pertinent laryngological examination. Journal of Otolaryngology 14: 151.

KLEINSASSER O (1968) Microlaryngoscopy and Endolaryngeal Microsurgery (transl. PW Hoffman). Philadelphia: WB Saunders.

KNOTT M, VOSS D (1963) Proprioceptive Muscular Facilitation. Philadelphia: Harper & Row.

KOBAYASHI T, NIIMI S, KUMADA M, KOSAKI H, HIROSE H (1993) Botulinum toxin treatment for spasmodic dysphonia. Acta Otolaryngologica Supplementum 504: 155-157.

KOIKE Y, HIRANO M, VON LEDEN H (1967) Vocal initiation: acoustic and aerodynamic investigations in normal subjects. Folia Phoniatrica 19: 173.

KOTBY N (1995) The Accent Method of Voice Therapy. San Diego: Singular Publishing Group Inc.

KOTBY MN, SHIROMOTO O, HIRANO M (1993) The accent method of voice therapy: effect of accentuations on F0, SPL, and airflow. Journal of Voice 7: 319-325.

KOTBY N, FADLEY E, MADKOUR O et al. (1992) Electromyography and neurography in neurolaryngology. Journal of Voice 6: 159-187.

KOUFMAN JA (1986) Laryngoplasty for vocal cord medialization: an alternative to Teflon. Laryngoscope 96: 726.

KOUFMAN J (1995) Reflux and voice disorders. In: Diagnosis and Treatment of Voice Disorders, Rubin J, Sataloff R, Korovin G, Gould W, eds. New York: Igaku-Shoin.

KOUFMAN JA, BLALOCK PD (1988) Vocal fatigue and dysphonia in the professional voice user: Bogart-Bacall syndrome. Laryngoscope 98: 493-499.

KOUFMAN JA, BLALOCK PD (1989) Is voice rest never indicated? Journal of Voice 3: 87-91.

KOUFMAN JA, BLALOCK PD (1991) Functional voice disorders. Otolaryngologic Clinics of North America 24(5): 1059-1073.

KOUFMAN JA, RADOMSKI TA, JOHARJI GM, RUSSELL GB, PILLSBURY DC (1995) Laryngeal biomechanics of the singing voice. Paper presented at the Annual Meeting of the American Academy of Otolaryngology Louisiana - Center for Voice Disorders of Wake Forest University September 18 1995. [http://www.bgsm.edu/voice/singing_voice.html]

KRAMARAC C (1982) Gender: how she speaks. In: Attitudes towards Language Variation, Ryan EB, Giles H, eds. London: Edward Arnold.

KREIMAN J, GERRATT B, KEMPSTER G, ERMAN A, BERKE G (1993) Perceptual evaluation of voice quality: review, tutorial, and a framework for future research. Journal of Speech and Hearing Research 36: 21-40.

KRIEBEL D, SAMA SR, COCANOUR B (1993) Reversible pulmonary responses to formaldehyde. A study of clinical anatomy students. American Review of Respiratory Diseases 148: 1509-1515.

LABARRAQUE ML (1952) Les phonophobies. Annales d'Otolaryngologie (Paris) 69: 200.

LADEFOGED P (1974) Respiration, laryngeal activity and linguistics. In: Ventilatory and Phonatory Control Systems, Wyke B, ed. Oxford: Oxford University Press.

LAGUAITE JK (1972) Adult voice screening. Journal of Speech and Hearing Disorders 37: 147-151.

LAGUAITE JK, WALDROP WF (1963) Acoustic analysis of fundamental frequency of voices before and after therapy. New Zealand Speech Therapy Journal 18: 23.

LAITMAN JT, REIDENBERG JS (1997) The human aerodigestive tract and gastroesophageal reflux: an evolutionary perspective. American Journal of Medicine 103(suppl 5): 2S-8S.

LALL M, EVISON G (1966) Voice production following laryngo-pharyngo-oesophagectomy. Journal of Laryngology 80: 1208.

LANCER JM, SYDER D, JONES AS, LeBOUTILLIER A (1988) The outcome of different management patterns for vocal cord nodules. Journal of Laryngology and Otology 102: 423-427.

LANDES BA (1977) Management of hyperfunctional dysphonia and vocal tension. In: Approaches to Vocal Rehabilitation, Cooper M, Cooper MH, eds. Springfield, IL: Thomas.

LANGLEY J (1988) Working with Swallowing Disorders. Winslow, Bucks: Winslow Press.

LANGLOIS A, BAKEN RJ, WILDER CN (1980) Pre-speech respiratory behaviour during the first year of life. In: Infant Communication: Cry and speech, Murry T, Murry J, eds. Houston, TX: College Hill Press:.

LANGLOIS A, WILDER CN, BAKEN RJ (1975) Pre-speech respiratory patterns in the infant. American Association for Speech and Hearing 17: 668.

LANGMORE SE, SCHATZ K, OLSEN N (1988) Fiberoptic endoscopic examination of swallowing safety. Dysphagia 2: 216-219.

LARSON CR (1988) The midbrain periaqueductal gray: a brainstem structure involved in vocalization. Journal of Speech and Hearing Research 28: 241-9.

LAST RJ (1984) Anatomy, Regional and Applied, 7th edn. Edinburgh: Churchill Livingstone.

LAUDER E (1968) The laryngectomee and the artificial larynx. Journal of Speech Disorders 33: 147.

LAVER JD (1980) The Phonetic Description of Voice Quality. Cambridge: Cambridge University Press.

LE QUESNE LP (1964) Pharyngeal repair by immediate pharyngogastric anastomosis. Proceedings of the Royal Society of Medicine 57: 1103.

LEDER SB, LERMAN JW (1985) Some acoustic evidence for vocal abuse in adult speakers with repaired cleft palate. Laryngoscope 95: 837.

LEE L, CHAMBERLAIN LG, LOUDON RG, STEMPLE JC (1988) Speech segment durations produced by healthy and asthmatic subjects. Journal of Speech and Hearing Disorders 53:186-193.

LEE STS, NIIMI S (1990) Vocal fold sulcus. Journal of Laryngology and Otology 104: 876-878.

LEHMANN QH (1965) Reverse phonation. A new manoeuvre for examining the larynx. Radiology 84: 215.

LEJSKA V (1967) Occupational voice disorders in teachers [Czech]. Pracovni Lekarstvi 19(3): 119-121.

LELL WA (1941) Diagnosis and direct laryngoscopy: treatment of functional dysphonia. Archives of Otolaryngology 34: 141.

LENNEBERG EH (1967) Biological Foundation of Language. New York: John Wiley & Sons, Inc.

LENNEBERG EH, REBELSKY F, NICHOLS I (1965) The vocalisation of infants born to deaf and hearing parents. Human Development 8: 23.

LEONARD JR, HOLT GP, MARAN AG (1972) Treatment of vocal cord carcinoma by vertical laryngectomy. Annals of Otology 81: 469.

LEOPOLD DA (1983) Laryngeal trauma: a historical comparison of treatment methods. Archives of Otolaryngology 109: 106.

LESKE MC (1981) Prevalence estimates of communicative disorders in the US. Speech disorders. ASHA 23: 217-225.

LEVI JN (1994) Language as evidence: the linguist as expert witness. North American Courts in Forensic Linguistics, The International Journal of Speech, Language and the Law 1: 1.

LEVIN NM (1962a) Esophageal speech. In: Voice and Speech Disorders: Medical aspects, Levin NM. Springfield, IL: Thomas.

LEWIS BI (1959) Hyperventilation syndrome. A clinical and physiological evaluation. California Medicine 91: 121.

LEWIS G, WESSELY S (1997) The Essentials of Postgraduate Psychiatry, 3rd edn. Cambridge: Cambridge University Press.

LEWIS MM (1936) Early Response to Speech and Babbling in Infant Speech. London: Kegan Paul.

LEWIS RS (1965) Pharyngeal reconstruction after pharyngolaryngectomy. Journal of Laryngology 79: 771.

LI SL (1985) Functional tracheoesophageal shunt for vocal rehabilitation after laryngectomy. Laryngoscope 95: 1267.

LIBERMAN AM (1957) Some results of research on speech perception. Journal of Acoustical Society of America 29: 117.

LIEBERMAN J (1998) Principles and techniques of manual therapy: applications in the management of dysphonia. In: The Voice Clinic Handbook, Harris T, Harris S, Rubin JS, Howard DM, eds. London: Whurr Publishers.

LIEBERMAN P (1967) Intonation in infant speech: physiologic, acoustic and perceptual criteria. In: Intonation, Perceptions and Language, Research Monograph No. 18. Cambridge, MA: MIT Press.

LINFORD REES WL (1982) A Short Textbook of Psychiatry, 3rd edn. London: Hodder & Stoughton.

LOCKART MS, PATON F, PEARSON L (1997) Targets and timescales: a study of dysphonia using objective assessment. Logopedics Phoniatrics Vocology 22: 15-24.

LOCKE JL (1995) More than words can say. New Scientist 18: 30-33.

LOFQVIST A, YOSHIOKA H (1980) Laryngeal activity in Swedish obstruent clusters. Journal of the Acoustical Society of America 68: 792-801.

LOGEMANN J (1983a) Evaluation and Treatment of Swallowing Disorders. San Diego: College Hill Press.

LOGEMANN J (1983b) Vocal rehabilitation after extensive surgery for post-cricoid carcinoma. In: Laryngectomy: Diagnosis to rehabilitation, Edels Y, ed. London: Croom Helm.

LOTZ WK, D'ANTONIO LL, CHAIT DH, NETSELL RW (1993) Successful nasoendoscopic and aerodynamic examinations of children with speech/voice disorders. International Journal of Pediatric Otorhinolaryngology 26: 165-172.

LUCHSINGER R (1962) Voice disorders on an endocrine basis. In: Voice and Speech Disorders: Medical aspects, Levin NM, ed. Springfield, IL: Thomas.

LUCHSINGER R (1965a) Physiology and pathology of respiration and phonation. The qualities of the voice. In: Voice, Speech and Language, Luchsinger R, Arnold E, eds. London: Constable.

LUCHSINGER R (1965b) Vocal disorders from laryngeal paralysis. Paralytic dysphonia. In: Voice, Speech and Language, Luchsinger R, Arnold E, eds. London: Constable.

LUCHSINGER R (1965c) Vocal disorders of emotional origin: psychogenic dysphonia. In: Voice, Speech and Language, Luchsinger R, Arnold E, eds. London: Constable.

LUCHSINGER R, ARNOLD E, eds (1965) Voice, Speech and Language. London: Constable.

LUDLOW CL, BASSICH CJ (1984) Relationship between perceptual ratings and acoustic measurements of hypokinetic speech. In: The dysarthrias: Physiology, acoustics, perception, management, McNeil MR, Rosenbek JC, Aronson AE, eds. San Diego: College Hill Press.

LUDLOW CL, CONNOR NP (1987) Spasmodic Dysphonia. Journal of Speech and Hearing Research 30: 197.

LUDLOW CL, BASSICH CJ, CONNOR NP, COULTER DC (1986) Phonatory characteristics of vocal fold tremor. Journal of Phonetics 14: 509-515.

LUDLOW CL, BAKER M, NAUNTON RF, HALLETT M (1987) Intrinsic laryngeal muscle activation in spasmodic dysphonia. In: Motor disturbances, vol I, Benecke R, Conrad B, Marsden CD, eds. New York: Academic Press.

LUDLOW CL, NAUNTON RF, SEDORY SE, SCHULZ GM, HALLETT M (1988) Effects of botulinum toxin injections on speech adductor spasmodic dysphonia. Neurology 38: 1220-1225.

LUDLOW C, BAGLEY J, YIN S-G, KODA JA (1992) Comparison of injection techniques using botulinum toxin injection for the treatment of the spasmodic dysphonias. Journal of Voice 6: 380-386.

LUDLOW CL, YEH J, COHEN LG, VAN PELT F, RHEW K, HALLET M (1993) Limitations of electromyography and magnetic stimulation for assessing laryngeal muscle control. Annals of Otology, Rhinology and Laryngology 103: 16-27.

LUM C (1976) The syndrome of habitual chronic hyperventilation. In: Modern Trends in Psychosomatic Medicine, Vol III. Hill O, ed. London: Butterworth.

LUM C (1981) Hyperventilation and anxiety state (Editorial). Journal of the Royal Society of Medicine 74: 1.

LUND WS (1990) Some thoughts on swallowing - normal, abnormal and bizarre. Journal of the Royal Society of Medicine 83: 138-142.

McCALL GN, SKOLNICK ML, BREWER DW (1971) A preliminary report of some atypical movement patterns in the tongue, palate, hypopharynx, and larynx of patients with spasmodic dysphonia. Journal of Speech and Hearing Disorders 36: 4.

McCLELLAND E (1994) Regina versus Neil Scobie. Forensic Linguistics, the International Journal of Speech, Language and the Law 1: 223-227.

McCROSKEY RL, MULLIGAN M (1963) The relative intelligibility of oesophageal speech and artificial larynx. Journal of Speech Disorders 28: 37-41.

MacCURTAIN F, FOURCIN AJ (1982) Applications of the electrolaryngograph wave form display. In: Transcripts of the Tenth Symposium on Care of the Professional Voice Ed. L. Van Lawrence Part 2: 51. The Voice Foundation, New York.

MacDONALD G (1994) The Alexander Technique. London: Hodder.

McGLONE RE, BROWN WS (1969) Identification of the shift between vocal registers. Journal of the Acoustical Society of America 46: 1033-1036.

McGLONE R, HOLLIEN H (1963) Vocal pitch characteristics of aged women. Journal of Speech Research 6: 164.

MACKENZIE C (1987) Communication disorders in Legionnaires' Disease. British Journal of Disorders of Communication 22: 253.

MACKENZIE K, DEARY IJ, SELLARS C, WILSON JA (1998) Patient reported benefit of the efficacy of speech therapy in dysphonia. Clinical Otolaryngology 23: 280-287.

McNEIL MR, ROSENBEK JC, ARONSON AE, eds (1984) The Dysarthrias: Physiology, acoustics, perception, management. San Diego, CA: College Hill Press.

McWILLIAMS BJ, BLUESTONE CD, MUSGROVE RH (1969) Diagnostic implications of vocal cord nodules in children with cleft palate. Laryngoscope 79: 2072.

McWILLIAMS BJ, LAVORATO AS, BLUESTONE CD (1973) Vocal cord abnormalities in children with velopharyngeal valving problems. Laryngoscope 83: 1745.

McWILLIAMS BJ, MORRIS HL, SHELTON RL (1984) Cleft Palate Speech. Philadelphia: BC Decker/Toronto: CV Mosby.

McWILLIAMS BJ, MORRIS HL, SHELTON RL (1990) Cleft Palate Speech, 2nd edn. Philadelphia: BC Decker.

MADDERN BR, CAMPBELL TF, STOOL S (1991) Pediatric voice disorders. Otolaryngologic Clinics of North America 24: 1125-1139.

MAGARIAN GJ (1983) Hyperventilation syndrome: infrequently recognised common expressions of anxiety and stress. Medicine 61: 219.

MALCOLMSON KG (1968) Globus hystericus velopharyngis. Journal of Laryngology 82: 219.

MARAN AGD (1988) Logan Turner's Diseases of the Nose, Throat and Ear, 10th edn. Sevenoaks, Kent: John Wright.

MARAN AG, HAAST NH, LEONARD JR (1968) Reconstruction surgery for improved glottic closure. Laryngoscope 78: 1916.

MARLAND PM (1952) The Treatment of Dysphonia Due to Recurrent Laryngeal Nerve Palsies. College of Speech Therapists' Oxford Conference Report.

MARLAND PM (1953) Speech therapy for cerebral palsy based on reflex inhibition. Speech 17: 65.

MARSDEN CD, QUINN LP (1990) The dystonias - neurological disorders affecting 20,000 people in Britain. British Medical Journal 300: 139-144.

MASSENGIL R (1972) Hypernasality. Springfield, IL: Thomas.

MATHIESON L (1993a) Vocal tract discomfort in hyperfunctional dysphonia. Voice 2: 40-48.

MATHIESON L (1993b) Disorders of voice. In: The Encyclopedia of Language and Linguistics, Asher RE, Simpson JMY, eds. London: Pergamon.

MATHIESON L (1997) Voice disorders following road traffic accidents. Journal of Laryngology and Otology 111: 903-906.

MATHIESON L (1999) Disorders of voice. In: Concise Encyclopedia of Language Pathology, Fabbro F, ed. London: Pergamon.

MATHIESON L (2000) The normal-disordered continuum. In: The Handbook of Voice Quality Measurement, Kent RD, Ball MJ, eds. San Diego: Singular.

MAX L, de BRUYN W, STEURS W (1997) Intelligibility of oesophageal and tracheo-oesophageal speech: preliminary observations. European Journal of Disorders of Communication 32: 429-440.

MEAD J, HIXON T, GOLDMAN N (1974) Configuration of the chest wall during speech. In: Ventilatory and Phonatory Control Systems, Wyke B, ed. Oxford: Oxford University Press, London.

MECHAM MJ (1987) Cerebral palsy. In: Studies in Communication Disorders. Halpern H, ed. Austin, TX: Pro-Ed.

MENDELSOHN MS, McCONNEL FMS (1987) Function in the pharyngoesophageal segment. Laryngoscope 97: 483.

MERWIN GE, GOLDSTEIN LP, ROTHMAN HB (1985) A comparison of speech using artificial larynx and tracheoesophageal puncture with valve in the same speaker. Laryngoscope 95: 730.

MICHEL J, HOLLIEN H, MOORE P (1966) Speaking fundamental characteristics of 15-, 16- and 17-year-old girls. Language and Speech 9: 46.

MICHELSSON K, SIRVIO P (1976) Cry analysis in congenital hypothyroidism. Folia Phoniatrica 28: 40.

MICHELSSON K, WASZ-HÖCKERT O (1980) The value of cry analysis in neonatology and early infancy. In: Infant Communication: Cry and early speech, Murry T, Murry J, eds. Houston, TX: College Hill Press.

MICHELSSON K, RAES J, RINNE A (1984) Cry score - an aid in infant diagnosis. Folia Phoniatrica 36: 219-224.

MICHELSSON K, RAES J, THODEN CJ, WASZ-HÖCKERT O (1982) Sound spectrographic cry analysis in neonatal diagnostics. An evaluative study. Journal of Phonetics 10: 79-88.

MIHASHI S, OKADA M, KURITA S, NAGATA K, ODA M, HIRANO M, NAKASHIMA T (1981) Vascular network of the vocal fold. In: Vocal Fold Physiology, Stevens KN, Hirano M, eds. Tokyo: University of Tokyo Press.

MILLER AH (1967) First experience with the Asai technique for vocal rehabilitation after total laryngectomy. Annals of Otology 76: 829.

MILLER AH (1968) First experience with the Asai Technique for vocal rehabilitation after total laryngectomy. In: Speech Rehabilitation of the Laryngectomised, 2nd edn. Snidecor JC, ed. Springfield, IL: Thomas.

MILLER RH (1992) Technique of percutaneous EMG-guided botulinum toxin injection of the larynx for spasmodic dysphonia. Journal of Voice 6: 377-379.

MILLER RH, WOODSON GE (1991) Treatment options in spasmodic dysphonia. Otolaryngologic Clinics of North America 24: 1227-1237.

MISTEREK M, KNOTHE M, JOHANNES E, HEIDELBACH JG, SCHEUCH K (1989) Studies of voice stress in teachers with functional voice disorders caused by teaching activity. Zeitschrift für die Gesamte Hygiene und Ihre Grenzgebiete 35: 415-416.

MOBEIREEK A, ALHAMAD A, AL-SUBAEI A, ALZEER A (1995) Psychogenic vocal cord dysfunction simulating bronchial asthma(abbrev. source). European Respiratory Journal 8: 1978-1981.

MOHR RM, QUENELLE DJ, SHUMRICK DA (1983) Vertico-frontolateral laryngectomy (hemilaryngectomy) - indications, technique and results. Archives of Otolaryngology 109: 384.

MOLONEY JR (1978) Relapsing polychondritis - its otolaryngological manifestations. Journal of Laryngology and Otology 92: 9-15.

MOLOY PJ, CHARTER R (1982) The globus symptom. Archives of Otolaryngology 108: 740.

MONOSON P, ZEMLIN WR (1984) Quantitative study of whisper. Folia Phoniatrica 36: 53.

MONRAD-KROHN GH (1947a) Dysprosody or altered melody of language. Brain 70: 405.

MONRAD-KROHN GH (1947b) The prosodic quality of speech and its disorders. Acta Psychiatrica et Neurologica 22: 255.

MONTGOMERY WW (1963) Cricoarytenoid arthritis. Laryngoscope 73: 801.

MOOLENAAR-BIJL AJ (1956) Voice correction under pathological conditions. Acta Physiologica Neerlandica 5: 85.

MOORE DM, BERKE GS, HANSON DG, WARD PH (1987) Videostroboscopy of the canine larynx: the effects of asymmetric laryngeal tension. Laryngoscope 97: 543.

MORRIS GH (1985) The remedial episode as a negotiation of rules. In: Sequence and Pattern in Communicative Behaviour, Street RL, Cappella JR, Cappella JN, eds. London: Edward Arnold.

MORRISON M, RAMMAGE L (1994) The Management of Voice Disorders. London: Chapman & Hall.

MORRISON MD, NICHOL H, RAMMAGE LA (1986) Diagnostic criteria in functional dysphonia. Laryngoscope 94: 1.

MORRISON M, RAMMAGE L, EMAMI AJ (1999) The irritable larynx syndrome. Journal of Voice 13: 447-455.

MOSES PJ (1954) The Voice of Neurosis. New York: Grune & Stratton.

MOSES PJ (1958) Rehabilitation of the post-laryngectomised patient. Annals of Otology 67: 538.

MOSES PJ (1959) The vocal expression of emotional disturbances. Kaiser Foundation Medical Bulletin 7: 107.

MOSES PJ (1960) The psychology of the castrato voice. Folia Phoniatrica 12: 204.

MUELLER PB (1971) Parkinson's Disease: motor speech behaviour in a selected group of patients. Folia Phoniatrica 23: 333.

MUELLER PB (1973) Paralytic dysphonia: a case presentation. Folia Phoniatrica 25: 104.

MUELLER PB (1978) Communicative Disorders in a Geriatric Population. Report - ASHA Convention, San Francisco.

MUELLER PB (1997) The aging voice. Seminars in Speech and Language 18: 159-169.

MUELLER PB, SWEENEY RJ, BARIBEAU LJ (1985) Senescence of the voice: morphology of excised male larynges. Folia Phoniatrica 37: 134.

MULTINOVIC Z (1994) Social environment and incidence of voice disturbances in children. Folia Phoniatrica 46: 135-138.

MURAKAMI Y, SAITO S, IKARI T, HARAGUCHI S, OKADA K, MARUYAMA T (1982) Esophageal reconstruction with a skin-grafted pectoralis major muscle flap. Archives of Otolaryngology 108: 719.

MURDOCH BE, THEODOROS DG, STOKES PD, CHENERY HJ (1993) Abnormal patterns of speech breathing in dysarthric speakers following severe closed head injury. Brain Injury 7: 295-308.

MURPHY GE, BOSNA AL, OGURA JH (1964) Determinants of rehabilitation following laryngectomy. Laryngoscope 74: 1535.

MURRAY J (1998) Chair, Clinical Standards Advisory Group - Cleft lip and/or palate report. London: The Stationery Office.

MURRAY R, HILL P, McGUFFIN P (1997) The Essentials of Postgraduate Psychiatry, 3rd edn. Cambridge: Cambridge University Press.

MURRY T (1980) Acoustic and perceptual characteristics of infant cries. In: Infant Communication: Cry and early speech, Murry T, Murry J, eds. Houston, TX: College Hill Press.

MURRY T, WOODSON G E (1995) Combined-modality treatment of adductor spasmodic dysphonia with botulinum toxin and voice therapy. Journal of Voice 9: 460-465.

MURRY T, HOIT DALGAAD J, GRACCO VL (1983) Infant vocalisation: a longitudinal study of acoustic and temporal parameters. Folia Phoniatrica 35: 245.

MURRY T, XU JJ, WOODSON GE (1998) Glottal configuration associated with fundamental frequency and vocal register. Journal of Voice 12: 44-49.

MUSGROVE J (1952) Nervous diseases of the larynx. In: Diseases of the Ear, Nose and Throat, Scott Brown WG, ed. Butterworth, London.

MYEARS DW, MARTIN RJ, ECKERT RC, SWEENEY MK (1985) Functional versus organic vocal cord paralysis: rapid diagnosis and decannulation. Laryngoscope 95: 1235.

MYERSON MC (1952) Smoker's larynx. Annals of Otology 59: 541.

MYSAK ED (1959a) Significance of neurophysiological orientation to cerebral palsy habilitation. Journal of Speech Disorders 24: 221.

MYSAK ED (1959b) Pitch and duration characteristics of older males. Journal of Speech Research 2: 46.

MYSAK ED (1968) Dysarthria and oropharyngeal reflexology. Journal of Speech and Hearing Disorders 28: 252.

MYSAK ED, HANLEY T (1959) Aging processes in speech: Pitch and duration characteristics. Journal of Gerontology 13: 309.

NAHUM MC (1967) Vocal rehabilitation for contact ulcer of the larynx. Archives of Otolaryngology 85: 41.

NARBAITZ R, STUMPF WE, SAR M (1980) Estrogen target cells in the larynx: autoradiographic studies with 3H-diethylstilbestrol in fetal mice. Hormone Research 12: 113-117.

NASSAR WY (1977) Polytef (Teflon) injection of the vocal cords: experience with 34 cases. Journal of Laryngology 91: 341.

NATIONAL ASSOCIATION OF TEACHERS OF SINGING (1992) The role of the Speech-Language Pathologist and Teacher of Singing in Remediation of Singers with Voice Disorders. The NATS Journal.

NATIONAL CENTER FOR VOICE AND SPEECH (1993) Occupation and Voice Data. New York: CIBA Foundation.

NEGUS VE (1931) Observations on Semon's Law derived from evidence of comparative anatomy and physiology. Journal of Laryngology 46:1.

NEGUS VE (1949) The Comparative Anatomy and Physiology of the Larynx. London: Heineman Medical.

NEGUS VE (1957a) The function of the paranasal sinuses. Archives of Otolaryngology 66: 430.

NEGUS VE (1957b) The mechanism of the larynx. Laryngoscope 67: 1961.

NEILS L, YAIRI E (1987) Effects of speaking in noise on vocal fatigue and vocal recovery. Folia Phoniatrica 39: 104-112.

NETSELL R, LOTZ W, PETERS JE, SCHUSTER L (1994) Developmental patterns of laryngeal and respiratory function for speech production. Journal of Voice 8: 123-131.

NETTER FH (1979) The CIBA Collection of Medical Illustrations, Vol. 7, Respiratory System. CIBA Foundation.

NEW GB, DEVINE KD (1949) Contact ulcer granuloma. Annals of Otology 58: 548.

NEWMAN J, NGUYEN A, ANDERSON R (1987) Lipo-suction of the head and neck. In: Otolaryngology, Vol 4, English GM, ed. Philadelphia: Harper & Row.

NEWMAN KB, MASON UG 3rd, SCHMALING KB (1995) Clinical features of vocal cord dysfunction. American Journal of Respiratory Critical Care Medicine 152(4 Pt 1): 1382-1386.

NEWSOM-DAVIS J (1970) Diseases of the nervous system: apraxia. In: The Respiratory Muscles: Mechanics and neural control, 2nd edn, Campbell EJM, Agostini E, Davis JN, eds. London: Lloyd-Luke Medical Books.

NIEBUHR E (1978) The cri du chat syndome - epidemiology, cytogenetics and clinical features. Human Genetics 44: 227-275.

NISHIJIMA W, TAKODA S, HASEGAWA M (1984) Occult gastrointestinal tract lesions associated with the globus symptom. Archives of Otolaryngology 110: 246.

NORGATE S (1984) Laryngectomy is not a Tragedy. Edinburgh: Churchill Livingstone.

NUTT JG, MUENTER MD, ARONSON A, KURLAND LT, MELTON LJ (1988) Epidemiology of focal and generalised dystonia in Rochester, Minnesota. Movement Disorders 3: 188-194.

OATES JM, DACAKIS G (1983) Speech pathology consideration in the management of transsexualism - a review. British Journal of Disorders of Communication 18: 3.

OLSON NR (1991) Laryngopharyngeal manifestations of gastroesophageal reflux disease. Otolaryngologic Clinics of North America 24: 1201-1213.

ORLIKOFF RE (1994) Anatomy and physiology of respiration. Current Opinion in Otolaryngology and Head and Neck Surgery 2: 220-225.

ORLIKOFF RF, BAKEN RJ (1993a) Clinical Speech and Voice Measurement. San Diego: Singular.

ORLIKOFF RF, BAKEN RJ (1993b) Clinical Speech and Voice Measurement Laboratory Exercises. San Diego: Singular Publishing Group Inc.

OSGOOD CE (1953) Method and Theory in Experimental Psychology. Oxford: Oxford University Press.

OSTWALD PF (1963) Soundmaking: The acoustic communication of emotion. Springfield, IL: Thomas.

OYER HJ, DEAL LV (1985) Temporal aspects of speech and the aging process. Folia Phoniatrica 37: 109.

PAGET R (1930) Human Speech. London: Kegan Paul.

PANNBACKER M (1998) Voice treatment techniques: a review and recommendations for outcome studies. American Journal of Speech-Language Pathology 7(3): 49-64.

PANTOJA E (1968) The laryngeal cartilages. Archives of Otolaryngology 87: 416.

PAPSIDERO MJ, PASHLEY NRJ (1980) Acquired stenosis of the upper airway in neonates:

an increasing problem. Annals of Otology 89: 512.

PARKER A (1974) Voice and intonation training for deaf children using laryngographic display. Proceedings of the 8th International Congress on Acoustics. London: Chapman & Hall.

PARKES CM (1975) The emotional impact of cancer on patients and their families. Journal of Laryngology 89: 1271.

PARNES SM, SATYA-MURTI S (1985) Predictive value of laryngeal electromyography in patients with vocal cord paralysis of neurogenic origin. Laryngoscope 95: 1323.

PATTIE MA, MURDOCH BE, THEODOROS D, FORBES K (1998) Voice changes in women treated for endometriosis and related conditions: the need for comprehensive vocal assessment. Journal of Voice 12: 366-371.

PEACHER WG (1949) Neurological factors in the etiology of delayed speech. Journal of Speech Disorders 14: 147.

PEACHER WG (1961) Vocal therapy for contact ulcer: a follow-up of 70 patients. Laryngoscope 71: 137.

PEACHER WG, HOLINGER P (1947) Contact ulcer of the larynx: the role of vocal re-education. Archives of Otolaryngology 46: 617.

PEMBERTON C, RUSSELL A, PRIESTLEY J, HAVAS T, HOOPER J, CLARK P (1993) Characteristics of normal larynges under flexible fiberscopic and stroboscopic examination: an Australian perspective. Journal of Voice 7: 382-389.

PERKINS WH, KENT RD (1986) Textbook of Functional Anatomy of Speech, Language and Hearing. San Diego: College Hill Press.

PERLMAN A (1994) Normal swallowing physiology and evaluation. Current Opinion in Otolaryngology and Head and Neck Surgery 2: 226-232.

PERRY A (1983) The speech therapist's role in surgical and prosthetic approaches to speech rehabilitation, with particular reference to the Blom-Singer and Panje techniques. In: Laryngectomy: Diagnosis to rehabilitation, Edels Y, ed. London: Croom Helm.

PERRY A (1987) Technical assistance for patients with voice disorders. In: Assistive Communication Aids for the Speech Impaired, Enderby P, ed. Edinburgh: Churchill Livingstone.

PERRY A, EDELS Y (1985) Recent advances in the assessment of failed oesophageal speakers. British Journal of Disorders of Communication 20: 229.

PETERSON HA (1973) A case report of speech and language training for a two-year-old laryngectomised child. Journal of Speech and Hearing Disorders 38: 275.

PIAGET J (1952) Play, Dreams and Imitation in Childhood (transl. C Gattegno, ME Hodgson). London: Heinemann.

PIGOTT RW (1977) The development of endoscopy of the palatopharyngeal isthmus. Proceedings of the Royal Society 195: 269.

PIGOTT RW (1980) Assessment of velopharyngeal function. In: Advances in Management of Cleft Palate, Edwards M, Watson ACH, eds. Edinburgh: Churchill Livingstone.

PIGOTT RW, MAKEPEACE APW (1975) The technique of recording nasal pharyngoscopy. British Journal of Plastic Surgery 28: 26.

POIRIER MP, PANCIOLI AM, DiGIULIO GA (1996) Vocal cord dysfunction presenting as acute asthma in a pediatric patient. Pediatric Emergency Care 12: 213-214.

POLLACK D (1952) Post arytenoidectomy voice therapy. Speech 16: 4.

PRESSMAN JJ, BAILEY BJ (1968) The surgery of cancer of the larynx with special reference to subtotal laryngectomy. In: Speech Rehabilitation of the Laryngectomized, Snidecor JC, ed. Springfield, IL: Thomas.

PROCTOR DF (1974) Glottic aerodynamics and phonation. In: Ventilatory and Phonatory Control Systems, Wyke B, ed. Oxford: Oxford University Press.

PROCTOR DF (1980) Breathing, Speech and Song. Vienna: Springer-Verlag.

PRONOVOST WL (1977) Voice therapy for the hearing impaired. In: Approaches to Vocal Rehabilitation, Cooper M, Cooper M, eds. Springfield, IL: Thomas.

PROSEK RA, MONTGOMERY AA, WALDEN BE, SCHWARTZ DM (1978) EMG biofeedback in the treatment of hyperfunctional voice disorders. Journal of Speech Disorders 43: 282.

PTACEK P, SANDER EK, MALONE WH, JACKSON CCR (1966) Phonatory and related changes with advanced age. Journal of Speech and Hearing Research 9: 353.

PUNT N (1968) Applied laryngology: singers and actors. Proceedings of the Royal Society of Medicine 61: 1152.

PUNT NA (1983) Laryngology applied to singers and actors. Journal of Laryngology and Otology (suppl 6).

RABBETT WF (1965) Juvenile laryngeal papillomatosis. The relation of irradiation and malignant degeneration. Annals of Otology 74: 1149.

RAES JPF, CLEMENT PAR (1996) Aerodynamic measurements of voice production. Acta Oto-Rhino-Laryngologica Belgica 50: 293-298.

RAES J, DEHAEN F (1998) Towards a standardized terminology and methodology for the identification of induced pain cries. Cry Reports Special Issue, 1987, Palmerston North, New Zealand: Massey University Press, pp. 49-52.

RAMIG L, DROMEY C (1996) Aerodynamic mechanisms underlying treatment-related changes in vocal intensity in patients with Parkinson disease. Journal of Speech and Hearing Research 39: 798-807.

RAMIG L, RINGEL R (1983) Effects of physiological aging on selected acoustic characteristics of voice. Journal of Speech and Hearing Research 26: 22-30.

RAMIG L, SHIPP T (1987) Comparative measures of vocal tremor and vibrator. Journal of Voice 1: 162-167.

RAMIG LO, SCHERER RC (1992) Speech therapy for neurological disorders of the larynx. In Neurologic Disorders of the Larynx, Blitzer A, Brin MF, Sasaki CT, Fahn S, Harris KS, eds. New York: Thième.

RAMIG LO, VERDOLINI K (1998) Treatment efficacy: voice disorders. Journal of Speech, Language and Hearing Research 41: S101-S116.

RAMIG LA, TITZE IR, SCHERER RC, RINGEL SP (1988) Acoustic analysis of voices of patients with neurologic disease: rationale and preliminary data. Annals of Otology, Rhinology and Laryngology 97: 164-172.

RAMIG LO, COUNTRYMAN S, THOMPSON LL, YOSHIYUKI H (1995) Comparison of two forms of intensive speech treatment for Parkinson disease. Journal of Speech and Hearing Research 38: 1232-1251.

RAMIG LO, COUNTRYMAN S, O'BRIEN C, HOEHN M, THOMPSON L (1996) Intensive speech treatment for patients with Parkinson disease: short- and long-term comparison of two techniques. Neurology 47: 1496-1504.

RANGER D (1964) Problems of repair after pharyngolaryngectomy. Proceedings of the Royal Society of Medicine 57: 1099.

RANGER D (1983) Extensive surgery for post-cricoid carcinoma. In: Laryngectomy: Diagnosis to rehabilitation, Edels Y, ed. London: Croom Helm.

RAVITS JM, ARONSON AE, DESANTO LW, DYCK PY (1979) No morphometric abnormality of recurrent laryngeal nerve in spastic dysphonia. Neurology 29: 1376-1382.

REICH AR, McHENRY MA (1987) Respiratory volumes in cheerleaders with a history of dysphonic episodes. Folia Phoniatrica 39: 71.

REMACLE M (1996) The contribution of videostroboscopy in daily ENT practice. Acta Oto-Rhino-Laryngologica Belgica 50: 265-281.

REMACLE M, DEGOLS JC, DELOS M (1996) Exudative lesions of Reinke's space. An anatomopathological correlation. Acta Oto-Rhino-Laryngologica Belgica 50: 253-264.

RETHI A (1963) L'innervation du larynx. Acta ORL Ibero-Amer 2: 43.

RICHARD I, GIRAUD M, PERROUIN-VERBE B, HIANCE D, MAUDUYT de la GREVE I, MATHE JF (1996) Laryngotracheal stenosis after intubation or tracheostomy in patients with neurological disease. Archives of Physical and Medical Rehabilitation 77: 493-496.

RINGEL R, CHODZKO-ZAJKO W (1987a) Some implications of current gerontological theory for the study of voice. Communication Sciences and Disorders and Aging. Washington DC: American Speech-Language-Hearing Association.

RINGEL RL, CHODZKO-ZAJKO WJ (1987b) Vocal indices of biological age. Journal of Voice 1: 31-37.

RINGEL R, KLUPPEL D (1964) Neonatal crying: A normative study. Folia Phoniatrica 16: 1.

RITTER FN (1967) The effects of hyperthyroidism upon the ear, nose and throat. Laryngoscope 77: 1427.

ROBB MP, SAXMAN JH (1985) Developmental trends in vocal fundamental frequency of young children. Journal of Speech and Hearing Research 28: 421.

ROBBINS J, FISHER HB, BLOM ED, SINGER MI (1984) Selected acoustic features of tracheoesophageal, esophageal and laryngeal speech. Archives of Otolaryngology 110: 670.

ROBBINS KT, HOWARD D (1983) Multiple laryngeal papillomatosis requiring laryngectomy. Archives of Otolaryngology 109: 765.

ROBE E, MOORE P, BRUMLIK J (1960) A study of spastic dysphonia. Laryngoscope 70: 219.

ROBE EY, MOORE P, ANDREWS AH, HOLINGER PH (1956a) A study of the role of certain factors in the development of speech after laryngectomy. 1. Type of operation. Laryngoscope 66: 173.

ROBE EY, MOORE P, ANDREWS AH, HOLINGER PH (1956b) A study of the role of certain factors in the development of speech after laryngectomy. 2. Site of pseudoglottis. Laryngoscope 66: 382.

ROBE EY, MOORE P, ANDREWS AH, HOLINGER PH (1956c) A study of the role of certain factors in the development of speech after laryngectomy. 3. Co-ordination of speech with respiration. Laryngoscope 66: 481.

ROBERTSON MS, ROBINSON JM (1984) Immediate pharyngoesophageal reconstruction. Archives of Otolaryngology 110: 386.

ROBERTSON SJ (1982) Dysarthria Profile. Manchester: Manchester Polytechnic.

ROBERTSON SJ, THOMSON F (1984) Speech therapy in Parkinson's Disease: a study of the efficacy and long term effects of intensive treatment. British Journal of Disorders of Communication 19: 213.

ROBERTSON SJ, THOMSON F (1986) Working with Dysarthrics: A practical guide to therapy for dysarthria. London: Winslow Press.

ROHLS, FAZZALARO W (1993) Transection of trachea due to improper application of automatic seat belt (submarine effect). Journal of Forensic Science 38: 972-977

ROMANO C, RAGUSA RM, SCILLATO F, GRECO D, AMATO G, BARLETTA C (1991) Phenotypic and phoniatric findings in mosaic cri du chat syndrome. American Journal of Medical Genetics 39: 391-395.

ROSENBEK JC, LaPOINTE L (1985) The dysarthrias. In: Clinical Management of Neurogenic Communicative Disorders, Johns DF, ed. Boston: Little, Brown & Co.

ROSENBERG W, DONALD A (1995) Evidence-based medicine: an approach to clinical problem solving. British Medical Journal 310: 1122-1126..

ROSS JA, NOORDZJI JP, WOO P (1998) Voice disorders in patients with suspected laryngo-pharyngeal reflux disease. Journal of Voice 12: 84-88.

ROTHSTEIN SG (1998) Reflux and vocal disorders in singers with bulimia. Journal of Voice 12: 89-90.

ROY N, LEEPER HA (1993) Effects of the manual laryngeal musculoskeletal tension reduction technique for functional voice disorders: perceptual and acoustic measures. Journal of Voice 7: 242-249.

ROY N, FORD CN, BLESS DM (1996) Muscle tension dysphonia and spasmodic dysphonia - the role of manual laryngeal tension reduction in diagnosis and management. Paper presented at the meeting of the American Laryngological Association Florida May 4-5 1996. <http://www.stic.net/users/ta2man/distonia.html>.

ROY N, FORD CN, BLESS DM (1998) The role of manual laryngeal tension reduction in diagnosis and management. Paper presented at the meeting of the American Laryngological Association, Orlando May 4-5 1996.

RYAN EB, GILES H, SEBASTIAN RJ (1982) An integrative perspective for the study of attitudes toward language variation. In: The Social Psychology of Language, Vol 1 - Attitudes towards Language Variation, Ryan EB, Giles H, eds. London: Edward Arnold.

RYAN WJ (1972) Acoustic aspects of aging voice. Journal of Gerontology 27: 265.

SABOL JW, LEE L, STEMPLE JC (1995) The value of vocal function exercises in the practice regimen of singers. Journal of Voice 9: 27-36.

SAKODA S (1993) Genetics in movement disorders. Nippon Rinsho 51: 2935-2939.

SALMON SJ (1978) Patients talk back. In: The Artificial Larynx Handbook, Salmon SJ, Goldstein LP, eds. New York: Grune & Stratton.

SAMUEL S, ADAMS FG (1976) The role of oesophageal and diaphragmatic movements in alaryngeal speech. Journal of Laryngology 90: 1105.

SAPIENZA CM, DUTKA J (1996) Glottal airflow characteristics of women's voice production along an aging continuum. Journal of Speech and Hearing Research 39: 322-328.

SAPIR S (1993) Vocal attrition in voice students: survey findings. Journal of Voice 7: 66-74.

SAPIR S (1994) Medical, surgical, and behavioral approaches to vocal therapeutics. Current Opinion in Otolaryngology and Head and Neck Surgery 2: 247-251.

SAPIR S, ARONSON AE (1985a) Aphonia after closed head injury: aetiologic considerations. British Journal of Disorders of Communication 20: 289.

SAPIR S, ARONSON AE (1985b) Clinician reliability in rating voice improvement after laryngeal nerve section for spastic dysphonia. Laryngoscope 95: 200.

SAPIR S, ARONSON AE (1987) Coexisting psychogenic and neurogenic dysphonia: a source of diagnostic confusion. British Journal of Disorders of Communication 22: 73-80.

SAPIR S, ARONSON AE, THOMAS JE (1986) Judgment of voice improvement after recurrent laryngeal nerve section for spastic dysphonia: clinicians versus patients. Annals of Otology, Rhinology and Laryngology 95: 137-141.

SAPIR S, ATIAS J, SHAHAR A (1990) Symptoms of vocal attrition in women army instructors and new recruits: results from a survey. Laryngoscope 100: 991-994.

SASAKI CT, WEAVER EM (1997) Physiology of the larynx. American Journal of Medicine 103: 9S-17S.

SATALOFF R (1981) Professional singers: the science and art of clinical care. American Journal of Otolarynology 3: 251-266.

SATALOFF RS, SPIEGEL JR, CARROLL LM, SCHIEBEL B-R, DARBY KS, RULNICK R (1988) Strobovideolaryngoscopy in professional voice users: results and clinical value. Journal of Voice 1: 359-364.

SATALOFF RT (1991) Professional Voice: The Science and Art of Clinical Care. New York: Raven Press.

SATALOFF RT, REINHARDT JH, O'CONNOR MJ (1984) Rehabilitation of a quadriplegic professional singer: Use of a device to provide abdominal muscle support. Archives of Otolaryngology 110: 682.

SATALOFF RT, SPIEGEL JR, CARROLL LM, DARBY KS, HAWKSHAW MJ, RULNICK RK (1990) The clinical voice laboratory: practical design and clinical application. Journal of Voice 4: 264-279.

SAWASHIMA M, HIROSE H (1983) Laryngeal gestures in speech production. In: The Production of Speech, MacNeilage PF, ed. New York: Springer-Verlag, pp. 11-37.

SCHAEFFER SD (1983) Neuropathology of spasmodic dysphonia. Laryngoscope 93: 1183.

SCHAEFFER SD, FREEMAN FJ (1987) Spasmodic dysphonia. Neurologic disorders in otolaryngology. Otolaryngologic Clinics of North America 20: 161-178.

SCHAEFFER SD, JOHNS DF (1982) Attaining functional oesophageal speech. Archives of Otolaryngology 108: 647.

SCHAEFFER SD, FINITZO-HIEBERT T, GERLING IJ, FREEMAN FJ (1983a) Brainstem conduction abnormalities in spasmodic dysphonia. In: Vocal Fold Physiology, Bless DM, Abbs JH, eds. San Diego: College Hill Press.

SCHAEFFER SD, FINITZO-HIEBERT T, GERLING IJ, FREEMAN FJ (1983b) Brainstem conduction abnormalities in spasmodic dysphonia. Annals of Otology Rhinology and Laryngology 92: 59.

SCHERER K (1995) Expression of emotion in voice and music. Journal of Voice 9: 235-248.

SCHERER KR (1978) Personality inference from voice quality: the loud voice of extroversion. European Journal of Social Psychology 8: 467.

SCHERER KR, GILES H (1979) Social Markers in Speech. Cambridge: Cambridge University Press.

SCHERER RC (1991) Physiology of phonation: a review of basic mechanics. In: Phonosurgery: Assessment and surgical management of voice disorders, Ford CN, Bless DM, eds. New York: Raven Press.

SCHERER RC, TITZE IR, RAPHAEL BN, WOOD RP, RAMIG LA, BLAGER RT (1986) Vocal fatigue in a trained and untrained voice user. In: Laryngeal Function in Phonation and Respiration, Baer T, Sasaki C, Harris K, eds. Boston: College Hill Press, pp. 533-555.

SCHOW RL, NERBONNE MA (1981) Hearing levels among elderly nursing home residents. Journal of Speech and Hearing Disorders 46: 124.

SCHULMAN R (1989) Articulatory dynamics of loud and normal speech. Journal of the Acoustical Society of America 85: 295-312.

SCHUTTE HK, SEIDNER W (1983) Recommendations by the Union of European Phoniatricians (UEP): standardizing voice area measurements/phonetography. Folia Phoniatrica 35: 286-8.

SCHUTTE HK, ŠVEC JC, SRAM F (1998) First results of clinical application of videoky-mography. Laryngoscope 108:1206-1210.

SCOTT S, CAIRD FI (1981) Speech therapy for patients with Parkinson's Disease. British Medical Journal 283: 1080.

SCOTT S, CAIRD FI (1983) Speech therapy for Parkinson's disease. Journal of Neurology, Neurosurgery, and Psychiatry 46: 140-146.

SCOTT S, CAIRD FI, WILLIAMS BO (1984) Evidence for an apparent sensory speech disorder in Parkinson's Disease. Journal of Neurology, Neurosurgery, and Psychiatry 47: 840.

SCOTT S, CAIRD FI, WILLIAMS BO (1985) Communication in Parkinson's Disease. London: Croom Helm.

SCOTT S, ROBINSON K, WILSON JA, MACKENZIE K (1997) Patient-reported problems associated with dysphonia. Clinical Otolaryngology 22: 37-40.

SEDLACKOVA E (1960) Les dysphonies hypercinétiques des enfants causées par surmenage vocal. Folia Phoniatrica 12: 48.

SEEMAN M (1922) Speech and voice without larynx. An experimental and clinical study of the development of speech without larynx. Casopis Lekaru Ceskych (Praha) 41: 369.

SEEMAN M (1959) Sprachstörungen bei Kindern. Marhold Saale.

SELIGER GM, ABRAMS GM, HORTON A (1992) Irish brogue after stroke. Stroke 23: 1655-1656.

SELL D, HARDING A, GRUNWELL P (1994) A screening assessment of cleft lip and palate speech (Great Ormond Street Speech Assessment). European Journal of Disorders of Communication 29: 1-15.

SELLEY NG (1979) Dental and technical aids for treatment of patients suffering from velopharyngeal disorders. In: Diagnosis and Treatment of Palatoglossal Malfunction, Ellis RE, Flack FC, eds. London: College of Speech Therapists.

SELLEY NG (1985) Swallowing difficulties in stroke patients: a new treatment. Age and Ageing 14: 361.

SENTURIA BH, WILSON FB (1968) Otorhinolaryngologic findings in children with voice deviations. Annals of Otology 77: 1027.

SESSIONS DG, MANESS GM, McSWAIN B (1965) Laryngofissure in the treatment of carcinoma of the vocal cord: a report of 40 cases and review of the literature. Laryngoscope 75: 490.

SETH G, GUTHRIE D (1953) Speech in Childhood. Oxford: Oxford University Press.

SHAW HJ (1966) Partial laryngectomy. Journal of Laryngology 80: 839.

SHAW HJ, FRIEDMAN I (1964) Diffuse keratosis of the larynx with multicentric malignant change and metastatic neuropathy. Journal of Laryngology 78: 757.

SHEPPARD WC, LANE HI (1968) Development of the prosodic features of infant vocalizing. Journal of Speech and Hearing Research 11: 94.

SHEPPERD HWH (1966) Androgenic hoarseness. Journal of Laryngology 80: 403.

SHERRINGTON C (1947) The Integrative Action of the Nervous System. Cambridge: Cambridge University Press.

SHIELS P, HAYES JP, FITZGERALD MX (1995) Paradoxical vocal cord adduction in an adolescent with cystic fibrosis. Thorax 50: 694-695.

SHINDO ML, HANSON DG (1990) Geriatric voice and laryngeal dysfunction. The Otolaryngologic Clinics of North America 23: 1035-1043.

SHIPP T (1975) Vertical laryngeal position during continuous and discrete vocal frequency change. Journal of Speech and Hearing Research 18: 707.

SHIPP T, HOLLIEN H (1969) Perception of the aging male voice. Journal of Speech and Hearing Research 12: 703.

SHIPP T, McGLONE RE (1971) Laryngeal dynamics associated with voice frequency change. Journal of Speech and Hearing Research 14: 761.

SIEGEL GM (1969) Vocal conditioning in infants. Journal of Speech Disorders 34: 3.

SIEGMAN AW (1987) The tell-tale voice: non-verbal messages of verbal communication. In: Non-verbal Behaviour and Communication, Siegman AW, Feldstein S, eds. New York: Laurence Erlbaum.

SILVER FM, GLUCKMAN JL, DONEGAN JO (1985) Operative complications of tracheoesophageal puncture. Laryngoscope 95: 1360.

SILVERMAN E, ZIMMER CH (1975) Incidence of chronic hoarseness among school age children. Journal of Speech Disorders 40: 211.

SIM M (1981) Psychopathia sexualis. In: Guide to Psychiatry. Edinburgh: Churchill Livingstone.

SIMPSON JC, SMITH JCS, GORDON MT (1972) Laryngectomy: the influence of muscle reconstruction on the mechanism of oesophageal voice production. Journal of Laryngology 86: 961.

SINGER MI, BLOM ED (1980) An endoscopic technique for restoration of voice after laryngectomy. Annals of Otology 89: 529.

SINGER MI, BLOM ED, HAMAKER RC (1983) Voice rehabilitation after total laryngectomy. Journal of Otolaryngology 12: 329.

SINGER MI, BLOM ED, HAMAKER RC (1986) Pharyngeal plexus neurectomy for alaryngeal speech rehabilitation. Laryngoscope 96: 50.

SINGER MI, HAMAKER RC, MILLER SM (1985) Restoration of the airway following bilateral recurrent laryngeal nerve paralysis. Laryngoscope 95: 1204.

SKINNER BF, VAUGHAN BF (1983) Enjoy Old Age: A programme of self management. New York: WW Norton.

SKYNNER ACR (1976) One Flesh, Separate Persons: Principles of family and marital psychotherapy. London: Constable.

SKYNNER R, CLEESE J (1983) Families and How to Survive Them. London: Methuen.

SLONIM NB, HAMILTON LH (1976) Respiratory Physiology. St Louis: CV Mosby.

SMITH ME, RAMIG LO, DROMEY C, PEREZ KS, SAMANDARI R (1995) Intensive voice-treatment in Parkinson disease: Laryngoendoscopic findings. Journal of Voice 9: 453-459.

SMITH PM (1979) Sex markers in speech. In: Social Markers in Speech, Scherer KR, Giles H, ed. Cambridge: Cambridge University Press.

SMITH S, THYME K (1976) Statistic research on changes in speech due to pedagogic treatment (the Accent Method). Folia Phoniatrica 28: 98.

SMITHERAN J, HIXON T (1981) A clinical method for estimating laryngeal airway resistance during vowel production. Journal of Speech and Hearing Disorders 46:138-146.

SMURTHWAITE H (1919) War neurosis of the larynx and speech mechanism. Journal of Laryngology 34: 13.

SNELL RS (1995) Clinical Anatomy for Medical Students, 5th edn. Boston: Little, Brown & Co. Inc.

SNIDECOR JC (1968) Speech Rehabilitation of the Laryngectomised, 2nd edn. Springfield, IL: Thomas.

SNIDECOR JC, CURRY ET (1959) Temporal pitch aspects of superior esophageal speech. Annals of Otology 68: 623.

SNIDECOR JC, CURRY ET (1960) How effectively may the laryngectomee speak? Proceedings of the 11th International Speech and Voice Conference, Stein L, ed. New York: Karger.

SNIDECOR JC, ISSHIKI N (1965) Air volume and air flow relationships of 6 male oesophageal speakers. Journal of Speech Disorders 30: 205.

SODERSTEN M, HERTEGARD S, HAMMARBERG B (1995) Glottal closure, transglottal airflow and voice quality in healthy middle-aged women. Journal of Voice 9: 182-197.

SOKOLOWSKY RR, JUNKERMANN EB (1944) War aphonia. Journal of Speech Disorders 9: 193.

SONIES B (1992) Oropharyngeal dysphagia in the elderly in oral and dental problems in the elderly. Clinics in Geriatric Medicine 8: 569-577.

SONNINEN A (1960) Laryngeal signs and symptoms of goitre. Folia Phoniatrica 12: 41.

SORENSEN H (1982) Laser surgery in benign laryngeal disease. Acta Otolaryngologica 94: 537.

SPARKS RW (1981) Melodic intonation therapy. In: Language Intervention Strategies in Adult Aphasia, Chapey R, ed. Baltimore: Williams & Wilkins.

SPARKS RW, HOLLAND A (1976) Method: melodic intonation therapy. Journal of Speech and Hearing Disorders 41: 287.

SPENCER PS, NUNN PB, HUGON J, LUDOLPH AC, ROSS SM, ROY DN, ROBERTSON RC (1987) Guam amyotrophic lateral sclerosis Parkinsonian-dementia linked to a plant excitant neurotoxin. Science 237: 517.

SPIEGEL JR, SATALOFF RT, GOULD WJ (1987) Treatment of vocal fold paralysis with injectable collagen: clinical concerns. Journal of Voice 1: 119.

STARK RE (1978) Features of infant sounds: the emergence of cooing. Journal of Child Language 5: 379.

STARK RE (1979) Pre-speech segmental feature development. In: Language Acquisition, Fletcher P, Garman M, eds. Cambridge: Cambridge University Press.

STARK RE, NATHANSON S (1975) Unusual features of cry in an infant dying suddenly and unexpectedly. In: Development of Upper Respiratory Anatomy and Function: Implications for SID, Bosma J, Showacre J, eds. Washington DC: US Department of Health and Education.

STARK RE, ROSE SN, McLAGAN M (1975) Features of infant sounds: the first eight weeks of life. Journal of Child Language 2: 205.

STATHOPOULOS ET, SAPIENZA C (1993) Respiratory and laryngeal function of women and men during vocal intensity variation. Journal of Speech and Hearing Research 36: 64-75.

STEER MD, HANLEY TD (1959) Instruments of diagnosis, therapy and research. In: Handbook of Speech Pathology, Travis LE, ed. London: Peter Owen.

STEINSCHNEIDER A (1972) Prolonged apnea and the sudden infant death syndrome:

clinical and laboratory observations. Pediatrics 50: 646.

STEINSCHNEIDER A, RABUZZI D (1976) Apnea and airway obstruction during feeding and sleep. Laryngoscope 86: 1359.

STEMPLE JC (1984) Clinical Voice Pathology: Theory and management. Columbus, OH: Merrill.

STEMPLE JC (1993) Voice Therapy: Clinical Studies. St Louis: Mosby Year Book.

STEMPLE JC, GLAZE LE, GERDMAN BK (1995) There is always a reason for a voice disorder. In: Clinical Voice Pathology: Theory and Management, 2nd edn. San Diego, CA: Singular Publishing Group Inc.

STEMPLE JC, STANLEY J, LEE L (1995) Objective measures of voice production in normal subjects following prolonged voice use. Journal of Voice 9: 127-33.

STEMPLE JC, WEILER E, WHITEHEAD W, KOMRAY R (1980) Electromyographic biofeedback training with patients exhibiting hyperfunctional voice disorder. Laryngoscope 90: 471-476.

STEMPLE JC, LEE L, DAMICO B, PICKUP B (1994) Efficacy of vocal function exercises as a method of improving voice production. Journal of Voice 8: 270-278.

STENGELHOFEN EJ (1993) Cleft Palate: Nature and remediation of communication problems. London: Whurr.

STETSON RH (1937) Esophageal speech for any laryngectomised patient. Archives of Otolaryngology 26: 132.

STEVENS KN, HIRANO M (1981) Vocal Fold Physiology. Tokyo: Tokyo University Press.

STOICHEFF ML (1981) Speaking fundamental frequency characteristics of non-smoking female adults. Journal of Speech and Hearing Research 24: 437.

STONES J, DRAKE TM (1984) An intensive course of therapy for patients with Parkinson's Disease. College of Speech Therapists' Bulletin 387.

STRAND EA, BUDER EH, YORKSTON KM, RAMIG LO (1994) Differential phonatory characteristics of four women with amyotrophic lateral sclerosis. Journal of Voice 8: 327-339.

STREET RL, HOPPER R (1982) A model of speech style evaluation. In: Attitudes towards Language Variation, Ryan EB, Giles H, eds. London: Edward Arnold.

STUART DW (1966) Surgery in cancer of the cervical oesophagus: plastic tube replacement. Journal of Laryngology 80: 382.

SUMMERS IR, MARTIN MC (1980) A tactile sound level monitor for the profoundly deaf. British Journal of Audiology 14: 30.

SUNDBERG J (1974) Articulatory interpretation of the singing formant. Journal of the Acoustical Society of America 55: 838.

SUNDBERG J (1977) The acoustics of the singing voice. Scientific American 236: 82.

SUNDBERG J (1995) Acoustic and psychoacoustic aspects of vocal vibrato. In: Vibrato, Dejonckere PH, Hirano M, Sundberg J, eds. San Diego: Singular Publishing Group, Inc.

SURUDA A, SCHULTE P, BOENIGER M et al. (1993) Cytogenetic effects of formaldehyde exposure in students of mortuary science. Cancer Epidemiology Biomarkers Prevention 2: 453-460.

ŠVEC JG, SCHUTTE HK (1996) Videokymography: High-speed line scanning of vocal fold vibration. Journal of Voice 10: 201-205.

SWENSON R, ZWIRNER P, MURRY T, WOODSON GE (1992) Medical evaluation of patients with spasmodic dysphonia. Journal of Voice 6: 320-324.

SWIFT AC, ROGERS J (1987) Vocal cord paralysis in children. Journal of Laryngology 101: 169.

TAKANO-STONE J (1987) Intervention for psychosocial problems associated with sensory disabilities in old age. In: Psychosocial Interventions with Sensorially Disabled Persons, Heller B, Flohr L, Zeagans LS, eds. New York: Grune & Stratton.

TANABE M, HONJO I, ISSHIKI N (1985) Neoglottic reconstruction following total laryngectomy. Archives of Otolaryngology 111: 39.

TANABE M, HAJI T, HONJO I, ISSHIKI N (1985) Surgical treatment for androphonia: an experimental study. Folia Phoniatrica 37: 15.

TANNEN D (1995) The power of talk: Who gets heard and why. Harvard Business Review 73: 138-148.

TARDY-MITZELL S, ANDREWS ML, BOWMAN SA (1985) Acceptability and intelligibility of tracheoesophageal speech. Archives of Otolaryngology 111: 213.

TARNEAUD J (1961) Traite Pratique de Phonologie et de Phoniatrie. Paris: Libraire Maloine.

TASHJIAN LS, PEACOCK JE (1984) Laryngeal candidiasis. Archives of Otolaryngology 110: 806.

TAUB S (1975) Air bypass prosthesis for vocal rehabilitation of laryngectomees. Annals of Otolaryngology 84: 45.

TEACHEY JC, KAHANE JC, BECKFORD NS (1991) Vocal mechanics in untrained professional singers. Journal of Voice 5: 51-56.

TEITEL AD, MACKENZIE CR, STERN R, PAGET SA (1992) Laryngeal involvement in systemic lupus erythematosus. Seminars in Arthritis and Rheumatism 22: 203-214.

TERRACOL J, GUERRIER Y, CAMPS F (1956) Le sphincter glottique; étude anatomo-clinique. Annals of Otolaryngology (Paris) 73: 451.

THOMSON St SC, NEGUS VE, BATEMAN GH (1955) Diseases of the Nose and Throat, 6th edn. London: Cassell.

THOMSON WJR (1976) Lungs. Black's Medical Dictionary, 31st edn. London: A & C Black.

THYME K (1980) Trials of the accent method. Proceedings of the XVIIIth IALP Congress, vol. 1. Washington, p. 633.

TITZE I (1981) The role of computational simulation in evaluation of physical properties of the vocal folds. In: Vocal Fold Physiology, Stevens KN, Hirano M. Tokyo: University of Tokyo Press.

TITZE IR (1990) Interpretation of the electroglottographic signal. Journal of Voice 4: 1-9.

TITZE I (1991) Phonation threshold pressure. A missing link for glottal aerodynamics.

In: Progress Report 1. Titze IR, ed. Iowa City: National Centre for Voice and Speech, pp 1-14.

TITZE IR (1992) Phonation threshold pressure: a missing link in glottal aerodynamics. Journal of the Acoustical Society of America 91: 2926-2935.

TITZE IR (1994a) Mechanical stress in phonation. Journal of Voice 8: 99-105.

TITZE IR (1994b) Principles of Voice Production. New Jersey: Prentice Hall.

TITZE IR (1994c) Towards standards in acoustic analysis of voice. Journal of Voice 8: 1-7.

TITZE I (1995) How do vibrating folds of moist skin generate exquisite operatic arias? New Scientist 23 September: 35-42.

TITZE IR, LEMKE J, MONTEQUIN D (1997) Populations in the US workforce who rely on voice as a primary tool of trade: a preliminary report. Journal of Voice 11: 254-259.

TOMODA H, SHIBASAKI H, KURODA Y, SHIN T (1987) Voice tremor: dysregulation of voluntary expiratory muscles. Neurology 37: 117-122.

TOSI O (1979) Voice Identification: Theory and legal applications. Baltimore, MA: University Park Press.

TRAVIS LW, HYBELS RL, NEWMAN MH (1976) Tuberculosis of the larynx. Laryngoscope 86: 549.

TRUDEAU MD, HIRSCH SM, SCHULLER DE (1986) Vocal restorative surgery: why wait? Laryngoscope 96: 975.

TUCKER HM (1976) Human laryngeal re-innervation. Laryngoscope 85: 769.

TUCKER HM (1978) Human laryngeal reinnervation: longterm experience with the nerve-muscle pedicle technique. Laryngoscope 85: 598.

TUCKER HM (1980) Laryngeal paralysis: etiology and management. In: Otolaryngology, vol. 3. English GM, ed. Philadelphia: Harper & Row.

TUCKER HM (1987a) Adductor spasmodic dysphonia. In: The Larynx, Tucker HM, ed. New York: Thième, pp. 152-154.

TUCKER HM (1987b) Neurological disorders. In: The Larynx, Tucker HM, ed. New York: Thième.

TUCKER HM, ed. (1987c) The Larynx. New York: Thième.

TUCKER HM (1988) Laryngeal framework surgery in the management of the aged larynx. Annals of Otology and Laryngology 97: 534-536.

TUCKER H (1993) The Larynx. New York: Thième.

TUCKER HM, LAVERTU P (1992) Paralysis and paresis of the vocal fold. In: Neurologic Disorders of the Larynx, Blitzer A, Sasaki M, Fahn S, Harris KS, eds. New York: Thième.

TUDOR C, SELLEY WG (1974) A palatal training appliance and a visual aid for use in treatment of hypernasal speech. British Journal of Disorders of Communication 9: 117.

TURNER L (1952) Chronic infective conditions of the larynx and tuberculosis of the larynx. In: Logan Turner's Diseases of the Nose, Throat and Ear, 5th edn, Guthrie D, ed. Bristol: John Wright/London: Simpkin Marshall.

URBANOVA O, UHROVA M (1987) Development of hyperfunctional voice disorders in teachers studied 1972-1985 at the phoniatric department of the Medical School Hospital in Bratislava. Ceskoslovenska Otolaryngologie 36: 295-299.

VALANNE E, VUORENKOSKI V, PARTANEN TJ, LIND J, WASZ-HÖCKERT O (1967) The ability of human mothers to identify the hunger cry signal of their own new-born infants during the lying-in period. Experimenta 23: 768.

VAN DEN BERG JW (1962) Modern research in experimental phonetics. Folia Phoniatrica 14: 81.

VAN GELDER L (1974) Psychosomatic aspects of endocrine disorders of the voice. Journal of Communication Disorders 7: 257.

VAN RIPER C (1947) Speech Correction. New York: Prentice Hall.

VAN RIPER C, IRWIN JV (1958) Voice and Articulation Drill Book. New York: Prentice Hall.

VAN THAL JH (1934) Cleft Palate Speech. London: Allen & Unwin.

VAN THAL JH (1961) Dysphonia. Speech Pathology and Therapy 4: 11.

VAN THAL JH (1962) Four generations of aphonia. Proceedings of the XIIth IALP Congress, Padua.

VENNARD W, VON LEDEN H (1967) The importance of intensity modulation in the perception of trill. Folia Phoniatrica 19: 19.

VERDOLINI K, SKINNER MW, PATTON T, WALKER PA (1985) Effect of amplification on the intelligibility of speech produced with an electrolarynx. Laryngoscope 95: 720.

VERDOLINI-MARSTON K, SANDAGE M, TITZE IR (1994) Effect of hydration treatments on laryngeal nodules and polyps and related voice measures. Journal of Voice 8: 30-47.

VERDOLINI-MARSTON K, BURKE MK, LESSAC A, GLAZE L, CALDWELL E (1995) Preliminary study of two methods of treatment for laryngeal nodules. Journal of Voice 9: 74-85.

VERMEULING VR (1966) Laryngeal carcinoma in the young. Laryngoscope 77: 1724.

VILKMAN E (1996) Occupational risk factors and voice disorders. Logopedics Phoniatrics Vocology 21: 137-141.

VON LEDEN H (1961) The mechanism of phonation. Archives of Otolaryngology 74: 660.

VON LEDEN H, MOORE P (1960) Contact ulcer of the larynx. Motion picture. Voice Research Lab, Northwestern Medical School, Chicago.

VON LEDEN H, MOORE P (1961) The mechanics of the cricoarytenoid joint. Archives of Otolaryngology 73: 541.

VOSS DE, IONTA MK, MYERS BJ (1985) Proprioceptive Neuromuscular Facilitation Patterns and Techniques. New York: Harper & Row.

VRABEC DP, DAVISON FW (1980) Inflammatory diseases of the larynx. In: Otolaryngology, vol. 3. English GM, ed. New York: Harper & Row.

VRTICKA K, SVOBODA M (1961) A clinical X-ray study of 100 laryngectomised speakers. Folia Phoniatrica 13: 174.

VRTICKA K, SVOBODA M (1963) Time changes in the X-ray picture of the hypopharynx, pseudoglottis and esophagus in the course of vocal rehabilitation in 70 laryngectomised speakers. Folia Phoniatrica 15: 1.

WALSHE FMR (1952) Anatomical or localising factors in diagnosis. In: Diseases of the Nervous System, 7th edn. Edinburgh: Churchill Livingstone.

WANG N-M, YEUNG KW, CHEN T-A (1986) Voice disorders in children with velopharyngeal valving problems. Proceedings of the XXth IALP Congress, Tokyo.

WARBURTON CJ, NIVEN RM, HIGGINS BG, PICKERING CAC (1996) Functional upper airways obstruction: two patients with persistent symptoms. Thorax 51: 965-966.

WARD PH, HANSON DG, ABEMAYER E (1985) Transcutaneous Teflon injection of the paralysed vocal cord: a new technique. Laryngoscope 95: 644.

WARD PH, COLTON R, McCONNELL F, MALMGREN L, KASHIMA H, WOODSON G (1989) Aging of the voice and swallowing. Otolaryngology Head and Neck Surgery 100: 283-285.

WASZ-HÖCKERT O, LIND J, VUORENSKI V, PARTENEN TJ, VALANNE E (1968) The infant cry: A spectrographic and auditory analysis. Clinics in Developmental Medicine, No. 29. Spastics International Medical Publication in association with Heinemann Medical.

WATANABE H, SHIN T, MATSUO H et al. (1994) Studies of vocal fold injection and changes in pitch associated with alcohol intake. Journal of Voice 8: 340-346.

WATKIN K, EWANOWSKI S (1985) Effects of aerosol corticosteroids on the voice: triamcinolone acetonide and beclomethasone dipropionate. Journal of Speech and Hearing Research 28: 301.

WAX MK, MYERS L, ANDERSEN PE, COHEN JI (1999) The effect of head and neck reconstruction on quality of life. Current Opinion in Otolaryngology and Head and Neck Surgery 7; 180-184.

WEDIN S (1972) Rehabilitation of speech in cases of palato-pharyngeal paresis with the aid of an obturator prosthesis. British Journal of Disorders of Communication 7: 117.

WEINBERG B, SHEDD DP, HORII Y (1978) Reed-fistula speech following pharyngolaryngectomy. Journal of Speech and Hearing Disorders 43: 401.

WEISBERG P (1963) Social and non social conditioning of infant vocalizations. Child Development 34: 377.

WEISMER G (1984) Articulatory characteristics of Parkinsonian dysarthria: segmental and phrase-level timing, spirantization and glottal-supraglottal co-ordination. In: The Dysarthrias: Physiology, acoustics, perception, management, McNeill MR, Rosenbek J, Aronson AE, eds. San Diego: College Hill Press.

WEISS DA (1950) The pubertal change of the human voice (mutation). Folia Phoniatrica 2: 126.

WEISS DA (1955) The psychological relations to one's own voice. Folia Phoniatrica 7: 209.

WEISS DA (1964) Cluttering. New York: Prentice Hall.

WENDLER J, ANDERS LC (1986) Hoarse voices: on the reliability of acoustic and auditory classifications. Proceedings of the XXth IALP Congress, Tokyo.

WEPMAN JM, McGAHAN JA, RICKARD JC, SHELTON NW (1953) The objective measurement of progressive esophageal speech development. Journal of Speech and Hearing Disorders 18: 247.

WEST JB (1979) Respiratory Physiology, 2nd edn. Baltimore, MA: William & Wilkins.

WEST R, ANSBERRY M, CARR A (1957) The Rehabilitation of Speech, 3rd edn. New York: Harper.

WETMORE SJ, KRUEGER K, WESSON K, BLESS-ING ML (1985) Long term results of the Blom-Singer speech rehabilitation procedure. Archives of Otolaryngology 3: 106.

WHITED RE (1985) A study of post-intubation laryngeal dysfunction. Laryngoscope 95: 727.

WIEMANN JM (1985) Interpersonal control and regulation in conversation. In: Sequence and Pattern in Communicative Behaviour, Street RL, Cappella JN. London: Edward Arnold.

WILDER C (1983) Chest wall preparation for phonation in female speakers. In: Vocal fold Physiology, Bless DM, Abbs J. San Diego: College Hill Press.

WILLIAMS GT, FARQUHARSON IM, ANTHONY J (1975) Fibreoptic laryngoscopy in the assessment of laryngeal disorder. Journal of Laryngology 89: 299.

WILLIAMS PL, BANNISTER LH, BERRY MM et al., eds (1995) Gray's Anatomy. London: Churchill Livingstone.

WILLIAMS SE, WATSON JB (1985) Differences in speaking proficiencies in three laryn-gectomee groups. Archives of Otolaryngology 3: 216.

WILLIAMS SE, WATSON JB (1987) Speaking proficiency variations according to method of alaryngeal voicing. Laryngoscope 97: 737.

WILLIAMSON J (1984) Drug induced Parkinson's Disease. British Medical Journal 288: 1457.

WILSON DK (1972) Voice Problems of Children. Baltimore, MA: Williams & Wilkins.

WILSON DK (1987) Voice Problems of Children, 3rd edn. Baltimore, MA: Williams & Wilkins.

WILSON F, OLDING DJ, MUELLER K (1980) Recurrent laryngeal nerve dissection. A case report involving return of spastic dysphonia after initial surgery. Journal of Speech and Hearing Disorders 45: 112.

WINITZ H (1969) Articulatory Acquisition and Behavior. New York: Prentice Hall.

WIRZ S (1986) The voice of the deaf. In: Voice disorders and their management, Fawcus M, ed. Croom Helm, London.

WIRZ S, SUBTELNY J, WHITEHEAD R (1980) A perceptual and spectrographic study of the tense voice in normal and deaf speak-ers. Folia Phoniatrica 33: 23.

WITTKOWER ED, MANDELBROTE BM (1955) Thyrotoxicosis. In: Psychosomatic Medicine, O'Neill D, ed. London: Butterworth.

WOLFE V, MARTIN D (1997) Acoustic corre-lates of dysphonia: type and severity. Journal of Communication Disorders 30: 403-416.

WOLMAN L, DORKE CS, YOUNG A (1965) The larynx in rheumatoid arthritis. Journal of Laryngology 79: 403.

WOO P, COLTON R, CASPER J, BREWER D (1991) Diagnostic value of stroboscopic examination in hoarse patients. Journal of Voice 5: 231-238.

WOO P, COLTON R, CASPER J, BREWER D (1992) Analysis of spasmodic dysphonia by aerodynamic and laryngostroboscopic measurements. Journal of Voice 6: 344-351.

WOODSON GE, MURRY T (1994) Botulinum toxin in the treatment of recalcitrant mutational dysphonia. Journal of Voice 8: 347-351.

WOODSON GE, SANTAMBROGIO G, MATTHEW OP, SANTAMBROGIO FB (1991) Responses to respiratory stimuli. In: Laryngeal Function in Phonation and Respiration, Baer T, Saski C, Harris KS, eds. San Diego: Singular Publishing Group Inc.

WOODSON GE, ZWIRNER P, MURRY T, SWEN-SON MR (1992) Journal of Voice 6: 338-343.

WORLD HEALTH ORGANIZATION (1971) The economics of health and disease. WHO Chronicles 25: 20-24.

WORLD HEALTH ORGANIZATION (1980) International Classification of Impairments, Disabilities and Handicaps (ICIDH). Geneva: WHO.

WORLD HEALTH ORGANIZATION (1992) ICD-10 Classification of Mental and Behavioural Disorders. Geneva: WHO.

WYKE B (1967) Recent advances in the neurology of phonation and reflex mechanisms in the larynx. British Journal of Disorders of Communication 2: 1.

WYKE B (1969) Deus ex machina vocis: an analysis of laryngeal reflexes in speech. British Journal of Disorders of Communication 4: 3.

WYKE B, ed. (1972) Ventilatory and Phonatory Control Systems. Oxford: Oxford University Press.

WYKE B (1983) Neuromuscular control systems in voice production. In: Vocal Fold Physiology, Bless DM, Abbs JH, eds. San Diego, CA: College Hill Press.

WYNDER EL, COVEY LS, MARBUCHI K, JOHNSON J, MUSCHINSKY M (1976) Environmental factors in cancer of the larynx, a second look. Cancer 38: 1591-1601.

WYNTER H, MARTIN S (1981) The classification of deviant voice quality through auditory memory. British Journal of Disorders of Communication 16: 204.

YAMAGUCHI H, YOTSUKRE Y, SATA H et al. (1993) Pushing exercise program to correct glottal incompetences. Journal of Voice 7: 250-256.

YANAGIHARA N (1967a) Hoarseness: investigation of the physiological mechanism. Annals of Otology 76: 472.

YANAGIHARA N (1967b) Significance of harmonic changes and noise components in hoarseness. Journal of Speech and Hearing Research 10: 531.

YANAGIHARA N, KOIKE Y (1967) The regulation of sustained phonation. Folia Phoniatrica 19: 1.

YANAGIHARA N, KOIKE Y, VON LEDEN H (1966) Phonation and respiration - Function study in normal subjects. Folia Phoniatrica 18: 323.

YEN PT, LEE HY, TSAI MH, CHAN ST, HUANG TS (1994) Clinical analysis of external laryngeal trauma. Journal of Laryngology and Otology 108: 221-225.

YOUNG E, HAWK SS (1955) Children with Delayed or Defective Speech: Motokinaesthetic factors in their training. Stanford: Stanford University Press/ London: Milfor.

YOUNG PE, BEASLEY NJ, HOUGHTON DJ et al. (1998) A new short practical quality of life questionnaire for use in head and neck oncology outpatient clinics. Laryngoscope 108: 1574-1577.

YUMOTO E (1983) The quantitative evaluation of hoarseness - a new harmonics to noise ratio method. Archives of Otolaryngology 109: 48.

YUMOTO E, SASAKI Y, OKAMURA H (1984) Harmonics-to-noise ratio and psychophysical measurement of the degree of hoarseness. Journal of Speech and Hearing Research 27: 2-6.

ZALIOUK A (1960) Falsetto voice in deaf children. In: Aktuelle Probleme der Phoniatrie und Logopedie, Vol 1. Zurich: Karger.

ZALIOUK A (1963) The tactile approach to voice placement. Folia Phoniatrica 15: 147.

ZEITELS SM, HOCHMAN I, HILLMAN RF (1998) Adduction arytenopexy: a new procedure for paralytic dysphonia with implications for implant medialization. Otology, Rhinology and Laryngology suppl 173: 2-24.

ZEITELS SM, HILLMAN RE, BUNTING GW, VAUGHN T (1997) Reinke's edema: phonatory mechanisms and management strategies. Annals of Otology, Rhinology and Laryngology 106: 533-543.

ZEMLIN WR, DAVIS P, GAZA C (1984) Fine morphology of the posterior cricoarytenoid muscle. Folia Phoniatrica 36: 233.

ZENKER W (1964) Vocal muscle fibres and their motor end-plates. In: Potentials in Voice Physiology, Brewer D, ed. New York: State University Press.

ZHANG SP, BANDLER R, DAVIS PJ (1995) Brain stem integration of vocalization: role of the nucleus retroambigualis. Journal of Neurophysiology 74: 2500-2512.

ZHANG SP, DAVIS PJ, BANDLER R, CARRIVE P (1994) Brain stem integration of vocalization: role of the midbrain periaqueductal gray. Journal of Neurophysiology 72: 1337-1356.

ZILSTORFF K (1968) Vocal disabilities of singers. Proceedings of the Royal Society of Medicine 61: 1147.

ZWITMAN DH (1979) Bilateral cord dysfunctions: abductor type spastic dysphonia. Journal of Speech and Hearing Disorders 44: 373.

ZYSKI BJ, BULL GL, McDONALD WE, JOHNS ME (1984) Perturbation analysis of normal and pathologic larynges. Folia Phoniatrica 36: 190-198.

Index

Page numbers printed in **bold** type refer to figures; those in *italic* to tables